Handbook of
Pediatric and Neonatal Transport Medicine

Edited by

David G. Jaimovich, MD
Assistant Professor, Department of Pediatrics
University of Illinois College of Medicine
Chicago Illinois
Section Chief, Division of Critical Care
Christ Hospital and Medical Center
Oak Lawn, Illinois

Dharmapuri Vidyasagar, MD, MSc
Professor, Department of Pediatrics
University of Illinois College of Medicine
Director of Neonatology,
University of Illinois Hospital
and Michael Reese Hospital
Chicago, Illinois

HANLEY & BELFUS, INC./ Philadelphia
MOSBY/ St. Louis • Baltimore • Boston • Carlsbad • Chicago • London
Madrid • Naples • New York • Philadelphia • Sydney • Tokyo • Toronto

Publisher: HANLEY & BELFUS, INC.
                  210 South 13th Street
                  Philadelphia, PA 19107
                  (215) 546-7293
                  FAX (215) 790-9330

North American and worldwide sales and distribution:

                  MOSBY
                  11830 Westline Industrial Drive
                  St. Louis, MO 63146

In Canada: Times Mirror Professional Publishing, Ltd.
                  130 Flaska Drive
                  Markham, Ontario L6G 1B8
                  Canada

Library of Congress Cataloging-in-Publication Data

Handbook of pediatric and neonatal transport medicine / [edited by] David Jaimovich,
Dharmapuri Vidyasagar
     p.   cm.
   Includes bibliographical references and index.
   ISBN 1-56053-060-X (soft : alk. paper)
   1. Pediatric emergencies.   2. Transport of sick and wounded.
I. Jaimovich, David, 1954- II. Vidyasagar, D.
   [DNLM: 1. Patient Transfer.   2. Transport of Patients–organization
& administration.   3. Critical care–in infancy & childhood.
   WX 215 H236 1995]
RJ370.H353 1995
618.92' –dc20
DNLM/DLC
for Library of Congress   95-47674
                                                                 CIP

HANDBOOK OF PEDIATRIC AND
NEONATAL TRANSPORT MEDICINE   ISBN 1-56053-060-X

Last digit is the print number: 9 8 7 6 5 4 3 2 1

Contents

Contributors

Barbara Atkin, R.N., B.S.N., M.B.A.
Department of Pediatrics, Christ Hospital and Medical Center, Oak Lawn, Illinois

Angel B. Bassuk, M.D.
Assistant Professor of Surgery, Rush-Presbyterian-St. Luke's Medical Center, Chicago, Illinois; Chief of Pediatric Surgery and Trauma, Christ Hospital and Medical Center, Oak Lawn, Illinois

Richard J. Berens, M.D.
Assistant Professor of Anesthesiology and Pediatrics, Medical College of Wisconsin, Wauwatosa, Wisconsin

Susan E. Day, M.D.
Associate Professor of Pediatrics, Medical College of Wisconsin; Medical Director, Transport Program, Children's Hospital of Wisconsin, Milwaukee, Wisconsin

Debra H. Fiser, M.D.
Professor of Pediatrics, Anesthesiology, and Psychiatry, University of Arkansas for Medical Sciences; Medical Director, Pediatric Intensive Care Unit, Arkansas Children's Hospital, Little Rock, Arkansas

Mark S. Gaylord, M.D.
Assistant Professor of Pediatrics, University of Tennessee Graduate School of Medicine, Knoxville, Tennessee

Mark G. Goetting, M.D.
Clinical Associate Professor of Pediatrics, Wayne State University, Detroit, Michigan; Director of Pediatric Critical Care, William Beaumont Hospital, Royal Oak, Michigan

Mary Gomez, R.N.
Transport Nurse, Children's Memorial Hospital, Chicago, Illinois

Mary Lou Gostisha, R.N., M.S.N.
Patient Care Manager, Pediatric Intensive Care Unit, Children's Hospital of Wisconsin, Milwaukee, Wisconsin

John W. Graneto, D.O., M.Ed.
Assistant Professor and Pediatric Residency Director, Departments of Pediatrics and Emergency Medicine, Chicago College of Osteopathic Medicine of Midwestern University, Chicago, Illinois

Yoon S. Hahn, M.D.
Professor of Neurological Surgery and Pediatrics, Chief of Pediatric Neurosurgery, Loyola University of Chicago Medical Center, Maywood, Illinois

Harriet S. Hawkins, R.N., C.C.R.N.
Neonatal/Pediatric Transport Nurse, Transport Team, Children's Memorial Hospital, Chicago, Illinois

Michel Nadim Ilbawi, M.D.
Associate Professor of Surgery, Northwestern University Medical School, Chicago, Illinois; Pediatric Cardiac Surgeon, Christ Hospital and Medical Center, Oak Lawn, Illinois

Ravi S. Iyer, M.D.
Fellow in Neonatology, University of Illinois at Chicago, Chicago, Illinois

David G. Jaimovich, M.D.
Assistant Professor, Department of Pediatrics, University of Illinois, Chicago, Illinois; Section Chief, Division of Critical Care, Christ Hospital and Medical Center, Oak Lawn, Illinois

Lucky Jain, M.D.
Associate Professor of Pediatrics and Director of Neonatology Fellowship Program, Emory University School of Medicine; Attending Neonatologist, Emory University Hospitals, Atlanta, Georgia

Alexander James Javois, Jr., M.D.
Pediatric Cardiologist, Christ Hospital and Medical Center, Oak Lawn, Illinois

Marilyn E. Jenkins, R.N., M.B.A., C.N.A.
Director of Nursing, Shriners Burns Institute, Cincinnati Unit; Clinical Faculty, College of Nursing and Health, University of Cincinnati, Cincinnati, Ohio

Richard J. Kagan, M.D.
Associate Professor of Surgery, University of Cincinnati College of Medicine; Staff Surgeon, Shriners Burns Institute; Director, Burn Special Care Unit, University Hospital, Cincinnati, Ohio

Steven E. Krug, M.D.
Associate Professor of Pediatrics, University of California, San Diego; Director, Pediatric Emergency Medicine, Children's Hospital, San Diego, California

Michael H. LeBlanc, M.D.
Professor of Pediatrics, University of Mississippi School of Medicine, Jackson, Mississippi

Steven Lestrud, M.D.
Instructor of Pediatrics, Northwestern University School of Medicine, Chicago, Illinois

Robert M. Levin, M.D.
Associate Professor of Pediatrics, Mount Sinai Hospital Medical Center; Chairman, Department of Pediatrics, Section Head, Pediatric Infectious Disease, Mount Sinai Hospital, Chicago, Illinois

Cheryl W. Major, R.S.N., B.S.N.
Associate in Pediatrics, Neonatal Outreach Coordinator, Newborn Regionalization Coordinator, Vanderbilt University School of Medicine, Nashville, Tennessee

Cynthia A. Michaluk, R.N., M.S.N.
Assistant Professor, Adjunct Faculty College of Nursing, Department of Pediatrics, University of Tennessee at Knoxville, Knoxville, Tennessee

Kenneth Miller, M.D.
Assistant Professor of Pediatrics, Rush Medical College, Chicago, Illinois; Section Chief, Pediatric Nephrology, Christ Hospital and Medical Center, Oak Lawn, Illinois

M. Michele Moss, M.D.
Associate Professor of Pediatrics, Division of Pediatric Critical Care and Cardiology, University of Arkansas for Medical Sciences; Attending Physician, Pediatric and Cardiovascular Intensive Care Units, Arkansas Children's Hospital, Little Rock, Arkansas

Paul L. Mueller, M.D.
Pediatric Endocrinologist, Christ Hospital and Medical Center, Oak Lawn, Illinois

Zehava L. Noah, M.D.
Assistant Professor of Pediatrics and Anesthesia, Northwestern University School of Medicine, Chicago, Illinois

Cindy I. O'Boyle, R.N.
Staff Nurse, Transport Nurse, Pediatric Intensive Care Unit, Christ Hospital and Medical Center, Oak Lawn, Illinois

Diane A. Ostrowski, R.N.C., M.Ed.
Neonatal Educator/Clinician, ECMO Coordinator, Christ Hospital and Medical Center, Oak Lawn, Illinois

Michael J. Painter, M.D.
Professor of Neurology and Pediatrics, University of Pittsburgh, School of Medicine; Chief, Division of Child Neurology, Children's Hospital of Pittsburgh, Pittsburgh, Pennsylvania

Anthony L. Pearson-Shaver, M.D.
Assistant Professor of Pediatrics, Medical College of Georgia; Medical Director, Pediatric Critical Care Transport Program, MCG Hospital and Clinics, Augusta, Georgia

Fernando P. Polack, M.D.
Department of Pediatrics, William Beaumont Hospital, Royal Oak, Michigan

Beth Ann Pope, M.D.
Private Practice of Child Neurology, Concord, New Hampshire

Karen S. Powers, M.D.
Assistant Professor of Pediatrics, University of Rochester School of Medicine and Dentistry; Associate Director, Strong Children's Critical Care Center, Rochester, New York

Gerardo Reyes, M.D.
Director, Critical Care Training, Department of Pediatrics, Christ Hospital and Medical Center, Oak Lawn, Illinois

Michael Scott Sabel, M.D.
Adjunct Attending and Instructor, Department of General Surgery, Rush-Presbyterian-St. Luke's Medical Center, Chicago, Illinois

Jeff E. Schunk, M.D.
Associate Professor of Pediatrics, University of Utah School of Medicine; Emergency Department, Primary Children's Medical Center, Salt Lake City, Utah

Lou M. Smith, M.D.
Trauma Surgeon, Good Samaritan Hospital, Downers Grove, Illinois

Philip Cooper Smith, M.D., Ph.D.
Assistant Professor of Surgery, University of Illinois, Chicago, Illinois; Pediatric Cardiac Surgeon, Christ Hospital and Medical Center, Oak Lawn, Illinois

David F. Soglin, M.D.
Assistant Professor of Pediatrics, Rush Medical College; Director, Pediatric Education, Cook County Children's Hospital, Chicago, Illinois

Curt M. Steinhart, M.D.
Associate Professor of Pediatrics, Surgery, and Anesthesiology, Medical College of Georgia; Medical Director, Pediatric ICU, MCG Hospital and Clinics; Medical Director, Pediatric ICU, University Hospital, Augusta, Georgia

Ascension Margarita Torres, M.D.
Assistant Professor of Pediatrics/Pediatric Surgery, Robert C. Byrd Health Sciences Center of West Virginia University, Charleston, West Virginia

Donald D. Vernon, M.D.
Associate Professor of Pediatrics, University of Utah School of Medicine; Director, Pediatric Intensive Care Unit, Primary Children's Medical Center, Salt Lake City, Utah

Dharmapuri Vidyasagar, M.D., M.Sc.
Professor of Pediatrics and Director of Neonatology, University of Illinois at Chicago; Director of Neonatology, University of Illinois Hospital and Michael Reese Hospital, Chicago, Illinois

Robert Wesolowski, E.M.T.-P.
Executive Administrator, Pediatric Criticare, Ltd., Oak Lawn, Illinois

George Anthony Woodward, M.D.
Assistant Professor of Pediatrics, University of Pennsylvania School of Medicine; Director of Transport Services, Children's Hospital of Philadelphia, Philadelphia, Pennsylvania

Melody J. Young, R.N.
Assistant Manager of Clinical Operations, Pediatric Intensive Care Unit, Christ Hospital and Medical Center, Oak Lawn, Illinois

Preface

The first organized documentation of medical transport was associated with warfare, when battle casualties were evacuated by horse-drawn vehicles. Later, in Europe, patients were air-lifted to hospitals by hot-air balloon. During World War I, casualties were transported to hospitals by fixed-wing aircraft.

In the 1950's, hospital-based Critical Care transport systems for adult civilian patients were initiated in Europe with anesthesia/intensive care teams transporting polio patients who required ventilatory support to the regional tertiary care centers. It was not until the 1970's that medical transport teams, composed of health care personnel from intensive care units and emergency rooms, were developed to provide patient care as an extension of the intensive care unit. Currently, more than 200 hospital-based prehospital and inter-hospital transport programs exist in the United States, including pediatric, neonatal, and adult teams.

The field of pediatric transport medicine, although new, has been evolving at a very rapid pace. We, the practitioners of pediatric, neonatal, emergency, and critical care medicine, have realized the need for training and experience in pediatric transport, recognizing that a well-trained and equipped pediatric/neonatal transport team will provide that infant or child with the best possible chances to improve their outcome. These teams are prepared for emergent circumstances that are unique to children; yet, due to the low pediatric patient volume, the practice of specialized teams has not fully developed throughout the country, but is mostly concentrated in major urban areas.

Neonates and children requiring tertiary critical care must be ensured an expeditious and safe transfer using the expertise of a dedicated neonatal or pediatric transport team.

The American Academy of Pediatrics recognized the need for a section dedicated to the transport of critically ill infants and children, and in 1990 the Transport Medicine Section of the Academy was officially formed to formulate guidelines and address the special needs of critically ill children requiring inter-hospital transport.

This book was planned to include information that has accumulated through the last two decades in pediatric/neonatal transport medicine. In developing an efficient transport program for pediatrics, several specific considerations need to be addressed. These are not just related to specific physical and mechanical designs for children but also to understanding the pathophysiology of pediatric and neonatal patients and disorders unique to this age group.

We are fortunate to have contributions from numerous experts in the field. We have attempted to provide the readers with information that will allow them to develop an efficient organization, to acquaint them with available modes of transportation, and to handle most commonly encountered medical problems in neonatology and pediatrics.

The chapters also include pathophysiology, clinical presentation, and management of neonatal and pediatric medical and surgical emergencies for emergency physicians and other healthcare professionals.

We have also provided a unique feature: a ready reference of algorithms for use by the transport team in the management of some common clinical problems encountered during pediatric and neonatal emergencies and a wealth of other tables, charts, graphs, and illustrations. We hope that these features will make the book more useful for all those involved in pediatric/neonatal transport.

This book is dedicated to the physicians, nurses, therapists, and paramedics involved in the care of critically ill neonates and children requiring prehospital and inter-hospital transport. Their skill, commitment, and dedication have saved and continue to save many lives.

We thank all of the authors for their contributions and acknowledge the support of the publisher.

David G. Jaimovich, M.D.
Dharmapuri Vidyasagar, M.D.

Dedication and Thanks

To healthcare professionals throughout the world who devote their lives to safely and effectively transporting critically ill infants and children.

To my parents, who guided and helped develop my career; to my wife and children, Lisa, Lauren, and Monica, who supported me in my endeavors.

To my father, Paul Jaimovich (1923–1994), who always taught me to reach for the stars.

D.G.J.

I am indeed indebted to my parents and the late Mrs. Vishnupuri Dharmapuri for their encouragement in my professional growth, and to my wife and children, Nagami, Sahana, Sadhana, and Sanjay, for their support in this endeavor.

D.V.

And we thank our editors, Linda Belfus and Bill Lamsback, for supporting the project, our secretarial staff for their efforts in making this project timely, and Gerry Walsh for her never-ending optimism and support.

D.G.J. and D.V.

CHAPTER 1

Organization of a Pediatric-Neonatal Transport Program

KAREN S. POWERS, M.D.

Morbidity and mortality in critically ill and injured infants and children will be decreased if they are cared for in a specialized intensive care unit.[20,22] Interhospital transport programs to facilitate the transfer of infants, children, and adolescents to these units have begun to evolve over the past two decades. As regionalization of these tertiary centers has occurred, so has the need to deliver expert intensive care to the referring institutions via a transport team. The goal of the transport team is to function as an extension of the intensive care unit (ICU), delivering the same quality of care whether in the referring institution or in an air or ground transport vehicle. This chapter focuses on the organization of a pediatric or neonatal transport program, including transport personnel, vehicles, equipment, communications, and record keeping.

REGIONAL CONSIDERATIONS

More than 100,000 childhood deaths occur each year; because most are widely scattered across the U.S., each community has only limited experience caring for the critically ill child.[6] Owing to advances in neonatology and pediatric critical care and refinements in technology, sophisticated ICUs devoted exclusively to children have been developed. The critical illness or injury often occurs far from an ICU, so the child requires stabilization and admission to the nearest hospital. If the child's needs exceed the capabilities of the local hospital, interhospital transport must be provided to maximize the likelihood of a good outcome.

Critical care for children is both expensive and labor intensive. Although transporting neonates and trauma victims to appropriate centers can improve outcome significantly,[9,11,29] national concerns for health care reform will force more efficient use of pediatric and neonatal intensive care resources and further regionalization of critical care units. This will require additional resources for transport systems.

Modes of transport vary from one geographic region to another and can depend on the distance to the receiving hospital, the number of referring and receiving institutions, terrain, weather patterns, and population density. The patient may be sent to the tertiary center via the local emergency medical services or in an ambulance accompanied by the referring physician or nurse. This option may save time, but the transport vehicles often have inadequate equipment—especially critical care equipment—and transporting personnel often are inexperienced in supporting infants and children. Also, many small communities are left understaffed while emergency personnel or physicians and nurses are temporarily displaced from their local duties. Therefore, a designated transport team not only may improve the outcome for the ill or injured child being transported, but has potential benefits for other community members who may require emergency services.

Distances to the accepting hospital may be great in rural communities. Therefore, fixed-wing or rotary-wing vehicles may be needed. (An intercity facility may need access only to ground vehicles.) As resources become limited, transport services may be shared by several institutions. A model of regionalization has been developed by the California Critical Care Coalition and District IX of the American Academy of Pediatrics. It encompasses the important components necessary for the care of the critically ill or injured child from the time of initial insult to his/her discharge from the hospital.[30]

Transport systems should encourage the return of children to the referring institution once they have had the maximal benefits of the tertiary institution. This is especially important for neonates.[1] This way, convalescence can be close to the patient's family. This plan also promotes efficient use of tertiary care beds and advances cooperative efforts among institutions.

PERSONNEL: ROLES AND SELECTION

Personnel are the most valuable component of a transport system.[2] These include the medical director, transport coordinator, medical control physician, transport physicians, transport nurses, paramedics, respiratory therapists, pilots, drivers, and dispatchers. All personnel should be trained formally in transport medicine. Their training should include the physiologic changes that occur at higher altitudes if the program is using air transport vehicles. Team members should be selected primarily for their clinical and diagnostic skills, interpersonal abilities, general physical condition, favorable response to stressful situations, ability to withstand fatigue, resistance to motion sickness, physical dexterity, enthusiasm, and commitment.[2]

The **medical director** for a pediatric/neonatal transport program should have specialty training in pediatric critical care, pediatric emergency medicine, or neonatology. Co-directors, one trained in neonatology and the other in pediatric critical care/emergency medicine, may be optimal for combined pediatric and neonatal transport programs. Programs that transport trauma victims need input from a pediatric surgeon. It is the responsibility of the medical director to oversee the program. Duties include selecting and training personnel, developing transport policies and protocols, approving equipment and medication lists, reviewing transport cases, establishing and implementing outreach programs, and managing quality improvement programs. The medical director or a designee must be available to the team 24 hours a day.[3]

The **transport coordinator** is responsible for the daily activities of the transport team: scheduling of transport team members; selection and maintenance of equipment; collection of transport data; budget management; and assisting the medical director. The transport coordinator usually is a registered nurse or paramedic. In some systems, the transport coordinator may receive the initial phone call and activate the team while the call is being forwarded to the medical control physician.

The **medical control physician**, available 24 hours a day, should have expertise in pediatric critical care, emergency medicine, pediatric surgery, or neonatology. This person also may function as medical director. The medical control physician is responsible for obtaining information about the patient, for offering the referring physician interim suggestions about patient management, determining the appropriate mode of transportation, defining the team composition, and maintaining supervisory contact with the team for the duration of the transport. It is also the medical control physician's responsibility to record demographic and clinical data in the appropriate data base or log.

The medical control physician must know the availability of beds and transport teams and should have the authority to accept patients without further consultation and to triage and to activate back-up systems as necessary. If other subspecialists (e.g., cardiology, surgery) are needed, the medical control physician is responsible for consulting with them. In some cases, the medical control physician may lack needed expertise and deem it more appropriate for the subspecialist to advise the referring physician or transport team about management issues.[7]

Transport physicians should be specifically certified for pediatric transport by the medical director. It is recommended by the American Academy of Pediatrics that such physicians be a postgraduate level III resident (PL-III) or higher, a fellow, or an attending physician.[2] Physicians should be selected for a transport team based on their clinical acumen and technical skills in managing critically ill children. They must have the ability to determine diagnostic and therapeutic priorities for pediatric patients, including interpreting roentgenograms in an emergent situation. Familiarity with pharmacology and skill and experience with endotracheal intubation, arterial and venous catheter placement, and chest tube insertion are mandatory.[25] If air transport is to be used, the transport physician must also be trained in flight physiology.

The **transport nurse** should be a registered nurse with pediatric or neonatal critical care experience. This person also should be chosen by the medical director for his/her medical skills and competence in managing airways, obtaining venous access, operating transport equipment with full understanding of its limitations, and using supplies. The transport nurse must deal sensitively with personnel and family members at the referring institution. Often the transport program will require that these nurses have inpatient care responsibilities when not actually on transport. It is recommended that the designated transport nurse have a patient assignment that will allow rapid transfer of his/her patient's care to another nurse to expedite departure.

On nurse-led teams, the nurse assumes the responsibility for coordinating patient stabilization, management, and monitoring during transport. Nurse team leaders may require facility with additional technical skills such as endotracheal intubation, intraosseous or central venous access, and evacuation of pneumothoraces. This nurse team leader must have the cognitive skills to assess patients accurately and to prioritize therapies appropriately.

A **transport paramedic** is part of many transport programs. The paramedic should be registered and should have received additional training and experience in pediatric patient management and interhospital transport. This person should be approved by the medical director on the basis of demonstrated cognitive and clinical skills. The paramedic usually assists the team leader with stabilization and management of the patient during the transport.

The **transport respiratory therapist** should be a registered therapist with additional training and experience in pediatric and neonatal critical care as well as in transport medicine. The respiratory therapist should be approved by the medical director for proven abilities in pulmonary stabilization and airway management. He or she should have expertise in transport respiratory equipment and portable ventilators, the oxygen delivery capabilities of various vehicles, and respiratory management at high altitudes. In many nurse-led transports, the respiratory therapist may be responsible for securing airways and endotracheal intubation. It is also helpful for the respiratory therapist to be able to assist the team leader in other duties deemed appropriate by the team leader.

The **pilots** and **drivers** should be trained appropriately and licensed in providing emergency medical transport services. The individual's safety records should be reviewed by the hospital's administration. The pilot should base the decision to fly solely on weather conditions, without coercion from the child's clinical status. Ambulance drivers should be discouraged from exceeding the speed limit or ignoring traffic signals; such time-saving risks rarely benefit the patient.

TEAM TRAINING

Until overseeing organizations approve guidelines for training of transport personnel, formal training programs must be designed and implemented by the program director. A few states may have specific minimum training requirements, such as the regulations for air transport teams legislated by Utah, and the program director must be aware of these.[26] Since each program differs in the types of patients transported, the location and abilities of referring institutions, and the transport vehicles and equipment used, training programs must be individualized. Nurses who transport without an accompanying physician should have more advanced training than nurses participating in physician-led teams. The course should cover all responsibilities related to the care and monitoring of pediatric and neonatal patients during transport. Such technical skills as endotracheal intubation, venous access, and evacuation of pneumothoraces should be taught. The team needs not only to understand clearly the indications and alternatives to these procedures; they should participate in a procedure laboratory using animal models, mannequins, or should witness supervised endotracheal intubations in the operating room. The Pediatric Advanced Life Support (PALS) course (American Heart Association, American Academy of Pediatrics, 1988), with an additional trauma module, and Advanced Pediatric Life Support (APLS) course (AAP/American College of Emergency Physicians, 1989) can serve as good educational models to be expanded upon.

In addition to airway management, the team should be trained in the technical skills needed for intraosseous or peripheral and central venous access. They also should become proficient in needle thoracostomies and chest tube placement for evacuation of pneumothoraces and life-threatening effusions and in pericardiocentesis.

Team members also need to be trained in transport medicine, including operation and maintenance of transport equipment, safety and survival skills for varying transport vehicles, and the physiologic consequences of altitude on the patient. Medical decision making and therapy triage can be emphasized via didactic lectures, mock transport scenarios, and team participation in devising protocols. The topics of the lectures should be skewed to the types of patients the program is likely to transport. Specific and detailed protocols should be developed by the program director, and each team member should be responsible for learning and complying with these protocols.

New transport team members initially should participate in supervised transports. Quality assurance processes can enhance the learning experience by using both immediate direct feedback from the medical control physician or medical director and frequent review of cases with the entire team. Continuing education should be included. Accurate records of the number of transports and procedures each team member participates in should be kept. A minimal number of procedures should be required to maintain skill levels. Mechanisms to refresh technical skills should be in place for team members not meeting these requirements.

The team also should receive suggestions for diplomatically dealing with conflicts that might arise at the referring institutions. Instructions in stress management are helpful.

TEAM COMPOSITION

Transport team composition for each mission usually is decided on an individual basis by the medical director or medical control physician based on the patient's condition and anticipated potential complications, length and mode of transport, and skills of the team members. The ultimate goal of the transport team is to maintain or improve the level of care that the child or infant receives at the referring institution. The Consolidated Omnibus Budget Reconciliation Act (COBRA) requires that patients must be transported by individuals qualified and trained to provide the appropriate treatment to maintain the patient's condition and to treat any reasonably foreseeable complication.[18]

The medical control physician or medical director usually can determine the need for a nurse, paramedic, and respiratory therapist based on the patient's pretransport condition. Much debate continues over whether or not to include a physician. Experience with neonatal transport suggests that the presence of a physician does not alter outcome.[28] However, studies dealing with pediatric and adult transports show that physician-based teams limit morbidity.[4,14] However, the presence of a physician untrained in pediatrics or transport medicine does not reduce the incidence of complications or improve outcome.[10,12]

Interhospital transport is expensive, and including a skilled transport physician contributes significantly to that expense. Some reports suggest that all interhospital transports do not require a physician.[16] Therefore, numerous studies have been performed to predict which children would benefit by a physician. Several have extrapolated the Pediatric Risk of Mortality (PRISM) illness severity scores into the interhospital transport setting to assess the need for a skilled physician. The results have been conflicting. One study demonstrated PRISM scores greater than 10 predicted physiologic deterioration;[12] other studies showed that the pretransport PRISM score did not predict the need for major interventions.[19,23] Detailed pretransport patient data have been used to predict the need for a physician-based transport team.[15] Despite all these efforts, there is still a need for a well-controlled study that stratifies patients by severity of illness or injury, probability of physiologic deterioration or complications, and pretransport stabilization, while taking into account the skills of the transport team. Until then, the role of a skilled pediatrician in pediatric transports will remain unclear.[31] Unfortunately, this leaves the composition of the optimal team up to the program director or medical control physician. Many transport systems thus feel committed to the highest level of care for all transports, leading to a potentially inefficient use of resources.

EQUIPMENT

The transport team must carry all necessary equipment, supplies, and medications with them. It is preferable that the equipment be dedicated solely to transport. The American Academy of Pediatrics Task Force on Interhospital Transport[3] recommends the following guidelines for transport equipment:

1. Provide the capability for life support in the transport setting.
2. Be lightweight (loadable by two persons), portable and self-contained, with a battery life of twice the expected transport duration.
3. Be durable enough to withstand altitude and thermal changes, acute decompression vibrations (4-G decelerative forces), and repeated use.
4. Be easily maintained and cleaned.
5. Have AC/DC capabilities.
6. Have no electromagnetic field interference.
7. Be able to fit through standard hospital doors and into transport vehicles and be secured easily to prevent shifting while en route.

In addition to a gurney, the transport team should have an isolette available to transport infants under 5 kg. Many teams will modify the equipment; e.g., the cardiorespiratory monitor, pulse oximeter, oxygen source, ventilator, and infusion pumps may be mounted on the gurney or isolette.[21] This can both free the hands of the transport team and secure the equipment. The cardiorespiratory monitor should have both invasive and noninvasive monitoring capabilities. A defibrillator/cardioverter must be available. Noninvasive automated blood pressure recording capabilities can be invaluable in children without indwelling arterial catheters. Digital measurement of pressures is helpful in a moving vehicle.

An electrically operated ventilator is recommended, since it will require lower air or oxygen flow. A pressure-driven ventilator can be substituted when the vehicle is not equipped with the appropriate electrical source. If the team is to transport neonates as well as older children, the ventilator must be able to deliver both small tidal volumes for the premature neonate and larger flows for adolescents. Some teams use separate ventilators for neonates. Ventilators should have the capability of delivering positive end-expiratory pressure (PEEP) and continuous positive airway pressures (CPAP). Adequate audio and visual alarms for pressure, volume, and flow should be available. Some teams may want capabilities to blend compressed air with oxygen; however, most transports can be managed safely on oxygen alone.

A temperature probe or thermometer is needed to insure that the neonate is maintained in a neutral environment. Some teams may wish to include transcutaneous O_2 and CO_2 monitors. Multichannel infusion pumps or syringe pumps are less bulky, especially when multiple infusions are needed.

Most teams will have supplies and medications organized into separate bags by patient size or by intended use, i.e., airway, vascular access, medications, etc. A special medication pack containing controlled substances and drugs that must be refrigerated should be properly stored in a place quickly accessible to the team. Tables 1 and 2 give examples of supplies and medication lists. Reference protocols and tables should be readily available to the team to determine appropriate equipment size and appropriate medications with correct dosages.

It is imperative that a current inventory of equipment, supplies, and medications be kept, assuring that medications and supplies are not outdated. Equipment should be inspected and tested before leaving for a transport. Medications and supplies used should be restocked as soon as possible following the completion of a transport.

TABLE 1.   Transport Supplies

Airway	Vascular Access	Additional Supplies
Bag-valve-mask system with oxygen reservoir	IV catheters (all sizes)	Thoracostomy set
	Central venous catheters	Thoracostomy tubes (all sizes)
Masks (all sizes)	Intraosseous needles	Closed chest drainage system
Oxygen tubing	IV tubing and connectors	Lumbar puncture set
Oral and nasopharyngeal airways (all sizes)	Needles/butterflies (all sizes)	Nasogastric tubes
	Three-way stopcocks	Salem sump tubes
Laryngoscope and blades (all sizes)	Alcohol and Betadine wipes	Razors
Stylets (adult and pediatric)	Arm boards	Chemstrips
Endotracheal tubes (all sizes)	Syringes (all sizes)	Lancets
Tracheostomy tubes (all sizes)	IV solutions	Tongue blades
End tidal CO_2 monitor	Sterile and nonsterile gloves (all sizes)	Cervical collars (all sizes)
Magill forceps		Backboard
10-ml syringes	Sterile gown	Restraints
Water-soluble lubricant	Caps/masks	Tape
Adhesive tape	Umbilical catheters	Dressings/bandages
Benzoin	Umbilical vessel introducer set	Splints
Heimlich valve	Umbilical tape	Blood pressure cuffs (all sizes)
Cricothyrotomy kit	Suture set	ECG electrodes (multiple sizes)
Nasal cannulas (all sizes)	Tourniquet	Defibrillator paddle gel
Simple oxygen masks (all sizes)	Tape measure	Stethoscope
Nonrebreather masks (all sizes)	Cutdown set	Scissors/clamps/forceps
Tracheostomy collars	Razors	Extra batteries
PEEP valve	Tape/Tagaderm	Extra bulbs
Manometer		Band-aids
Tonsil suction		Vaseline gauze
Suction catheters (all sizes)		4 × 4 sponges
DeLee suction with mucus trap		2 × 2 sponges
Bulb syringe		Rubber bands
Humidification units		Safety pins
Nebulizers		Blood tubes
		Urinary catheters (all sizes)
		Urine bags
		Pacifier
		Stocking caps
		Penlight/flashlight
		Saran wrap

TRANSPORT VEHICLES

A number of factors should be considered in selecting the mode of transportation. These include (1) severity and stability of injury or illness, (2) urgency to provide advanced care, (3) transportation time between hospitals, (4) availability of carrier, (5) availability and capability of personnel, (6) weather and traffic conditions, (7) geography, (8) safety, and (9) cost. Current modes of medical transport include ground ambulances, rotor-wing (helicopter) aircraft, and fixed-wing (airplane or jet) aircraft. In rural areas, all three modes usually are needed, while urban areas typically require only ground vehicles and rotor-wing aircraft.

The main determinant for the mode of transport is the patient's diagnosis and condition. Information obtained from the referring hospital can help the medical control physician determine the level of care the patient is now receiving and the urgency for transport. If the patient is at an institution with capabilities to diagnose and treat an ill or injured child, an expeditious transport may be a lower priority. However, a child with an epidural hematoma, or an injured child still at the scene, will warrant expeditious transport to the tertiary institution, such as by helicopter. However, if the helicopter cannot land on the hospital

TABLE 2.   Transport Medications

Emergency Drugs	Cardiovascular Medications (cont.)	Intubation Medications	Antibiotics
Atropine	Procainamide	Atropine	Ampicillin
Bretylium	Propranolol	Ketamine	Ceftriaxone
Calcium chloride	Prostaglandin E_1[1]	Pancuronium[1]	Chloramphenicol
Dextrose	Tolazoline	Succinylcholine[1]	Gentamicin
Epinephrine		Thiopental[2]	Nafcillin
Lidocaine	**Neurologic Medications**	Vecuronium	Penicillin G
Naloxone	Diazepam[2]		
Sodium bicarbonate	Lorazepam[1]		**Miscellaneous**
	Mannitol	**Analgesia/Muscle**	Albumin (5%)
Cardiovascular Medications	Phenobarbital[2]	**Relaxation**	Dexamethasone
Adenosine	Phenytoin	Diazepam[2]	Diphenhydramine
Amrinone		Fentanyl[2]	Furosemide
Diazoxide	**Respiratory Medications**	Lorazepam[1]	Glucagon
Digoxin	Albuterol	Midazolam[2]	Heparin
Dobutamine	Aminophylline	Morphine sulfate[2]	Hydrocortisone
Dopamine	Atropine	Pancuronium[1]	Insulin[1]
Epinephrine	Epinephrine	Vecuronium	Kayexalate
Hydralazine	Isoproterenol		Potassium chloride
Isoproterenol	Solumedrol		Racemic epinephrine
Nitroprusside	Terbutaline		Vitamin K
Norepinephrine			

[1] Kept in special refrigerated medication pack.
[2] Kept in special controlled substance medication pack.

grounds and if multiple transfers from the hospital to a ground ambulance to the helicopter are necessary, overall transport time may not be reduced.

Second, the safety of the transport team must be given high priority. The decision to fly should be made by the pilot, based solely on weather conditions and the geography to be covered. Similarly, the decision to use a ground vehicle should be based on traffic and road conditions at the time of transport. Back-up vehicles should be available, particularly ground ambulances, in the event of mechanical problems or the need for simultaneous transports.

The advantages and disadvantages for each type of transport vehicle are summarized in Table 3. Ground ambulances are most frequently used. They can provide door-to-door service, with the patient placed on a stretcher at the referring hospital and then directly delivered to the receiving institution. If an emergency arises en route, the vehicle can be stopped, allowing the transport team to perform any necessary therapies while stationary. Also, an ambulance can easily be detoured to a nearer hospital, if necessary for stabilization or to replenish exhausted supplies. There are few weather or weight restrictions for the use of ground vehicles. Therefore, several team members as well as family members usually can be accommodated as long as there are enough seat belts. In addition, ground vehicles are the most economical to purchase or lease as well as to operate, fuel, insure, and service.

Motion sickness is commonly encountered in ground vehicles.[13] If this occurs, caring for the patient can be extremely difficult. Motion sickness often can be alleviated by premedication prior to departure, by keeping the cabin cool, and visually fixating on stationary objects. Transport by ground ambulance usually entails lengthier and more tiring transports. The ground vehicle is restricted to roads and highways, so unforseen traffic congestion can significantly lengthen transport times, which may impact battery life of the equipment. Poor rear suspension with a narrow wheel base and high center of gravity, as well as

TABLE 3.   Transport Vehicles: Advantages and Disadvantages

Ground Ambulance	Fixed-Wing Aircraft	Rotor-Wing Aircraft
Advantages		
Available	Rapid transpoert over longer distances	Rapid transport time
Can be used in most weather conditions	Can fly around or above inclement weather	Can reach otherwise unaccessible areas
Requires only two transfers of child	Pressurized cabins	
Adequate cabin space	Larger cabin to carry more passengers or equipment	
Minimal weight restrictions for number of passengers		
Easily diverted		
Relatively low cost to own, lease, or maintain		
Disadvantages		
Longer transit times	Requires airport runway	Requires unobstructed landing site
Mobility limited by road and traffic conditions	Requires multiple patient transfers	Small cabin space
May lack needed power, suction, and gas flow sources	High costs	Weight limits
		May require multiple patient transfers
		Limited fuel capacity which limits range
		Restricted by weather
		Noise and vibration interference
		No cabin pressurization
		Safety concerns
		Increased costs

poor road conditions, can lead to uncomfortable bouncing. This may be detrimental to some patients, especially those with orthopedic injuries. Such movement may increase the risk of dislodging lines and tubes and, combined with a noisy environment, may make continuous patient monitoring difficult.

The obvious advantage of rotor-wing aircraft is rapid transport time, usually one-half to one-third the time of ground vehicles. In addition, the helicopter can reach locations inaccessible by ground ambulances. Despite common belief, helicopters are generally safe as long as foul weather guidelines are strictly followed.[24]

The rotor-wing aircraft requires either a helipad or an unobstructed landing site, which may not be available at all referring hospitals. If not available, transferring the patient from the hospital to an ambulance and then to the helicopter may be necessary. Besides increasing transport time, this also may put the patient at increased risk—especially of dislodging lines and tubes. Space and weight are restricted in a helicopter, limiting the number of transport personnel. Noise and vibration often can interfere with adequate patient monitoring. Motion sickness also can be a problem.

Weather conditions that decrease visibility can limit flights. Altitude, especially in helicopters that fly higher than 8000 feet, can lead to hypoxia and dysbarism.[5] Finally, operating costs for rotor-wing aircraft are significantly higher than for ground transport vehicles.

The main advantage of fixed-wing aircraft is rapid transport over longer distances, usually greater than 150–200 miles. Interestingly, the transport group from Salt Lake City reported that helicopter transports were 400% more expensive than fixed-wing aircraft (with their associated ground transport) for distances between 100 and 150 miles, with no significant difference in transport time.[27] Fixed-wing aircraft have fewer restrictions on weight and numbers of personnel, owing to larger cabin space, and can fly above or around inclement weather.

Fixed-wing aircraft require runways of specified length and may be delayed by airport traffic. Atmospheric changes remain a concern; some smaller aircraft are not pressurized, and even larger aircraft may only be pressurized to 7000–8000 feet. Using fixed-wing aircraft also requires multiple moves for the patient to reach the airplane and is substantially more expensive than ground vehicles.

COMMUNICATIONS

Communication is an essential component of a successful transport program. The referring institution needs to be in prompt contact with the medical control physician, who can accept or decline the referral and make interim recommendations for patient management. This is best done via a dedicated "hot line" to direct calls to a center where a trained dispatcher can process the transport request and dispatch the appropriate personnel according to protocols established by the medical director.[3] Many programs have toll-free numbers available for their referral area.[8] These services need to be operable 24 hours a day, and seven days a week.

Dispatchers should be able to contact transport personnel rapidly via telephone, pager, or radio. The dispatcher should have access to maps with estimated travel times, current weather conditions, and bed availabilities. The speed with which the team can be located and assembled can be of vital importance. Once the team has been dispatched, continuous communications between the team, the medical control physician, and the referring hospital should be established. The communication center must have radio (UHF or VHF) frequencies to communicate with cellular phones aboard the ground ambulances or aircraft. Radio and telephone patching capabilities are also vital to avoid unnecessary additional calls. Fixed-wing aircraft using VHF frequencies may quickly go out of range; thus, contact between control towers and hospitals may become necessary.[24] The communication center also should be able to contact appropriate fire and police departments, especially when arrangements for helicopter landings on undesignated sites must be made.

Ideally, all communications should be recorded on tape, If this is not possible, careful logs and documentation of all communications should be kept. All medical advice should be entered on the patient's hospital chart. These transactions should be reviewed routinely by the medical director both for quality assurance and as potential teaching tools.

The receiving institution should provide follow-up to referring personnel. This may also facilitate the transfer of the infant or child back to the referring hospital once the services of the receiving hospital are no longer needed.[17] The referring personnel often are eager for feedback about their stabilization and management of the patient. Thus, receiving institutions can informally or even formally educate them about current concepts for care of seriously ill children and neonates and the use of specialized resources.

RECORD KEEPING

Complete records should be an integral part of all transport programs. The data collected should include such data as patient name, age, and referring hospital; operational information about mode of transport and team members; such clinical data as diagnosis, severity of illness, and procedures performed; and, finally, financial information for billing and reimbursement. A computer may be helpful in storing this information, especially if the program transports a large number of children. The computer also can allow integration of information into pre-existing hospital billing and record systems.

As mentioned above, such data can facilitate quality assurance of the transport program. The demographics also can be helpful in identifying and then targeting referral patterns. Pertinent information can be incorporated into a patient summary for the referring physicians and can provide statistical information to referring hospitals. Finally, the data collected can document trends to be used for future planning and budgeting.

SUMMARY

The success of a transport program depends on a sound organization. This organization involves determining regional needs and resources, selecting and training transport personnel, acquiring transport equipment, selecting transport vehicles, and establishing a communication center. The transport team can then function successfully as an extension of the neonatal or pediatric ICUs to reduce morbidity and mortality in ill or injured neonates or children.

REFERENCES

1. American Academy of Pediatrics, The American College of Obstetricians and Gynecologists: Interhospital care of the perinatal patient. In Guidelines for Perinatal Care, 2nd ed. Elk Grove Village, IL, AAP, and Washington: ACOG; 1988, p 209.
2. American Academy of Pediatrics, Committee on Hospital Care: Guidelines for air and ground transportation of pediatric patients. Pediatrics 78:943, 1986.
3. American Academy of Pediatrics, Task Force on Interhospital Transport: Guidelines for Air and Ground Transport of Neonatal and Pediatric Patients. Elk Grove Village, IL, AAP, 1993.
4. Baxt WG, Moody P: The impact of a physician as part of the aeromedical prehospital team in patients with blunt trauma. JAMA 257:3246, 1987.
5. Blumen IJ, Abernethy MK, Dunne MJ: Flight physiology. Clinical considerations. Crit Care Clin 8:597, 1992.
6. Campbell PM: Transportation of the critically ill and injured child. Crit Care Q 8:1, 1985.
7. Day S, McCloskey K, Orr R, et al: Pediatric interhospital critical care transport: Consensus of a national leadership conference. Pediatrics 88:696, 1991.
8. Dobrin RS, Block B, Gilman JI, Massaro TA: The development of a pediatric emergency transport system. Pediatr Clin North Am 27:633, 1980.
9. Ferrara A, Schwartz M, Page H, et al: Effectiveness of neonatal transport in New York City in neonates less than 2500 grams—a population study. J Community Health 13:3, 1988.
10. Hamman BL, Cue JI, Miller FB, et al: Helicopter transport of trauma victims: Does a physician make a difference? J Trauma 31:490, 1991.
11. Hood JL, Cross A, Hulka B, Lawson EE: Effectiveness of the neonatal transport team. Crit Care Med 11:419, 1983.
12. Kanter RK, Tompkins JM: Adverse events during interhospital transport: Physiologic deterioration associated with pretransport severity of illness. Pediatrics 84:43, 1989.
13. Lachenmyer J: Physiological aspects of transport. Inter Anesthesiol Clin 25:15, 1987.
14. Macnab AJ: Optimal escort for interhospital transport of pediatric emergencies. J Trauma 31:205, 1991.
15. McCloskey KA, Johnston C: Critical care interhospital transports: Predictability of the need for a pediatrician. Pediatr Emerg Care 6:89, 1990.
16. McCloskey KA, King WD, Byron L: Pediatric critical care transport: Is a physician always needed on the team? Ann Emerg Med 18:247, 1989.
17. McCloskey KA, Orr RA: Pediatric transport issues in emergency medicine. Emerg Med Clin North Am 9:475, 1991.
18. Omnibus Budget Reconciliation Act of 1989, Section 6018 42 USC 1395 cc (West Supp 1990).
19. Orr RA, Venkataraman ST, Singleton CA: Pediatric risk of mortality score (PRISM): A poor predictor in triage of patients for pediatric interhospital transport [abstract]. Ann Emerg Med 18:170, 1989.
20. Paneth N, Kiely JL, Wallenstein S, et al: Newborn intensive care and neonatal mortality in low-birth-weight infants. A population study. N Engl J Med 307:149, 1982.
21. Petre JH, Bazaral MG, Estafanous FG: Patient transport: An organized method with direct clinical benefits. Biomed Instrum Technol 23:100, 1989.

22. Pollack MM, Alexander SR, Clarke N, et al: Improved outcomes from tertiary center pediatric intensive care: A statewide comparison of tertiary and nontertiary care facilities. Crit Care Med 19:150, 1991.
23. Rubenstein JS, Gomez MA, Rybicki L, Noah ZL: Can the need for a physician as part of the pediatric transport team be predicted? A prospective study. Crit Care Med 20:1657, 1992.
24. Schneider C, Gomez M, Lee R: Evaluation of ground ambulance, rotor-wing, and fixed-wing aircraft services. Crit Care Clin 8:533, 1992.
25. Smith DF, Hackel A: Selection criteria for pediatric critical care transport teams. Crit Care Med 11:10, 1983.
26. Thomas F, Gibbons H, Clemmer TP: Air ambulance regulations: A model. Aviat Space Environ Med 57:699, 1986.
27. Thomas F, Wisham J, Clemmer TP, et al: Outcome, transport times, and costs of patients evacuated by helicopter versus fixed-wing aircraft. West J Med 153:40, 1990.
28. Thompson TR: Neonatal transport nurses: An analysis of their role in the transport of newborn infants. Pediatrics 65:887, 1980.
29. Trunkey D: Regionalization of trauma care. Top Emerg Med 3:91, 1981.
30. White Paper: Pediatric critical care systems. San Francisco, District IX, American Academy of Pediatrics, 1989.,
31. Zaritsky A, Beyer AJ: MD or not MD: Is that the question? Crit Care Med 20:1633, 1992.

CHAPTER 2

Transport Management Considerations

HARRIET S. HAWKINS, R.N., C.C.R.N.

PRETRANSPORT ARRANGEMENTS (INTERHOSPITAL TRANSPORT)

Interhospital transport of the critically ill pediatric patient requires excellent communication between the referring hospital, the transport team, and the receiving hospital. This communication begins with the initial phone call from the referring hospital and does not end until the patient has been safely admitted to the receiving hospital.

DATA GATHERING AND DOCUMENTATION

In order to provide a safe and suitable transport, including equipment, medications, staff, and mode, it is the responsibility of the transport team to obtain adequate information about the patient during the initial phone call. This includes a brief incident-related history, current vital signs, the child's weight, pertinent physical findings, relevant laboratory results, and any treatment modalities instituted.

A standardized form, filled out during the initial phone call, will enable all members of the transport team to locate necessary information as they prepare for the transport.[2] It can also guide the questions asked of the referring hospital, ensuring that all important information is obtained. This form should be considered a part of the patient's permanent hospital record (Fig. 1). The information obtained at this time will help determine the mode of transport as well as team composition.

The responsibility of the receiving hospital begins when the referring facility makes the initial contact and increases greatly when the patient has been accepted for admission.[2,17] It is therefore of utmost importance that accurate documentation of all communication be an ongoing part of interhospital transports. All recommendations for care, including who gave the recommendations and who received them, must be recorded.

TEAM COMPOSITION

Interhospital transports may be done by transport teams from the receiving facility, by free-standing critical care transport teams, or by independent ambulance services. Many tertiary care facilities have transport teams staffed by physicians, nurses, respiratory therapists, and/or paramedics. Free-standing critical care transport programs may also use a similar mix of personnel. A

DATE	TIME	CALL TAKEN BY

PATIENT NAME	BIRTHDATE	AGE

REFERRING HOSPITAL	REFERRING HOSP. PHONE NO. ( )	PATIENT'S HOSP. LOCATION

REFERRING PHYSICIAN	REFERRING PHY. PHONE NO. ( )	INSURANCE	HMO APPROVAL ☐ YES ☐ NO	HMO MD

CMH ATTENDING ACCEPTING TRANSPORT	CMH ATTENDING APPROVED TRANSPORT TEAM	PREVIOUS CMH ADMISSIONS	SERVICE/ATTENDING FOR PREV. ADMISSIONS

HISTORY/PHYSICAL EXAM/DIAGNOSIS

PRESENT WT. | BIRTH WT. (kgs)
GESTATIONAL AGE | AGE IN HOURS
APGARS ( )₁ ( )₅ ( )₁₀

PATIENT DATA BASE

TIME	TEMP.	HR	RR	B/P

RESPIRATORY | LAST ORAL INTAKE

INTUBATED/TRACHED ___ TUBE SIZE	VENTILATED PARAMETERS	RENAL	GI

CARDIAC | PERFUSION

NEUROLOGICAL

MEDICATIONS GIVEN (INCLUDE TIME) | IV FLUIDS/SITES/RATES

LABORATORY DATA

TIME	HGB	HCT	WBC	DIFFERENTIAL P B E B L M	PLTS	COAGS

TIME	NA	K	CL	CO₂	BUN	CR	CA	GLUCOSE	OTHER LABS

BLOOD GASES
TYPE	TIME	PH	PCO₂	PO₂	BE	HCO₃	O₂ SAT	VENT SETTINGS
TYPE	TIME	PH	PCO₂	PO₂	BE	HCO₃	O₂ SAT	VENT SETTINGS

XRAY/CT SCAN RESULTS | C-SPINE IMMOBILIZATION

510 REQ PRIOR TO ARRIVAL OF TRANS TEAM

ALL PATIENTS
☐ HAVE CHARTS & X-RAYS COPIED (INC. CT SCANS)
☐ INFORM REFERRING HOSPITAL OF MODE OF TRANSPORT & ESTIMATED TIME OF ARRIVAL
☐ HAVE FAMILY AVAILABLE FOR CONSENT

NEONATES ONLY
☐ HAVE MOTHER'S CHART COPIED
☐ OBTAIN CORD BLOOD & MOTHER'S BLOOD IF POSSIBLE
☐ OBTAIN PLACENTA & PLACE IN A TRANSPORTABLE CONTAINER IF POSSIBLE

PHONE ORDERS/SUGGESTIONS
1.   4.
2.   5.
3.   6.

MODE OF TRANSPORT ☐ AMBULANCE ☐ HELICOPTER ☐ FIXED WING	INDIVIDUAL RECEIVING ORDERS/SUGGESTIONS NAME TITLE	SIGNATURE OF INDIVIDUAL GIVING ORDERS/SUGGESTIONS NAME TITLE

FIGURE 1.   Transport telephone call record (The Children's Memorial Hospital of Chicago).

decision regarding team composition will be made based on patient condition, team protocols, and staff experience.[9,11,14,16] When an independent ambulance service is to be used for interhospital transport, it is imperative that the transporting personnel be able to provide the care needed by the child. This requires good assessment by the referring staff, the receiving staff, and the paramedics actually doing the transport. Ambulance services must have protocols for interhospital transport which dictate the variety of pediatric patients that they can safely transport. An example would be a service without an isolette asked to transport a two-week-old infant during the winter in extremely cold conditions. This infant's needs for temperature control might be better served by transport in a prewarmed isolette. Another example is the child who is receiving an intravenous medicated drip. If this child is dependent on the continuous infusion of a medication, the child must be transported with the intravenous drip on a pump. Many private ambulance services do not have a pump and are not familiar with their use. In this case a pump would need to be made available for the transport, and a staff member from the referring facility would have to accompany the patient on transport.

The interhospital transport team will be challenged by a variety of medical and surgical diagnoses. Studies have shown that the most frequent problems encountered in the pediatric patient are related to respiratory and neurologic problems.[2,5,9,10,13] These problems are often described in general, nonspecific terms and the detailed work-up necessary to provide a specific diagnosis usually is not available prior to transport. The diagnosis of seizures is the most common reason for transport in almost all studies. Although there are multiple causes for seizures in the pediatric patient, the exact cause often will not be obvious at the time of the initial phone call, and perhaps not even on team arrival. The transport team must begin evaluation of possible causes as soon as the patient is referred and must be able to provide treatment as necessary.

COMMUNICATION

Both hospital-based and free-standing critical care transport teams must have a mechanism for efficient handling of emergent calls. The referral community should be able to call 24 hours a day and receive immediate contact with an individual who can triage the emergent call and rapidly access stabilization advice as necessary.[1,2]

In order to prevent the need for a second transport, it is the responsibility of the transport team to ascertain that an appropriate bed is available at the receiving hospital. This includes consideration of intensive care bedspace availability, potential isolation needs, and the presence of specialists and subspecialists. To facilitate a smooth transition of patient care, the receiving facility must be aware of the estimated time of team arrival, thereby assuring that medical, nursing, and ancillary personnel will be readily available to provide care for the patient.[5]

Communication with the referring facility must continue while the transport team is en route from the base hospital. A designated contact person, one familiar with the current transport as well as transport protocols and guidelines, should be readily available to continue stabilization advice as necessary. This contact person also should be able to access the transport team to inform them of changes in patient status.

STABILIZATION ADVICE (INTERHOSPITAL)

Stabilization advice from the receiving hospital or base facility is focused on maintenance of airway, breathing (ventilation), and circulation. All patients must have a stable airway for transport; adequate ventilation, whether spontaneous or assisted; and vascular access. If any of these parameters are recognized as deficient at the time of the initial contact with the referring facility, the receiving hospital or base facility should make recommendations for care. A patient who does not have a stable airway for transport requires intubation. Intubation prior to transport team arrival will shorten the amount of time that the team spends in the referring facility and encourages a timely return to the receiving hospital. Although it is certainly true that all necessary interventions may not be anticipated at the time of the initial and subsequent phone calls, any problems that are recognized should have treatment recommended. Certainly, many necessary treatments may be available only at the receiving hospital, but the basics of airway maintenance, ventilation, and vascular access should be available at all facilities that provide care to children.

Additional interventions necessary prior to transport, such as drug therapy (antibiotics, anticonvulsants, sedation) or tube placement (gastric tube or urinary catheter), should be recommended for initiation prior to team arrival at the referring facility. Any procedure performed by the referring staff that will facilitate a shorter stay at the referring facility and, therefore, a more rapid return to the receiving hospital should be recommended during the pretransport phone calls. Transport protocols can assist in determining transport recommendations for both specific and nonspecific diagnoses.

TRANSPORT TEAM ASSESSMENT AND INITIAL STABILIZATION

When the transport team arrives at the referring facility, their initial responsibility is to perform a rapid assessment of the patient, focusing initially on airway, breathing, and circulation. In addition, they should receive current information from the referring staff. Laboratory tests that may have been requested at the time of the initial phone call can be reviewed, the chest x-ray and other pertinent films can be examined, and procedures performed by the referring staff can be assessed.

In a transport setting, urgent therapy and the management of life-threatening problems is the priority. If the patient is in severe respiratory distress on arrival of the team, a blood pressure may not be a priority. The priority is airway management and ventilation, and the recording of blood pressure may be delayed 15–20 minutes. Diagnosis-specific evaluations may not be done until after arrival in the Pediatric Intensive Care Unit.[2] Although the whole patient should be assessed, in-depth examination should be deferred until after the transport. For example, a two-year-old drug ingestion does not need an ear examination on transport.

The goal of the transport is to provide a safe and timely transport to the receiving hospital. Because ambulances and helicopters are noisy, bumpy, and cramped, anticipated stabilization procedures should be performed at the referring facility. Many patients may never be quite "stable" prior to transport, but the goal is to have the patient as stable as possible before loading into the transport vehicle.

Interhospital transport teams may be considered extensions of the Pediatric Intensive Care Unit, with that quality of care beginning when the transport team assumes care of the patient. In addition to providing care for life-threatening problems, the transport team must secure all tubes and lines before loading into the transport vehicle.[2,17]

AIRWAY

As mentioned previously, a patent, maintainable airway is a necessity for transport. All patients should be assessed for their ability to continue to maintain their airway for the duration of the transport. Patients with a decreased level of consciousness should be positioned appropriately, using a jaw thrust or head tilt, chin lift as necessary. Positioning the airway of the somnolent infant and toddler may be facilitated by the use of a shoulder roll. Upper airway secretions should be suctioned as needed. Airway adjuncts, such as oropharyngeal or naso- pharyngeal airways, may be considered. A patient with decreased airway control due to a postictal phase may be quite well managed with the use of one of these adjuncts.

Children who are awake and in respiratory distress should be allowed to remain in a position of comfort. This may include sitting on the lap of the primary caregiver during the assessment.

Infants and children with severe respiratory distress, respiratory failure, unresponsive patients who have lost the ability to protect their airway, and patients with increased intracranial pressure are candidates for elective intubation prior to transport. Intubation may have been performed prior to transport team arrival. The initial assessment of the transport team includes examination of breath sounds and chest expansion with assisted ventilation as well as assessment of ETT position on the chest film.[6] If the patient is not intubated, airway assess- ment again includes examination of breath sounds and chest expansion with spontaneous ventilation, level of consciousness, and perhaps blood gas analysis.

A major decision of the transport team is whether to intubate prior to transport. No one parameter can answer this question, and the patient's entire status must be considered. This includes the trends in assessment—Is the patient improving or deteriorating based on vital signs, history, and mental status? Other considerations are the mode of transport planned and the length of time in the transport vehicle. If the decision is made to intubate, the most experienced person available should perform the procedure. This may be the anesthesia staff from the referring hospital, or it may be a member of the transport team, depending on their expertise. Appropriate sedation should be provided prior to the intubation.

After intubation and assessment of breath sounds and chest expansion, a chest film may be requested. The endotracheal tube must be well secured prior to transport. It is the prerogative of the transport team to retape an existing endo- tracheal tube. Since it is the responsibility of the team to maintain an artificial airway for the duration of the transport, team members should feel comfortable resecuring the tube to their satisfaction.

BREATHING

The initial assessments of airway and breathing actually occur simultane- ously. The full examination of respiratory status includes assessment of respiratory rate, breath sounds (quality and quantity), accessory muscle use (work of breath- ing), color, and level of consciousness. The use of oxygen saturation monitors and end-tidal carbon dioxide monitors can provide noninvasive evaluation of ventilatory status. Arterial blood gas analysis can give definitive information about oxygenation and ventilation, but should never be considered independent of patient status.

All patients with respiratory distress or with any problem that might in- crease oxygen consumption should receive supplemental oxygen. Although the ideal is to deliver a high concentration of oxygen, the method of delivery is not critical in patients who require low F_IO_2, and a variety of methods will provide some supplemental oxygen. The hypoxic patient must, however, receive 100% oxygen, and it is vital that appropriate methods be available to do this. Head hoods can effectively deliver 90%[3] or higher and are well tolerated by infants.

Head hoods are available in sizes that can accommodate larger infants, not just newborns, and these can be used for the duration of the transport. Infant partial rebreathing masks and pediatric nonrebreathing masks can deliver high concentrations of oxygen (80–95%), but the masks themselves may not be tolerated by the irritable toddler. A face tent can provide 40–50% oxygen and has the advantage of also providing humidity (Fig. 2). This method is frequently well tolerated and should be considered as a method for delivery of supplemental oxygen.

A patient in obvious respiratory failure on physical examination does not need an arterial blood gas to document this fact. As soon as respiratory failure is recognized, the patient should be ventilated manually using a bag and mask, and arrangements should be made to intubate. After intubation and initiation of controlled ventilation, a blood gas can be obtained to assess current status and direct further ventilatory efforts. Since most transport vehicles do not have systems to blend compressed air and 100% oxygen, thereby providing a lower F_1O_2, ventilation with 100% oxygen during transport is acceptable. Although a definitive diagnosis of the cause of respiratory failure is not a necessary part of transport, the chest x-ray, taken to confirm placement of the endotracheal tube, may provide valuable insight into the problem.

Reactive airway disease is a common diagnosis of the 90s. Nebulized treatments should be started as soon as the diagnosis of reactive airway disease is noted. Continuous nebulized beta-2 agonist treatments may prevent the need for ventilatory support.[4,15] The transport team should be able to provide continuous nebulizer treatments for the duration of the transport, if needed. Since patients

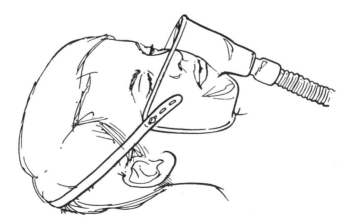

FIGURE 2. Face tent.

with this diagnosis often are difficult to ventilate mechanically and are at high risk for barotrauma, intubation should be considered only if deterioration is present in spite of maximal pharmacologic therapy.[2,5]

CIRCULATION

The patient's circulatory status is assessed, documenting heart rate, skin perfusion (capillary refill, quality of peripheral vs. central pulses, color, temperature of the skin), blood pressure, urine output, hydration status (skin turgor, mucous membranes), and level of consciousness. All critically ill or potentially critically ill patients should have at least one well-secured site of vascular access for transport. This may be a peripheral intravenous line, a central line, or an intraosseous line. Although the ideal is to have two sites, this may not always be necessary. The determination of need rests with the transport team.

The heart rate is assessed and compared with normal rates for the age of the child. Sinus tachycardia may be due to a variety of factors, such as pain, fever, fear, and crying, or may be due to respiratory distress or shock. Again, the assessment of parameters is made by looking at the entire child, not just one parameter.[8]

Hypovolemic shock is the most common type of shock seen in children.[3] Early signs of shock should be recognized and treatment initiated immediately. The combination of history and presentation will usually facilitate the differential diagnosis of type of shock. Fluid therapy for the treatment of shock consists of bolus fluids of 20 ml/kg of lactated Ringer's or normal saline. The bolus should be drawn up in syringes and manually pushed into the patient. Using 20-ml syringes provides less resistance when pushing through the small intravenous catheters usually placed in the child. This size syringe also enables easy calculation of the amount of fluid given. An 8-kg child would receive 8–20 ml syringes of fluid. After the bolus has been pushed, all vital sign parameters are reassessed, and repeated boluses are given as necessary. Albumin, 5%, should be available during transport and may be pushed as a fluid bolus, depending on the suspected etiology of the shock.

Although the initial bolus should be given while at the referring hospital, bolus fluid administration is something that can be easily done in any transport vehicle. If a stopcock is placed in line with the intravenous tubing, fluids can be safely pushed in transit without the use of needles. Inotropic therapy, if needed, should be started at the referring hospital. Although a transport team may certainly be able to initiate such therapy en route, it is physically much easier to do in the stable, nonmoving environment of the referring facility. All transport teams must have pumps available that can deliver medicated drips at the low flow rates frequently required in the pediatric patient.

Although cardiac dysrhythmias are uncommon in pediatrics,[2] the transport team must have the ability to monitor and treat any dysrhythmias. A cardiac monitor should be used on all transports, and a monitor/defibrillator unit should be available. The defibrillator must be capable of delivering the lower levels of energy necessary for the pediatric patient, and pediatric paddles must be available.[3] In addition, resuscitation medications such as epinephrine, lidocaine, atropine, and adenosine should be carried by the team.

NEUROLOGIC STATUS

Evaluation of the level of consciousness is an ongoing assessment, performed together with the stabilization of airway, breathing, and circulation. In the responsive child, age-appropriate behavior should be assessed, asking the parents or primary caregiver for their evaluation of the child's behavior. Pupillary response should be assessed in the child with a diminished level of consciousness. In addition, a brief ongoing neurologic assessment can be performed using the **AVPU** scale: **A**lert; responsive to **V**erbal stimuli; responsive only to **P**ainful stimuli; or **U**nresponsive.[7]

Seizure activity, a common pediatric diagnosis, may have a variety of causes. Initial stabilization includes oxygen delivery and administration of an anticonvulsant intravenously. Accurate recording of seizure activity, describing both the type of seizure and the duration, is important. The importance of airway maintenance and adequate ventilation cannot be overemphasized.[5]

Patients with suspected or known increased intracranial pressure are treated with the goal of preventing secondary injury. The patient's head should be elevated 30° and positioned midline. Mechanical ventilation is performed with the goal of controlled hyperventilation using the lowest effective setting of positive end-expiratory pressure. Mannitol should be available for use if necessary.

TEMPERATURE CONTROL

Temperature regulation is a key concern when discussing the pediatric patient. In the child, the high ratio of surface area to body mass encourages rapid heat loss. During the initial assessment and stabilization by the referring facility, the child may have been undressed and exposed, and hypothermia may result. The smaller the child, the more rapidly hypothermia can develop. Infants utilize brown fat as a source of heat, and this increases oxygen consumption by increasing the metabolic load. In the stressed infant, this may result in lactic acidosis and hypoxemia.[7,8,12]

Equipment such as heat lamps or warming blankets may be used in the emergency department environment to help rewarm the child. Although radiant warmers are an effective warming device for the small infant, they may not be readily available in the emergency department, and the staff may not be familiar with their use. Other adjuncts, such as heat packs, warm water in gloves, warmed inhaled oxygen, and warmed intravenous fluids, also may assist in temperature control in the infant and child. A temperature must be a part of the ongoing assessment of vital signs. A rectal temperature is preferred in the infant, toddler, and unconscious child, assuming they are not immunocompromised.

The transport team must consider temperature control as an important factor during the actual transport. Warm blankets should be available, especially in cold climates. Mylar "space" blankets are excellent to help insulate the patient and conserve body temperature.[5] Covering the head with a hat or blanket also can prevent heat loss. Pediatric critical care transport teams should have a transport isolette to use for infants. Most available transport isolettes can accommodate an infant up to 5 kg. The isolette should be prewarmed because they often take 20–30 minutes to reach the desired temperature. In addition to providing a warm environment, the isolette allows for better observation of the infant, who need not be bundled.

Fever increases metabolic demands and should be reduced when possible. Antipyretics can be given at the referring facility and excess bundling avoided. Extreme cooling must be avoided; it causes shivering, increasing the metabolic rate.[2]

HISTORY

Prior to leaving the referring facility, the transport staff should quickly review the history, asking questions of the parent or primary caregiver. Immunizations, allergies, past medical history (including medications), and recent exposure to communicable disease must be noted. An accurate recording of the events and treatment at the referring facility must accompany the patient on transport. This should include any work-up done, as well as the dose and time of all medications given.

HEAD-TO-TOE ASSESSMENT

The team should do a brief head-to-toe assessment, especially in the unconscious or postarrest infant or child. This may alert the team to other problems that may not have been identified. Unusual bruises, rashes, or skin markings should be documented and reported.

MISCELLANEOUS INTERVENTIONS

A gastric tube should be inserted in any patient with gastric distention or any patient being ventilated for transport. Either a nasogastric or orogastric tube is appropriate. For transport, the tube can be secured and placed to an open mucus trap or to a syringe and manually aspirated as necessary.

When appropriate, an indwelling urinary catheter should be placed. Not all patients will need this intervention, but any patient presenting with signs of shock and/or a postarrest patient will require ongoing assessment of urine output.

Infants and small children have decreased stores of glycogen in the liver. Stress may cause hypoglycemia, and a bedside glucose should be evaluated in all infants, regardless of the diagnosis. Children will require a bedside glucose if the presentation included seizures or dehydration—and in the postarrest patient of any age. Maintenance intravenous fluids should be calculated and all solutions titrated so that the child is receiving the appropriate hourly fluid rate. The fluid to be infused will depend on the presentation and on any available laboratory work as well as the results of the bedside glucose.

Oral food and fluids should be restricted or withheld prior to transport, depending on the condition of the child. Occasionally, a child will develop motion sickness, especially if riding backward in an ambulance. If the child is awake and insisting on oral fluids, the amounts should be limited. Sedation may be necessary in the intubated patient, both to facilitate effective ventilation and to prevent agitation and possible extubation.[5] A short-acting drug, such as midazolam, morphine, or fentanyl, can be used to accomplish this task. The short duration of these drugs allows for intermittent reevaluation of neurologic status.

PARENTS

The parents should remain at the referring facility until the transport team arrives. This enables the team to discuss the care of the child, obtain the necessary history, and obtain consents. It is important that the team discuss the patient with the family. The family may have misconceptions about the potential diagnosis or probable outcome, and these should be clarified by the team before they leave with the child.[18] Each team is different, and not all require that the parents/guardian give permission for transport. If this is a requirement, however, and the parents are no longer present, a delay in returning to the receiving hospital may result.

Although the general rule is that parents are not allowed to ride in the transport vehicle, there may be flexibility, depending on the mode of transport, distance of transport, team composition and number, status of the child, and parent behavior. Most alert toddlers and preschoolers are better cared for in the presence of a parent or caregiver. It is much more appropriate to allow the parent to accompany the child than it is to have the child crying throughout the transport. The less responsive the child, the less they need their parents, and it is appropriate for the parents to find transportation to the receiving hospital by some other means. Parents must be assessed for their ability to remain compliant and calm during the transport. Handling an emergency in the transport vehicle is challenging enough without the added burden of a stressed parent.

DOCUMENTATION

Ongoing assessment of the patient should occur at regular intervals throughout the transport. Vital signs must be recorded and all interventions documented. A flow sheet geared especially for the transport team will make this ongoing documentation easier, both to record at the time of transport and to read and understand later. The time of any changes in status should be noted on the transport record as well as the time of interventions and assessments (Fig. 3).

SAFETY RESTRAINTS

All stretchers used in the transport environment will have safety belts affixed. Infants and toddlers, however, may not be effectively restrained on such a stretcher. Varying the configuration of the safety belts may result in increased security, but it is rarely optimal. Crisscrossing the two belts over the child is certainly more effective than the standard procedure of each belt going from side to side.[5] A car seat is the preferred safety restraint system and should be used whenever possible. A standard commercial car seat may be used effectively. The Tumbleforms is an excellent safety restraint system and is adaptable for small infants as well as children. It is easily washed after each use as it is covered in soft plastic.

SUMMARY

It must be remembered that special skills, knowledge, and equipment are necessary to transport infants and children. There are many variables in the transport environment and all of them can affect the outcome of the patient. Assessment and stabilization during transport are geared toward the most emergent issues. Because any hospital is better than an ambulance, helicopter, or airplane, the "swoop and scoop" philosophy of scene response does not apply to the pediatric critical care transport setting. The goal is to provide a timely and safe transport of the patient so that definitive care can be provided at the receiving hospital.

MEDICAL RECORD NO.		PT. ACCT. NO.	
DATE TRANSPORT	TOTAL TRANSPORT TIME	PATIENT NAME	
TRANSFER FROM: HOSPITAL/UNIT		BIRTHDATE	TIME OF BIRTH	AGE AT REFERRAL
TRANSFER TO: HOSPITAL/UNIT		G.A.	BIRTH WEIGHT	PRESENT WEIGHT
REFERRING MD	MD PHONE	HOSP. PHONE	REASON FOR TRANSPORT

EQUIPMENT	MODE	TRANSPORT LOG
☐ PORTABLE ISOLETTE 3600	☐ Helicopter	CALL
☐ PEDS MONITOR 3601		DEPART CMH
☐ PORTABLE VENTILATOR 3602	☐ Fixed Wing	ARRIVE HOSP.
☐ PULSE OXIMETER 3606		DEPART HOSP.
☐ O₂ 3604 ☐ AIR 3605	☐ Ambulance	ARRIVE CMH
☐ NEO TRANSPORT MONITOR 3607		RespTherapist:

ARRIVAL / **ADM.**

TIME / T / P / R / BP / COLOR / O₂ SAT / FIO₂ / C/6 / Perfusion

NEUROLOGICAL — MODIFIED GLASGOW COMA SCALE

EYES OPEN: 4-SPONTANEOUSLY 3-TO SPEECH 2-TO PAIN 1-NONE

PUPILS: 2 3 4 5 6 7 8

BEST MOTOR RESPONSE: 6-OBEYS COMMANDS 5-LOCALIZES PAIN 4-WITHDRAWAL 3-FLEXION ABNORMAL 2-EXTENSION 1-NONE

BEST VERBAL RESPONSE:
5 - Oriented/Social smile, orients to sound, follows objects, cooing, jargon, converses. Interacts appropriately with environment.
4 - Confused/Disoriented/Consolable cries. Aware of environment, uncooperative interactions.
3 - Inappropriate Words/Inappropriate persistant cries, moaning, inconsistantly aware of environment, inconsistantly consolable.
2 - Incomprehensible Sounds/Agitated, restless, inconsolable cries. Unaware of environment.
1 - No response/No response

MEDICATIONS

MEDICATION	DOSE	ROUTE	TIME

RESPIRATORY THERAPY

TIME / MODE / FIO₂ / CPAP / IMV/RATE / INSP.TIME / TUBE/TRACH. SIZE / TIME / pH / pCO₂ / pO₂ / HCO₃ / B.D. / O₂ SAT

CHECKLIST	Y	N
VIT K		
EYE CARE		
C-SPINE IMMOBILIZED		
BAG & MASK		
GAG PRESENT		
SWALLOW PRESENT		

IV FLUIDS   **TRANSPORT PERSONNEL**

OUTPUT

URINE	
STOOL	
G.I.	
OTHER	

FIGURE 3.   Transport record (The Children's Memorial Hospital of Chicago).

REFERENCES

1. American Academy of Pediatrics Task Force on Interhospital Transport: Guidelines for Air and Ground Transport of Neonatal and Pediatric Patients. Elk Grove Village, IL, 1993.
2. Aoki BY, McCloskey K: Evaluation, Stabilization, and Transport of the Critically Ill Child. Chicago, Mosby, 1992.
3. Chameides L, Hazinski MF (eds): Textbook of Pediatric Life Support. Dallas, American Heart Association, 1994.
4. Colacone A, Wolkove N, Stern E, et al: Continuous nebulization of albuterol (salbutamol) in acute asthma. Chest 97:693, 1990.
5. Day SE: Intra-transport stabilization and management of the pediatric patient. Pediatr Clin North Am 40:2, 1993.

6. Fuller J, Frewen T, Lee R: Acute airway management in the critically ill child requiring transport. Can J Anaesth 38:252, 1991.
7. Haley K, Baker R (eds): Emergency Nursing Pediatric Course. Park Ridge, IL, Emergency Nurses Association, 1993.
8. Hazinksi MF: Nursing Care of the Critically Ill Child, 2nd ed. St. Louis, Mosby, 1992.
9. Kanter RK, Tompkins JM: Adverse events during interhospital transport: Physiologic deterioration associated with pretransport severity of illness. Pediatrics 84:43, 1989.
10. Kissoon N, Frewen TC, Kronick JB, et al: The child requiring transport: Lessons and implications for the pediatric emergency physician. Pediatr Emerg Care 4:1, 1988.
11. MacNab AJ: Optimal escort for interhospital transport of pediatric emergencies. J Trauma 31:205–209, 1991.
12. Mayer K, Cunningham J: Pediatric medical emergencies. In Lee G (ed): Flight Nursing Principles and Practice. St. Louis, Mosby, 1991.
13. Mayer TA, Walker ML: Severity of illness and injury in pediatric air transport. Ann Emerg Med 13:108, 1984.
14. McCloskey KA, Johnston C: Critical care interhospital transports: Predictability of the need for a pediatrician. Pediatr Emerg Care 6:89–92, 1990.
15. Moler FW, Hurwitz ME, Custer JR: Improvement in clinical asthma score and $PaCo_2$ in children with severe asthma treated with continuously nebulized terbutaline. J Allergy Clin Immunol 81:1101, 1988.
16. Orr RA, Venkataraman ST, Singleton CA: Pediatric Risk of Mortality Score (PRISM): A poor predictor in triage of patients for pediatric interhospital transport [abstract]. Ann Emerg Med 18:170, 1989.
17. Venkataraman ST, Rubenstein JS, Orr RA: Interhospital transport: A pediatric perspective. Crit Care Clin 8:3, 1992.
18. Youngberg BJ: Medical-legal considerations involved in the transport of critically ill patients. Crit Care Clin 8:3, 1992.

CHAPTER 3

Organization of a Neonatal Transport Program

CHERYL W. MAJOR, RNC, BSN

All hospitals that accept neonatal patients in transfer (outborn admissions) either should have a transport system of their own or should have an arrangement with another transport program. This service must provide the appropriate equipment, supplies, and personnel needed to handle any clinical situation that might develop, both upon arrival of the team at the referring hospital and during the actual transport. The overall goal is to try to continue whatever care is required in the hospital during the transport.[1]

Most hospitals that operate a transport service or are considering the creation of such a program already have been serving as a secondary (level II) or tertiary (level III) facility. Hospitals, whether nearby or in a remote area of the community or state, have a relationship with the physicians who direct specialized neonatal and pediatric services. This relationship or network may be prompted or encouraged by educational affiliations, state or locally mandated maternal and child health programs, or third-party contracts. In order for the transport service to operate promptly and efficiently, the referring community must be informed of the process for consultation and referral of patients, the pretransport care they are expected to provide, and the information that must be prepared to accompany the patient being transferred.

A written protocol should be developed to explain what patients should be considered for consultation and possible transfer. This would include a direct phone number so that unnecessary operator delays can be avoided. Information or specimens that should accompany the patient in transport also should be included in the protocol. It should be posted in the labor and delivery department, nursery, emergency department, and in referring physician offices within the network.

The outreach education program, usually an aspect of the network, must continually update referring hospital staff on necessary stabilization and pretransport care. In-service programs to enhance skills of airway management, including endotracheal intubation and suctioning, oxygen administration, monitoring, and assisted ventilation; chest compression; emergency administration of drugs and fluids; and maintenance of thermal stability should be available to all members of the health care team. Additional skills such as evaluation and management of sepsis and tension pneumothorax would also be appropriate to include.

The identification of an individual to serve as a "liaison" between the receiving and referring hospital facilitates prompt communication and dissemination of information. This person should be designated by the referring facility as the appropriate nurse or manager to direct mail or phone calls regarding patient information, educational offerings, or transport-related questions or concerns.

TRANSPORT PERSONNEL

The decision as to who should accompany the neonate during transport should be made jointly by the referring and receiving physicians based on the clinical condition. The team must have the collective expertise to provide the necessary observation and monitoring as well as specific interventions required in critical situations. Additional knowledge of the transport equipment and vehicle is also necessary.[1,6,7,11]

Potential Team Members
1. Neonatologist
2. Neonatology fellow
3. Pediatric resident
4. Neonatal nurse practitioner
5. Neonatal transport nurse
6. Neonatal staff nurse
7. Flight nurse/pilot
8. Respiratory therapist
9. EMT/paramedic
10. Neonatal transport driver-assistant

In selecting the team members, the following should be considered:
1. Existing state, local, and program standards
2. The amount of supervision required and available to the transport team
3. The degree of illness of the neonate
4. The distance and estimated length of transport
5. The legal scope of practice

Special courses and competency testing should be provided to confirm the educational preparation of the individual team members. The actual content will vary depending on the role of the team member. The course objectives should include, but not be limited to, the ability of the team member to:[1,11,15]

1. Obtain a pregnancy, labor, delivery, and nursery history and utilize data to anticipate problems.

2. Collaborate with other team members in performing a thorough physical and gestational age assessment prior to and throughout transport.

3. Perform a designated role in the performance of a complete resuscitation.

4. Describe the effect of environmental factors, e.g., humidity, ambient temperature, and velocity of air flow, on the neonate's thermal status and methods of promoting a neutral thermal environment during transport.

5. Describe the effects of speed acceleration and deceleration on gastrointestinal (GI) function and methods of reducing such stressors during transport.[5]

6. Utilize safe, efficient measures to limit complications of intravascular therapy during transport.

7. Describe the effects of altering atmospheric pressure, altitude, temperature, and humidity on neonatal respiratory function and measures to minimize these effects.[2]

8. Set up and correctly utilize respiratory support and monitoring equipment used during transport.

9. Identify the special techniques and measures required to limit the side effects of respiratory distress, GI obstructions, abdominal wall defects, and cardiac disease during transport.

10. Develop and implement procedures that will enhance prevention of infection and use of universal precautions in transport situations.

11. Describe and utilize measures that will enhance a positive relationship between parents and health care personnel in the referring and receiving centers.[9,10]

12. Collaborate with members of the neonatal network in developing transport plans that provide comprehensive, continuous, and expert care.

A transport service that performs more than 300 transports per year might find it desirable to have a dedicated transport team. The advantages include the development of transport expertise due to regular transport activity, development of a personalized relationship with the referring hospital staff, including knowledge of the level of care that can be provided, and readily available staff when a request for transport is received. When newborn nursery staff are used to perform transports, the NICU service may become disrupted; if the nursery is unable to admit additional patients owing to excessive census, an independent transport staff could more easily transport the patient to an alternate secondary or tertiary facility. Many transport programs with a dedicated staff are more easily able to expand their service to include back-transport of the newborns after their NICU stay. In units where maternal transports are encouraged when high-risk neonates are identified prenatally, the number of back-transported infants might equal or exceed the number of incoming "critical" transports.

TRANSPORT VEHICLE

The choice of a ground ambulance, rotary-wing aircraft, or fixed-wing aircraft as the transport vehicle is largely determined by the distance between hospitals and the local resources. Distances greater than 150 miles usually require the availability of air transport to reduce transport time. However, ground transport must be arranged to supplement air transport when weather conditions compromise transport safety or the landing location is too remote from the hospital. Ground transport also permits stopping the vehicle when an acute situation develops requiring evaluation and intervention, such as extubation or a pneumothorax.

The ambulance used for neonatal transport should, at a minimum, meet the requirements for a basic life support ambulance.[14,16] In order to accommodate neonates, the ambulance also must provide:

1. Secure fixation of the transport incubator to the cot rails.

2. Secure fastening of other equipment (e.g., oxygen and air tanks, monitoring equipment).

3. Independent power source to supplement equipment batteries to guarantee uninterrupted and fail-safe operation of the incubator and other monitoring and supportive equipment. Necessary adapters to access the ambulance power source should be readily available.

4. Environmental conditions that reduce the risk of temperature instability, excessive noise and vibration, and lack of cleanliness.[4]

5. Rapid and safe transport without compromising safety. The team leader should indicate the speed necessary since the neonate in most cases will be stable prior to beginning the transport, thus not requiring "emergency" speeds.

When using fixed-wing or rotary-wing aircraft for neonatal transport, knowledge of and compliance with the recommendations of the Commissions on Accreditation of Air Medical Services (CAAMS) is necessary.[2,3,11]

Tertiary neonatal units that admit a large number of neonates in transfer (outborns) often invest in a dedicated specialty neonatal intensive care ambulance. For such a vehicle to be licensed, each state must waive requirements to offer full-service ALS. Accomplishing this waiver may require modification of an existing EMS regulation. Kentucky and Tennessee are two states that have accomplished this regulatory adjustment.[14,16]

TRANSPORT EQUIPMENT AND SUPPLIES

The organization and maintenance of neonatal transport equipment and supplies are the responsibility of the transporting service.[16] If any equipment will be shared between the transporting hospital and the ambulance service, a plan should be in place to guarantee that it will be properly maintained and readily available when needed. A checklist should be in place to guarantee that all necessary equipment is available and in working order at all times and a posttransport checklist prepared to ensure replacement of supplies and recharging of equipment. When more than one patient requires transport, e.g., twins, duplicate equipment and supplies must be available.

Although the transporting team should bring all the equipment and supplies required to care for the neonate during stabilization and transport, the referring hospital should be able to provide a radiant warmer for thermal support while the team is assessing and stabilizing the neonate. The referring hospital also might provide laboratory tests such as arterial blood gases and radiographs for endotracheal tube or umbilical catheter placement prior to the team's departure.

When selecting specific equipment, weight and size should be considered in addition to the clinical function. When the transporter and supportive equipment exceed 200 pounds, a hydraulic lift may be required for ease of loading and unloading.

Thermal Support Equipment and Supplies

1. Transport incubator
2. Radiant warmer
3. Thermometer and/or temperature monitor and probes
4. Plastic wrap
5. Insulating blankets
6. Heat shield
7. Chemically activated heat packs or mattresses
8. Blankets

A transport incubator is required to provide a suitable thermal and protected environment during transport. The heat source should be adequate enough to provide the desired ambient temperature when preheating and recovery from being opened in a minimum of time. A servo-controlled heat mechanism with readily accessible and readable controls and temperature indicators is helpful. In extremely cold weather or with very premature and/or cold-stressed neonates, additional heat support may be necessary. A heat shield, covering the neonate's body with plastic wrap, using chemically activated heat packs or mattresses, or covering the exterior of the incubator with an insulating blanket are possible aids to reducing heat loss due to evaporation, conduction, convection, and radiation.

Care must be taken, however, to protect the infant from possible scalding injury and not to reduce the visibility.

The transport incubator must also provide:

1. A compartment in which portable oxygen and air cylinders may be locked securely

2. Unrestricted visibility from at least two sides

3. A light source in or on the incubator to guarantee uninterrupted illumination

4. Portability and adequate support by a frame that can be modified to accommodate necessary monitoring and supportive equipment

5. A frame that securely locks during transit

6. Safety restraint devices to secure infants inside the incubator while in motion

7. Easy accessibility to neonate via portholes that reduce loss of heat and oxygen

8. Adapters for connection to necessary AC/DC power sources in referring hospitals as well as in ambulance

A servo-controlled overhead radiant warmer should be available for neonates with special procedural needs and when frequent access is necessary. To promote safety while in motion, however, the warmer should be a feature of the transport incubator, not a free-standing open bed warmer.

Intermittent axillary and/or rectal temperature monitoring with rigid instruments can injure patients during transport. Newer incubators and vital signs monitors have the capability of providing continuous measurement and display of skin, axillary, or rectal temperatures by way of flexible and soft probes.

Respiratory Support Equipment and Supplies

1. Oxygen and air tanks with appropriate indicators of in-line pressure and gas content

2. Flowmeters

3. Oxygen blender

4. Oxygen analyzer

5. Oxygen tubings and adapters

6. Oxygen hood

7. Neonatal oxygen masks, nasal cannula

8. Neonatal/infant positive pressure bags and masks with manometer

9. Continuous positive airway pressure apparatus: nasal prongs; endotracheal tube

10. Mechanical ventilator with back-up circuit

11. Endotracheal tubes: 2.5, 3.0, 3.5, and 4.0 mm

12. Laryngoscope with size 0 and 1 straight blades

13. Laryngoscope batteries and extra lamps

14. Endotracheal tube holders or tape to secure ET tube

15. Blood gas analyzer

16. Transcutaneous O_2 and CO_2 monitor

17. Oxygen saturation monitor

18. End-tidal CO_2 monitor

19. Equipment for diagnosis and management of air leak syndromes: transilluminator; angiocaths #18, #20; thoracic catheters #10, #12, #14; chest tube drainage system; Heimlich drain

20. Surfactant administration supplies; endotracheal adapter

Most newborns require supplementary O_2 and/or respiratory support during transport. Even if a newborn is adequately oxygenated on room air prior to transport, the availability of oxygen and positive pressure ventilation by mask must be assured. The following guidelines offer assistance in the provision of O_2 and respiratory support during the pretransport and transport period.

1. The oxygen/air system must be able to deliver specific O_2 concentrations (FiO_2) throughout the entire transport. Surplus should be available to cover unexpected needs and delays (Table 1).

2. All gas cylinders must be appropriately secured to the incubator as well as the oxygen compartment of the ambulance.

3. The ambient O_2 concentration should be monitored with a calibrated analyzer and documented at least every 15–30 minutes.

4. Free flow O_2 should be administered via an appropriately sized mask or oxygen hood. A mask may interfere with oropharyngeal suctioning and the monitoring of the FiO_2, suggesting a preference for the oxyhood. Administration of O_2 into the entire incubator is not recommended owing to the inability to maintain necessary ambient O_2 when portholes are opened for care.

5. Nasal or endotracheal continuous positive airway pressure (CPAP) may be necessary to assist the neonate with alveolar instability and/or pulmonary edema. An anesthesia bag or mechanical ventilator may be used to administer O_2 and positive pressure. The protocol should be similar to that used in the receiving NICU. An orogastric tube open to the atmosphere should be considered to reduce gastric distention during nasal CPAP. The administration of the same FiO_2 via nasal prongs and an oxyhood has been found to reduce O_2 loss due to mouth breathing during nasal CPAP.

6. A neonatal or infant positive pressure bag and mask with appropriate safety features including a manometer should be available for short-term ventilation prior to placement on a ventilator or in case an acute need develops during transport. A portable ventilator should be available to provide uninterrupted mechanical ventilation when such assisted ventilation is needed. The management of a neonate requiring mechanical ventilation during transport should be per protocol approved by the medical director of the transport program. The ventilator must be securely mounted on the transport incubator with appropriate adapters to the medical gases. To conserve the oxygen/air tanks on the transporter, it is recommended that the ventilator be switched to the

TABLE 1. Oxygen Consumption Data

Cylinder Size/Type	Approx Weight (lbs)		Length (in) Incl Valve	Diameter (in)	Capacity		Inhalation @ 8 LPM (Approx Usage Mins)
	Empty	Full			Cu Ft	Liters	
D-Lightweight Steel	10	11	20	4½	12.7	360	45
D-Aluminum	5.7	6.8	19½	4⅜	15	414	52
E-Lightweight Steel	15	17	30	4½	22	625	78
E-Aluminum	8.2	10.2	28¾	4⅜	24	682	85
45 Cubic Feet	20.5	24.5	23	6¾	45	1278	159 (2.7 hr)
M-Steel	68	70	47	7	107	3030	378 (6.4 hr)
M-Aluminum	40	42	47	7¼	122	3458	432 (7.2 hr)
G-Steel	100	115	55	8½	187	5300	662 (11 hr)
H-Steel	110	130	55	9	244	6912	864 (14.4 hr)

Tennessee Perinatal Care System Guidelines for Transportation (September, 1985).

hospital's source of air and oxygen during the pretransport period. This may require the verification of oxygen/air adapter compatibility between the transporter and the hospital's medical gas gauges.

7. A system to provide heated humidification of oxygen is recommended. Technical difficulties are sometimes encountered in maintaining the heat with resultant condensation and evaporative cold stress of the neonate. There are devices that can be used in conjunction with a ventilator to raise the humidity without electricity or an external water supply.

8. A blood gas analyzer to verify blood gases is desirable. Technical difficulties due to vibration and motion often interfere with calibration, reducing its reliability during transport. State regulations also may forbid its use in some mobile intensive care units. A blood gas should be analyzed in the referring hosptial's laboratory if such information is needed to plan infant management.

9. Transcutaneous O_2 and CO_2 monitors should be considered to assess the infant during transport. Miniaturization of the monitor and reduction in calibration time have made the instrument more attractive to transport teams. Unless the neonate is extremely premature or poorly perfused, the heated sensor should not burn if the transport is completed within 2–4 hours.

10. Oxygen saturation monitoring using a pulse oximeter has become the principal oxygenation monitor during transport. Its portability and immediate read-out of pulse and O_2 saturation within seconds are definite advantages over transcutaneous monitoring. Limitations of its accuracy are related primarily to the difficulty in positioning the sensor on certain neonates and interference by activity and motion of the extremity during transport. Improved sensor design and variable sizes address these concerns.

11. End-tidal CO_2 monitoring is available to assess exhaled CO_2 via an endotracheal tube. Its application during neonatal transport has been helpful in identifying endotracheal extubation and changes in pulmonary CO_2 gas exchange. In the absence of arterial blood gas information, end-tidal CO_2 monitoring might permit more confident adjustments in ventilatory assistance by the transport team.

12. A protocol by the transport medical director for the evaluation and management of air leak syndromes must be followed by the transport team. The need for acute evacuation of a pneumothorax, pneumopericardium, or pneumoperitoneum may occur before transport in the referring hospital or during transit. A fiberoptic light to transilluminate the chest should be available in the ambulance when x-ray verification is not possible.

13. Surfactant replacement therapy may be beneficial in situations of greater distance between the referring and receiving hospitals. A protocol must clarify the indication for surfactant administration and the monitoring of the pulmonary response. The team must be qualified and experienced in mechanical ventilation and endotracheal intubation.

Suction Equipment and Supplies
1. Bulb syringe
2. Regulated suction with gauge limiting <100 mmHg or <4 inches Hg
3. Suction catheters with whistle tip and finger control (#5, 6½, 8, and 10 Fr)
4. Feeding tube (#8 Fr) and 20-ml syringe for orogastric decompression
5. Sterile gloves
6. Sterile water for irrigation
7. Meconium aspirator for use with endotracheal tubes for evacuation of meconium if attending delivery

Monitoring Equipment and Supplies

1. Cardiac monitor and leads to permit continuous heart rate surveillance. Alarm limits should be set to detect rates <100/minute or >200/minute. Limb leads or chest leads may be used as long as there is no interference with pulmonary and cardiac auscultation. A back-up battery should be fully charged prior to transport to guarantee uninterrupted cardiac monitoring.

2. A stethoscope must be available for auscultation of cardiac and breath sounds. Noises during transport, however, may interfere with auscultation, requiring that the ground ambulance be stopped if acute deterioration of the newborn occurs.

3. A peripheral blood pressure monitor and appropriate cuffs must be available for evaluation of the neonate prior to and during transport. Hypotension, most commonly due to hypovolemia, is relatively frequent in the sick neonate.

4. Central arterial and/or venous blood pressure monitoring would be recommended for unstable newborns. During transport, intermittent peripheral blood pressure monitoring may be technically difficult owing to vibration and motion.

5. Blood sugar evaluation should be done upon arrival of the transport team for planning of the appropriate glucose infusion. During transport, a method of glucose monitoring must be available. Reagant strips or instruments that do not require water rinsing are best suited to the transport situation.

Parenteral Infusion Equipment and Supplies

Most infants require parenteral therapy during transport. An infusion pump should be used that is portable, battery-powered, and calibrated to ensure accurate delivery of fluid volumes. Syringe pumps avoid problems related to temperature extremes and hanging tubing. Critically ill infants may require more than one infusion and two or more infusion pumps, e.g., cardiac patients requiring prostaglandin infusion. Supplies necessary for peripheral and umbilical infusions include:

1. Intravenous catheters (#22, 23, 24, 25, 26 gauge)
2. Syringes (1 ml, 3 ml, 6 ml, 12 ml, 20 ml, 35 ml)
3. Pediatric armboards, tape, or transparent dressings
4. Three-way stopcocks
5. Intravenous administration tubing compatible with infusion pump
6. Umbilical catheter tray
7. Umbilical catheters (#3.5 Fr and #5 Fr)

Peripheral infusions or umbilical catheters may already be in place on arrival of the transport team. Continuation or initiation of fluid therapy is the responsibility of the transport team. Umbilical venous catheters may be used if peripheral intravenous therapy is not successful and when umbilical artery catheters are not needed for blood gas monitoring and/or continuous blood pressure.

Supplies for Sepsis Work-up and Treatment

Many referring hospitals will already have collected the appropriate cultures and initiated antibiotic therapy prior to the transport team's arrival. If difficulties prevented the cultures from being collected or if the risk of infection was not appreciated, the transport team should be prepared to follow a medical protocol for a sepsis work-up with immediate antibiotic therapy before leaving the referring hospital.

1. Blood culture media should be available for aerobic and anaerobic cultures.

2. Pediatric lumbar puncture (LP) trays are needed for the evaluation of spinal fluid. In unstable or very serious clinical states, the LP may be postponed.

3. Bladder tap or catheterization for urine culture or antigen testing is preferable to the use of urine bags. A #5 Fr feeding tube is recommended for catheterization.

4. Nasopharyngeal cultures in nonintubated infants and tracheal cultures if intubated along with a chest radiograph will assist in evaluation of possible pneumonia.

5. A complete blood count and differential should be performed by the referring hospital laboratory if possible. To prevent delay in transport departure, the results should be phoned to the receiving hospital physician.

6. Superficial cultures such as axillae, ear, umbilicus, and gastric aspirate may be of assistance in identifying a potential pathogen.

Medications

All medications that might be necessary to stabilize or resuscitate a newborn prior to or during transport should be organized and portable for easy access at all times. This may be accomplished by an incubator frame with drawers or a separate bag or tackle box. A checklist of the required inventory should be completed at least daily with special attention paid to solution concentrations and expiration dates. Drugs such as phenobarbital and fentanyl require special pharmacy-directed security and documentation measures. A cooler is necessary for temperature-sensitive medications such as prostaglandin E_1. Written guidelines and phone consultation with the receiving hospital's designated physician, if necessary, should direct the transport team's administration of medications.

1. Sterile water for injection (preservative-free)
2. Normal saline (preservative-free)
3. Intravenous dextrose solution (10%, 50%)
4. Heparin (1000 units/ml)
5. Plasma expander: 5% albumin or plasma protein fraction
6. Sodium bicarbonate (0.5 mEq/ml) prefilled syringes
7. Tris(hydroxymethyl)aminomethane (THAM)
8. Epinephrine (1:10,000) prefilled syringes
9. Atropine
10. Dopamine
11. Dobutamine
12. Tolazoline
13. Prostaglandin E_1
14. Calcium gluconate 10%
15. Pavulon
16. Phenobarbital
17. Fentanyl
18. Dilantin
19. Narcan (0.4 mg/ml or 1.0 mg/ml)
20. Furosemide
21. Decadron
22. Digoxin
23. Surfactant (Exosurf, Survanta)
24. Broad-spectrum antibiotics: ampicillin and gentamicin

NEONATAL CONSULTATION AND TRANSPORT DOCUMENTATION

Records are essential for continuing care of the neonate and for the evaluation of the referral process. The referring hospital, transport team, and receiving hospital share responsibility for adequate documentation of clinical data.

Referring hospital responsibilities include provision of:

1. A copy of the complete maternal prenatal record
2. A copy of the current maternal medical record
3. A copy of the newborn's medical record, including all nurses' notes
4. A completed infant referral (Fig. 1). Not all receiving centers request such a form.

Transport team responsibilities include provision of:

1. A transport history, assessment, and admission note summarizing care of infant by the referring hospital and transport team. This is written by the transport team leader. Historical information in the medical record is supplemented by an interview with the parent(s) and family prior to leaving the referring hospital.

2. A neonatal transport worksheet. This is completed by the transport nurse. Vital signs are recorded every 15–30 minutes as well as other pertinent clinical information, including assessment and procedures done prior to and during transport.

3. A signed legal consent for neonatal transport, treatment during transport, and admission to the receiving hospital.

Some transport teams also complete a form summarizing the transport care, which is mailed to the designated referring hospital "liaison" for dissemination to the appropriate perinatal staff. Comments regarding the pretransport care are also included. This serves as an opportunity to reinforce good management and suggest specific interventions for the future.

Receiving center responsibilities include:

1. Maintenance of a record of all consultation and/or referral calls. The times of the transport request and team notification in conjunction with actual departure times permit calculation of program response times.

2. Maintenance of a record of the actual medical or nursing consultation or transfer conversations. Both the historical information received during the interview and the advice given by the receiving center should be documented.

3. Record of any follow-up conversations with the referring physician.

4. Arranging for an admission letter and discharge summary to be sent to the referring physician.

Communication

Phone communication by a direct number is essential for direct access to the transport team. A neonatologist, fellow, pediatrician, or nurse practitioner should be assigned responsibility for responding to such calls on a rotating basis. The consultation will aid in the development of a treatment plan resulting in one of three possible dispositions:

1. The required neonatal care can be provided by the referring hospital resulting in a simple consultation. A follow-up call within 24 hours should verify the appropriateness of the decision.

2. The transport is necessary, but the condition of the neonate does not require a team to be dispatched. The referring hospital is authorized to bring the patient after discussion of transport management. Preparation is made for the admission.

INFANT REFERRAL HISTORY

I. Identification

Baby's name: _____ Sex: _____ Race: _____
Date of birth: _____ Time of birth: _____
Place of birth: _____ Referring hospital: _____
Father's name: _____ Occupation: _____
Address: _____ Home phone: _____
County of residence: _____ Work phone: _____
Referring physician: _____

II. Maternal History

Mother's name: _____ Age: _____ Birthdate: _____
          Last, First, Middle, Maiden
Mother's social security number: _____
Prepregnant weight: _____ Height: _____ Weight at delivery: _____
Smoking: No/Yes (_____ cig/day) Drugs: No/Yes What? _____
Alcohol: No/Yes Hypertension: No/Yes Chronic or PIH
Chronic renal disease: No/Yes Diabetes: No/Yes (class: _____)
Chronic pulmonary disease: No/Yes
Heart disease: No/Yes
Married: No/Yes Occupation: _____
Blood type: _____ G: __ P: __ Term: __ Premature: __ Ab: __ Stillbirths: _____

III. Previous Pregnancies

Year Birthweight Gestational Age Sex VAG/C-Section VTX/Breech Special Care Required
1. _____
2. _____
3. _____
4. _____

IV. Present Pregnancy

Planned/unplanned LMP: _____ Sure/Unsure
EDC by dates: _____ EDC by ultrasound: _____
Prenatal care began: _____ I/II/III trimester
          Month/Day/Year
Number of prenatal visits: _____ Prenatal physician: _____
Antibody screen: _____ PPD: _____
GC: _____ VDRL: _____
Problems during pregnancy:
    Infections: _____ Premature labor (dates): _____
    Bleeding: _____ Glycosuria: _____
    Blood pressure: _____ Edema: _____
    Illnesses: _____ Proteinuria: _____

V. Labor and Delivery

Labor: Spontaneous/Induced Indication for induction: _____
Duration: 1st stage _____ 2nd stage _____
Rupture of membranes: Spontaneous/Artificial
Date and time of ROM: _____ Duration PTD: _____
Amniotic fluid: Polyhydramnios/Oligohydramnios/Foul smelling/Clear/Meconium-stained
          Cloudy/Bloody
Amniotic fluid culture: Yes/No
Vaginal bleeding (Amount, Pain, When): _____
Medications: Time Amount Mode
  Analgesic: _____
  Antibiotics: _____
  Pitocin: _____
  Other: _____
Fetal monitoring: Decreased FHT variability
          Extended fetal bradycardia
          Extended fetal tachycardia
          Late deceleration
          Variable deceleration

FIGURE 1 *(Continued on following page)*

VI. Delivery
Delivering physician: _____
Anesthesia: _____
Vaginal presentation: VTX, Breech, Face, Brow
Assisted delivery: Low forceps, mid forceps, vacuum extraction, rotation
C-Section: _____ Indication: _____ Type of incision: _____
Problems during delivery: _____
Placenta description: Weight:
       Abruption: Present (%)/Absent   Calcification: Present/Absent

VII. Infant At Birth
Time of birth: _____   Birth weight: _____
Gestational age by dates: _____ By exam: _____ By ultrasound: _____

APGAR Score: 1 min   5 min   min _____

____ Heart rate _____
____ Resp effort _____
____ Muscle tone _____
____ Reflex irritability _____
____ Color _____
            Total: _____

Resuscitation:
       Oxygen (Method Used) _____
       Suction: Oropharynx/Endotracheal   Meconium: No/Yes
       Endotracheal intubation: No/Yes   How long: _____
       Positive Pressure Ventilation: No/Yes   How long: _____
                              Manual/Ventilator
       Medications: Time _____ Type _____ Amount _____ Mode _____

VIII. Infant After Birth
Problems: _____
Pretransport stabilization:
       Oxygen (Mode and %): _____
       Intubation: No/Yes
       Bagging/ventilator: _____ Rate: _____ Pressures: _____
       IV fluids: Type: _____ Rate/Hr: _____
       Mode of IV administration: UA/ UV/Peripheral _____
       Medications:
              Eye prophylaxis: _____
              Vitamin K (Amt): _____
              Antibiotics: Time _____ Type _____ Amount _____ Mode _____
       Other: _____
Blood studies:
       Hematocrit: _____% (Central/Peripheral)
       Hemoglobin: _____
       Blood type: _____ Coombs: _____
       Blood count: _____
       Blood gases: _____
              Time   Source   pH   PO$_2$ PCO$_2$ BE   Respiratory management
       Chest x-ray: _____
       Has baby voided: No/Yes   Stool: No/Yes

IX. Comments:_____
_____
_____
_____
_____
_____

FIGURE 1 *(Continued from previous page)*

3. Transport by a specialized team is necessary. The supportive care that should be provided as well as the estimated time of team arrival is discussed.

During the transport, the team should have direct access to the receiving and referring centers by way of a mobile phone. This permits communication with the referring hospital in case there is a need for further assistance with pretransport care. The receiving hospital also can be reached when returning with the patient; thus, admission preparations can be made based on the most recent patient parameters, e.g., ventilator settings. All ambulances are required to have radio communications, but these usually are relayed by way of emergency departments, not directly into the neonatal patient care area.

Weekly progress letters are recommended to continue communication and to help prepare the referring physician for the possible back transport or home discharge of the patient. Copies of these progress letters might also be sent to the delivering physician or midwife and nursery staff.

Family Support

A newborn who requires transport to a facility for specialized care causes a variety of emotional responses within the family. Shock, denial, anger, sadness, and fear of the unknown all may be encountered by the referring hospital staff, transport team, and receiving center when dealing with the mother, father, grandparents, and other family support persons. Interventions to reduce the stress and support the grief response must be incorporated into the transport process.[9,10]

1. Allow parents to see and touch their child or children prior to transport. If the mother cannot be moved, the transporter with the neonate should be taken to the mother's room.

2. Thorough explanation ought to be given of the clinical problems and anticipated transport care by the referring physician and again by the transport team.

3. Information about the receiving hospital should be given to the parents, including location, parking rules, visiting policies, and general NICU facts. Some nurseries have created video tapes that personalize the NICU and its staff, removing some of the fear of the unknown that parents experience.

4. At least two Polaroid photographs should be taken of the patient and given to the mother.

5. Consider maternal transfer if the condition of the neonate is extremely critical.

6. Consider a phone call to the parents shortly after admission of the infant.

BACK TRANSPORT

In a regionalized system of care there is an emphasis on providing cost-effective appropriate care. Consequently, when a newborn infant no longer requires the resources of the tertiary or level III facility, plans should be made to return the patient to an appropriate level I or level II neonatal unit if home discharge is not yet possible. This is advantageous to the tertiary center as well as the family and other community hospitals.

The discharge planner or back transport coordinator is often a nurse who is familiar with the community hospitals and resources and may actually be the nurse who performs the transport. Arranging the back transport involves:

1. Assessment of the level of care required by the infant
2. Talking with parents regarding their choice of follow-up physician

3. Gaining acceptance of medical responsibility by the chosen community physician

4. Obtaining parental consent for transport

5. Communication and planning of care with the community nurses

6. Coordinating the discharge documentation, including the nursing and medical discharge summary.

The clinical care during transport will depend on the needs of the patient. Necessary therapy such as oxygen delivery, intravenous fluids, and cardiorespiratory monitoring must be continued throughout transport. At a minimum, the patient should be transported in a battery-supported incubator with cardiac monitoring, with a positive pressure bag and mask and oxygen source in case of acute deterioration.

REFERENCES

1. Accreditation Standards of the Commission on Accreditation of Air Medical Services (CAAMS), 2nd ed, Anderson, SC, 1993.
2. American Academy of Pediatrics and American College of Obstetricians and Gynecologists: Guidelines for Perinatal Care, 3rd ed. Elk Grove Village, IL, March of Dimes, 1992, p 35.
3. ASHBEAMS: Minimum Quality Standards. January 1987.
4. Bose CL: The transport environment. In MacDonald MG, Miller MK (eds): Emergency Transport of the Perinatal Patient. Boston, Little, Brown, 1989, p 194.
5. Campbell AN, Lightstone AD, Smith JM, et al: Mechanical vibration and sound levels experienced in neonatal transport. Am J Dis Child 138:967, 1984.
6. Danzig D: Neonatal transport teams: A survey of functions and roles. Neonatal Network 3:2, 1984.
7. Dunn N: Nursing practice in neonatal transport. Neonatal Network 1:16, 1983.
8. Ferrara A, Harin A: Emergency Transfer of the High-Risk Neonate. St. Louis, Mosby, 1980.
9. Hubner L: Neonatal transport: The psychosocial impact on the family. Neonatal Network 1:10, 1983.
10. McBurney B: The role of the community hospital nurse in supporting parents of transported infants. Neonatal Network 6:60, 1988.
11. National Association of Neonatal Nurses (NANN): Neonatal Transport Standards and Guidelines, 2nd ed, 1994.
12. Shenai JP: Sound levels for neonates in transit. J Pediatr 90:811, 1977.
13. Shenai JP, Johnson GE, Varney RV: Mechanical vibration in neonatal transport. Pediatrics 68:55, 1981.
14. State of Tennessee: EMS Rules and Regulations, 1988.
15. State of Tennessee: Tennessee Perinatal Care System, Educational Objectives for Nurses Levels I, II, II, IV. Neonatal Transport Nurses, 1993.
16. State of Tennessee: Tennessee Perinatal Care System Guidelines for Transportation, 1985.
17. Thompson TR: Neonatal transport nurses: An analysis of their role in the transport of newborn infants. Pediatrics 64:887, 1980.
18. U.S. Department of Transportation and the American Medical Association Commission on Emergency Medical Services: Air Ambulance Guidelines, Washington, DC, 1986.
19. Wright D, Einhorn T, Margulie RA: Ensuring safety during air transport. In MacDonald MG, Miller MK (eds): Emergency Transport of the Perinatal Patieint. Boston, Little, Brown, 1989, p 234.

CHAPTER 4

Aviation Physiology in Pediatric Transport

GEORGE A. WOODWARD, M.D.
DONALD D. VERNON, M.D.

Air transport greatly improves the speed of specialized care delivery. Undoubtedly, much morbidity and mortality has been avoided or circumvented thanks to this expedient mode of transport. Flying, however, is not free of complications. Catastrophic equipment failures or weather-related accidents are public knowledge, but many caretakers are unaware of the stresses air travel can have on a transported patient. It is well known that hypoxia, noise, vibration, cold, lack of humidity, hyperventilation, visual difficulties, and gas- or pressure-related events may affect pilots and flight personnel who otherwise are in good health. Acutely or chronically ill patients, however, may be compromised in their ability to acclimate to the stresses that flight imposes. While a healthy adult or child may ascend to 10,000–12,000 feet above mean sea level with only a mild increase in heart and ventilation rate, patients with pulmonary disease or other illnesses may have much less tolerance for an increase in altitude.[19] This chapter will review aviation physiology to remind the medical caretaker of problems one may encounter during air transport. Preparation prior to flight and recognition of potential difficulties during transport can help prevent some untoward sequelae.

GAS LAWS

To understand the effects of aviation on a patient, one must have an awareness and understanding of simple gas laws. Many laws dictate the behavior of gases at different pressures and temperatures, but the ones most relevant to routine air transport are Boyle's law and Dalton's law.[4,19] Boyle's law states that, with a constant temperature, the volume of a gas varies inversely with pressure. This can be stated as $P_1V_1 = P_2V_2$, where P_1 and V_1 represent initial pressure and volume and P_2 and V_2 resultant pressure and volume. For example, as barometric pressure decreases (with an increase in altitude), the volume of the gas will increase (Fig. 1). Conversely, on descent from altitude the barometric pressure will increase and the gaseous volume will decrease. The results of these changes are usually not severe during flight, although a fatality has been reported.[11]

Dalton's law (law of partial pressure) states that the total pressure of a gaseous mixture is the sum of the individual or partial pressures of all the gases in the mixture. Therefore, the total pressure of a gas (P_T) is the sum of the partial pressures ($P_1 + P_2 + P_3 \ldots$) contained in that mixture. For example, the total

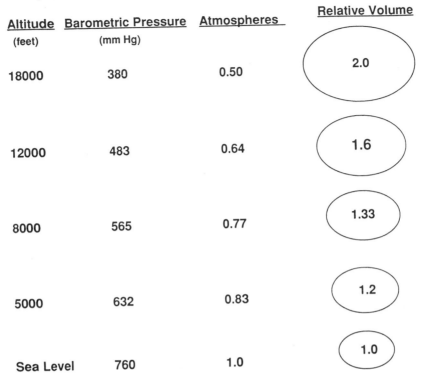

Altitude (feet)	Barometric Pressure (mm Hg)	Atmospheres	Relative Volume
18000	380	0.50	2.0
12000	483	0.64	1.6
8000	565	0.77	1.33
5000	632	0.83	1.2
Sea Level	760	1.0	1.0

FIGURE 1. Boyle's law ($P_1V_1 = P_2V_2$ or $P_1/P_2 = V_1/V_2$). As altitude increases, barometric pressure decreases and volume of gas increases. Diagram illustrates enclosed gas expansion at specific altitudes. "Atmospheres" is comparison to the amount of pressure exerted by the overlying one square inch air column. At sea level, this equals 14.7 pounds per square inch (psi) and one-half that amount (7.35 psi) at 18,000 feet.

pressure of air equals 1, with partial pressures being made up of nitrogen (0.78), oxygen (0.21), and other gases (0.1) (Fig. 2). The partial pressure of oxygen does not change with an increase or decrease in altitude and is always approximately 21% of the total volume of air. With air at altitude being less dense, however, oxygen molecules are farther apart and therefore less available to the patient. Barometric pressure does change with altitude and determines the amount of oxygen available for inspiration. As Table 1 demonstrates, one can predict the available PO_2 at each altitude by knowing the barometric pressure.

There are several other important gas laws, but their effects during routine air transport are negligible.

PRESSURE AND VOLUME EFFECTS ON THE PATIENT AND EQUIPMENT

These two gas laws are important to remember when preparing a patient for air transport and during the actual transport. One must consider if air (gas) is trapped within a space that may compromise a patient when the volume enlarges with an increase in altitude. Routine air spaces in the human body include the middle ear, sinuses, bowel, and occasionally the teeth.[1,4,19] A rapid ascent with decreased barometric pressure without venting of this increased volume of air can lead to disturbing and painful sequelae. The signs and symptoms of air

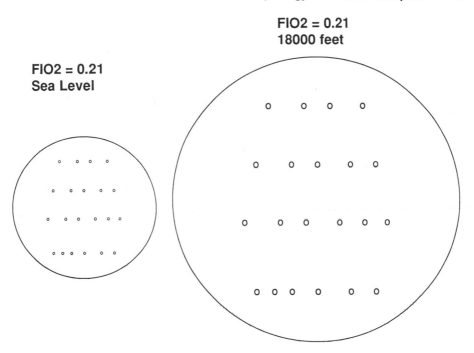

FIGURE 2. Dalton's law (law of partial pressures): $(P_T = P_1 + P_2 + P_3 \ldots)$. The total pressure of a gas is the sum of its component gases. Diagram illustrates that the percentages of air components (oxygen illustrated and represents 21% of air) at different altitudes does not change, although air is less dense at a higher altitude.

trapping and increased volume often can be alleviated by such simple procedures as swallowing, yawning, or Valsalva maneuver for middle ear air; awakening patients on descent to allow for equilibration of air in the eustachian tube; giving decongestants prior to flight for sinus congestion; belching or passing flatus for increased intestinal air; and descent if problems are not abated.[1,4,8,19] Aoki and McCloskey expand on these difficulties and treatments in their recent text.[1] One must be diligent to avoid sequelae from artificial air pockets, as in the external ear canal when tight ear plugs are used for noise control. While these pressure-related problems can be painful, they often lead only to a minor inconvenience

TABLE 1. The Effects of Altitude and Decreased Barometric Pressure on Oxygen Availability

	Altitude (1000 feet)			
	0	10	20	30
Barometric pressure	760	523	349	225
PO_2	160	110	73	47
H_2O vapor pressure	47	47	47	47
"Dry BP"	713	476	302	178
$PaCO_2$	40	40	40	40
PaO_2				
FIO_2 0.21	100	50	13	0
FIO_2 0.5	307	194	107	45
FIO_2 1.0	663	436	262	138

to the crew unless they distract attention from other more important tasks. In the patient, however, they can lead increased anxiety and distress, with hyperventilation and related physiologic changes. Alert, awake patients should be advised of potential pressure-related changes during ascent and descent and options for therapy reviewed. Sicker patients, however, may not be able to avoid these volume-related changes nor implement routine therapies. Sicker or acutely ill patients also may have areas of air trapped where increased volume with ascent will lead to more serious consequences. Emphysematous blebs or bullae may burst with an increase in volume, resulting in pneumothorax. A small pneumothorax, asymptomatic at sea level, may develop tension and cause serious problems on ascent to an 8000-foot cabin altitude. A patient with pneumocephalus from an open skull fracture may have difficulties if this air space increases. Expansion of the trapped intracranial air could lead to development or progression of increased intracranial pressure from the mass effect. Air trapped in a penetrating intraocular injury may cause pressure on the inner eye, resulting in vitreous extrusion with an increase in volume. The patient with a bowel obstruction or increased intraintestinal air may vomit or aspirate (gastric air); increase the size of the bowel leading to local ischemia, necrosis, or perforation (intestinal air); or may compress the diaphragm and decrease effective vital capacity (intraintestinal or intraabdominal air). Decreased vital capacity along with diminished oxygen availability will lead to poor tissue oxygenation and the signs and symptoms of hypoxemia[19] (Table 2). Trapped gastrointestinal tract gas also can lead to severe pain and a decrease in blood pressure, with syncope and shock secondary to vascular compression.[19] Gastric and rectal tubes should be considered when appropriate in the management of these patients. Open wounds may have air trapped in the soft tissues, but do not usually present a problem unless expansion is limited by a circumferential splint or cast. Cast bivalving may be necessary before ascent to altitude.[8]

Air volume and pressure in pneumatic devices such as MAST trousers, blood pressure cuffs, air splints, or intravenous bottles will be affected by pressure changes during ascent and descent as well.[1,17] The air in MAST trousers will increase in volume and pressure with ascent to the limits of the pop-off valves within the trousers and will diminish in volume and pressure with descent.[16] The same will occur with blood pressure cuffs and air splints. These require constant monitoring to avoid an inadvertent tourniquet effect on an extremity with the increased pressure and volume. On descent added volume may be needed for pneumatic devices if there was a volume leak or if air was removed during ascent. Air in intravenous glass bottles will expand with an increase in altitude, raising the pressure on intravenous fluids.[8] This will increase the rate of the pressure-related flow and can be detrimental if fluid or drug administration must be carefully rate-limited. The opposite will happen on descent. With less

TABLE 2.   Signs and Symptoms of Hypoxemia

Headache	Tingling or warm sensation, sweating	Performance deterioration
Fatigue	Behavioral changes	Muscle incoordination
Tachypnea	Agitation	Numbness
Tachycardia	Confusion	Reduced, blurry vision
Air hunger	Irritability	Cyanosis
Dullness, drowsiness	Feeling of well-being (euphoria)	Syncope
Listlessness	Impairment of judgment	Unconsciousness
Light-headedness or dizzy	Faulty memory	Convulsions

pressure, the fluid flow will be slower. For these and other reasons, one should not use glass intravenous bottles during air transport. Intravenous pumps and plastic intravenous bags are most useful in avoiding rate variability secondary to pressure changes during ascent and descent.

Air in balloons (cuffs), as on endotracheal tubes or Foley catheters, also can lead to problems during ascent and descent. While the bladder usually is large enough to accommodate an increase of several fold in Foley catheter balloon size, the trachea cannot increase in size to accommodate an expanding balloon. Tracheal mucosal ischemia could result from a prolonged flight with a balloon that is tightly inflated.[8] An endotracheal balloon that loses volume during descent could lead to ineffective ventilation secondary to increased air leak around the balloon. These problems can be avoided by routinely assessing the balloon to ensure that it is properly inflated or by using water or saline rather than air, as the change in pressure with altitude will not affect liquid as it does gas.[1] Large-volume, low-pressure cuffs may be useful in these situations.[8]

One must be careful with air transport for a patient involved in a diving accident. A small increase in altitude can cause large increases in the volume of trapped air. This is especially dangerous with an air embolism in the cardiovascular or central nervous system.[19] A patient who has been subjected to the increased barometric pressure under water is particularly susceptible to pressure-related sequelae during air transport. In fact, a flight to 8000 feet after SCUBA diving actually places the diver at the same barometric pressure risks as a nondiver would experience at 40,000 feet in a nonpressurized aircraft.[4]

OXYGENATION AND VENTILATION

Hypoxia is the most dangerous stressor for air transport. Atmospheric PO_2 decreases linearly with barometric pressure (see Table 1). The result is a decrease in oxygen available for exchange in the lungs at what may seem to be rather modest altitudes. Oxygen tension in the alveoli (PAO_2) can be calculated using the alveolar gas equation. Note that Dalton's law requires that the total pressure be equal to the sum of all the component gases; therefore, one must account for the vapor pressure of water, 47 torr at body temperature, since air in the lungs is always completely saturated with water vapor. This can be stated by the alveolar gas equation, $PAO_2 = (BP - PH_2O) \times FIO_2 - (PCO_2 \times 1/R)$, where BP is barometric pressure and R is the respiratory quotient, usually about 0.8. For a normal individual breathing "room air," this can be further simplified as $PAO_2 = (BP - 47) \times 0.21 - (50)$.

The effect of increasing altitude on PAO_2 is also shown in Table 1. One can see that increasing altitude (decreasing barometric pressure) can profoundly reduce PAO_2 and that administration of supplemental oxygen can provide adequate O_2 for gas exchange, even at very reduced barometric pressures.

Thus, both increasing barometric pressure and supplying supplemental O_2 can effectively treat hypoxemia due to transport-related changes in barometric pressure. The simplest way to avoid hypoxia is with supplemental O_2. For most air-transported patients (other than premature newborns), the use of 100% O_2 via nasal prongs, face mask, or intubation is preferred. For patients with significant diffusion difficulties, however, even 100% O_2 may not be sufficient for adequate oxygenation. For example, a patient with pulmonary disease who is receiving 100% O_2 with a PaO_2 of 75 at sea level would not be a good candidate for routine air transport. An increase in altitude would decrease the available O_2 which would lead to a further decrease in PaO_2 and O_2 delivery.

Consideration of the alveolar gas equation suggests that a reduction in $PACO_2$ should also increase PAO_2. Indeed, hyperventilation is a natural compensation for hypoxemia in the normal situation. This mechanism can significantly improve the PAO_2 by decreasing $PACO_2$, as noted in Table 3. Uncontrolled hyperventilation, however, can be detrimental.

The signs and symptoms of hyperventilation can be confused with those of hypoxia.[4,19] The onset of hyperventilation is usually more gradual, however, and may be associated with muscle spasm or tetany. Hyperventilation may accompany anxiety or fear concerning the medical condition or the transport itself. An increase in supplemental delivered O_2 can help distinguish between hypoxia and hyperventilation. The symptoms of hypoxia should improve after four or five breaths of 100% O_2, whereas hyperventilation symptoms will continue. If hyperventilation continues, one should attempt to slow the respiratory rate by talking to or distracting the patient.

It may also seem reasonable that an increase in the barometric pressure by application of positive end-expiratory pressure (PEEP) might increase PAO_2. Although PEEP may be very useful in the treatment of arterial hypoxemia due to acute lung disease, such as the adult respiratory distress syndrome, it does not act via changes in barometric pressure. A consideration of the actual pressures involved will indicate why. For instance, PEEP of 30 cm H_2O is considered a very high level of PEEP, but a barometric pressure of 30 torr is equivalent to an altitude change of only about 1500 feet. Thus, application of even this very high level of PEEP will yield a change in PAO_2 of only about 5%, or about 6 torr for an individual breathing air at sea level, when considering only the changes in barometric pressure. For the individual with severe acute lung disease, who has improvement in arterial oxygenation with the application of PEEP, this therapy is obviously beneficial, but it will not effectively compensate for changes in barometric pressure.

EFFECTS OF PREEXISTING ILLNESS

It is important to consider that the physiologic effects of changes in barometric pressure do not act in isolation, but are superimposed on disease processes that are ongoing in each patient. The patient with severe lung disease probably presents the greatest problem. Adult respiratory distress syndrome, for instance, may result in lung disease of such severity that proper oxygenation is nearly impossible even at sea level in the ICU. Indeed, an inability to oxygenate such patients properly may be the reason to arrange for transport, perhaps to a facility that can provide higher-level care or such specialized therapy as extracorporeal membrane oxygenation. In some cases, even modest changes in barometric pressure associated with air transport may be poorly tolerated. Waggoner

TABLE 3. Oxygen Availability with Changes in Ventilation (PCO_2) at Inspired Oxygen Concentrations (FIO_2) of 21 and 100 Percent

Barometric Pressure	PCO_2	PAO_2 ($FIO_2 = 0.21$)	PAO_2 ($FIO_2 = 1.0$)
760	40	100	673
760	20	125	693
760	60	75	653
523	40	50	483
523	20	75	503
523	60	25	463

reported the case of a child with significant lung disease who experienced severe hypoxemia on transport and arrived at the receiving institution with a PaO_2 of 21 torr.[19] Interestingly, Grant and coworkers examined the question of transport of the patient with severe hypoxemic respiratory failure using a computer model. They concluded that most gas exchange problems caused by decreases in barometric pressure could be overcome by breathing oxygen.[6] Any patient who requires oxygen at sea level will require larger amounts at altitude. Furthermore, patients who are compensating for their lung disease at sea level may require supplemental O_2 during transport. As mentioned, the clinical signs of hypoxemia are fairly nonspecific, but include tachycardia, tachypnea, anxiety, agitation, headache, and confusion[4,19] (Table 2). The pulse oximeter is invaluable in monitoring arterial oxygenation during transport.

One must also consider aspects of the patient's condition that may not seem related to changes in barometric pressure, at least at first glance. Primary among these are changes in blood hemoglobin concentration, since many patients are transported after experiencing trauma, associated bleeding, and anemia. Hemoglobin is essential to O_2 transport; virtually all O_2 carried by the blood is bound to this protein. A 50% drop in hemoglobin will result in approximately a 50% drop in O_2 carrying capacity. Even fairly severe anemia, with a hemoglobin of 7 gm/dl blood, might be tolerated if oxygen tension were maintained. However, such a patient has little reserve, and might not tolerate decreased PAO_2 related to changes in barometric pressure if any arterial desaturation resulted. A hemoglobin level of 7 gm/dl represents a reasonable lower limit for safe air transport, although a patient who is compensating for anemia at sea level while breathing "room air" probably can be transported safely if supplemental O_2 is provided.

A patient with a decreased cardiac output also will react unfavorably to a decrease in available O_2. Patients with metabolic difficulties, such as methemoglobinemia or carbon monoxide poisoning, will not benefit from a decrease in available O_2. As the delivery of O_2 is of vital importance during a high-altitude air transport, it is important to reassess continually the O_2 delivery system and the response of the patient to the delivered oxygen. It is important to realize that one will not appreciate cyanosis in a patient with a normal hemoglobin level until the O_2 saturation is 75% or less.

Changes in barometric pressure also may affect the flight team. Hypoxia is the most obvious and important such effect, but other interesting phenomena may be observed. For instance, Flynn and coworkers studied the effects of barometric pressure on contact lens wearers and found that changes in altitude as slight as 6000 feet caused bubbles underneath the lens, although no effects on vision could be demonstrated.[5]

AIRCRAFT AND ENVIRONMENTAL ISSUES

Pressure-related problems often do not occur at usual air medical flight altitudes or in pressurized aircraft. Pressurization effectively subjects a patient to a lower altitude (higher barometric pressure) than the outside environment.[1] Helicopters generally do not have pressurized cabins, but seldom fly at high altitudes, so these patients are not commonly subjected to great changes in air pressure. In areas such as the U.S. mountain West, however, adverse pressure effects might occur when transport originates from an area of lower altitude and the aircraft must ascend to cross a mountain range. Fixed-wing aircraft, on the other hand, fly at high altitudes. Although cabins are pressurized in these aircraft, this does not necessarily protect patients from dysbarism. Air pressure in the cabin is routinely equivalent to the barometric pressure at 8000 feet elevation ("cabin altitude"), which is approximately 565 torr[8] (Fig. 1). According to Boyle's law, this will lead to a 33% increase in volume of gas in an enclosed space—conceivably enough to be problematic (in the form of a pneumothorax, for instance). Cabin pressurization is limited by the ability of the aircraft structure to maintain a pressure differential, which can range from 5.5–10.5 psi.[8] Thus, cabin altitude is determined both by the characteristics of the specific aircraft and by the flight altitude. If the patient cannot tolerate the effects of decreased air pressure, it is possible to compensate by pressurizing the cabin or descending to a lower altitude, where a lesser pressure differential between the cabin and atmospheric pressure yields a higher cabin pressure (lower cabin altitude). However, in most cases, the cabin pressure, and hence the PO_2, will be lower than that at sea level when the aircraft is above 22,500 feet.[8] It might seem ideal for every medical transport to fly at altitudes low enough to allow a sea-level cabin altitude; however, low-altitude flight has several serious drawbacks, including increased fuel consumption, lower speed, and increased turbulence.[8] Reduced-altitude flights have been used in special cases, such as that of a six-year-old boy with severe chronic lung disease who had lost consciousness on commercial flights (cabin altitude 8000 feet), but who tolerated a long transport where the cabin altitude was maintained below 3700 feet. This flight required extensive planning and extra fuel stops.[9]

Modern transport aircraft reliably maintain cabin pressurization, and loss of cabin pressure rarely occurs during civilian peacetime flights. However, should this occur, the results may be disastrous.[19] The risk is possibly greater for the flight team than for the patient, as most patients are transported on supplemental O_2, while the crew is breathing cabin air at $FIO_2 = 0.21$. Loss of cabin pressure will rapidly produce unconsciousness from hypoxemia.[4] At 30,000 feet, useful consciousness is estimated at 90 seconds, decreasing to 30–60 seconds at 35,000 feet.[4,19] As noted previously, supplemental O_2 can protect against hypoxemia due to low barometric pressure, but the time required to begin oxygen is critical.[4] Marotte and coworkers noted that even a brief delay in donning oxygen masks (3–8 seconds) following rapid decompression from cabin altitude 8000 feet to 30–39,000 feet resulted in severe desaturation in experimental subjects, producing hemoglobin saturation levels as low as 63%.[10]

While hypoxia, pressure, and volume changes are the main concerns of the effects of air transport on a patient, one also must consider the changes presented by noise, vibration, motion, gravitational forces, temperature, and humidity.[1,2,4,17,19] The temperature decreases with altitude, as does the humidity.[17] While temperature is easily controlled in an aircraft, pressurized air, which is compressed and forced into the cabin has humidity identical to the outside air. In a typical prop aeromedical transport plane, this varies between 10–25%, although it can be as low as 5–10% at 30–40,000 feet.[8,19] For the patient this should be addressed with fluid intake and humidified O_2 delivery when applicable. While the cabin temperature in the plane is usually comfortable, one must be prepared for the possibility of decompression and a rapid decrease in temperature. The temperature at altitude can be calculated by remembering that the lapse rate for temperature change is minus 2°C for each 1000 feet increase in altitude.[8] There should be warming blankets available for the patient if needed.

Rapid decompression also can predispose one, especially if intubated, to pneumothroax or air embolism.[17] The probability of significant sequelae from decompression depends on the speed at which the decompression takes place.[4,19]

This in turn is related to the size of the space being decompressed, the area of decompression, and the pressure differential.[19] In most civil air transports this is not a grave concern. If decompression is slower than 0.5 seconds, the risk of the above sequelae is minimal.[4]

The gravitational forces associated with rapid acceleration and deceleration can lead to a pooling of blood, with decreased oxygen and nutrient delivery as well as variations in cardiac output.[8] These are more theoretical concerns, as it is usually impractical to reposition patients during transport to avoid these forces completely. The linear acceleration with most civil transport aircraft is limited to 0.5 g and is not strong enough, nor of sufficient duration, to cause significant problems to the patient.[8,19] Acute deceleration, however, may be more likely with rapid braking and perhaps is more relevant to patient positioning.[18] A head-injured patient, for example, could be positioned with the head forward on take-off and aft on landing to avoid blood pooling with the linear acceleration and deceleration. Most likely, however, the patient's position will not adversely affect outcome in routine air transports. One must also be aware that forces present during transport (linear, centrifugal, turbulence) will adversely affect traction weights and other free devices; therefore, these should not be used. The forces presented may change the position of the patient in relation to securing straps, which may become loosened or misconnected. This is especially important in an immobilized patient with straps across the bony prominences of the shoulder and pelvis, which, owing to positional changes, may have moved to put pressure on the abdomen and chest. One can appreciate how this could lead to respiratory insufficiency in an already-compromised patient. Shifting of the patient with motion or vibration could be disastrous for one who has a cervical spine injury and has moved from a neutral immobilization position to hyperextension or hyperflexion.[20] One should request that aeromedical pilots avoid steep (short field) takeoffs, steep banking turns, and rapid decelerations, when possible, to avoid increased linear and centrifugal (change in direction) forces that may lead to deterioration of an already compromised patient.

Vibration and noise can be disconcerting to the patient, lead to increased anxiety, and be manifested physiologically by increased blood pressure, heart rate, diaphoresis, and combativeness.[4,19] One should anticipate these changes, prepare the patient, provide ear protection, vibration dampening, and reassurance. Noise and vibration also affect the capability of the caretaker to assess the patient in a routine manner.[13] Stethoscopes are virtually worthless in a loud aircraft environment for auscultation of breath sounds, heart sounds, or blood pressure measurement.[8,13] Use of electronic devices such as Doppler, EKG, pulse oximetry, and capnography may provide better clues for the moment-by-moment evaluation of vital functions. Blood pressure determination by palpation also can be useful if the vibration is not excessive. Visual alarms for vital sign abnormality or equipment malfunction will be more useful than auditory alarms in noisy aircraft. Auditory clues to patient condition such as air leak around an endotracheal tube cuff and grunting respirations will be less helpful to the caretaker. Communication between crew members and the patient will be impeded by the loud background environment, but can be improved with the use of aviation headsets and intercoms.

Noise exposure is a problem outside the aircraft and can cause significant problems for both the crew and the patient. This may be especially important in a tenuous neonatal patient at risk of altered physiologic parameters with an increase in noise and vibration during air transport.[3,17,19] Neonates are generally transported in some type of isolette or incubator to help control some of the physiologic stresses of flight, particularly thermal stress. However, such attempts can have unexpected effects. All medical equipment generates electromagnetic interference, and Nish and coworkers reported that 70% of neonatal incubators, monitors, and ventilators generate excessive electromagnetic interference by military standards.[12] The potential for catastrophic interference with aircraft electronics exists, although no accidents are documented to have resulted from this cause.

Turbulence is also a potential problem for both the crew and the patient. Objects, personnel, and patients who are not secured can become projectiles or be hit by one in a turbulent aircraft.[8] This problem can be avoided easily by ensuring that all patients and cargo are securely fastened to the aircraft prior to movement. Not only can turbulence make care of the patient difficult, it can also predispose all occupants, even seasoned flight crew members, to motion sickness.

One must be prepared to treat air (motion) sickness in a patient or accompanying family member during a flight. Air sickness can be manifested by anxiety, diaphoresis, increased salivation, nausea, vomiting, hyperventilation, headache, pallor, and decreased attention.[8] This represents an inconvenience in a seated passenger, but may lead to more significant sequelae, such as aspiration and hypoxia, in a secured patient who is supine. Treatment options for motion sickness can include oxygen, concentration on a stationary object, and cooling of the environment, as well as prophylactic medication.[8]

Other issues that should be considered for the patient (and crew) with air transport are the possibilities of carbon monoxide or gas fume inhalation while working in the vicinity of a helicopter, prop, or jet plane.[15] This can be a problem with helicopter flights in a relatively enclosed area where the medical team and patient are close to the aircraft and its fumes for a prolonged period. Symptoms of nausea, headache, rhinorrhea, light-headedness, cough, sleepiness, and eye tearing can be secondary to exhaust or jet fuel fumes.[15] It is important to remember that carbon monoxide has more than a 200 times greater affinity for hemoglobin than does oxygen and that the patient who has problems with hypoxia, anemia, poor perfusion, acute blood loss, or low hemoglobin may be especially susceptible to the effects of carbon monoxide exposure during evaluation next to a running helicopter. These symptoms should abate with removal of the offending source and supplemental O_2. It is important to remember that these symptoms also can affect the healthy members of the medical team. Their effect, however, is probably much more pronounced in the compromised patient.

Care should be given to preparation of the crew and patient in case of aircraft malfunction and crash or landing in an off-airport location. Crews should be trained and properly equipped for survival with water landings, mountainous, uninhabited, climate extremes, or other hostile terrain.[4] Passengers should be briefed on emergency procedures before the transport.

SUMMARY

Patients who undergo aeromedical transport obviously suffer from a wide variety of diseases and physiologic derangements. It is impossible to describe every possible situation related to changes in barometric pressure or other transport-related stresses that might be encountered during transport. However, one can anticipate many problems by carefully considering the patient's specific disease process and how it may interact with changes encountered during air transport. Proper preparation and anticipation of the effects of air transport for each patient will help ensure a safe and uneventful transport.

REFERENCES

1. Aoki BY, McCloskey K: Physiology of Air Transport. Evaluation, Stabilization, and Transport of the Critically Ill Child. St. Louis, Mosby, 1992.
2. Browne L, Bodenstedt R, Campbell P, Nehrenz G: The nine stresses of flight. J Emerg Nurs 13:232–234, 1987.
3. Campbell AN, Lightstone AD, Smith JM, et al: Mechanical vibration and sound levels experienced in neonatal transport. Am J Dis Child 138:967–970, 1984.
4. Department of Transportation, Federal Aviation Administration: Physiology Training. Oklahoma City, 1980.
5. Flynn WJ, Miller RE II, Tredici TJ, et al: Contact lens wear at altitude: Subcontact lens bubble formation. Aviat Space Environ Med 58:1115–1118, 1987.
6. Grant BJB, Bencowitz HZ, Aquilina AT, et al: Air transportation of patients with acute respirtory failure: Theory. Aviat Space Environ Med 58:645–651, 1987.
7. Howard RP, Rivera O: Biomedical aspects of neonatal transport. In MacDonald MG, Miller MK (eds): Emergency Transport of the Perinatal Patient. Boston, Little, Brown, 1989.
8. Lachenmyer J: Physiological aspects of transport. Int Anesthesiol Clin 25(2):15–41, 1987.
9. Macnab AJ, Vachon J, Susak LE, Pirie GE: In-flight stabilization of oxygen saturation by control of altitude for severe respiratory insufficiency. Aviat Space Environ Med 61:829–832, 1990.
10. Marotte H, Toure C, Clere JM, Vieillefond H: Rapid decompression of a transport aircraft cabin: Protection against hypoxia. Aviat Space Environ Med 61:21–27, 1990.
11. Neubauer JC, Dixon JP, Herndon CM: Fatal pulmonary decompression sickness: A case report. Aviat Space Environ Med 59:1181–1184, 1988.
12. Nish WA, Walsh WF, Land P, Swedenburg M: Effect of electromagnetic interference by neonatal transport equipment on aircraft operation. Aviat Space Environ Med 60:599–600, 1989.
13. Pasic TB, Poulton TJ: The hospital-based helicopter: A threat to hearing? Arch Otolaryngol 111:507–508, 1985.
14. Poulton TJ: Helicopter downdraft: A wind chill hazard. Ann Emerg Med 15:103–104, 1986.
15. Poulton TJ: Medical helicopters: Carbon monoxide risk? Aviat Space Environ Med 58:166–168, 1987.
16. Sanders AB, Meislin HW: Effect of altitude change on MAST suit pressure. Ann Emerg Med 12:140–144, 1983.
17. Task Force on Interhospital Transport: Guides for Air and Ground Transport of Neonatal and Pediatric Patients. American Academy of Pediatrics, 1993, pp 99–102.
18. Vernon DD, Woodward GA, Skjonsberg AK: Management of the patient with head injury during transport. Crit Care Clin 8:619–631, 1992.
19. Waggoner RR: Flight physiology. In Lee G (ed): Flight Nursing, Principles and Practice. St. Louis, Mosby, 1991, pp 2–27.
20. Woodward GA: Neck trauma. In Fleisher GR, Ludwig S (eds): Textbook of Pediatric Emergency Medicine, 3rd ed. Philadelphia, Williams & Wilkins, 1993.

CHAPTER 5

General Neonatal Physiologic Considerations

MARK S. GAYLORD, M.D.
CINDY A. MICHALUK, R.N., M.S.N.

The successful completion of a neonatal transport requires an understanding of the unique physiology of the newborn infant and the adverse conditions of the transport environment. The immediate newborn period is characterized by rapid physiologic changes in temperature, sleep state, and respiration. This transitional period often is adversely affected by various disease states, environmental conditions, and treatment practices that can seriously complicate transport. In this chapter, we will discuss this transitional period, temperature regulation, and the effects of adverse environmental conditions, and fluid and metabolic requirements during transport. We will also describe two conditions unique to neonatal transport: the management of the extremely low birthweight infant and the hydropic neonate.

TRANSITION

The unique physiologic changes associated with the birth process remain a marvel to the complex human physiologic nature. At no other time do such dramatic changes in environment, organ function (i.e., onset of respiration; rerouting of the fetal cardiovascular system; rapid maturation of hepatic, renal, and bowel function), and reorganization of metabolic processes occur.[1,2] This period of almost instantaneous transition must be traversed by all newborn infants, whether small or large, premature or mature. The clinician must be able to distinguish these normal physiologic changes from disease states and aid those infants where transition is delayed or nonexistent. The inability to recognize an abnormal transition period can cause complications in an infant with existing disease or endanger an otherwise healthy infant.

With birth and the clamping of the umbilical cord, the cardiovascular system of the infant almost instantaneously switches from one characterized by the low-resistance parallel circulation of the fetus (Fig. 1) to the higher systemic resistance series circulation of the infant.[1] Unlike the infant's series system, where deoxygenated blood returns via the right heart to a low-resistance pulmonary system and ejects oxygenated blood from the left heart to a high-resistance systemic circulation, the fetal circulation is a more complex parallel system. Oxygenated blood (25–30 mmHg) returns from the placenta via the ductus venosus (Fig. 1) of the liver to the right heart.[2] Only 10–12% of this blood (just enough for lung growth and metabolism) perfuses the lungs; the majority

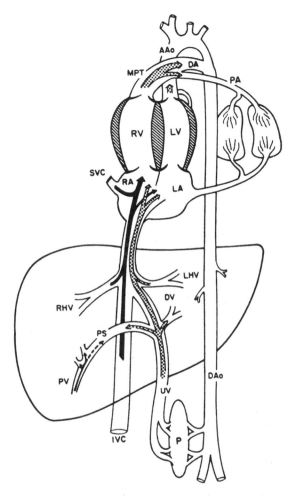

FIGURE 1. Diagrammatic representation of the normal fetal circulation. QP, pulmonary flow; QS, systemic flow. (From Klaus MH, Fanaroff AA: Care of the High-Risk Neonate, 3rd ed. Philadelphia, W.B. Saunders, 1986, with permission.)

is ejected by the right ventricle via the patent ductus arteriosus, bypassing the pulmonary circulation to the aorta and the body and eventually returning to the placenta for recirculation. Although the fetal body receives blood from both ventricles, the right ventricle is the most dominant and ejects 65% of the combined output. The left ventricular output is distributed primarily to the brain (20% of combined ventricular output), the myocardium (3%), and the rest (10%) across the aorta to the body. The fetal circulation is characterized by a high-resistance pulmonary circulation, maintained by the active constriction of the muscular arteries (secondary to the low fetal oxygen tension and complex interactions of endogenous chemical mediators) and the low-resistance placental circulation. With the onset of respiration, the removal of the low-resistance placenta, the dramatic fall in the pulmonary vascular resistance, and the addition of the higher systemic resistance, the fetal circulation functionally switches to the series, adult one characterized by the functional and eventually permanent closure of the ductus venosus, ductus arteriosus, and foramen ovale. These changes are thought to be mediated by the dilatation of resistant pulmonary arterial vessels by the higher oxygen environment, release of vasodilatory substances (nitric oxide, bradykinin, prostacyclin), and the fall of vasoconstrictive substances.[2] Adverse environmental conditions and disease states present at birth can alter this normal transition and lead to the persistence of the fetal circulation represented by high pulmonary resistance, low pulmonary blood flow, maintenance of the patency of the ductus ateriosus or foramen ovale, and low systemic oxygen tensions. Without proper treatment this state can lead to persistent hypoxia and death.[3]

Within a few breaths at birth, the newborn infant quickly transforms the lung from its fluid-filled state to an organ of gas exchange. The onset of vigorous respirations is initiated by many factors, such as cold, tactile stimulation, and chemoreceptors. Within a few breaths lung fluid is removed and expansion approaches normal.[2]

The infant's thermal transition must be facilitated by care providers. Although the stress of being born wet in a cold environment may help initiate respirations, without proper warming (radiant warmer, warm blankets, mother's abdomen) an infant's core temperature may drop 2-3°C and jeopardize a normal transition.[2]

Since the birth process profoundly affects the fetus, close surveillance during the first hours after birth is critical. The stress and stimuli of labor have been compared to a surgical procedure with massive sympathetic outpouring. In the normal, full-term infant following an uneventful labor, an abrupt increase in heart rate (160-180 bpm) is noticed for up to one hour after birth. This first period of reactivity is associated with rapid and irregular respirations (60-90 per minute), transient retractions and nasal alar flaring, active crying, alert exploratory behavior, spontaneous startles and moro reflexes, tremors, increased muscle tone, and purposeless movements. After this period of increased reactivity and alertness, the infant passes into an unresponsive or sleep period for one to two hours. By this time color should be pink, heart rate slowed to 120-140 bpm, and respirations observed of 40-60 per minute. Occasional myoclonic jerks may occur during this period, with rapid return to sleep. Between two and six hours of age the infant again becomes active (second period of reactivity), with resultant tachycardia and periods of rapid respirations (> 60 breaths/minute). Abrupt changes in color, tone, heart rate (less than 100 bpm to greater than 160 bpm), and respirations (irregular with apneic pauses) are not unusual.[4] Therefore, the clinician must be cognizant of the changing transitional state in order to distinguish a disease condition from normal transition.

Processes that disturb normal transition such as birth asphyxia, maternal narcotics and anesthesia, prematurity, cold stress, and acidosis may delay or eliminate the transition period and lead to the persistence of the fetal cardiovascular state characterized by tachycardia, low oxygen tensions, and need for ventilatory support.[3] All infants, regardless of size, therefore must be observed and aided through this critical period. All births should be attended by a person specifically assigned to care for the newborn. The infant is immediately dried, warmed (usually by an overhead radiant warmer), and its airway gently suctioned. The infant must then be closely observed by trained personnel aware of the transitional state until vital signs are stable. Any alteration in this process requires immediate treatment to avert the persistent fetal circulation state.[5]

THERMOREGULATION DURING NEONATAL TRANSPORT

One of the primary clinical responsibilities of the transport team during neonatal transport is to keep the infant warm. Maintaining the infant's temperature within the normal range by providing warmth and minimizing heat loss is essential to the survival of the sick infant. Personnel who perform neonatal transport should have a clear understanding of the process of thermoregulation in infants, mechanisms of heat loss, practical methods of keeping infants warm, and the consequences of cold and heat stress. The following sections will address the differences between infants and adults in thermoregulation, the concept of the neutral thermal environment, mechanisms of heat loss, means of monitoring body temperature, methods of maintaining body heat and reducing heat loss during transport, and the effects of cold and heat stress on the infant.

Heat produced by metabolism during normal body processes must be dissipated through the transfer of heat from the body to the environment. A balance of heat production and heat loss, therefore, is essential to maintain normal body temperature. When an infant is exposed to a cold environment heat production increases. Unlike in adults, shivering in newborn infants is an ineffective method of heat production when exposed to cold stress; therefore, heat is generated by the metabolism of brown fat tissue. This unique metabolism generates heat that is transferred via the circulation to other parts of the body. Brown fat is stored in the body beginning at 26–30 weeks of gestation. Once brown fat is utilized, it is not replenished. The metabolism of brown fat is highly oxygen-dependent, and disorders impairing oxygenation will impair the infant's ability to respond to cold stress.[6]

Infants' unique characteristics result in excessive heat losses and difficulty in maintaining normal body temperature during changing environmental conditions. Secondary to an increased body surface area in relation to body mass, infants have a larger area available for heat loss.[7] In addition, infants have less adipose thermal insulation and an inability to change posture to conserve heat in response to cold stress.[8] Since preterm infants have even less total adipose tissue, they are at even greater risk for excessive heat loss. With decreasing gestational age total body water content increases from 69% seen in full-term infants to 86% observed in very low birthweight infants. This increases heat loss from evaporation, especially in very tiny infants.[6]

An infant's neutral thermal environment is the temperature range necessary in the environment to maintain heat balance with minimal expenditure of energy. The temperature of the surrounding environment of the infant, whether it be the nursery itself or inside a transport incubator, must be adjusted to provide a neutral thermal environment (usually 33–36.5°C). Some infants are particularly at risk for thermal instability, despite the maintenance of a neutral thermal environment. These include preterm infants, infants small for gestational age, and infants with central nervous system disease and/or any type of stress. Temperature instability alone may be an indication of a more serious disease process.[6]

The normal body temperature of an infant should be between 36.3° and 36.9°C.[10] Monitoring an infant's body temperature during transport is crucial. Many devices for monitoring temperature are available, including mercury, electronic digital, and tympanic thermometers. The tympanic thermometer has not been shown to be accurate for newborn infants.[11,12] Mercury thermometers are easily broken during the routine movement of transport, and spilled mercury is considered an environmental hazard since the inhalation of mercury vapors is potentially toxic to infants.[13,14] In addition, spilled mercury is corrosive and may damage aircraft controls. Because of the corrosive properties and danger of spillage, a mercury thermometer should not be carried inside an aircraft.[15] If a mercury thermometer is used, it should not be left anywhere inside the incubator.[13,14]

The measurement of temperature via the axilla in infants is preferred to eliminate the risk of rectal perforation. If taken properly, axillary temperatures adequately reflect rectal temperatures in both term and preterm infants.[10,16] Axillary temperature should be taken by placing the thermometer tip deep in the axilla for a full five minutes or until the electronic thermometer indicates the temperature reading is complete. Some of the newer electronic thermometers do not require a full five minutes for an accurate reading. The infant's temperature should be monitored frequently during transport. If continuous monitoring is unavailable, then temperature should be monitored intermittently, on arrival of the transport team, after placement in the incubator for a period of 10 minutes, and then every 30–60 minutes.

There are four mechanisms of heat transfer that must be controlled to minimize heat losses in newborn infants: radiation; evaporation; conduction; and convection. During radiation an object losses heat to a cooler object placed nearby.[17] In the Intensive Care Nursery (ICN), an infant in an open warmer may lose heat to any nearby cooler surfaces (i.e., windows, walls). Transport vehicles, especially ambulances, are poorly insulated. During transport, an infant may lose heat to the cooler walls of the transport vehicle. Therefore, the transport incubator may be required to increase heat production dramatically, thus increasing power demands on the battery and decreasing battery life. During cold temperatures the transfer of the infant from the hospital into the transport vehicle may produce a sudden decrease in temperature, with the infant losing heat to the incubator walls despite the use of double-walled transport incubators.[9]

Heat loss through conduction occurs when an object loses heat to a cooler object that it directly contacts.[17] Infants lose heat through conduction if placed in a transport incubator not sufficiently prewarmed. Placing the infant on any cool surface, such as a scale or an x-ray table, will result in heat loss through conduction.

Evaporative heat loss results when moisture from an object evaporates into the cooler ambient air and occurs in a variety of ways.[17] At delivery the infant emerges from a warm, wet environment into a cool, dry one. Rapid cooling (2–3°C) occurs if the infant is not dried immediately.[2] Wet blankets left under the infant further increase heat loss. All infants at delivery should be dried thoroughly with warm blankets. Any wet blankets should be removed immediately away from direct contact with the infant. If the infant is born outside the hospital, drying and reducing heat loss becomes even more critical. Blankets or towels can be warmed under the heater of the transport vehicle and then used next to the infant. The transport vehicle's heat should be turned on to warm the cabin, and the dry infant can be placed next to or on the mother's abdomen and both covered with blankets.

Evaporative heat loss also occurs via the respiratory tract. As air enters the upper respiratory tract, it is warmed and humidified. Warmed air inside transport incubators has a lower relative humidity than ambient air. Humidity cannot be added to the incubator owing to the risk of colonization with bacterial organisms, such as *Pseudomonas aeruginosa* and *Klebsiella pneumoniae*. Infants who require oxygen via hood, mask, or assisted ventilation should have all gases warmed and humidified. Since air bypasses the upper respiratory tract in intubated infants, gases delivered to the endotracheal tube should be warmed to 35° or 36°C and maximally humidified to reduce heat loss.[18] During transport humidity can be given to infants who are intubated by adding a hydroscopic condenser humidifier directly to the adaptor for the endotracheal tube.[19]

Heat loss secondary to convection occurs when cooler air flows over a warmer object.[17] Infants in open radiant warmers near an air vent may lose heat as air currents flow over them. Convective heat losses occur during transport in a similar fashion. In a helicopter or fixed-wing aircraft, air vents designed for passenger comfort are commonly positioned to blow directly on the incubator, resulting in heat loss from the infant. If caring for the infant requires opening of the portholes or removing the infant from the incubator, care must be taken to close or redirect all air vents. Hot unloads (unloading while the rotor blades are in motion) should be avoided in order to reduce additional convective heat losses. The infant should not be removed from the incubator while the rotor blades are in motion unless an aircraft emergency is declared. Under these emergency circumstances, the infant should be wrapped in a blanket or placed against the chest of the transport team member, and secured inside the flight suit.

Cold stress in transported infants is not unusual, because the transport team initially is focused on resuscitative measures and procedures. Cold stress is defined as a body temperature less than 36°C skin or 36.5°C rectal or axillary temperature.[10] Sheldon and coworkers reported the mean temperature of transported infants less than 1500 grams was below 35.9°C, with some as low as 32°C. Inadequate drying of the infant, leaving wet blankets in the bed, and improper use of the radiant warmer contributed to this problem in infants born at referring hospitals.[20] Signs and symptoms of cold stress include poor perfusion, acrocyanosis, lethargy, skin cool to the touch, poor feeding, apnea, and/or bradycardia.[6] Cold stress can produce hypoglycemia, respiratory distress, persistent acidosis, poor perfusion, clotting disorders, shock, hypoxia, and death.[10] Upon detection of cold stress, slow rewarming should be initiated immediately. Fast rewarming increases oxygen consumption and may result in apnea.[10,18] In addition to close monitoring of the incubator and body temperature, blood pressure, blood sugar, and arterial blood gases should be closely monitored.

A neutral thermal environment is maintained by transporting the infant in a specifically designed neonatal transport incubator. Most transport incubators available today can accommodate any infant less than 5 kilograms. Some of the newer models are designed for infants up to 10 kilograms. With few exceptions, an infant requiring neonatal transport should be transported in a transport incubator. Exceptions might include the unanticipated transfer of two or more infants from the same referring hospital by using the same incubator or an incubator plus a radiant warmer. Use of a car seat for neonatal transport is permitted if the infant is term, clinically stable without need for oxygen and/or ventilation, is able to maintain normal body temperature in the transport vehicle, and monitoring of heart rate, respiratory rate, and noninvasive oxygen is available. Placing twins in one incubator is an option, if both will fit easily without obstruction of air flow inside the incubator.

Prior to loading the infant, the incubator should be prewarmed, with the air temperature set to approximate the neutral thermal environment. Table 1 may be used for guidance while prewarming the incubator.[17] Incubator covers may reduce heat loss when moving from the hospital to the transport vehicle during cold weather. Reflective sheets impregnated with aluminum help to reduce heat loss further.[17] Large, adult-sized blankets can be thrown over the incubator and are readily available in most hospitals. Regardless of the type of cover used, adequate visibility of the infant must be maintained throughout the transport process.

Since the cranium represents a large part of an infant's total body surface area, commercially manufactured or homemade hats also can significantly

TABLE 1.   Suggested Initial Incubator Temperature Settings for Newborns
with Normal Body Temperature*

| Birth Weight (gm) | Temperature Setting (°C) | |
	Clothed	Exposed
>2500	28	33
1501–2500	31	35.5
<1500	33	36.5

* Assumed conditions are an environmental relative humidity of approximately 50%, ambulance temperature of 25°–28°C, and protection against radiant heat loss for infants of <1500 gm birth weight. If environmental humidification is not used, add 1°C for all weight groups.
From Oliver TK: Temperature regulation and heat production in the newborn. Pediatr Clin North Am 12:765–779, 1965, with permission.

decrease heat loss. Caps lined with polyurethane reduce evaporative heat loss even further.[21,22] Cotton stocking-knit caps, composed of material typically used to line orthopedic casts, also reduce heat loss, but are less effective than thinsulate caps.[22] Stocking-knit material is readily available in most hospitals. Caps can be made by tying one end with a string or rubber band and placing it on the infant's head. Caps should cover most of the head without covering the face, allowing adequate visualization of the infant's color. Any material available, such as towels or cloth drapes, can be modified for use as a cap. If a homemade cap is used, lining the cap with a plastic wrap will improve its effectiveness, especially in very low birthweight infants.

Most sick infants transported in incubators are left unclothed for easy accessibility and constant observation of color, respiratory effort, intravenous lines, monitor wires, and activity. In infants at higher risk for cold stress (i.e., abdominal wall defects, very low birthweight infants, or during incubator heater or battery failure), heat loss may be reduced by covering the infant with a blanket inside the incubator. Use of a small blanket should not interfere with the normal flow of warmed air. Commercially available blankets made of flexible aluminum wrap reduce radiant heat loss, but also significantly reduce visibility. These can be used in normal full-term infants born outside the hospital who are stable clinically. In very low birthweight infants, clear plastic wrap is also effective in reducing heat loss from evaporation and convection and decreasing evaporative insensible water losses.[9] Plastic wraps do not interfere with visibility, although they must be removed or folded back to provide access to the infant. Placing a very low birthweight infant into a plastic bag up to the neck also can reduce heat and insensible water loss while allowing visibility. Plexiglass heat shields may reduce heat loss, but restrict access to the infant and are cumbersome for use inside a transport incubator.[23]

Chemical warming packs can be useful in prewarming the transport incubator during extremely cold ambient temperatures.[24] If chemical warming packs are used, they should not be placed against the skin of the infant. Some packs can heat to 40°C, exposing the infant's delicate skin to the possibility of extensive burns.[9] Placing a blanket or sheepskin between the infant and the chemical pack will reduce the risk of burns. When these packs are used, the temperature of the infant should be monitored very closely—continuously, if possible. Inspection of the skin should occur at least every 30 minutes. If the skin becomes reddened, the chemical pack should be removed. The use of surgical gloves with warmed water also may cause burns and should be avoided.

To assist thermal regulation during neonatal transport, the temperature inside the transport vehicle itself should be maintained at 25°–28°C. During cold ambient temperatures the transport vehicle's heater should always function to prevent cooling of the walls. All doors and windows should be closed until immediately before loading the incubator.[9]

Infants with abdominal wall defects (i.e., gastroschisis, omphalocele) are at increased risk for cold stress due to all types of heat loss. Sterile, soft roller gauze soaked with sterile warmed normal saline should cover the exposed viscera. Gauze can be wrapped around the trunk and the exposed viscera in a figure-8 fashion, giving support to the exposed viscera and reducing heat loss.[25] Because of the threat of significant evaporative heat loss from the moist gauze, the defect should also be enclosed in a similar figure-8 fashion with clear plastic wrap or by placing the infant's lower torso in a bowel bag. A bowel bag reduces heat loss, provides adequate visibility, and protects the viscera from bacterial microorganisms by maintaining a sterile environment.[20] If the infant is in a radiant warmer at the referring hospital, heat loss may be further reduced by placing the infant in the incubator in an expeditious manner.[26]

Very low birthweight (VLBW) infants (less than 1250 gm) are at greater risk for cold stress, especially during transport. Because of their smaller body size these infants have an even greater body surface area than term infants. Since VLBW infants do not have sufficient stores of body fat, they depend almost completely on external heat sources to maintain body warmth and usually will need even additional heat sources—e.g., hats, plastic wrap, and/or chemical packs—to maintain their temperature.[10]

The prevention of overheating during warm ambient temperatures also may be a problem in some areas. Heat stress results in increased heart rate, respiratory rate, oxygen consumption, glucose utilization, and insensible water losses. Peripheral vasodilation may lead to hypotension.[6] In addition, heat stress may produce central nervous system damage due to hypernatremic dehydration, heatstroke, and may even cause death.[8] The most common causes of heat stress in the transported infant are improperly regulated radiant warmers and incubators. For infants nursed in a radiant warmer, immediate assessment of the infant's temperature, the temperature setting of the warmer, and whether the servo or manual control is chosen and the heat probe is functioning properly is necessary to avoid overheating as the team prepares for departure. Overheating can easily occur in the transport incubator as well. Elevated temperature due to fever is uncommon in newborn infants. Temperature elevation secondary to fever can be differentiated from iatrogenic heat stress by measuring skin temperature simultaneously with core temperature via the rectum. If the source of the elevated temperature is environmental (iatrogenic), the core temperature will be less than the skin temperature.[10] Since direct sunlight on the incubator for prolonged periods can lead to additional heat stress, avoiding prolonged periods in the sun is recommended. If this is unavoidable, covering a portion of the incubator with a blanket to provide shade and/or moving into a shaded area will help prevent heat stress.

Since heat stress increases the metabolic demands of the infant and increases oxygen requirements, the source of the heat, once identified, should be quickly removed.[10] Overheating by malfunction of the external source should be treated by immediately removing the infant from the incubator or warmer and placing the infant in another. If the infant's temperature is 37.5°–39°C, remove any clothes, hats, or blankets and expose to room temperature until the temperature falls. If the temperature exceeds 39°C, sponging with tepid water at approximately 35°C until the skin temperature is below 38°C is helpful. Opening the incubator doors may reduce the temperature of the inside air; however, the temperature probe may sense this cooling and paradoxically increase heat production, negating this cooling method.

FLUID AND ELECTROLYTES

Most infants ill enough to require neonatal transport are unable to tolerate enteral feedings and must be supplied with parenteral fluids to maintain fluid homeostasis. Management of fluid and electrolyte balance requires a basic knowledge of the normal mechanisms regulating water and electrolyte balance in term and preterm infants, the effects of insensible water losses, and of specific conditions that affect fluid balance. The careful administration of parenteral fluid and electrolytes is essential for the completion of a successful transport.

The goal of fluid and electrolyte management is to replace ongoing losses of water and electrolytes and to restore the body to normal fluid and electrolyte balance, thus facilitating recovery from illness and, ultimately, aiding growth.[27] In the fetus, fluid homeostasis is maintained by the placenta. With birth, the neonate assumes this vital role while handicapped by immature skin and renal function. Therefore, the maintenance of fluid and electrolyte equilibrium becomes a great challenge for all caregivers of sick infants.

During the immediate postnatal period, a contraction of the extracellular fluid compartment normally occurs. Therefore, the goal of initial fluid therapy is to maintain normal serum electrolytes while allowing the loss of this extracellular water. Fluids administered at a rate of 60-90 ml/kg/day usually allow for this contraction of the extracellular compartment. A 10% dextrose solution at this rate will supply 4-6 mg/kg/min of glucose, maintaining the serum glucose within the desired range of 60-120 mg/dl. Infants less than 1250 grams at birth frequently do not tolerate a 10% dextrose solution, and 5% dextrose should be chosen. Regardless of the concentration of dextrose chosen, frequent monitoring of the infant's glucose should be performed during transport. The administration of supplemental electrolytes, such as sodium, chloride, and potassium, usually is not necessary during the period of transport. The administration of calcium may be necessary for infants at risk for hypocalcemia (e.g., VLBW infants) and can be supplied as 2 mEq/100 ml as Ca gluconate.[28]

After the immediate postnatal period, the goal of fluid therapy is to replace fluid and electrolyte losses and maintain fluid balance. Fluids administered at a rate of 90-150 ml/kg/day, sodium (2-3 mmol/kg/day, administered as sodium chloride), and potassium (1-3 mmol/kg/day, as potassium chloride) are necessary.[21]

Precise calculation of fluid rates and accurate delivery of the desired rates are essential during transport. The rate of fluid administration can be calculated by the following formula:

$$\frac{\text{weight in kilograms} \times \text{desired fluid intake over 24 hours}}{24} = \text{ml/hr}$$

For example, if an infant weighed 2.6 gm at birth and a desired fluid volume of 80 ml/kg/day was desired, then a fluid rate of 8.7 ml/hr would be calculated.

$$\frac{22.6 \times 80}{24} = 8.7 \text{ ml/hr}$$

In the first week of life infants will lose 1-3% of their body weight daily, owing to the contraction of the extracellular fluid compartment. Since weight may fluctuate significantly during this time, birth weight should be used as a consistent point of reference to calculate fluid rates until the infant's fluid balance is stable and the infant consumes sufficient calories for growth.[27]

The accuracy of parenteral fluid administration is essential to avoid fluid overload. Fluids must be administered on an intravenous infusion pump approved for use in infants. We recommend an intravenous pump adjustable to tenths of a ml. Most programs now use light-weight syringe pumps for transport. If a syringe pump is unavailable, a buretrol should be used and no more than 12 hours' worth of fluids allowed in the buretrol to prevent inadvertent fluid overload due to pump malfunction.

Ongoing monitoring of fluid therapy during transport is essential as a guide to further management. Since the physical signs of fluid abnormalities are neither specific nor sensitive, and since laboratory information often is not available to assist in guiding fluid management in newborn infants, the selection of the initial rate and composition of fluid is based primarily on the infant's birthweight, gestational age, and disease process. In addition, information collected by the transport team is invaluable in assessing the infant for further fluid and electrolyte management. Accurate recording of the birthweight and gestational age is essential. Other important information include pertinent maternal history, records of urine and stool output prior to transport, measurement of identifiable losses (e.g., stool, gastric, vomitus, etc.) and estimated insensible water losses.

For infants over 12 hours of age, documentation of birthweight, current weight, and past urine and stool output are even more critical. With neonates at high risk for fluid imbalance (e.g., VLBW infants and gastrointestinal surgical conditions), a measurement of serum electrolytes prior to transport may be helpful. These tests can be drawn before the transport team arrives. Hopefully, results will be available upon arrival. A legible copy of all nurses' notes and all laboratory values are necessary to accurately assess past urine output, stool, vomitus, gastric drainage, and laboratory results.

Intake and output during transport should be accurately documented in the transport record. Total fluid intake, including fluids administered prior to arrival of the transport team (including volume expansion), and fluids subsequently administered by the transport team must be recorded. The amount of fluid infused each hour and total fluid volume since birth should be documented. Significant fluid volume administered with medications also should be recorded. If the infant had been feeding prior to transport, enteral intake, including an estimate of breastfeeding volumes, should be noted. All output, including urine, stool, gastric, vomitus, and blood loss, should be documented as accurately as possible. Wet diapers, marked with their dry weight, can be folded and taped closed to be weighed upon arrival at the receiving hospital.

Special Problems

Some infants (e.g., VLBW, abdominal wall defects) experience excessive fluid losses and require meticulous fluid management. VLBW infants have tremendous insensible water losses via their skin and quickly become dehydrated with potential serum hypertonicity and metabolic acidosis.[29] Application of a semipermeable polyurethane membrane, such as Op-site or Tegaderm, to the exposed areas of the chest and abdomen has been shown to reduce insensible water loss.[30] Since EKG pads can be positioned on the polyurethane membrane and both left in place for several days, its application does not interfere with observation or monitoring of the patient nor does it result in skin injury. The use of a flexible plastic blanket also has been shown to reduce insensible water losses and decrease oxygen consumption in VLBW infants in radiant warmers.[31] These plastic blankets are easily adaptable to transport and also help maintain body temperature by decreasing convective air currents. Even though external measures are used to decrease excessive losses, VLBW infants still need additional fluids to compensate for these losses at a rate of 90–120 ml/kg/d, depending on birth weight (Table 2). As noted before, VLBW infants may demonstrate glucose intolerance at higher rates of fluid administration, and a 5% dextrose solution should be utilized.

Infants with exposed viscera secondary to an abdominal wall defect will have excessive fluid losses from the exposed organs, third spacing, and aggressive gastric drainage. To reduce evaporative water loss, the exposed viscera should be wrapped with sterile gauze in a figure-8 fashion and moistened with warmed sterile normal saline. The infant should also be placed in a sterile bowel bag up to the level of the chest to reduce evaporative losses and help conserve body temperature.[25] The maintenance of adequate circulating fluid volume is essential in these infants to maintain perfusion to the viscera, prevent dehydration from excessive insensible losses, and avoid hypovolemic shock. Once intravenous access is obtained, infants should be given a fluid bolus of 20 ml/kg of normal saline, 5% albumin, or fresh-frozen plasma.[26] Subsequent fluid administration is recommended to be 5% dextrose in lactated Ringer's solution at a rate of at least 120 ml/kg/day (5 ml/kg/hr).[25] Frequent reassessment of perfusion is necessary because additional volume expansion may be required. Since vasopressor agents can decrease perfusion to the abdominal viscera, these agents are not recommended unless hypotension persists after generous volume replacement.

MANAGEMENT OF THE EXTREMELY LOW BIRTHWEIGHT INFANT

Recent technologic advances and regionalization of perinatal care have led to the improved survival of preterm infants.[32,33] With the advent of surfactants the survival of the extremely low birthweight (ELBW) infant (<1000 gm) has improved even further, though concern for excessive morbidity remains.[34] Therefore, the neonatal transport team often is summoned to manage and transport these tiny infants.

Often the first concern of the referring caregiver is whether active resuscitation should be begun on these extremely tiny infants. Most institutions agree that all infants ≥ 750 gm or 25–26 weeks' completed gestation should have full resuscitation.[35,36] Whether to intervene actively in an infant less than 25 weeks has created much debate. This controversy is fueled by the difficulty of accurately assessing gestational age, as organ maturity at birth is the ultimate determinant of outcome. Though obstetric management with accurate prenatal histories and early ultrasound evaluation has improved the antenatal assessment of gestational age, many women (up to 20% in some series) threatening to deliver preterm infants have inadequate or no prenatal care, making the accurate assessment very difficult.[37]

TABLE 2. Fluid Management in Infants with Very Low Birthweight

Weight (gm)	Fluid (ml/kg/day)		
	Day 1	Day 2	Day 3
≤600–1,000	120	140	140–180
1,001–1,250	100	120	120–140
1,251–1,500	90	100	120–130
1,501–2,000	80	90	100–120
≥2,000	70	80	90–120

In addition, for the infant less than 28 weeks' gestational age, postnatal assessment may be unreliable.[38] In general, the postnatal assessment of gestational age tends to be an overestimate[39] and, in the opinion of Yu and coworkers, futile when less than 28 weeks.[40] Recently, Allen and associates suggested that infants born at 22 weeks' gestation or less, with a birthweight less than 500 gm, be offered only comfort care. For those born at 23 or 24 weeks, they suggest flexibility with resuscitation, considering the views of the family and the condition of the infant at birth; and all infants born at 25–26 weeks should have full resuscitation (Fig. 2). However, owing to the difficulty of accurately assessing gestational age, we have modified this strategy for our newborn transports. We recommend that all infants be immediately weighed in the delivery room. If their birthweight exceeds 500 grams, we advise resuscitation, at least until the neonatal team arrives. If the infant is less than 600 grams, our resuscitation will entail only intubation, ventilation, and thermal stabilization. Infants over 600 grams are given a trial of full resuscitation, including chest compressions and cardiopulmonary medications. Though we realize that the outcome of CPR in small infants is guarded,[42] we feel uncomfortable asking the referring physician or transport team to make a decision to forego the resuscitation of >600-gm infants in the field and will reserve the decision about further treatment until full evaluation can be made in the receiving institution.

Once the decision is made to actively care for the ELBW infant, delivery room resuscitation proceeds in a manner similar to that for all preterm births.[43]

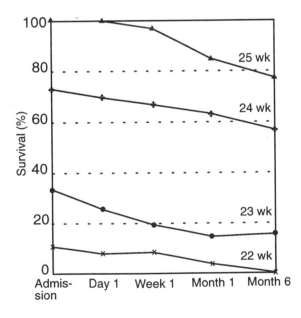

FIGURE 2. Survival of infants born at 22–25 weeks' gestation, according to gestational age. Survival was studied from the time of infants' admission into the neonatal intensive care unit to six months after birth. Gestational ages were based on the best obstetrical estimate. (From Allen MC: N Engl J Med 329:1597–1601, 1993, with permission.)

The infant must be warmed, dried, and the airway/breathing assessed. Most ELBW infants will require intubation in the delivery room, and only rarely will we transport an ELBW infant without an endotracheal tube. We recommend that all ELBW infants be stabilized, if at all possible, prior to transport. This stabilization usually includes thermal regulation in a radiant warmer with the use of a thermal cap,[22] plastic blanket,[31] or Porta-Warm Mattress (Marion Scientific Co., Kansas City, MO)[24]; placement of an umbilical artery or vein catheter; placement of a pulse oximeter; radiographic confirmation of endotracheal tube and umbilical catheter placement; and an arterial blood gas study. Parenteral fluid is begun with D5W after serum glucose assessment at 100–150 ml/kg/day; 10% dextrose is chosen if the initial serum glucose is $\leq$50 mg/100 ml. Fluid rate is estimated depending on the gestational age, with more immature neonates (23–25 weeks) requiring higher fluid volumes (see Table 2). Owing to their susceptibility to early and severe barotrauma, we select ventilator settings with the lowest peak inspiratory pressure (PIP) as possible and adjust the rate, FIO_2, and liter flow to give adequate oxygenation and ventilation. We recommend the lowest liter per minute flow to give the required PIP. Higher flows increase airway resistance.[43]

The use of surfactants during transport has recently been reported.[44] Owing to the unpredictability of pulmonary compliance changes and the need for stringent ventilation management, we have elected only to administer surfactant to infants who will require a long transport period (greater than 6 hours). In addition, we recommend the administration of surfactants prior to transport only to those referring institutions with established experience with their use.

Secondary to the extreme fragility and lability of these infants, the transport team should consider the most rapid mode of transport (ground, fixed-wing, or rotary) with minimal external environmental factors (sound, vibration, cold). Therefore, most of these infants are best served by ground or fixed-wing vehicles. To minimize the stresses inherent to these transport vehicles, we often sedate ELBW infants with 10 mg/kg of intravenous phenobarbital.

Though the safe transport of ELBW infants can be achieved, infants of high-risk pregnancies have improved survival when delivered in a Level Three regional center.[45] In fact, transport of these infants is often considered a failure of a regionalized perinatal program.[32] Therefore, if at all possible, we recommend that mothers be transported to the nearest Level Three center where all care for her ELBW infant can be provided.

MANAGEMENT OF HYDROPS FETALIS

With the declining frequency of Rh isoimmunization,[46,47] the incidence and etiology of hydrops fetalis has also changed. With an estimated incidence of 1 in 3748 births, nonimmune hydrops fetalis (NIHF) has become the most common cause of hydrops.[48] NIHF is a disease of multifactorial etiologies (Table 3) characterized by obstetric complications of polyhydraminos (75%); maternal anemia (45%); preeclampsia (29%); postpartum hemorrhage and retained placenta (64%); preterm birth (mean gestational age of 27.3 $\pm$ 5.7 weeks) and a fetal/neonatal mortality of 50–98%.[48,49] A recent series has described the increasing frequency of genetic etiologies in NIHF (35%), with only 10% secondary to isoimmunization and 29% idiopathic.[50]

Infants with fetal hydrops may be diagnosed by their extreme degree of generalized edema; hypoproteinemia; respiratory distress associated with hyaline membrane disease; pulmonary hypoplasia or pleural effusions; ascites; pericardial effusions; anemia; and hepatosplenomegaly. The major symptoms of generalized

TABLE 3.   Etiologies of Nonimmune Hydrops Fetalis

Fetal

1. *Hematologic*
   Homozygous thalassemia
   Chronic fetomaternal transfusion
   Twin-to-twin transfusion
   Multiple gestation with "parasitic" fetus

2. *Cardiovascular*
   Severe congenital heart disease
      (atrial septal defect, ventricular septal
      defect, hypoplastic left heart, pulmo-
      nary valve insufficiency, Ebstein's
      anomaly, subaortic stenosis)
   Premature closure of foramen ovale
   Myocarditis
   Large arteriovenous malformation
   Tachyarrhythmias: paroxysmal SVT,
      atrial flutter
   Bradyarrhythmias: heart block
   Fibroelastosis

3. *Pulmonary*
   Cystic adenomatoid malformation of lung
   Pulmonary lymphangiectasia
   Pulmonary hypoplasia (diaphragmatic
      hernia)

4. *Renal*
   Congenital nephrosis
   Renal vein thrombosis

5. *Intrauterine infections*
   Syphilis
   Toxoplasmosis
   Cytomegalovirus
   Leptospirosis
   Chagas disease
   Congenital hepatitis

6. *Congenital anomalies (genetic)*
   Achondroplasia
   Trisomy 18, 21
   Multiple anomalies
   Turner syndrome

7. *Miscellaneous*
   Meconium peritonitis
   Lymphatic malformations
   Dysmaturity
   Tuberous sclerosis
   Storage disease
   Small bowel volvulus

8. *Placental*
   Umbilical vein thrombosis
   Chorionic vein thrombosis
   Chorioangioma

9. *Maternal*
   Diabetes mellitus
   Toxemia

10. *Idiopathic*

edema and body cavity effusions are theorized to be secondary to (1) congestive heart failure; (2) decreased colloid osmotic pressure; (3) anemia.[49] Optimal management of these infants requires early recognition and aggressive obstetric and neonatal management. Once an antenatal diagnosis of hydrops fetalis is entertained, frequent evaluations of fetal well-being should be made, antenatal steroids should be initiated, and plans for a possible early cesarean section delivery in a tertiary center made. If referral to a tertiary facility cannot be arranged, the transport team must be prepared for emergent resuscitation and stabilization, including immediate paracentesis and thoracentesis.[49]

Since birth asphyxia is almost universal (77%), the delivery room management of hydrops fetalis often requires immediate intubation of a depressed infant.[49] Intubation may be difficult secondary to the infant's generalized edema, rendering positioning difficult, and glottic edema. Several large-bore (16–18 gauge) over-the-needle intravenous catheters should be available to perform paracentesis (left lower abdominal quadrant or midline one-half the distance between the umbilicus and pubis symphysis) or thoracentesis (midaxillary line, 4th–6th intercostal space).[48] We elect to tap the abdomen first prior to thoracentesis. Since hyaline membrane disease, pulmonary effusions, and pulmonary hypoplasia are common, high ventilatory pressures (20–40 cm H_2O) and rates (40–70 bpm) may be required for adequate oxygenation and ventilation.[49,51] The pretransport use of surfactants in these critically ill infants may aid pulmonary management and enable a more stable transport. Umbilical artery and venous catheters for central arterial and venous pressure monitoring should be placed. Despite the increase in total body water and extracellular fluid, these infants usually have normal or reduced blood volumes[52,53]; therefore, volume expansion may be necessary if peripheral perfusion is compromised. Disseminated intravascular coagulopathy is common in the first 24 hours, and infusions of fresh frozen plasma or cryoprecipitate may be required.[49]

Once pulmonary stabilization has been obtained, these infants require transport to a tertiary care center experienced in managing severely ill neonates. Centers with high-frequency ventilation and/or extracorporeal membrane oxygenation should be considered. Transport of these infants usually will require chest tube suction systems, means to vigorously ventilate the infant, and the quickest mode of transport. Additional volume and inotropic medications may be necessary to support blood pressure. Since hydrops fetalis is associated with high mortality, pictures of the infant prior to transport should be taken and the family encouraged to spend time with their infant. If mortality appears imminent, blood for chromosome study should be obtained.[50] The successful transport of an infant with hydrops fetalis requires the flawless participation of all members of the transport team and is a challenge not often forgotten.

REFERENCES

1. Adams FH: Fetal circulation and alterations at birth. In Moss AJ, Adams FH, Emmanouilides CG (eds): Heart Disease in Infants, Children and Adolescents. Baltimore, Williams & Wilkins, 1977, pp 11–13.
2. Rudolph AJ, Garcia-Prats JA: Anticipation, recognition and transitional care of the high risk infant. In Klaus MH, Fanaroff AA (eds): Care of the High Risk Neonate. Philadelphia, W.B. Saunders, 1986, pp 51–68.
3. Fox WW, Dura S: Persistent pulmonary hypertension in the neonate: Diagnosis and management. J Pediatr 103:505–514, 1983.
4. Desmond M, Franklin R, Valbona C, et al: The clinical behavior of the newly born. I. The term baby. J Pediatr 62:307, 1965.
5. Desmond M, Rudolph A, Phitaksphraiwon P: The transitional care nursery. Pediatr Clin North Am 13:651, 1966.
6. Streeter NS: High-risk Neonatal Care. Rockville, MD, Aspen, 1986, pp 87–106.
7. Adamsons K: The role of thermal factors in fetal and neonatal life. Pediatr Clin North Am 13:599–619, 1966.
8. Hey E: Thermoregulation. In Avery GB (ed): Neonatology, 4th ed. Philadelphia, JB Lippincott, 1993, pp 357–365.
9. Chance GW: Thermal environment in transport. In Sinclair JC (ed): Temperature Regulation and Energy Metabolism in the Newborn. New York, Grune & Stratton, 1978, pp 227–240.
10. Frigoletto FD, Little GA (eds): Guidelines for Perinatal Care, 2nd ed. American Academy of Pediatrics, American College of Obstetricians and Gynecologists, 1988, p 274.
11. Selfridge J, Shea SS: The accuracy of the tympanic membrane thermometer in detecting fever in infants aged 3 months and younger in the emergency department setting. J Emerg Nurs 19:127–130, 1993.
12. Davis K: The accuracy of tympanic membrane measurement in children. Pediatr Nurs 19:267–272, 1993.
13. McLaughlin JF, Telzrow RW, Scott CM: Neonatal mercury vapor exposure in an infant incubator. Pediatrics 66:988–990, 1982.
14. Waffarn F, Hodgman J: Mercury vapor contamination of infant incubators: A potential hazard. Pediatrics 64:640–642, 1992.
15. Code of Federal Regulations of Transportation, 49 CFR 1751, October 1992.
16. Mayfield SR, Bhatia J, Nakamura KT, Rios GR, Bell EF: Temperature measurement in term and preterm neonates. J Pediatr 104:271–275, 1984.
17. Oliver TK: Temperature regulation and heat production in the newborn. Pediatr Clin North Am 12:765–779, 1965.
18. Perlstein PH, Edwards NK, Sutherland JM: Apnea in premature infants and incubator-air-temperature changes. N Engl J Med 282:461–466, 1970.
19. Gedeon S, Mebius C, Palmer K: Neonatal hygroscopic condenser humidifier. Crit Care Med 15:51–54, 1987.
20. Sheldon RE: The bowel bag: A sterile transportable method for warming infant. Pediatrics 53:267, 1974.
21. Rowe MI, Weinberg GH, Andrews W: Reduction of neonatal heat loss by an insulated heat cover. J Pediatr Surg 18:909–913, 1983.
22. Marks KH, Devenyi AG, Bello ME, et al: Thermal head wrap for infants. J Pediatr 107:956–959, 1985.

23. LeBlanc MH: Evaluation of two devices for improving thermal control of premature infants in transport. Crit Care Med 12:593-595, 1984.
24. Nielson HC, Jung AL, Atherton SO: Evaluation of the Porta-Warm Mattress as a source of heat for neonatal transport. Pediatrics 58:500-504, 1976.
25. Filston HC, Izant RJ: Management outline of common pediatric surgical problems. In The Surgical Neonate, 2nd ed. Norwalk, CN, Appleton-Century-Crofts, 1985, p 235.
26. Richey DA: Transporting the infant with an abdominal wall defect. Neonatal Network 9:53-56, 1990.
27. Bell EF, Oh W: Fluid and electrolyte management. In Avery GB, Fletcher MA, McDonald MG (eds): Neonatology, 4th ed. Philadelphia, JB Lippincott, 1993, pp 312-329.
28. Shaffer SG, Weismann DN: Fluid requirements in the preterm infant. Clin Perinatol 19:233-250, 1992.
29. Doyle LW, Sinclair JC: Insensible water loss in newborn infants. Clin Perinatol 9:453-482, 1982.
30. Knauth AL, Gordin M, McNelis W, Baumgart S: Semipermeable polyurethane membrane as an artifical skin for the premature neonate. Pediatrics 83:945-950, 1989.
31. Baumgart S: Reduction of oxygen consumption, insensible water loss, and radiant heat demand with use of a plastic blanket for low-birth-weight infants under radiant warmers. Pediatrics 74:1022-1028, 1984.
32. Shenai JP, Major CW, Gaylord MS, et al: A successful decade of regionalized perinatal care in Tennessee: The neonatal experience. J Perinatol 1:137-143, 1991.
33. Hack M, Horbar JD, Malloy MH, et al: Very low birth weight outcomes of the National Institute of Child Health and Human Development Neonatal Network. Pediatrics 87:587-597, 1991.
34. Liechty EA, Donovan E, Purohit B, et al: Reduction of neonatal mortality after multiple doses of bovine surfactant in low birth weight neonates with respiratory distress syndrome. Pediatrics 88:19-28, 1991.
35. Hack M, Fanaroff AA: Outcome of extremely-low-birth-weight infants between 1982 and 1988. N Engl J Med 321:1642-1647, 1989.
36. Hack M, Fanaroff AA: How small is too small? Considerations in evaluating the outcome of the tiny infant. Clin Perinatol 15:773-788, 1988.
37. Ott WJ: Accurate gestational dating. Obstet Gynecol 66:311-315, 1985.
38. Spinnato JA, Sibai BM, Shaver DC, Anderson GD: Inaccuracy of Dubowitz gestational age in low birth weight infants. Obstet Gynecol 63:491-495, 1984.
39. Dillon WD, Egan EA: Aggressive obstetric management in late second trimester deliveries. Obstet Gynecol 58:685-690, 1981.
40. Yu VYH, Loke JL, Bajuk B, et al: Prognosis for infants born at 23-28 weeks gestation. Br Med J 293:1200-1205, 1986.
41. Allen MC, Donohue PK, Dugman AE: The limit of viability—neonatal outcome of infants born at 22-25 weeks gestation. N Engl J Med 329:1597-1601, 1993.
42. Lantos JD, Miles SH, Silverstein MD, Stocking CB: Survival after cardiopulmonary resuscitation in babies of very low birth weight. N Engl J Med 348:91-95, 1988.
43. Bhat R, Zikos-Labropoulou E: Resuscitation and respiratory management of infants weighing less than 1000 grams. Clin Perinatol 13:285-297, 1986.
44. Manchanda M, Kenyon CF, Kronick JB: Use of bovine surfactant during interhospital transport of premature infants with respiratory distress syndrome. Abstrat: American Academy of Pediatrics meeting, New Orleans, 1992.
45. Gortmaher S, Soboi A, Clark C, et al: The survival of very low-birth-weight infants by level of hospital by birth: A population study of perinatal systems in four states. Am J Obstet Gynecol 152:517-524, 1985.
46. Freda VJ, Gorman JG, Pollach W, et al: Prevention of Rh hemolytic disease—Ten years' clinical experience with Rh immune globulin. N Engl J Med 292:1014, 1975.
47. Pollach W, Freda VJ, Gorman JG: Ten years of Rh disease prevention. Perinatal Care 2:8, 1978.
48. Hutchison AA, Drew JH, Yu VY, et al: Nonimmune hydrops fetalis: A review of 61 cases. Obstet Gynecol 59:347-352, 1982.
49. Etches PC, Lemons JA: Nonimmune hydrops fetalis: A report of 22 cases including three siblings. Pediatrics 64:326-332, 1979.
50. Maldergem LV, Janiaux E, Fournean C, Gillerot Y: Genetic causes of hydrops fetalis. Pediatrics 89:81-86, 1992.
51. Wertz AW, Heeren MM: Delivery room resuscitation. In Pomerance JJ, Richardson CJ (eds): Neonatology for the Clinician. Norwalk, CT, Appleton & Lange, 1993, p 93.
52. Brans YW, Milstead RR, Bailey PE, et al: Blood volume estimates in coombs-test positive infants. N Engl J Med 290:1450, 1974.
53. Phibbs RH, Johnson P, Tooley WH: Cardiorespiratory status of erythroblastotic newborn infants: II. Blood volume, hematocrit and serum albumin concentration in relation to hydrops fetalis. Pediatrics 3:13, 1974.

CHAPTER 6

Transport Safety

GERARDO REYES, M.D., F.A.A.P.
ROBERT WESOLOWSKI, E.M.T.-P.

Safety is defined in Webster's dictionary as "freedom from hurt, injury, or loss." With the rapidly expanding use of air and ground medical transport systems throughout the country, safety has become an important issue in transport medicine. In 1973, the Public Health Services Act was made into law. The emergency medical services (EMS) systems portion of the act addressed issues and concerns regarding medical transport safety and was the first nationwide comprehensive effort leading to a sophisticated EMS system.[11] It is calculated that more than 1 million patients have been transported by air medical programs since the first hospital-based helicopter transport system was created at St. Anthony's Hospital in Denver, Colorado, in 1972.[2,9] The latest statistics for 1994 reveal more than 170,000 patients transported by more than 200 air transport programs.[5]

The increased use of transport systems has led to an increased number of EMS vehicle accidents and unnecessary fatalities. Studies in New York and Arizona reveal that, on average, one ambulance accident resulting in injury or death occurs every day. Extrapolation from those results yields an estimated 5,400 injuries and 17 deaths annually as a consequence of ground EMS vehicle accidents in the United States.[4] Statistics published by the Aviation Safety Institute in 1986 demonstrated that medical helicopters had a fatal accident rate three times the national average for commercial helicopters; the primary causes were adverse weather conditions, engine problems, and obstacle strikes.[6]

This chapter discusses safety issues regarding both land and air EMS transport and ways to prevent accidents and minimize injuries to the patient and medical personnel.

SAFETY ISSUES IN AIR AND GROUND TRANSPORT OF PEDIATRIC PATIENTS

Over the last 20 years, medical transportation systems have changed dramatically in their efficiency and sophistication. As these systems have evolved, the priority issue in their development has been safety. A pediatric transport system should be capable of rapidly delivering advanced pediatric skills and critical care to the patient at the referring hospital and maintaining that level of care during transport to the tertiary care facility. The method used to transport a critically ill child, be it by ground vehicle, helicopter, or fixed-wing aircraft, is a crucial factor in providing expedient and quality health care. The decision as to the most appropriate vehicle for transport should be made prior to utilizing the available resources, thus saving precious time for the transport team and patient. Today's most sophisticated pediatric transport systems should have available both air and ground ambulances.

It is our hope that the information following in this chapter will help you focus the attention of your transport team into developing safe practices. Safety is not just a matter of rights and wrongs—it is a process that involves a transport team which is controlled by protocols, well-trained personnel, the best equipment, a definitive process of choosing the proper mode of transportation, and an on-going quality-assurance program. If all of these factors are controlled by a strong medical command, a safe and workable environment exists.

PERSONNEL COMPOSITION OF A PEDIATRIC AIR/GROUND TRANSPORT SYSTEM

The most important issues in establishing an efficient pediatric transport system are (1) medical control by a dedicated pediatric specialist and (2) a transport team that is composed of qualified individuals.

Safety concerns can be kept to a minimum by ensuring that the personnel assigned to a transport team are well-trained, not only in the care of the critically ill patient but also in the use and maintenance of their equipment and the safety devices on all vehicles utilized for transportation.

The transport team should be able to continue or improve the level of medical care initiated at the referring facility. The Consolidated Omnibus Reconciliation Act (COBRA) mandates that patients be transported by medical personnel trained and qualified to provide whatever treatment is necessary or required to maintain the patient's condition and treat any possible complications.[5] Factors critical in the selection of medical transport personnel include[1]:

1. Formal training and competence in pediatric surface and air transport

2. General physical condition (limitations must be considered because these may be hazardous to the team member and his or her ability to function as a team member)

3. Emotional and physical limitations (response to stress, ability to withstand fatigue, susceptibility to motion sickness)

4. Weight and height requirements (a priority, especially in air transport)

5. Tactfulness and sensitivity (not only must the individuals be capable of handling the patient medically, but they also must be tactful and sensitive to the needs of the patient as well as the receiving hospital)

6. Leadership (teaching, good communication skills)

7. Enthusiasm and motivation

The transport team should be familiar with the use and location of all essential equipment or other vital supplies on their transport vehicle. All members should review how to secure and release mounting systems, evacuate the patient and crew if an accident or fire should occur, and locate and use the fire extinguisher and communication equipment.

A pediatric transport system must maintain the skills of the team members by 1) transporting enough critical patients to maintain those skills and 2) having in place a quality continuing education program and a continuous quality-assurance program that cover all the operations for the transport system. Although transport teams vary immensely in composition, the training of the transport team is an important component that directly affects the success or failure of all transports. Each institution should develop a philosophy that mirrors that of the individual taking responsibility as medical control of the transport team.

The debate continues over the choice of team members who will achieve the greatest decrease in mortality and morbidity. The data remain inconclusive, with some programs requiring a physician and others stating that a well-trained nurse combination team can also affect patient care. The latter programs claim that no advantage is seen in patient care or outcome when a team includes a physician. Regardless of the composition of the transport team, selection of team members should be made from a pool of personnel who are specifically trained in pediatric transport. This can include teams of nurse–paramedic, nurse–physician, nurse–respiratory therapist, and nurse–nurse. Ninety-seven percent of helicopter air medical services provide two medical crew members. Of these, 53% are nurse–paramedic teams, 11% are nurse–physician, 11% are nurse–nurse, 20% are nurse–other, and 5% are other combinations.[2]

SELECTING A MODE OF TRANSPORTATION

In choosing the mode of transportation for the patient, many factors become involved. The information gathered from the referring hospital must be quickly considered, and a determination made by a qualified individual as to the best mode of transportation. A formal process of gathering this information from the referring hospital must be consistent with all tranports. The general indications for accepting a referral include the medical conditions of the patient and, in the referring physician's judgment, the lack of personnel and/or facilities at the referring hospital to provide optimal medical care. The accepting hospital should have a standard protocol for accepting patients and a formal information sheet that must be filled out before accepting a referral (Fig. 1).

Many considerations are important in selecting the mode of transportation and should be analyzed before determining what vehicle to use. The first consideration should be the diagnosis and stability of the patient. This determination affects the urgency of care and determines which vehicle is safest to transport the individual. The American Academy of Pediatrics Guidelines for Air and Ground Transportation state, "If a patient's medical condition is unstable, even a minimal shortening of the transport time to the referring hospital by one mode of transportation rather than another may be life-saving."[1]

The second consideration is safety. Prevention is not a foreign concept to health professionals. Unfortunately, safety programs are frequently modified or eliminated first when budget reductions are required. In general, safety operations in and around ground and air vehicles share several common features. First and foremost is the evaluation of weather and road conditions. In heavily populated areas, peak traffic times, construction zones, and any existing detours must also be considered. Each of these conditions can delay the transport of a patient, thus putting unnecessary stress on the transport team.

GROUND TRANSPORT SAFETY

There are many advantages in using ground ambulance systems. The most obvious is direct service of a ground ambulance. The ground ambulance can specifically pick up the transport team at their facility and deliver them to the referral hospital. The patient is put directly on the stretcher or isolette and then put directly into the ground ambulance for transport. There is no need for concern about landing zones and/or runways, and there is no need to transfer the patient from one car to another as may be necessary in air transport.

TRANSPORT INFORMATION SHEET

Date   Time   Call taken by:

Patient Name | Birthdate | Age | Weight

Referring Hospital | Phone | Hospital Location

Referring Physician | Insurance | HMO Approved

Attending Accepting Transport | Patient's Private MD

Story/Physical Exam/Diagnosis

Patient Data Base

Time   Temp   Hr   RR   B/P   Last Oral Intake

Respiratory | Renal | O_2

Intubated/Trached   Vent Parameters

Cardiac   Perfusion

Neurological

Medications Given: Include Time   IV Fluids/Sites/Rates

Laboratory Data

Time   HGB   HGT   WBC   DIFF: P B S E L M   PLTS   COAG

TIME   NA   K   CL CO_2 BUN   CR   CA   GLU   Other

Blood Gas

Time   Type   Ph PCO_2 PO_2 HCO_3 BE O_2SAT   Vent Settings

Time   Type   Ph PCO_2 PO_2 HCO_3 BE O_2SAT   Vent Settings

X-ray/CT Scan Results   C-Spine Immobilization

None Order Suggestion:

Have Family Available for Consent   _____Our Transport
Have Charts and X-rays Copied   _____Their Transport
                                          _____Helicopter

FIGURE 1.   Transport information sheet.

VITAL SIGNS

TIME	TEMP	HR	RR	BP	MAP

RESPIRATORY CARE

TIME	FIO₂	IMV	CPATH/PIP	TV	O₂ SAT	SUCT	SECR	RATE

BLOOD GASES

TIME	TYPE	PH/PCO₂	PO₂/HCO	BE/0₂

HEMATOLOGY

WBC/RBC	HB/HCT	PLTS

MEDICATION/IVF

TIME	DOSE	RATE	ROUTE	GIVEN BY

NURSING SUMMARY _____

_____

RN SIGNATURE _____

INPUT   OUTPUT

TIME	IV	PO	URINE

NAME: _____
DIAGNOSIS: _____
AGE: _____ SEX: _____ WT.: _____
PARENTS NAME & PHONE #: _____

REFERRING HOSPITAL: _____

INITIAL CALL: _____
PT. ACCEPTED: _____
AMBULANCE CALLED: _____
AMBULANCE ARRIVED: _____
DEPARTED SMMHC: _____
ARRIVED REF. HOSP: _____
DEPARTED REF. HOSP: _____
ARRIVED SMMHC: _____

PROCEDURES: _____
CXR: _____
INTUBATION: _____
ETT RETAPED: _____
NG: _____
FOLEY: _____
PIV: _____
CUTDOWN: _____
INTRAOSSEOUS: _____
OTHER: _____

ETT: SIZE _____
        LANDMARK
        TYPE _____
AIRWAY: SIZE _____
        TYPE _____

KEY: RT ___ TYPE OF RESP. TREATMENT GIVEN

FIGURE 1 *(Cont.).*   Transport information sheet.

An additional advantage to ground transport is that they can divert at any time to the closest hospital facility should the need arise. In addition, for training and safety purposes, ground ambulances are more readily available for training personnel. Such training and orientation to the location of all the supplies and equipment on a ground ambulance will make team members more comfortable when working in the environment of the ground ambulance. Inversely, the more limited availability of air transport units does not allow the transport team an opportunity to develop the same level of comfort as they will with a ground transport unit.

The most utilized type of vehicle in medical transports is the ground ambulance. The U.S. Department of Transportation has developed specifications regulating the manufacture and design of vehicles used as ambulances. The Federal regulation that governs ambulances is KKK-A-1822-C, and it establishes the minimum standards and equipment for a vehicle to qualify as an ambulance, including the required basic life support (BLS) and advanced life support (ALS) equipment.[7] In the transport of pediatric patients, it is advisable to use primarily ALS vehicles. Obviously, with more knowledgeable personnel and more advanced equipment available to the transport team, better care can be provided for the patient.

Each ground transport vehicle must also be equipped with safety devices such as emergency lights, sirens, air horn, and public address system. These devices are to be used to alert pedestrians and other vehicles of your presence, but these warning devices do not give the ambulance operator the strict right of way. Most states have regulations governing the use of these warning devices. While operating these warning devices, the ground ambulance operator must continue to obey traffic laws. Although some states may exempt emergency vehicles from certain traffic laws, abuse of these exemptions tends to lead to unsafe driving practices. Some exemptions to traffic laws for emergency vehicles include proceeding through red lights or stop signs after slowing and giving other motorists an opportunity to clear the intersection, exceeding the posted speed limit, and, in some states, moving in the opposite direction of flow of traffic if no other vehicles are present.

Despite these exemptions, all ambulance operators must exhibit extreme caution at all times. Unfortunately, overuse of the siren may occur, in which individuals believe that it is not only a warning device but also allows them the right of way regardless of traffic volume or the situation. Such careless operation can lead to accidents. When accidents occur, not only is the transport delayed, but also there is potential for injury to bystanders, the ambulance crew, transport team, and patient.

The overuse of warning devices can be minimized by categorizing patients simply into two groups: Code 1 and Code 2. Patients in Code 1 are in an immediate life-threatening situation, and speed is essential. Thus, use of warning devices will expedite transport. However, in this situation, air transport would be the wiser choice to transport a patient in such critical conditions because it is statistically safer than ground transport. The second category is Code 2 and includes patients who are stable but require transfer from the referral hospital for any number of reasons (e.g., the hospital lacks facilities to treat the patient at the present level or lacks the ability to treat the patient for a long time). These patients are picked up by the transport team in an ambulance and transported back to the tertiary hospital in accordance with all traffic laws.

During transport of a Code 1 patient, the use of warning devices does not justify recklessness. With use of these warning devices, transport time can be reduced, but the focus should be on safe transport.

There are few weather restrictions on ground transports, which in itself is an advantage when choosing the type of transport to use. All transport team members and/or family members who ride in the ambulance must be safely secured. In addition, all equipment must be secured in the event an accident or a defensive maneuver that would cause equipment to drift in the back of the ambulance. Other concerns for ground transports are the potential for motion sickness, rough ride due to the poor suspension systems on ambulances, and a repetitive acceleration and deceleration of the vehicle. Despite these few disadvantages, most hospital-based transport teams are more comfortable working in the ground ambulance, simply because most transports are done by ground vehicles. The comfort level of the transport team, not only in the treatment of the patient but also in the safe operation of the vehicle, tends to improve success of the transport program.

If any transport is going to be 60–90 minutes, it would be advisable to consider air transport. Ground ambulances are limited by the amount of power they can provide for any adjunct equipment that may be needed for the care of the patient. Also, communication problems may arise with transport times over 90 minutes.

In summary, ground transport is the most utilized means of transporting patients. In addition, it is the most economical means.

HELICOPTER TRANSPORT SAFETY

Helicopter medical transport systems have gained in popularity since 1972 when the first hospital-based system was established.[9] However, helicopter transportation is not a panacea, and its benefits must be weighted against its inherent risks, such as crashes or emergency landings because of poor weather or engine failure. Basic safety issues include[3]:
1. Appropriate indications for use of helicopters
2. Providing a safe landing zone
3. Use of protective eye and head gear
4. Proper procedure on approaching the aircraft
5. Orientation to the aircraft's safety features

Helicopter transport is indicated when a patient must be transported over a long distance in a short time, especially in rural areas where distances are great, road systems are poor, and access to ground transportation is minimal. Also, certain terrain features, such as mountains or forests, may make helicopter evacuation of the patient better and more efficient than ground transportation.

Loading and Unloading

The most important safety issue during the loading and unloading of a patient is following the pilot's instructions. The pilot is ultimately responsible for the safety of the patient and medical personnel, and his or her instructions should be followed carefully. When approaching the aircraft, follow the safety approach zones (Fig. 2), and always wait for the pilot's instructions. Exceptions to these safety zones are allowed with the MBB-B0105 and MBB-BK117 helicopters, both of which have the access doors in the back.

In most cases, loading and unloading of the patients is done when the engine is off and the blades are not turning. If the patient is in critical condition, the pilot may allow the medical personnel to load or unload the patient while the engine is on and the blades are turning. If this is the case, two hazards must be taken into consideration, noise and wind. Rotating blades are capable of

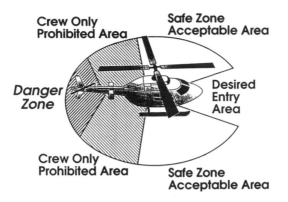

Crew Only
Prohibited Area

Safe Zone
Acceptable Area

*Danger
Zone*

Desired
Entry
Area

Crew Only
Prohibited Area

Safe Zone
Acceptable Area

FIGURE 2.   Helicopter approach areas. (Adapted from Klein K, Bills DM: Transport safety. In Byron A, McCloskey K (eds): Evaluation, Stabilization, and Transport of Critically Ill Child. St. Louis, Mosby, 1992, p 648; with permission.)

generating winds up to 50 mph, and noise from the engine can reach 100 decibels.[10] To prevent ear damage, protective head gear must be worn at all times by the medical personnel and patient when approaching the aircraft and during flight. The head gear also has a built-in microphone and speakers for intrahelicopter communications.

The wind from the rotating blades can generate a mini-storm in the landing zone. For this reason, precautions must be taken to avoid damage or injury from flying objects. Loose equipment, such as stethoscopes, blankets, loose clothing, and charts, must be properly secured. The landing zone should be free of litter or debris, and protective glasses should be worn, including by the patient.

Although most helicopters' rotors are 7–10 feet above the ground, precautions must be taken to avoid contact with blades, especially by intravenous poles and antennas. When the landing zone is in uneven or sloping ground, the helicopter should be approached from the downhill side if possible.[7]

In-Flight Safety

After loading the patient, the medical personnel should become familiar with the safety features of the helicopter. It is the pilot's duty to orient the passengers regarding the use of oxygen, emergency exits, seatbelts, intrahelicopter communications, emergency landing procedures, and fire extinguishers, among other things. The stretcher and the patient, as well as all medical equipment, must be properly secured to avoid damage during turbulent flight conditions.

Before departure, a careful and thorough examination of the patient is mandatory, with special emphasis to the airway and circulation. If the patient is intubated, the endotracheal tube must be properly secured to avoid an accidental extubation during airborne transport, an event that can seriously compromise the patient; in addition, the mechanical ventilator must be properly strapped to the helicopter. Care must also be given to the intravenous lines to avoid displacement during the flight. If the patient has broken bones, make sure the extremities or the neck are fully immobilized before take-off. Sedation may be appropriate for patients on mechanical ventilation and/or patients who are combative or agitated.

Helicopter safety involves common sense and adherence to the safety procedures and protocols as explained by the pilot. Safety standards and guidelines are available from the Helicopter Association International, the Federal Aviation Administration, the Department of Transportation, and the Association of Air Medical Services.

FIXED-WING AIRCRAFT SAFETY

Fixed-wing aircraft is the third component of the medical transport system. Because of its high cost and maintenance and the need for a runway, fixed-wing medical transport is mostly limited to the transport of patients between cities or towns.

Like helicopters, airplanes require that the medical personnel follow proper safety procedures. Again, the pilot has ultimate responsibility for the safety of the passengers and medical personnel. His or her instructions should be followed very closely.

When approaching the aircraft, keep a safe distance from the engines and exhaust system. The fumes from the exhaust can be toxic, and the wind created by the jet engines or propellers can create similar hazards as rotating helicopter blades. The exhaust system can reach temperatures of 600°C, and even brief contact with these hot surfaces can cause third-degree burns. While on the runway, keep an eye on other planes that could be landing or taxiing.[10]

In-flight safety protocols are similar to those of helicopter flights. Rapid decompression is one hazard not commonly encountered in helicopters that can be quite dangerous in fixed-wing aircraft. During rapid decompression, oxygen masks should be worn immediately by all passengers. The medical crew should don their masks before attending to the needs of the patient so that they may provide care for the patient while the cabin is decompressed. Flying objects and debris can be a cause of serious injury and sometimes death.[10] Common sense and proper adherence to the safety instructions of the pilot should minimize any dangers to the patient or medical personnel.

COMMUNICATION

An additional focus for a safe transport system is a superior communication system. Communication begins with the initial contact from the referring hospital and must continue once the transport team leaves the hospital, picks up the patient, and returns to the accepting hospital. At all times, the transport team should have the means to communicate with either hospital (or for that matter, with any hospital that they deem necessary to contact). This requires the transport vehicle to have a radio or cellular phone.

Communication is the key to a successful transport system. Communications can be accomplished through a central dispatcher, who can coordinate all transmissions, or communications can be direct between the individuals involved. In any event, the transport vehicle must always have a means to communicate, in case of emergency or just to notify the hospital of a change in condition of a patient. The transport team should be trained in the proper use of the communication equipment. They should also check all communication equipment before venturing out on the transport.

VENDORS

The choice a hospital must make when starting a transport system program is whether to purchase and operate their own ambulance or to seek out an already existing ambulance vendor. The advantages of owning and operating one's own ambulance are controlling its availability, stocking specific equipment deemed necessary for your transport program, and hiring personnel specifically trained in the needs of your program. The initial cost of vehicles and equipment as well as the additional liability must be weighed heavily before making this decision. Utilization of existing vendors does minimize the initial cost, and contracts can be devised so that vendor ambulances are available per each institution's specifications with fees based on actual usage. In selecting a vendor, a very specific and comprehensive checklist must be met by the vendor of choice. A suggested vendor checklist is outlined in a recent article by Schneider et al.[8]

A comprehensive quality-assurance program should be on-going in the evaluation of any vendor that is chosen by the hospital. Since the vendor is contracted to provide the services specifically outlined by your hospital, it is important that an individual oversee the operation of that vendor with the hospital's concern as the focus. With many vendors in the market today, the pediatric specialists responsible for the program should be able to outline the specifics needed of the vendor, thus requiring that vendor to uphold all the needs of the particular program. The vendor must fulfill many specific criteria and continue an ongoing quality-assurance program of their own. A strong relationship between the vendor and project director will enhance success of the transport team.

SUMMARY

The establishment of a medical transport team by a hospital or medical center must focus on the safety issues. As the number of transports increases yearly, by ground and air, ambulance manufacturers are constantly improving the safety of their vehicles. In addition, it is imperative that medical transport personnel undergo continuous training and education. Trade publications, such as *Hospital Aviation, Air Medical Journal, The Journal of Air Medical Transport*, and *Air Medical Safety Quarterly*, can be a source of useful information and guidelines regarding safety issues and concerns. Transport teams should also update their safety protocols by following publications from such national organizations as the American Academy of Pediatrics, the Federal Aviation Administration, and the Federal Emergency Management Agency.

Statistics illustrate the continued increase in use of patient transport systems to provide patients the best care available. It is our responsibility to ensure that this process succeeds in a responsible and safe environment.

REFERENCES

1. American Academy of Pediatrics Committee on Hospital Care: Guidelines for air and ground transportation of pediatric patients. Pediatrics 78:943–950, 1986.
2. Collett HM: Annual transport statistics. Air Med Transport 10(3):11, 1991.
3. Federal Emergency Management Agency, United States Fire Administration: EMS safety, techniques and applications. Washington, DC, U.S. Fire Administration, Apr 1994.
4. Klein K, Bills DM: Transport safety. In Byron A, McCloskey K (eds): Evaluation, Stabilization, and Transport of the Critically Ill Child. St. Louis, Mosby, 1992, p 648.
5. Myfield T: 1994 Annual transport statistics and transport fees survey. Air Med 13(4):132–135, 1994.
6. Mrochek P, Sorenson P: Missing aircraft—If disaster strikes, is your program prepared? Air Med Transport 12:17–19, 1989.
7. Peto G, Medwe WJ: EMS Driving the Safe Way. Englewood, NY, Brady, 1992.
8. Schneider C, Gomez M, Lee R: Evaluation of ground ambulance, rotor-wing, and fixed-wing aircraft services. Crit Care Clin North Am 8(3):533–563, 1992.
9. Scholl MD, Geshekter CL: The Zed expedition: The world's first air ambulance? J R Soc Med 81:679–680, 1989.
10. Scott PM, Broady JH, Hunt B, et al: Aircraft safety. In Lee G (ed): Flight Nursing: Principles and Practice. St. Louis, Mosby, 1991, pp 597–610.
11. Stohler S, Jacobs BB: Interhospital transfer of the critical patient. Emerg Care Q 4(4):66–78, 1989.

CHAPTER 7

Administrative Pearls

MARY LOU GOSTISHA, R.N., M.S.N.

TEAM COMPOSITION

Transport of critically ill pediatric patients requires stabilization and care from caregivers with the knowledge and understanding of the unique needs of the pediatric population. Careful selection of team members and proper training are essential. The transport environment is an uncontrolled environment, requiring personnel of high skill. Familiarity with pediatric disease states is necessary to assess the status of the patient, to note subtle changes in condition, and to anticipate potential problems or status changes. Staff transporting these patients should have the cognitive and technical skills necessary to provide adequate care and sufficient experience to maintain those skills.[4] The exact amount of experience in pediatric critical care required of potential team members will depend on the goals and needs of individual teams.[1] If team members do not have pediatric critical care experience, education and training must be provided.

The ideal composition of the pediatric transport team remains controversial.[2] Depending on the resources available within the system, team members may be registered nurses, physicians, respiratory therapists, paramedics, or emergency medical technicians.[11] The transport team should contain at least one member experienced in diagnosis and management of pediatric illnesses or injuries and who is able to recognize potential deterioration in the patient's condition.[1] Team selection should focus more on the individual's skills and ability to manage patient care than on specific titles or degrees.

Personnel may come from various areas within the institution, bringing with them a varied background of knowledge and experience. Transport team members must be flexible and emotionally stable, able to act independently, and possess good interpersonal skills.[1]

Communication skills become an essential component of transport. Communication within the team is important in providing care, but communication with the referral staff is another key component. When the transport team enters the referral facility, the nature of the situation is such that the potential for misunderstanding is great. Team members must be sensitive to the need for all communications to be on the highest professional level.[1]

It is impossible to identify the ideal personnel profile or team composition for every transport team in every situation. Team composition must be individualized to the needs of the patient population likely to be transported and based on the resources available within the institution.[15]

TEAM TRAINING

Whether the team does exclusively pediatric transports or both adult and pediatric transports, training for pediatric transport must be comprehensive.[2] Whatever the team composition, the team members must be well prepared and highly competent in managing emergencies in children.[1] Competence can be gained through a variety of means; the specifics depend on the experience of team members and the goals of the transport program.

No standard curriculum for training has been established for pediatric transport. Guidelines for training have been suggested by the American Academy of Pediatrics' Task Force on Interhospital Transport. The Association of Air Medical Services does not specifically address the issue of pediatric transport education but does support training and experience commensurate with the specialty-care air environment.[7]

Formal training of transport team members should be coordinated by the medical director and team coordinator/manager. Learning needs should be clearly identified based on the patient population likely to be transported.

Training should include a didactic component focusing on physiology and management relative to the patient population to be transported and disease entities likely to be encountered. Flight physiology can be incorporated if air transports are to be performed. Other possible components may include, but are not limited to, specific instruction on transport operations particular to the institution, documentation requirements, medications, and communication on transport.

The technical component of team training should focus on equipment operation and trouble-shooting and on procedural skills such as airway management and intravenous access. Skill laboratories, operating room experience, and animal laboratories can be used effectively to teach technical skills. Teams that do not utilize physicians as part of the team may require additional skills and training.

Certification in Pediatric Advanced Life Support (PALS), Advanced Pediatric Life Support (APLS), or the Neonatal Resuscitation Program may also be considered as part of team training.[1] Certification must be accompanied by practical experience to maintain the knowledge and skills acquired.

Training and education must be individualized to the team experience level and in consort with role expectations that have been established for team members. Additional topics that may be included are safety, communication, and the role of public relations in transport.

A preceptor program can be very helpful in providing practical experience. New transport personnel accompany experienced team members on several transports, gaining firsthand knowledge of the transport experience. This provides learning opportunities that cannot be taught in a classroom.[5]

Team members must be familiar with any protocols or care guidelines that have been established by the program. Recurrency training or some other means of evaluating knowledge should be established as part of the educational program.[3] This can be incorporated in the quality improvement monitoring activities of the team.

NURSING RESPONSIBILITIES

Responsibilities of the nurse on transport vary depending on the team composition and the resources available to the transport team. In light of the wide variance in possible responsibilities, the role of the Transport Nurse

Clinician (TNC) at Children's Hospital of Wisconsin will be used to describe possible functions.

The transport team at Children's Hospital is primarily a physician-led team. There is the ability to staff with an R.N. only, M.D.-R.N.-R.T., M.D.-R.N., or R.N.-R.T., depending on the specific needs of the patient. The decision on team composition is a collaborative decision made by the TNC and medical control physician.

There is no central dispatch center at Childrens Hospital of Wisconsin. The TNC is responsible for taking patient information from the referral facility. If stabilization assistance is required, a pediatric intensivist is contacted to speak with the referring physician. The TNC then begins making arrangements for the transport and for admission of the patient to the hospital. Team members, vehicle vendors, and the admitting department must be contacted to facilitate the transport.

The TNC is generally responsible for assembling equipment and supplies necessary for transport. Communication en route to the referral facility is accomplished via cellular phone in the ground vehicles and via radio in the helicopter and fixed-wing aircraft.

Upon the team's arrival at the referral facility, patient care becomes the priority. The TNC is responsible for providing total nursing care to the patient. As the patient is stabilized and prepared for transport, monitoring equipment must be connected and secured. Consent for transport of the patient to the receiving facility should be obtained from the legal guardian. Parents are allowed to see and touch their child prior to transport and are given maps and directions to the hospital. Specific tasks may be delegated to other team members, but ensuring their completion is the responsibility of the transport nurse.

Communication with the receiving facility is done prior to leaving the referral facility. The TNC also communicates with the nurse who will be caring for the patient at the receiving hospital. This helps ensure that necessary equipment and supplies are available upon arrival and provides for a smoother transition from transport to inpatient care.

Upon arrival at Children's Hospital, the TNC transfers care of the patient and ensures that all documentation is complete. Patient billing for the transport is completed at this time. Equipment and supplies are restocked and readied for future transports.

Many other responsibilities may be incorporated into the role of the transport nurse. Maintenance of supplies and equipment, patient follow-up and call back to the referral facility staff, outreach activities, as well as educational responsibilites are all important functions that can be part of the transport nurse's role.

DOCUMENTATION

Documentation of care provided on transport is best accomplished with data forms specifically designed for the transport program. This ensures documentation of consistent information in an organized manner. This documentation becomes an essential link between the referral facility, transport team, and receiving facility. The medical record serves as a basis for planning patient care and continuity in evaluation of the patient's condition and treatment; it supplies documentary evidence of the course of the patient's evaluation, treatment, and any changes in condition. It also documents communication between the health care professionals who provide care for the patient and assists in protecting the legal interests of the patient.[1]

Information in the transport record should include, but not be limited to, data such as team configuration and notification times, mode of transport, and time of departure; clinical data such as reason for transport, patient assessment data, and procedures performed; and demographic data such as patient age, sex, and location of the referring hospital. This information becomes part of the patient medical record, documenting care provided during stabilization and transport (Fig. 1).

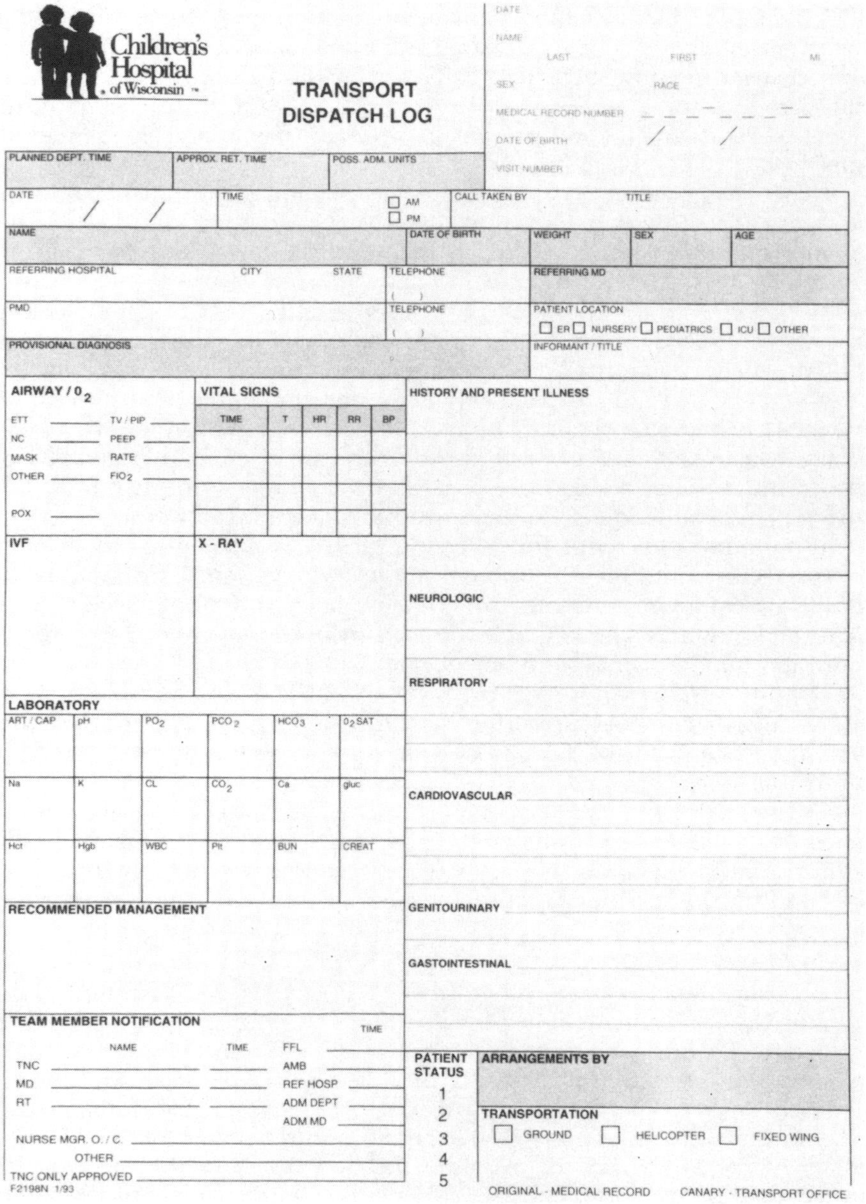

Children's Hospital of Wisconsin ™

TRANSPORT DISPATCH LOG

DATE
NAME LAST FIRST MI
SEX RACE
MEDICAL RECORD NUMBER
DATE OF BIRTH / /
VISIT NUMBER

PLANNED DEPT. TIME	APPROX. RET. TIME	POSS. ADM. UNITS

DATE / / | TIME ☐ AM ☐ PM | CALL TAKEN BY | TITLE

NAME | DATE OF BIRTH | WEIGHT | SEX | AGE

REFERRING HOSPITAL | CITY | STATE | TELEPHONE ( ) | REFERRING MD

PMD | TELEPHONE ( ) | PATIENT LOCATION ☐ ER ☐ NURSERY ☐ PEDIATRICS ☐ ICU ☐ OTHER

PROVISIONAL DIAGNOSIS | INFORMANT / TITLE

AIRWAY / O_2
ETT ____ TV / PIP ____
NC ____ PEEP ____
MASK ____ RATE ____
OTHER ____ FIO_2 ____
POX ____

VITAL SIGNS

TIME	T	HR	RR	BP

HISTORY AND PRESENT ILLNESS

IVF

X - RAY

NEUROLOGIC

RESPIRATORY

LABORATORY

ART / CAP	pH	PO_2	PCO_2	HCO_3	O_2 SAT
Na	K	CL	CO_2	Ca	gluc
Hct	Hgb	WBC	Plt	BUN	CREAT

CARDIOVASCULAR

RECOMMENDED MANAGEMENT

GENITOURINARY

GASTOINTESTINAL

TEAM MEMBER NOTIFICATION

	NAME	TIME		TIME
TNC			FFL	
MD			AMB	
RT			REF HOSP	
			ADM DEPT	
			ADM MD	

NURSE MGR. O. / C.
OTHER
TNC ONLY APPROVED
F2198N 1/93

PATIENT STATUS
1
2
3
4
5

ARRANGEMENTS BY

TRANSPORTATION
☐ GROUND ☐ HELICOPTER ☐ FIXED WING

ORIGINAL - MEDICAL RECORD CANARY - TRANSPORT OFFICE

FIGURE 1. Transport dispatch log used at Children's Hospital of Wisconsin.

Incorporation of the documentation system with a computerized data-management system is not essential but can provide a means of storing and retrieving data to monitor trends in the transport patient population. Referral patterns can be evaluated for development of marketing strategies. Planning and budgetary needs can be identified.[11] Computerization also allows participation in data exchange with an interfacility network via a standardized national database.[4]

Documentation not only provides a means of recording care but provides a means of evaluating care and patient outcomes through the quality improvement process. It is an essential element in the transport process, providing data to quantify care provided while assisting in gathering data useful for assessment, planning, and improvement of the program.

QUALITY IMPROVEMENT

Monitoring the quality and effectiveness of the care delivered on transport is a key factor in providing a high-quality transport service. Quality improvement (QI) implies the distinguishing of characteristics that determine the value or degree of excellence of the transport program and provides a mechanism to effectively monitor the care provided.[1]

At this time, the Joint Commission on Accreditation of Healthcare Organizations (JCAHO) has not specifically addressed QI for transport programs. Quality guidelines for transport programs have been established by the American Academy of Pediatrics' Task Force on Interhospital Transport, the National Flight Nurse Association, and the Association of Aeromedical Services.

Quality Improvement should be viewed as an ongoing process, not an end in itself. The focus of the QI process is monitoring and improving patient care. Specific outcomes of care provided on transport may be complex to assess. Transport care may be provided for short periods of time or the patient may be transported to another hospital, making follow-up difficult.[14]

The QI program should utilize the expertise of the team members, medical director, transport coordinator/manager, and hospital risk manager to evaluate problems or potential problems when they are identified.[12] All team disciplines should be included in monitoring activities to provide comprehensive review and problem-solving. This can provide learning opportunities as well as a format for improving patient care. The composition of the group and reporting relationships vary for individual programs.

The monitoring program utilized in the transport program should be designed to meet the standards of the QI monitoring program established within the hospital. Examples of the factors influencing transport care that may be part of a monitoring program are guidelines for care, team education, and problems or potential problems identified on transport. Monitors focus on the degree to which the guidelines have been followed and how these contributed to the outcomes of care. This is generally accomplished through documentation review, although group or committee case reviews may also be an effective means of monitoring care. QI monitors must be designed to gather data that reflect that the established quality of care was provided during the transport.

Identifying essential aspects of care for the patient population transported is the first step in the monitoring process. Monitoring may focus on specific patient populations, i.e., intubated patients or neonates, or on specific interventions, i.e., intubations or intraosseous needle insertions. A combination of both methods may also be employed.

QI data should be used as an educational tool to provide proactive problem-solving rather than as a punitive means of review. Group review of transport cases can ensure that all team members participate in the QI process. This provides a means of problem-solving that also ensures that individuals not directly involved in the transport learn from the experience.[3] Trending of problems and issues noted in the monitoring activity provides the ability to develop a plan of action to correct identified problems and alleviate future problems.

QI remains a vital component of the transport program. Development of a systematic, multidisciplinary QI review process for all facets of the transport program can help ensure that care is optimal.

FAMILY SUPPORT

The transport team has many important roles and responsibilities while on transport. One of the most important and often very difficult aspects of transport is the need for emotional support of parents and family. The literature provides very little information and few guidelines for transport team members regarding the emotional state of the parents during this critical period of time.[6] It is far easier to focus on the technical aspects of care than it is to deal with the emotional chaos of parents in crisis.[16] Hospitalization and the need for transport of a child following a traumatic injury or illness can precipitate a crisis for the entire family. The transport team is in a key position to assist the family; however, time constraints and the patient's immediate medical needs can lead to the family being overlooked. Many of the same principles utilized in helping families of patients hospitalized in the intensive care environment can be used in transport. Intervention for families should be based on principles of crisis intervention.

An important aspect of crisis intervention is timing. When an individual's tension rises, he or she begins to mobilize resources and elicit help from others. The individual is more susceptible to outside influence than when in a state of equilibrium.[10] This is important to realize when dealing with the family of a patient who is about to be transported. It is a crucial time to intervene and assist the family to cope with the situation.

Studies have shown that initially all parents go through a period of overwhelming shock and disbelief accompanied by feelings of helplessness.[13] The shock and disbelief may be intensified by the physical appearance of the child as a result of trauma, bandages, endotracheal tubes, and monitoring lines.

Parents have been suddenly and unexpectedly thrust into a crisis, and their reactions can often be difficult to cope with. Parents may use coping methods such as aggression, regression, withdrawal, and repression. These may be manifested by verbal hostility, pacing, wringing of hands, or crying.[16] A multitude of other responses may be noted and are not outside the realm of normalcy. Although coping is generally defined from the point of view of the individual in stress, an important component of coping includes the responses of professionals and others in the situation that may enhance the coping response.[8] Verbal expressions of anger, guilt or animosity should be met with acceptance and reassurance. Accepting emotional outbursts calmly and reassuring the parents that their child is being cared for and is being comforted can help reduce parental anxiety.[16]

The loss of physical control that is often imposed may be difficult for parents to cope with. The care of their child is in the hands of strangers. The transport environment only intensifies these feelings. It is imperative that parents be given access to the transport team to ask questions and be able to trust that their child is in competent hands.

During the initial crisis, parental concerns center on the immediate health status of their child. The parents' need for information about their child's condition ranks very high among the stressors reported by parents.[16] Providing them with information and explanations of what is happening can help restore feelings of control to the parents. The team should assess the parents' perceptions of the illness or injury and the congruence with reality.[16] Sometimes, despite reassurances that the child is stable, parents still may fear that the child is in imminent danger. Isolation from the child can feed these fears and heighten parental anxiety.

Communication gaps often occur when explanations are given in medical jargon. It is important to give explanations in a manner that is understandable to the parent. Even though the parents may not remember all or any of the information, its provision at this time is crucial. At no time during the interactions should the critical nature of the child's condition be minimized. It is unfair to parents and destructive to trust to give false hopes and reassurances.[16] It is imperative that each member of the team be aware of what is happening to the child so that the parents receive the same information from all individuals. If parents feel that they are being misled or that information is being withheld, they will lose trust in the team.[13]

Other common stressors reported by parents were seeing their child in pain, seeing the child frightened and sad, dealing with the child's inability to communicate with the parent, feeling unable to protect the child, and not knowing how best to help the child.[9] Being aware of the stressors that parents are exposed to in this situation can greatly enhance the transport members' ability to meet the needs of the family as well as of the child.

A quick assessment of the emotional status of the family and their current coping strategies can guide the team in helping the family cope with the transport situation. Utilizing the referral facility staff and the relationships they have established with the family members can help facilitate communication and rapport building with the family.

Some additional interventions that can help lessen parental anxiety include seeing and touching their child prior to transport. Providing the parents with directions to the receiving facility and parking information can assist the parents in getting to the receiving facility, allowing them to be reunited with their child.

During transport, the care of the child is paramount; however, the parental and family needs cannot be neglected. The child is an integral part of a family unit, and the needs of the entire unit must be met. Supporting the parents through this immediate crisis period can contribute to the long term well-being of both the child and parents.

REFERENCES

1. American Academy of Pediatrics Taskforce on Interhospital Transport: Guidelines for Air and Ground Transport of Neonatal and Pediatric Patients. Elk Grove Village, Il, American Academy of Pediatrics, 1993.
2. Blumen I, Tressa J: Transporting the critical care child. Emergency 22:36, 1990.
3. Connolly H, Fetcho S, Hageman J: Education of personnel involved in the transport program. Crit Care Clin 8:481, 1992.
4. Day S, McCloskey K, Orr R, et al: Pediatric interhospital critical care transport: Consensus of a national leadership conference. Pediatrics 88:696, 1991.
5. Dyer L: Training and development of the ICU nurse for critical care transport. Crit Care Nurs 9:71, 1989.

6. Frischer L, Gutterman D: Emotional impact on parents of transported babies: Considerations for meeting parents' needs. Crit Care Clin 8:649, 1992.
7. Lumpe D: Association of air medical services publishes new voluntary standards. JEMS 17:28, 1992.
8. Miles M, Carter M: Coping strategies used by parents during their child's hospitalization in an intensive care unit. Child Health Care 14:14, 1985.
9. Miles M, Carter M, Elberly T, et al: Toward an understanding of parent stress in the pediatric intensive care unit: Overview of the program of research. MCN 18:181, 1989.
10. Moore A: Crisis intervention: A care plan for families of hospitalized children. Pediatr Nurs 15:234, 1989.
11. Pon S, Notterman D: The organization of a pediatric critical care transport program. Pediatr Clin North Am 40:241, 1993.
12. Reynolds M, Thomsen C, Black L, et al: The nuts and bolts of organizing and initiating a pediatric transport team. The Sutter Memorial experience. Crit Care Clin 8:465, 1992.
13. Rothstein P: Psychological stress in families of children in a pediatric intensive care unit. Pediatr Clin North Am 27:613, 1980.
14. Steenson M, Erdman T: A comprehensive QA structured transport system: A qualitative and quantitative approach to improving patient care. J Nurs Qual Assur 3:64, 1989.
15. Venkataraman S, Rubenstein J, Orr R: Interhospital transport: A pediatric perspective. Crit Care Clin 8:515, 1992.
16. Wolterman M, Miller M: Caring for parents in crisis. Nurs Forum 22:34, 1985.

CHAPTER 8

Pediatric Cardiology in Transport Medicine

ALEXANDER J. JAVOIS, M.D.

Heart disease in the pediatric transport patient can be classified into four categories:
1. Known cardiac defects
2. Unknown or suspected cyanotic defects
3. Arrhythmias
4. Shock

A brief description of endocarditis and empiric treatment for suspected cases is presented at the end of the chapter; this diagnosis is often suspected in febrile patients with known congenital heart disease. Tables are also provided for age-specific normal heart rates and blood pressures.

PATIENTS WITH KNOWN CARDIAC DEFECTS

The critically ill child with a known congenital heart defect can be classified as follows: totally repaired, palliated, or unrepaired. The assessment of an ill child with a known cardiac defect must consider the extent of repair in order to develop an appropriate differential diagnosis.

The details of pre- and postoperative considerations for each known defect will be presented. A general category of "Postoperative Complications" will address problems in patients who have undergone recent cardiac surgery (issues that arise usually within six to eight weeks after surgery); this topic will immediately follow the discussion of specific congenital heart defects.

Aortic Stenosis

Unrepaired

There may be poor cardiac output due to severe fixed obstruction. Chronically strained myocardium needs inotropic support.

Neonatal. Critical aortic stenosis (AS) in the neonate is a ductal-dependent lesion. When the ductus closes, systemic output is suddenly limited to flow across the stenotic valve and results in severe metabolic acidosis, which compounds heart failure. Clinically, left heart failure is evident: poor pulses, gallop rhythm, tachypnea, retractions, and rales. **Prostaglandin E_1** is indicated.

Childhood. Usually asymptomatic until the stenosis becomes critical, at which time there is a history of fatigability, exertional dyspnea, and possibly syncope. Severe left heart failure may result with poor pulses, gallop rhythm, tachypnea, and rales. **Inotropic support and diuresis** are indicated.

S/P Total Repair
The child may have significant restenosis and/or have developed severe aortic insufficiency (AI), which is synonymous with chronic volume overload. Signs and symtoms of left heart failure will be evident. Both severe AS and AI will respond to **inotropic support and diuresis.**

Atrial Septal Defect

Unrepaired
There is a pure volume overload on the right side of the heart and the lungs. Congestive heart failure (CHF) from simple (even large) secundum atrial septal defect (ASD) in infancy is uncommon; also consider bacterial pneumonia in the differential diagnosis of tachypnea. Large primum ASDs may cause CHF in infancy. Intravenous (IV) **diuresis and inotropic support** are indicated in CHF.

S/P Total Repair
Secundum ASD: rare atrial arrhythmia. Primum ASD: rare atrial arrhythmia. Also consider mitral regurgitation with secondary pulmonary edema (this is also rare and would likely occur many years postop).

AV Canal (Atrioventricular Canal or Endocardial Cushion Defect)
Absence of the lower portion of the atrial septum and the upper portion of the ventricular septum resulting in a large "hole" in the center of the heart. Mitral and tricuspid valves are also malformed.

Unrepaired
There is almost always excessive flow to the lungs. There is volume and pressure overload on the right ventricle and, to some extent, on the left ventricle. Congestive heart failure is common and may be seen early in infancy. **Diuresis and inotropic support** are indicated in CHF.

S/P Palliative Surgery
Pulmonary artery banding reduces the volume overload on the lungs. The "band" is a synthetic strip of material (much like a shoelace or umbilical tie) that is wrapped around the main pulmonary artery and tied down, narrowing the diameter of the vessel. The patient may "outgrow" the band, resulting in too little pulmonary blood flow and thus marked cyanosis (with no respiratory distress). This problem may be seen within weeks of surgery if the band was placed too tight. Oxygen won't help but won't hurt. If the band is too loose, it will not sufficiently restrict blood flow. Tachypnea with pulmonary edema on chest radiograph (CXR) are the clues. Diuresis and inotropic support are needed in this rare case.

S/P Total Repair
Residual ASD and/or ventricular septal defect (VSD) components of the original defect usually provide only small left-to-right shunts, which do not produce symptoms. An early problem (weeks to months) may be subaortic stenosis (related to complex mitral valve anatomy); there may be signs of left-sided CHF. If so, IV diuresis and inotropic support are necessary. Left-sided CHF may also be due to severe mitral regurgitation. This is typically a late postop problem (months to years). **Diuresis and inotropic support** are indicated.

Coarctation of Aorta

Unrepaired
Neonatal.   Severe coarctation of the aorta (COA) results in ductal-dependent blood flow to the abdominal viscera and lower extremities (LE). Spontaneous closure of the ductus arteriosus will result in reduced flow to the LE and viscera with sudden left heart failure developing; the neonate will appear "septic" secondary to low cardiac output and consequent severe metabolic acidosis. In this case, all pulses may be equally weak due to the poor output state. To promote reopening of the ductus, PGE_1 is indicated. Acidosis will depress myocardial funtion; **inotropic support** is indicated.

Childhood.   Coarctation of the aorta is generally asymptomatic and may progress gradually, resulting in weak or absent femoral pulses. Acidosis beyond the neonatal period is rare. Upper extremity hypertension is present but hypertensive crisis is not typical.

S/P Total Repair
Persistent hypertension (HTN) is uncommon in infants or children, reflecting recoarctation, which can gradually develop at any age. It is not uncommon in those for whom surgical repair was done late in childhood. Subaortic stenosis, not present at the time of surgery, may develop months or years later; if severe enough, left-sided CHF may develop. **Diuresis and inotropic support** may be indicated.

Hypoplastic Left Heart Syndrome
Marked underdevelopment of the left ventricle, due to severe mitral and/or aortic stenosis or atresia with negligible or absent forward blood flow into the ascending aorta; blood flow into the aorta is dependent on a widely patent ductus arteriosus (PDA)[7]

Unrepaired
As the PDA closes, systemic output is compromised and severe metabolic acidosis develops. Inotropes and PGE_1 are emergently indicated. Pulmonary edema, often present, responds to IV diuretics. Other measures are instituted to decrease pulmonary blood flow,[1] thereby increasing flow across the PDA to the aorta; these measures include intubation, hypoventilation, and no supplemental oxygen (or bleeding in nitrogen or carbon dioxide)[11] to keep $PaCO_2$ in the 50-55 mmHg range and oxygen saturation (O_2) in the 70s. Sedation and paralysis help minimize oxygen consumption and acidosis.

S/P Palliative Surgery
Stage I Norwood Procedure.   The end result is that the right ventricle becomes the systemic rather than the pulmonary pump. A new or "neo" aorta is created by enlarging the existing hypoplastic aorta with either synthetic material (gortex) or cryopreserved human tissue (aortic homograft) along with the main pulmonary artery. The right and left pulmonary arteries, which were separated from the main pulmonary artery, now receive blood flow through an aortic-to-pulmonary shunt (a gortex tube). Cyanosis is a sign that the shunt is not providing enough blood flow to the lungs; conversely, high O_2 saturations may indicate excessive pulmonary flow. In this situation oxygen will be of little help. Right ventricular (RV) dysfunction after the Norwood procedure is common and may result in arrhythmias and/or CHF; cardiac output may be preload-dependent and dehydration may compromise flow through the shunt. Weak pulses should be treated with **inotropes, and dehydration should be corrected.**

Glenn Shunt.   Approximately 6–12 months after the Stage I Norwood procedure, a Glenn shunt typically is placed. The superior vena cava (SVC) is transected and connected directly to the right pulmonary artery. The previous shunt is left in place. Patients may develop CHF due to progressive RV dysfunction.

S/P Total Repair
Fontan Procedure.   This results in all blue (systemic venous) blood entering directly into the pulmonary arteries, and all oxygenated (pulmonary venous) blood going to the systemic circulation. The typical surgery after the Glenn shunt involves attaching the superior portion of the right atrium (where the SVC used to come in) to the underside of the right pulmonary artery and partitioning the right atrium so that all inferior vena cava (IVC) blood flow is channeled directly into the pulmonary artery; the previously placed aortic-to-pulmonary-artery shunt is then ligated.

Dysfunction of the RV over time is common;[10] the architecture of the RV is not designed to pump against systemic vascular resistance. Inotropes and diuretics may be needed to treat CHF (poor pulses, tachypnea, pulmonary edema, peripheral edema). Arrhythmias may develop and are likely secondary to ventricular dysfunction and previous atrial surgery.

Patent Ductus Arteriosus

Unrepaired
Premature Infants.   Pulmonary vascular resistance (PVR) is low in newborn premature infants (intraacinar arteries develop relatively late in fetal life and continue to form even after birth of a term infant as the alveolar ducts and alveoli continue to develop);[9] a symptomatic, large left-to-right shunt may occur early. Oxygen promotes a drop in pulmonary vascular resistance, thereby further increasing left-to-right shunting and pulmonary overcirculation. Unnecessary FIO_2 should be avoided in cases of a known large PDA.

Term Infants.   In the first few days of life, when there is elevated PVR, there will be little increase in pulmonary blood flow. As PVR drops, left-to-right shunting increases. A large PDA in a neonate may cause respiratory distress and poor feeding.

All Ages.   With any turbulent blood flow the risk for endocarditis increases. Small PDAs often seen in older children can produce high velocity flow into the pulmonary artery; bacteremia may lead to endothelial colonization where the turbulent jet strikes the lumen of the pulmonary artery. A PDA is the most commonly associated lesion in children with endocarditis. See endocarditis discussion at end of chapter.

S/P Total Repair
Generally, this is an uncomplicated procedure with an unremarkable postop course unless the surgeon inadvertently ligates the left pulmonary artery instead of the ductus; in this rare case, a left-to-right shunt persists into the right pulmonary artery with no flow into the left pulmonary artery. Within months, potentially irreversible changes to the pulmonary vascular bed of the right lung may cause pulmonary hypertension and reversal of shunt at the ductal level.

Pulmonary Stenosis

Unrepaired
Neonatal critical pulmonary stenosis is a ductal-dependent lesion if there is little forward flow across the valve. These patients require a PGE_1 infusion. Cyanosis is due to atrial right-to-left shunting. Ventricular dysfunction may require inotropic support.

Progressive pulmonary stenosis in older children can lead to RV failure; the most common symptoms are dyspnea and fatigue. Cyanosis is uncommon; when present it is usually due to right-to-left shunt across an ASD. Symptomatic children require **inotropic support and diuresis.** Endocarditis should be considered in febrile patients.

S/P Total Repair

Relief of stenosis through surgery or cardiac catheterization (balloon valvuloplasty) can relieve some or all of the obstruction but the dysplastic valve tissue always will create turbulent flow into the pulmonary artery, posing a risk for endocarditis. Febrile patients after relief of obstruction should have blood cultured and IV antibiotics started prior to or during transport.

Transposition of the Great Arteries

Transposition of the great arteries (TGA) is the most common cyanotic congenital heart defect. In this condition, the parallel blood circuits preferentially keep deoxygenated blood in the systemic circulation. Survival depends on adequate mixing at the atrial and ductal levels. The diagnosis may be suspected if a differential cyanosis is present: *blue upper extremities and pink lower extremities.* In TGA the differential cyanosis occurs because the RV pumps red blood into the main pulmonary artery with resultant flow across a patent ductus into the descending aorta (legs). Marked diffuse cyanosis is compatible with poor mixing at the ductal or atrial levels.

Unrepaired

Progressive cyanosis is common, and there is little response to 100% oxygen. The patient will require PGE_1 to improve upon atrial mixing. Older neonates, however, may not respond to PGE_1. Atrial septostomy may be urgently required to produce adequate mixing. Congestive heart failure with pulmonary overcirculation is more common when there is an associated VSD. Inotropic support and diuresis are often needed in critically ill neonates.

S/P Palliative Surgery

Palliative surgery is rarely performed today. However, many older patients have undergone atrial baffle procedures (Mustard and Senning procedures) when they were infants. This surgery does not correct the transposition anatomy but merely redirects the systemic and pulmonary venous return into the appropriate circulation. A "baffle," or partitioning, of the atria is created such that pulmonary venous return is directed toward the tricuspid valve (thus to the RV, aorta, and systemic circulation), and systemic venous return is directed toward the mitral valve (thus to the LV, main pulmonary artery, and pulmonary circulation). The PDA is ligated. The end result is "normal," or physiologic, circulation with no mixing of blood at any level. With time (years), the RV begins to fail because it is pumping against systemic vascular resistance (which it was never designed to do). Typically the right-sided failure is slow to develop, and there is a history of progressive fatigue, exercise intolerance, and exertional dyspnea. Diuretics and inotropic support are inicated in symptomatic patients. Ventricular arrhythmias from RV failure also may develop.

S/P Total Repair

The arterial switch is the state-of-the-art repair. Potential problems after the switch include:

1. Twisting of reimplanted coronary arteries with resultant ischemia and/or infarction, dysfunction, and arrhythmia. Inotropic support should be used

cautiously so as not to aggravate potential arrhythmias and increase myocardial oxygen demand (in a state of impaired coronary perfusion/oxygen delivery).

2. Supravalvar pulmonary stenosis.

3. Progressive aortic insufficiency.

The stenosis and insufficiency develop slowly over months to years but may progress. Severe AI may cause CHF and require anticongestive therapy.

Truncus Arteriosus

Truncus arteriosus (TA) results from a developmental arrest in which the common great artery, the TA, fails to divide into separate great arteries. This "trunk" sits atop both ventricles; there is a large VSD.

Unrepaired

Neonatal CHF is common because the pulmonary arteries, which come off the common "trunk," are exposed to systemic pressure and therefore have unrestricted flow (a hugh left-to-right shunt). Severe cyanosis is uncommon because of this large pulmonary blood flow. Progressive CHF (tachypnea, rales, and poor feeding) develops within weeks after birth as pulmonary vascular resistance drops and pulmonary flow increases. Congestive heart failure should be treated with IV **inotropes and diuretics.**

S/P Palliative Surgery

Pulmonary artery banding is, on very rare occasions, done to control the excessive pulmonary flow. See discussion of possible complications under "Atrioventricular Canal."

S/P Total Repair

Total repair involves using a valved conduit that attaches the right ventricle to the pulmonary arteries; the VSD is also closed. Problems include the following:

Conduit stenosis. This may occur since the conduit is not living tissue; it is chemically treated and freeze treated and therefore does not grow with the child. Stenosis develops over time and, if undetected, can result in severe right heart failure. The valve within the conduit may also become stenotic and calcified, and become incompetent. If significant insufficiency is present, it may hasten the onset of CHF.

Truncal insufficiency or stenosis. The native valve of the truncus is left in the aortic position. This is a congenitally abnormal valve (often quadricuspid) and is susceptible to progressive insufficiency, but stenosis may also occur. Either of these problems may lead to left-sided CHF.

Tetralogy of Fallot

Tetralogy of Fallot (TOF) consists of:

1. ventricular septal defect (VSD);

2. malposition of the aorta such that it sits on top of (overrides) the VSD;

3. pulmonary stenosis: a combination of single or multilevel obstruction situated below, at, or above the valve;

4. right ventricular hypertrophy (RVH), which is secondary to the pressure and volume overload from the VSD and stenosis.

Pentalogy of Fallot includes a fifth defect, an atrial septal defect (seen in about 15% of TOF).

Unrepaired

Pink Tetralogy. This is common in the neonatal period and represents the physiology of a large VSD with minimal or mild obstruction to right ventricular outflow. With time, as the infundibular muscle bundles hypertrophy, the obstruction to RV outflow progresses (see discussion of "Tet Spells" below). Initially there is little right-to-left shunting across the VSD, since blood follows the path of least resistance (to the pulmonary vascular bed). Thus, the patient may be referred to as a "pink tet" and may present with CHF from pulmonary overcirculation. **Fluid restriction and diuresis** are indicated. Inotropic support must be used with caution, since it may accentuate the outflow obstruction by inducing spasm of the infundibular (subpulmonary) muscle.

Cyanotic TOF with or without "Tet Spells." The systolic murmur in a patient with TOF is chiefly due to right ventricular outlet obstruction, typically from subpulmonary muscle bundles. These bundles become more obstructive with time (weeks to months), and right-to-left shunting across the VSD develops and increases; this is why a patient with TOF may be initially pink as a newborn but become progressively cyanotic. Sudden severe cyanosis or "tet spells" are due to spasm or contraction of the hypertrophied and obstructive subpulmonary muscles, resulting in a sudden drop in pulmonary flow and marked increase in right-to-left shunting across the VSD. The systolic murmur will be much softer and may even disappear during a "tet spell" because there is little flow across the narrowed RV outflow tract and therefore little turbulence (which is what creates the murmur).

Treatment of "Tet Spells." Treatment is designed to (1) reduce the spasm and (2) increase systemic vascular resistance (SVR), thereby shifting the path of least resistance toward the pulmonary bed. Infants can be physically manipulated into the **knee-chest** position to simulate the squatting position, which increases systemic resistance. Pharmacologic intervention includes (A) **morphine**, 0.2 mg/kg/dose subcutaneous or IM to reduce the spasm (or the noxious stimuli that is provoking the spasm—i.e., agitation, pain, or crying); (B) **phenylephrine**, 0.1–0.5 mg/kg/min for systemic vasoconstriction. **Volume**, a bolus of IV fluids (10 ml/kg, which may be repeated once), will also increase systemic pressure. The benefits from **oxygen** are limited by the fixed obstruction to pulmonary flow. Always consider endocarditis in a febrile patient with TOF. Patients may be on oral **propranolol** prior to repair; this is given to prevent spasms. Propranolol IV, for acute treatment of spasm, has been used but is very dangerous as it may induce life-threatening hypotension.

S/P Palliative Surgery

Severe obstruction to pulmonary blood flow in utero may result in hypoplastic main and branch pulmonary arteries. Before total repair can be performed in such cases, growth of the pulmonary arteries is stimulated by increasing blood flow into the arteries from a systemic-to-pulmonary-artery shunt. Two commonly used shunts are (1) a modified Blalock-Taussig shunt, which is a gortex tube extending from the subclavian to the pulmonary artery, and (2) a central shunt, which is a gortex tube from the ascending aorta to the main or a branch pulmonary artery.

A shunt may be too large, thereby causing pulmonary overcirculation, tachypnea, and rales; too small, thereby limiting pulmonary flow and resulting in persistent cyanosis; or clotted, thereby causing severe cyanosis. Only overcirculation can be medically treated (with diuresis). All three problems with a systemic-to-pulmonary-artery shunt may require urgent surgical correction.

S/P Total Repair

Outcome after total repair of TOF usually depends on the type and severity of the inital RV outflow obstruction. Residual stenoses may be present (subvalvar, valvar, or supravalvar). Progressive pulmonary insufficiency along with stenosis may occur, resulting in RV failure (fatigue, peripheral edema, etc.). Diuresis and inotropic support are indicated. The surgical relief[1] of the subpulmonary obstruction involves resection of RV muscle and occasionally a transmural incision with placement of a synthetic patch to enlarge the RV outflow tract. These procedures result in scar tissue formation within the RV myocardium that can be a focus for later ventricular ectopy. Stenosis and insufficiency may strain the RV and may induce ventricular tachycardia. Frequent single premature ventricular contractions (PVCs) or couplets do not require treatment, but runs of PVCs in the presence of heart failure should be treated **lidocaine:** loading dose 1 mg/kg over 10 minutes, maintenance infusion of 20–50 mg/kg/min.

Anomalous Pulmonary Venous Return (APVR)

Unrepaired

The clinical findings depend on the number of anomalous connections, their location, and whether stenosis is present at the connection.

Partial APVR. If only a single vein is involved and there is no venous obstruction, there are typically no symptoms in childhood. Multiple anomalous veins present a significant volume load to the RV and pulmonary bed (similar to the physiology of an ASD). Cyanosis is uncommon but fatigue and dyspnea may occur in adulthood. Frequent respiratory infections are particularly associated with complete right-sided APVR to the inferior vena cava as there are associated parenchymal changes to the entire right lung (small right hemithorax may be seen on CXR). Pulmonary venous stenosis is typically seen with subdiaphragmatic connections and present in the neonatal period; there is associated pulmonary edema with respiratory distress.

Total APVR. The degree of cyanosis depends upon the pulmonary vascular resistance and the amount of pulmonary blood flow. Initial cyanosis at birth may disappear as PVR drops and pulmonary blood flow increases. The typical infant with TAPVR has three to four times more pulmonary than systemic blood flow. Because of this, cyanosis may only be minimal, and the systemic O_2 saturations are in the upper 80s or even 90%. Right-sided heart failure from pulmonary overcirculation in most infants occurs before 6 months of age. Inotropic support and diuresis are needed in the acute presentation.

Obstruction with TAPVR (at either the venous connection or the interatrial communication—i.e., small/restrictive patent foramen ovale or ASD) presents clinical symptoms in the first days of life and requires urgent surgical intervention. **Avoid** volume-overloading these patients since this will increase pulmonary edema. Do not expect improvement in oxygen saturations with initiation of PGE_1; typically there is equalization of saturations in all four chambers of the heart and therefore great arteries. The clinical status may improve with PGE_1 in a baby with restricted atrial communication (blood that cannot get to the left side of the heart through a small ASD/PFO can reach systemic circulation across the PDA into the aorta).

S/P Total Repair

Direct anastomosis of a pulmonary vein to the left atrium can result in stenosis and obstruction of pulmonary venous return. Chest radiograph will reveal segmental pulmonary congestion. Treatment is primarily surgical, but, if there is extensive obstruction and pulmonary edema, fluid restriction is indicated. Multiple pulmonary veins may also become obstructed at their entrance into the left atrium, hours to days or weeks after surgery. Clinically the patient will present with severe respiratory distress and diffuse pulmonary edema (even "white-out") on CXR.

Ventricular Septal Defect

Unrepaired

Neonatal.   Moderate or even large defects may be asymptomatic in the first few weeks of life because of elevated PVR. There is a significant rise in pulmonary blood flow as PVR drops and symptoms of pulmonary overcirculation develop: poor feeding, poor weight gain, tachypnea, retractions, lethargy. Acutely ill neonates require inotropic support and diuresis. Patients should be NPO with mild fluid restriction (80–100 ml/kg/day) until heart failure is controlled. Severe failure requiring intubation may respond to systemic afterload reduction; as resistance to blood flow drops, more blood flows across the aortic valve into systemic circulation and less across the VSD into the pulmonary bed. **Amrinone**, 5–15 mg/kg/min, can be used as both an inotropic agent and a systemic vasodilator.

Infant or Child.   An infant with a very large unrestricted VSD will present with CHF early in life. If the VSD is of moderate size, CHF may present later in infancy. Poor growth may be the chronic sign of CHF, with more acute signs consisting of poor feeding, tachypnea, and perhaps lethargy. Physical findings include tachycardia, tachypnea, hyperdynamic precordium, holosystolic murmur, and likely an apical diastolic rumble. Cardiomegaly and increased pulmonary vascular markings will be seen on CXR. The electrocardiogram (EKG) usually reveals biventricular hypertrophy. In the older child with VSD, RVH is an ominous sign of severe pulmonary hypertension from long-standing left-to-right shunt. The pulmonary hypertension may result in cyanosis owing to right-to-left shunting across the VSD. **Initial treatment** is with **IV diuresis** and **inotropic support.** The patient should be kept **NPO** in the initial treatment of CHF. Oxygen desaturation is unlikely in the young child since the problem is excessive pulmonary blood flow. However, if pulmonary edema or other lung disease is present, there will be impaired gas exchange at the alveolar level.

Oxygen therapy in the tachypneic child with a VSD may aggravate CHF by dropping pulmonary vascular resistance, thereby further increasing the left-to-right shunt/pulmonary overcirculation. **Fluid restriction** should also be used in the acute management of the normovolemic child in CHF (i.e., two-thirds maintenance).

S/P Palliative Surgery

Palliation of the large VSD is reserved for preterm infants who cannot tolerate open heart surgery or for children with other more serious associated cardiac defects that demand earlier surgical correction and the VSD repair left for later. The palliative procedure is pulmonary artery banding, which restricts pulmonary blood flow. See discussion of banding under "Atrioventricular Canal."

S/P Total Repair

Total repair of VSD involves the placement of a synthetic patch, usually gortex, on the right ventricular surface of the septum. The previous surgical approach consisted of right ventriculotomy, which usually leaves extensive scar tissue in the RV and may become a source for ventricular ectopy. Right bundle branch block is a common sequela from this ventriculotomy. Complaints of palpitations, chest pain, presyncope, or syncope, with evidence for frequent PVCs or ventricular tachycardia, should prompt consideration for IV lidocaine. Current surgical approach[3] is through a right atrial incision; the tricuspid valve is pushed open and the gortex patch is sutured in place, occluding the VSD. Ventricular tachycardia is rare and RBBB is far less common from this atrial approach. It typically takes 6–12 months for the gortex to completely endothelialize; before this, there is the risk for seeding the gortex if bacteremia is present.

Febrile, ill-appearing children who are less than one year postop VSD repair should be placed on treatment for endocarditis after blood cultures are obtained (preferably from two separate sites).

EVALUATION OF THE CYANOTIC NEWBORN

A frequent reason for referring a newborn to a tertiary care nursery is for management and evaluation of systemic arterial desaturation with or without respiratory distress. The diagnostic dilemma typically addresses the question, "Is the baby's cyanosis due to pulmonary or cardiac pathology?" This issue is often complicated by the consideration that the cyanosis may be due to a combination of both respiratory and cardiovascular problems.[18] The distinction can often be made by obtaining a detailed perinatal and postnatal history as well a thorough physical exam. Specific lab data can confirm one's suspicion and help conclude whether or not an echocardiogram is ultimately needed.

Recognition of cyanosis in the newborn is not solely dependent upon the experience and skill of the observer. Multiple factors play a role in the detection of cyanosis. The physiologic basis for cyanosis does not depend on the level of desaturation of hemoglobin but rather on the absolute concentration of deoxygenated hemoglobin. Cyanosis is apparent when there is 3 gm of reduced (deoxygenated) hemoglobin per deciliter of blood. Therefore, the oxygen saturation, when cyanosis becomes evident, also depends on the hemoglobin concentration. An anemic newborn with a hemoglobin concentration of 8 gm/dl will appear cyanotic only when the oxygen saturation drops toward 62% (= [8-3]/8), whereas a polycythemic newborn with a hemoglobin of 23 gm/dl will demonstrate cyanosis when the saturation drops to only 87% (= [23-3]/23).

The principal clinical concern regarding cyanosis is not the degree of cyanosis (which we demonstrated is dependent on hemoglobin concentration) or level of desaturation but the actual oxygen content of the blood. If the oxygen content is low, the metabolic demands of the tissues may not be met.

Acrocyanosis or peripheral cyanosis of the hands and feet is common in the neonate. Acrocyanosis is true cyanosis in that there are 3 or more gm/dl of unoxygenated hemoglobin, but this cyanosis is related to the sensitive, vasoreactive beds in the periphery. Cold environment or cold skin temperature results in clamped down vasculature with resultant sluggish blood flow and higher extraction of oxygen from each gram of hemoglobin. Often the exact cause of acrocyanosis in the newborn is not readily obvious. The clinical importance is to distinguish this from central cyanosis which involves the mucous membranes.

The following categories address issues that should raise suspicion that a child's central cyanosis is cardiac in etiology rather than respiratory.

History

The transport team should quickly assess the family history for congenital heart defects, birth defects, syndromes, and early infant deaths. The perinatal history should be assessed for exposure to rubella or coxsackie, radiation exposure, diabetes, or any general concerns of the obstetrician. Birth history should include noting the method of delivery (C-sections are more prone to transient tachypnea), maternal infection risk factors (temperature or prolonged rupture), and Apgar scores (evidence for asphyxia). Neonatal history should include the timing of the onset of respiratory distress or cyanosis, a description of the general appearance of the child and how it changed over time (onset of symptoms may not be related to simply the development of sepsis but may be related to spontaneous closure of the ductus arteriosus in lesions where systemic circulation depends on its patency).

Physical Examination

General. Is the child vigorous or lethargic and nonresponsive? Is cyanosis central or peripheral? Is the cyanosis differential? Cyanotic lower extremities and pink upper extremities are consistent with a right-to-left ductal shunt compatible with either severe pulmonary hypertension from lung disease or persistent fetal circulation (high pulmonary vascular resistance), or from critical juxtaductal coarctation of the aorta in which descending aortic flow depends upon ductal patency. Blue upper extremities with pink lower extremities is highly suggestive of pulmonary hypertension and congential heart disease. This type of differential cyanosis is most commonly associated with TGA and pulmonary hypertension (deoxygenated blood from RV to ascending aorta to head and arms; oxygenated blood from LV to main pulmonary artery through a PDA to descending aorta, to legs). Pre- and postductal oxygen saturations may help determine if mild differential cyanosis is present.

Pulmonary. It is important to critically assess the breathing pattern of the infant. Pulmonary disease generally will result in an increased work of breathing; this may include to varying degrees nasal flaring, retractions, and grunting. Persistent tachypnea is more common in respiratory disease but may also be seen in congenital heart disease. More common in cardiac disease, however, is hyperpnea or increased tidal volume. Stridor, most commonly associated with tracheomalacia, can be consistent with a vascular ring.

Pulses. Four extremity pulses should be routinely palpated. Weakened pulses in all four extremities should prompt palpation of neck pulses. Equally weak pulses everywhere may be consistent with critical aortic stenosis as well as sepsis. Decreased pedal or femoral pulses should raise the suspicion for coarctation of the aorta. Differential pulses between the upper extremities is also suggestive of coarctation (right arm pulse usually greater than left arm pulse unless the right subclavian has an anomalous origin from the descending aorta; in this case neck pulses will be stronger than those of all four extremities, which may be equally weak).

Heart Rate. Normal range for the newborn is between 70 and 180. Greater than 230 is highly suggestive of supraventricular tachycardia, which is more commonly seen in Ebstein's anomaly (downward displacement of the tricuspid valve with a right-to-left atrial shunt) than any other congenital heart defect.

Cardiac. Palpation of a thrill in the newborn is most commonly associated with significant semilunar valve stenosis (AS and PS). Prominent ventricular impluse is typically associated with lesions that result in pulmonary overcirculation. Auscultation of heart tones includes characterization of:

1. S1 and S2: loud and snappy S2 is consistent with pulmonary hypertension; single S2 is consistent with a single semilunar valve (pulmonary atresia, aortic atresia, truncus arteriosus); widely split S2 is consistent with an ASD.

2. Presence of S3 or S4 (gallop rhythm) may be consistent with Ebstein's anomaly; in patients with cardiogenic shock these are associated with poor ventricular compliance; an isolated S3, unless unusually loud, may be a normal finding.

3. Very loud, harsh systolic ejection murmurs in the newborn are associated with severe or critical semilunar valve stenosis; critical pulmonary stenosis (PS) is more likely to be associated with cyanosis due to significant right-to-left atrial shunt; critical AS may also present with cyanosis from right-to-left ductal flow

and will develop poor pulses and metabolic acidosis as the ductus closes. Both lesions are ductal dependent.

Decompensation in a neonate who was described to previously have a loud murmur (possible critical AS or PS) demands immediate infusion of PGE_1(as the ductus closes and cardiac function deteriorates, the murmur may get much softer owing to diminished cardiac output).

4. "Normal" exam with no murmur but perhaps the suggestion of a single S2 in light of marked cyanosis is consistent with TGA.

5. Loud systolic murmur which was not present at birth but which got progressively louder may be consistent with a VSD (as pulmonary vascular resistance drops over the first days of life, the RV pressures will fall, resulting in a greater pressure difference between left and right ventricles and therefore greater turbulent flow).

Laboratory Evaluations

Chest X-ray. Findings suggestive of cardiac disease include:
1. Cyanosis with clear lung fields;
2. Cardiomegaly; objective data include a cardiothoracic ratio > 0.55;
3. Prominent or diminished pulmonary vascular markings;
4. Isolated levocardia (apex of heart to left with stomach bubble on right and liver on left) is believed to have nearly a 100% association with complex congential heart defects.

Electrocardiogram. Is often unrewarding as a single diagnostic tool. Highly associated findings include LVH and left axis deviation in tricuspid atresia; RVH and left axis deviation with endocardial cushion defects (AV canal defects).

CBC. To rule out anemia, polycythemia, and leukocytosis.

Serum Glucose and Electrolytes. Hypoglycemia may be a cause of cyanosis. Chronic hypoglycemia may be associated with cardiomegaly, myocardial dysfunction, and right-to-left atrial shunting. An IV infusion of glucose provides a rapid clinical response. A rare cause of hypotension and cyanosis is adrenal failure; hyperkalemia and hyponatremia are seen. Hypocalcemia is associated with DiGeorge syndrome (conotruncal abnormalities such as truncus arteriosus, tetralogy of Fallot, and aortic arch anomalies).

Hyperoxia Test. This test is used to help discern the etiology of hypoxemia which is defined as an arterial partial pressure of oxygen (PaO_2) < 60 mmHg. The initial determination of PaO_2 is done on room air; then FiO_2 is increased to 1.0 for at least 5–10 minutes. A second arterial blood gas is obtained. The results can be divided into four general categories[14]: alveolar hypoventilation, ventilation-perfusion mismatch, and right-to-left shunting, which may be subdivided into the fourth category of likely cyanotic heart disease if there is little evidence for pulmonary disease (Table 1).

TABLE 1. Hyperoxia Test for Cyanotic Congenital Heart Disease

	PaO_2 $FIO_2 = .21$	$PaCO_2$ $FIO_2 = .21$	PaO_2 $FIO_2 = 1.0$
Alveolar hypoventilation	< 60	> 50	> 300
V-Q mismatch	< 60	35–45	> 300
R-L shunting	< 60	35–45	< 200
Likely cardiac	< 60	35–45	< 50

There are several caveats to this guideline:

Persistent fetal circulation.   Clinically, PFC may manifest features of all the categories; marked elevation of pulmonary vascular resistance (idiopathic, secondary to surfactant deficiency, or diffuse parenchymal disease from sepsis or aspiration) may lead to marked elevation of RV and RA pressures with right-to-left shunting at both the atrial and ductal levels.

Total anomalous pulmonary venous return.   TAPVR associated with significant increase in pulmonary blood flow and therefore may show a modest response to the hyperoxia test. In general, however, PaO_2 is in the range of 75–200 mmHg.

Methemoglobinemia.   The diagnosis is suspected by the general appearance of a lavender or gray-slate blue color to the patient.

Intervention in Suspected Cyanotic Congenital Heart Disease

Useful guidelines for defining when intervention[14]is indicated in cyanotic newborns include:

- pH $<$ 7.32 or $PaCO_2$ $>$ 42 or PaO_2 $<$ 60 on FiO_2 = 0.21. Repeat ABG in 15 to 60 minutes to determine if child is improving or deteriorating. Consider hyperoxia test.
- pH $<$ 7.28 or $PaCo_2$ $>$ 50 or PaO_2 $<$ 50 on FiO_2 = 0.5. Intervention is indicated, increase FiO_2, endotracheal intubation and assisted ventilation or PGE_1.
- pH $<$ 7.25 or $PaCO_2$ $>$ 60 or PaO_2 $<$ 40 on FiO_2 = 1.0. Immediate intervention indicated.

Prostaglandin E_1: PGE_1 should be used when there is a high index of suspicion for congenital heart disease with obligatory ductal flow. The infusion is typically begun at 0.1 $\mu g/kg/min$. Lesions with ductal-dependent systemic blood flow include: (1) hypoplastic left heart syndrome, (2) critical aortic valve stenosis, (3) severe juxtaductal coarctation of the aorta, and (4) interrupted aortic arch.

The common lesions with ductal dependent pulmonary blood flow are those with obstruction to right heart outflow: (1) tricuspid atresia with intact ventricular septum, (2) pulmonary atresia with intact ventricular septum, (3) critical pulmonary valve stenosis.

Even though TGA is a ductal-dependent cardiac lesion and PGE_1 is indicated, the response is variable depending upon the status of the pulmonary vascular resistance (PVR); high PVR (pulmonary hypertension) will result in oxygenated blood entering systemic circulation (but primarily to the lower extremities). As the infant ages from day to day, however, PVR will begin to fall and there may be less shunting of oxygenated blood into systemic circulation by way of the ductal pulmonary-aortic shunting. On the other hand, reversal of the ductal shunt (aorto-pulmonary shunting) results in greater pulmonary flow and left atrial distention, with consequent greater LA-RA shunting. Severely cyanotic infants with TGA (PaO_2 $<$ 30, saturations $<$ 70) with a patent ductus arteriosus on PGE_1 need urgent cardiac catheterization for atrial balloon septostomy; mixing of blood is much more efficient at the atrial level and also results in higher oxygenated blood reaching the brain.

There are a number of complications associated with PGE_1 infusion (Table 2). All infants on PGE_1 should be intubated for transport to avoid apneic episodes and perhaps further (life-threatening) desaturation. An intubated infant may also be appropriately sedated for transport, thereby reducing demand for oxygen delivery in a system that may already be stressed by hypoxemia. Other maneuvers to reduce metabolic demands include providing a neutral thermal environment.

Preparation for Transport.   (Which can be arranged by phone prior to arrival of transport team).

TABLE 2.   Complications Associated with PGE_1

Apnea, seen in approximately 10% of patients
Systemic hypotension
Inhibition of platelet aggregation
Fever
Mottling or hyperemia of skin

1. Maximize oxygen carrying capacity by adjusting hematocrit above 40%. **Blood transfusions** in cases of suspected congenital heart disease whether **cyanotic or acyanotic** should be done with **CMV negative and irradiated** washed packed RBCs. DiGeorge syndrome is associated with conotruncal anomalies and carries with it the risk of immunodeficiency due to partial or complete underdevelopment of the thymus; lesions particularly associated with DiGeorge syndrome include truncus arteriosus, Tetralogy of Fallot, and interrupted aortic arch. Also, in patients with hypoplastic left heart syndrome, the surgical intervention chosen by some families is cardiac transplantation. Even in those families who do not initially choose transplantation, it may be later indicated if the outcome from the first stage Norwood operation is poor. Irradiated, CMV-negative blood reduces the posttransplant risk of host-versus-graft rejection (from transfused WBCs) and overwhelming CMV infection associated with immunosuppression.

2. Provide a neutral thermal environment. Use head covering (greatest source of heat loss) and swaddling, and an isolette with a radiant heat source is indicated. Prevention of heat loss also limits metabolic demands and oxygen consumption.

3. Appropriate IV access and fluids. Particularly if PGE_1 is being infused, more than one IV site may be indicated. Always mix your own PGE_1; you are likely more accustomed to using PGE_1 than the referring hospital. Depending upon the age of the child and presence of congestive heart failure, dextrose-containing fluids may be infused at 80–100 ml/kg/day.

4. Assess recent CXR for endotracheal tube position before transport. Make sure ETT is secure. Suction ETT before leaving.

5. Check ABG before leaving to make sure oxygenation and ventilation are adequate. Be aware of even mild metabolic acidosis as it may be a sign of ductal closure particularly in lesions with ductal-dependent systemic flow.

6. Ventilator parameters: Avoid supraphysiologic PEEP in cyanotic congenital heart defects; in these cases there is typically decreased pulmonary blood flow and PEEP may further reduce pulmonary circulation, resulting in a further decrease in systemic saturation. However, in lesions with ductal-dependent systemic blood flow an increase in PEEP to 8–10 cm H_2O will enhance flow from the pulmonary artery into systemic circulation.

Postoperative Complications[5,12]

Postpericardiotomy Syndrome. This is a febrile illness which has its onset as early as 1 week after surgery in which the pericardium has been opened; onset may be delayed until two or more weeks after surgery. The syndrome is characterized by a pericardial and pleural reaction with effusion. Occasionally there is also pulmonary parenchymal involvement. Etiology is unclear but autoantibodies have been implicated in the pathogenesis. Along with fever, there are other signs of inflammation; elevation of sedimentation rate and leukocytosis may be seen.

The clinically important manifestation of the postpericardiotomy syndrome is the potential for tamponade from a large pericardial effusion. A child with this entity may have chest pain that develops after resolution of the usual postoperative pain. Pain may radiate to the left shoulder and worsen with inspiration or supine position. The pain becomes less intense as the pericardial fluid increases, separating the pericardial surfaces. Signs of pericarditis may be seen on EKG (ST segment elevation and/or T wave changes/inversion). With a very large effusion, there may be diffuse low voltage QRS complexes. Chest x-ray will show cardiomegaly with significant pericardial effusion; cardiomegaly should not always be assumed to be congestive heart failure, as treatment modalities are quite different. Echocardiography can quickly determine the presence of significant pericardial effusion. Pleural effusions may also be seen on CXR.

Pericardial effusion that is causing hemodynamic compromise (tamponade) should be urgently treated with pericardiocentesis. Signs of compromise include distended jugular veins, tachycardia, weak pulses with narrow pulse pressure (progressive drop in systolic BP with rise in diastolic BP), paradoxical pulse (profoundly weak pulses during inspiration and stronger pulses during expiration), pallor, tachypnea, muffled heart tones, irritability, or listlessness in the infant.

In a febrile postoperative patient, endocarditis should also be considered in the differential diagnosis. Blood cultures should be drawn and antibiotics started prior to transport.

Postoperative Anemia. This is associated with mechanical trauma to red blood cells from perfusion through the tubing and membrane oxygenator of the heart-lung bypass machine. The intravascular life span of transfused blood and blood traumatized by the bypass machine is shortened. Falling hematocrit may be seen for seven to ten days postop. Significant anemia beyond this period may be related to an intravascular mechanical hemolytic anemia; in this case, blood is traumatized or even fragmented as it is forced through a tiny hole usually within or at the edge of a synthetic patch. This may be associated with profound anemia requiring transfusion.

Postperfusion Syndrome. Typically occurs 4–6 weeks after surgery which utilizes extracorporeal (heart-lung bypass) circulation. There is usually fever, splenomegaly, and atypical lymphocytes. There may also be hepatomegaly, lymphadenopathy, and nonspecific rash. Clinically there is no hemodynamic significance to this syndrome; it needs to be differentiated from endocarditis and postpericardiotomy syndrome, which have specific treatments and sequelae. Etiology may be viral or autoimmune related.

SHOCK

Shock is a condition in which there is inadequate perfusion of vital organs. The etiology can be quite specific (i.e., cardiogenic, hemorrhagic, septic, anaphylactic, or neurogenic) but may be unknown to the transport team who is assessing the patient for the first time. Physical findings rather than laboratory data are the most reliable and rapid way of diagnosing shock and following the efficacy of therapy.

Initially with moderately diminished cardiac output, there is tachycardia with maintenance of blood pressure due to peripheral vasoconstriction.[15] This results in cool extremities, poor capillary refill, and weakening of peripheral pulses; urine output will fall. With progression of shock, mesenteric hypoperfusion develops which results in underactive or absent bowel sounds and even distention. As cardiac output falls further, only central pulses may be felt (carotid, femoral, axillary). The hands and feet may be cyanotic from increased oxygen extraction from sluggish flow through peripheral beds. Hyperpnea and tachypnea develop as a compensatory mechanism to metabolic acidosis. Changes in mentation may develop; initially the child may be agitated or restless and then lethargic or obtunded. As shock progresses and compensatory mechanisms can no longer maintain vital perfusion; significant drop in blood pressure with narrowing of pulse pressure will be seen.

Initial treatment is directed at improving tissue perfusion. Intravascular access is essential; this may be accomplished by as large an intravenous catheter as possible or intraosseous access if necessary (avoid 24G catheters whenever possible, as this limits rapid infusion for resuscitation). Isotonic solutions (normal saline or Ringer's lactate) are likely the most available (and least expensive) fluids for the transport team. Initial resuscitation volume is 10–20 ml/kg by IV or IO push over 5–10 minutes. This dose is repeated until improved circulation (pulses and perfusion) is noted or signs of circulatory congestion are evident (jugular venous distention or pulmonary congestion). Once perfusion is reestablished, it may be necessary to continue to provide generous (2–3 times maintenance) IV fluids to compensate for ongoing losses (hemorrhagic or extracellular).

Oxygen should be administered even if there are normal saturations by pulse oximetry. Metabolic demand is increased particularly if there is fever or tachycardia. Supplemental oxygen may improve oxygen tissue delivery even if it is only by increasing the dissolved component. Oxygen should be used with caution in the neonate where ductal-dependent systemic blood flow may exist; serial exams that demonstrate deterioration with oxygen therapy should warrant discontinuation of oxygen. Prostaglandin therapy should be considered in all neonates with shock.

If tachycardia persists and significant augmentation of intravascular volume does not enhance perfusion, inotropic agents may be used to enhance the contractility of the myocardium. The specific choice must be tailored to the clinical situation. Each agent may enhance perfusion but agent-specific side effects should be monitored. Infusions should be started at low doses and slowly increased, observing for deleterious effects. Dobutamine, amrinone, and isoproterenol may cause systemic vasodilation and make underlying hypotension worse. Dopamine and epinephrine increase systemic vascular resistance, which may worsen myocardial dysfunction. Amrinone is particularly useful in cardiogenic shock as it enhances myocardial contractility with concomitant reduction in afterload.

Creation of an inotropic drip is most easily calculated by the "rule of six;" the drip is created by adding a specific number of milligrams of inotrope with 100 ml of an appropriate IV fluid. The number of milligrams of inotrope to add to 100 ml of IV fluid is calculated as follows:

$$6 \times \text{weight in kg} \times \text{drip dosage in } \mu g/kg/min \div \text{drip rate in ml/hr}$$

The most common inotropes, typical infusion dosage, and compatibilities are listed in Table 3.

Efforts should also be directed at reducing oxygen consumption/metabolic demands in the patient in shock. A thermoneutral environment should be

TABLE 3. Commonly Administered Inotropes in Critically Ill Infants and Children

Inotrope	Range of Infusion	Compatible IV Fluid for Preparation of Drip
Amrinone	5–20 μg/kg/min	Not compatible with dextrose
Dobutamine	5–20 μg/kg/min	D5W, D10W, NS
Dopamine	5–20 μg/kg/min	D5W, D10W, NS
Epinephrine	0.05–0.5 μg/kg/min	D5W, D10W, NS
Isoproterenol	0.05–0.5 μg/kg/min	D5W, D10W, NS

maintained; oxygen consumption is increased in febrile conditions as well as shivering and nonshivering thermogenesis. Oxygen consumption can also be decreased by controlling the work of breathing. Mechanical ventilation, although it will reduce the energy expended by the patient, carries risks; positive pressure ventilation can adversely affect venous return, particularly in the hypovolemic patient. Correcting anemia will increase oxygen-carrying capacity as well as reduce tachycardia and the oxygen demand of the myocardium.

MANAGEMENT OF ARRHYTHMIAS

The transport team should primarily be interested in managing arrhythmias that are causing or may potentially cause hemodynamic instability. The transport monitor must be equipped with a recording device to print rhythm strips. All arrhythmias should be recorded and saved for evaluation by a pediatric cardiologist. Continuous EKG strips should *always* be obtained during any attempts at terminating an arrhythmia—e.g., vagal maneuvers or infusions of antiarrhythmics such as adenosine (the onset and termination of arrhythmias give vital clues to the exact arrhythmia diagnosis and most successful form of management).

In general, lead II is most appropriate for single-lead monitoring because it gives an easily identifiable upright P wave during sinus rhythm. The placement of electrodes for lead II is easily remembered by associating the standard color codes of the electrodes as follows: **white** is right (arm), **black** is opposite white (therefore left arm), and **red** means "stop," so the red lead is placed on the left leg (which is the location of the brake pedal in a car). If tiny or nearly flat P waves are seen in this configuration of electrodes, try switching the left leg electrode to the right leg. A fourth lead, **green**, is placed on the right leg (remember that the right leg is used for the accelerator pedal in a car).

The common arrhythmias will be presented with EKG rhythm strips (as you will not have capability to obtain a 12-lead EKG). In all cases, the mentioned medical intervention is indicated if there is hemodynamic instability—that is, weak pulses, poor perfusion, hypotension, disorientation in older children, and chest pain as described by older children (the sensation of palpitation is not an indication in itself for intervention).

Wandering Atrial Pacemaker

Changing P wave morphology is caused by electrical impulses originating from different sites in the atria. It is a benign finding and not indicative of progressive sinoatrial or atrioventricular node block (Fig. 1).

Extrasystoles

Premature Atrial Contractions (PACs)

This is the most common form of ectopy in the newborn. In general, this is a benign arrhythmia. Sometimes it can be associated with supraventricular

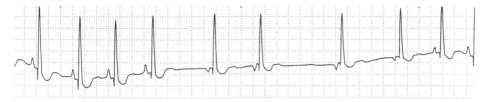

FIGURE 1

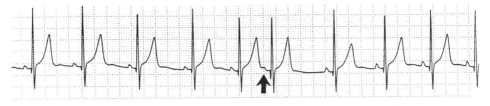

FIGURE 2

tachycardia (SVT), but PACs do not predispose to SVT unless there is an underlying anatomic substrate (e.g., an accessory bypass tract). The (PACs) may be as frequent as every other beat and still not cause hemodynamic compromise unless there are other cardiovascular problems. These PACs are usually identified as complexes that arise earlier than expected within the underlying sinus rhythm with a P wave morphology that is usually different from that of the sinus beats; most commonly the QRS morphology is identical in appearance to the normal sinus QRS morphology (Fig. 2).

However, if a PAC comes early enough, two different circumstances may arise: (1) The PAC may be aberrantly conducted, resulting in a wide QRS morphology (because the depolarization arrives at the bundle of HIS and ventricular myocardium when it is relatively refractory). This wide QRS is differentiated from a PVC by the presence of a P wave (often within the T wave (Fig 3). (2) If a PAC occurs when the HIS is absolutely refractory, there will be no conduction (no QRS). However, a pause in the normal sinus P-wave interval may be seen due to the PAC resetting (depolarizing) the sinus node. The small, broad arrows in Figure 4 demonstrate nonconducted PACs. The long, narrow arrow points out an aberrantly conducted PAC; note that it is not a wide QRS morphology as seen in Figure 3 but the morphology differs from the normal QRS morphology (Fig. 4).

The PACs may be seen in short runs but are not predictive of SVT. This does not warrant treatment (Fig 5).

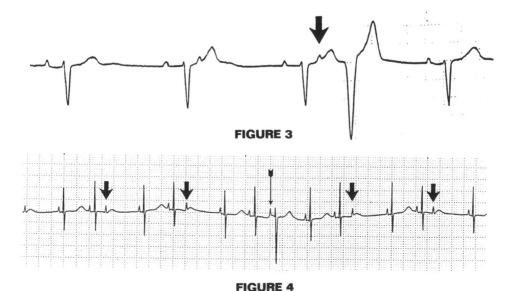

FIGURE 3

FIGURE 4

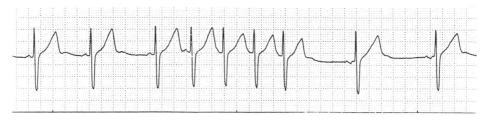

FIGURE 5

Premature Ventricular Complexes

A PVC can generally be differentiated from PACs or PACs with aberrant ventricular conduction because they not only are premature wide QRS complexes, but also are generally not preceded by P waves and are associated with ST-T wave morphologies that are also different from sinus/generated ST-T morphologies. PVCs were generally thought to produce a "fully compensatory pause," meaning the sum of the RR interval before the beat plus the RR interval after the beat is equal to the sum of two basic RR intervals. However, PACs can cause a fully compensatory pause and PVCs may cause less than a fully compensatory pause[8] (Fig. 6).

Isolated PVCs, like PACs may be as frequent as every other beat; this regular occurrence is called bigeminy. Bigeminy is not indicative of progressive ventricular arrhythmia or tachycardia (Fig. 7).

Every third systole as a PVC is referrred to as trigeminy (Fig. 8).

Two PVCs in a row are called a couplet. Couplets are usually not predictive of imminent ventricular tachycardia but warrrant further evaluation after transport (holter evaluation) (Fig. 9).

Bradyarrhythmias

The most common etiology for bradycardia in infants, particularly neonates, is hypoxemia. The upper airway should be quickly assessed for obstruction

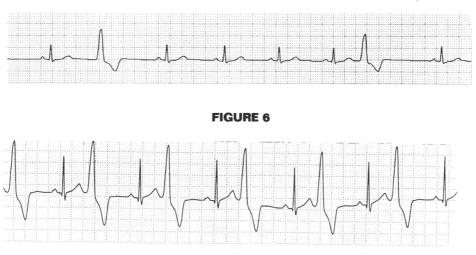

FIGURE 6

FIGURE 7

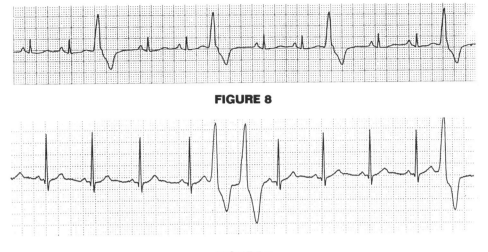

FIGURE 8

FIGURE 9

either from secretions, tongue and soft tissue positioning, or foreign body. If hypoventilation is the cause for hypoxemia, endotracheal intubation should be performed. Metabolic derangements may also result in symptomatic AV block or sinus node dysfunction[6].

Symptomatic bradycardia may require initiation of cardiopulmonary resuscitation while intravenous agents are being prepared. Intravenous administration of agents used to modify the autonomic nervous system in severe bradycardia include atropine (10–40 μg/kg/min), epinephrine (0.1–1.0 μg/kg/min), or isoproterenol (0.05–0.50 μg/kg/min).

Temporary pacing may be difficult for the transport team to accomplish but should be considered for patients with severe bradycardia unresponsive to intravenous agents. Transcutaneous/transthoracic pacing is likely the most available pacing modality to the transport team and can be performed with the aid of a specially modified defibrillator/monitor pack. Transvenous pacing of the right ventricle can be accomplished without fluoroscopy with bipolar catheters and inflatable balloon tips (flow-directed catheters); the catheters are available in 3 Fr and 5 Fr calibers and can be successfully placed from femoral, subclavian or jugular approaches. Transesophageal temporary pacing (capturing the atria) can be performed as well but will be useful only if AV nodal conduction is intact.

Tachyarrhythmias

Ectopic Atrial Tachycardia[16]

This atrial arrhythmia is characterized by a narrow complex QRS tachycardia preceded by P waves which originate from an atrial site other than the sinus node. Therefore, the P waves may not be upright in II or may be an unusual shape (wide or narrow). The danger with this arrhythmia is not that there is hemodynamic compromise with the onset of the tachycardia but that there is myocardial dysfunction with long-standing tachycardia (usually of many hours or days duration). A dilated cardiomyopathy may result from many days of tachycardia, and there may be signs of both left and right heart failure (pulmonary congestion and peripheral edema). Treatment for both the tachycardia and myocardial dysfunction is the same, termination of the tachycardia. Ectopic atrial tachycardia

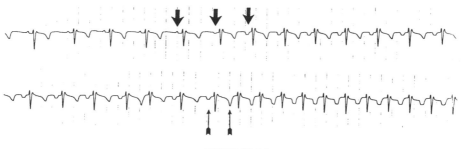

FIGURE 10

typically responds to a beta blocker; a good first line therapy is esmolol, which can be titrated from 25 μg/kg/min up to 200 μg/kg/min. Digoxin may also be used but is often ineffective; it will have the added benefit of enhancing myocardial contractility. Inotropes and stimulants should be avoided as they may act to aggravate the tachycardia.

In Figure 10 the wide arrows mark the onset of the ectopic atrial tachycardia; note the P wave morphology changes. In the second tracing, the ectopic atrial tachycardia begins to accelerate and the P waves are superimposed on the T wave; note the T wave morphology changes due to the superimposition of the P wave.

Supraventricular Tachycardia[13]

The most common presentation is in the infant, typically under 4 months of age. Presenting signs often include poor feeding, fussiness, tachypnea, and pallor. Heart rates are typically > 220. In older children and teenagers the rates may only be just greater than 160. The typical EKG features a narrow QRS tachycardia with no identifiable P waves (occasionally an astute observer will note in some leads a retrograde P which comes shortly after the S wave) (Fig. 11).

Vagal maneuvers in infants are typically unsuccessful but may be attempted; the most successful maneuver is usually the dive reflex, which involves suddenly covering the entire face of the infant with a plastic bag full of ice water (more ice than water is best). This also may be tried on older children. Cooperative older children can also be taught how to gag themselves (not recommended in hemodynamically unstable patients as they may not be able to protect their airway if they vomit); older children may also be instructed on the Valsalva maneuver (which typically must be a prolonged forceful strain).

Management of infants or children with *hemodynamically unstable SVT* is synchronized DC cardioversion. Synchronization discharges the energy at the peak of the QRS complex. Random cardioversion may result in discharge of energy on the T wave, which could result in ventricular fibrillation. Initial dose is 1 joule/kg; if this is unsuccessful, subsequent synchronized cardioversion is at 2 joules/kg. Semielective DC cardioversion should be preceded by adequate

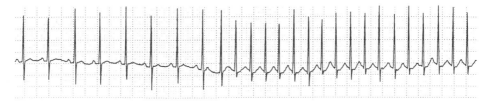

FIGURE 11

sedation and analgesia. Transthoracic cardioversion should not be performed in the awake patient. We typically administer a combination of midazolam, 0.1 mg/kg/dose IV, and fentanyl, 1–2 µg/kg/dose IV. If severe hemodynamic compromise is present, do not wait for sedation to be drawn up; it is likely that the patient is obtunded anyway. An amnestic sedative should be given immediately after cardioversion to the semiconscious patient. After successful cardioversion, IV digoxin can be given to prevent recurrence unless underlying preexcitation exists suggestive of Wolf-Parkinson-White (see below).

Medical management of *hemodynamically stable SVT* in descending order of preference:

Adenosine: 50–300 µg/kg/dose, 6 mg max IV dose. Method of action is cessation of conduction through the SA and AV nodal tissue; conduction through the AV node is an integral part of the reentrant pathway in the majority of SVT. The half-life of adenosine is less than 10 seconds. Therefore, the infusion has to be rapidly given by IV push in as large a vein as possible (central venous access is not necessary, but a brachial vein is preferred to a foot or hand vein). This is best accomplished by attaching a three-way stopcock directly to the hub of the IV catheter. In one port attach the syringe with adenosine; in the other port attach a 5–10 ml normal saline flush. Rapidly push in the adenosine; then rapidly turn the stopcock valve and push in the flush. Record a continuous EKG during the infusion; there may be a many-second "pause" (no QRS complexes). The initial recovery rhythm may be a junctional rhythm. Sinus rhythm typically follows within seconds to minutes. If tachycardia immediately resumes, examine the area of "pause"; 1:1 conduction of atrial flutter can appear to be SVT (flutter waves buried in the T waves) but adenosine will not terminate the flutter, just the AV conduction (no QRS complexes). Therefore, the flutter waves will become quite evident during the "pause."

Side effects of adenosine are rare but include **bronchospasm** and **cardiac arrest** (flat line). The competitive antagonist for adenosine is aminophylline. A rescue bolus of 0.5–1.0 mg/kg should be considered with cardiac arrest. Adenosine should be used with caution in patients with known sinus node dysfunction, severe reactive airway disease, or after cardiac transplantation.

Digoxin. Do not use prior to cardioversion as it may increase the risk of ventricular fibrillation. Digitalization dose is based on age and weight (Table 4). The initial dose is ½ the total loading dose. Two subsequent doses (each ¼ the total loading dose) are given at 8 and 16 hours after the initial dose. Digoxin is not used as a first-line drug to terminate SVT because it is *contraindicated in SVT with underlying Wolff-Parkinson-White (WPW) syndrome;* digoxin acts to slow conduction at the AV node. In WPW this will then preferentially increase

TABLE 4. Digitalizing Dose in Infants, Children, and Adolescents

Age/Weight	Total PO Digitalizing Dose*
Preterm infant	20 µg/kg PO
Term infant	30 µg/kg PO
1 mo–2 years	40–50 µg/kg PO
> 2 years	30–40 µg/kg PO
5–10 years	20–30 µg/kg PO
Adults	10–15 µg/kg PO

* IV dose is 75–80% of PO dose)
Note: IV digoxin is infused over five minutes.

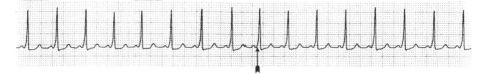

FIGURE 12

conduction down the accessory Kent bundle. If the patient develops an atrial tachycardia or atrial fibrillation, all impulses may be transmitted preferentially down the Kent bundle leading to a hemodynamically unstable ventricular response (ventricular tachycardia or fibrillation).[4]

The preexcitation seen in WPW is demonstrated in Figure 12; the arrow points out the "delta wave," which is the early activation of the ventricles through the accessory pathway. Note that the PR interval is very short because the delta wave begins at the end of the P wave.

Procainamide: 2–3 mg/kg over 5 minutes repeated q 10–30 min prn (max 100 mg). Maintenance 20–80 μg/kg/min (max 2 gm/24 hr).

Esmolol: See discussion of esmolol under ectopic atrial tachycardia.

Propranolol: rarely used IV as it can result in life-threatening hypotension.

Verapamil: rarely used in infants as it can cause life-threatening hypotension. In older children and adults there is much more successful experience but hypotension is always a concern. The dose is 0.1 mg/kg IV over a 60-second period. The dose may be repeated once if there has been no hypotension five minutes after the first dose. Atropine, isoproterenol and calcium chloride should be available to reverse severe hypotension from verapamil. It is *contraindicated* in patients who have received propranolol or other beta blockers as well as quinidine or disopyramide in the previous 48 hours. Verapamil is also contraindicated if there is any aberrance to the QRS complex (widening or changing morphology); the arrhythmia may actually be a ventricular arrhythmia in which case verapamil could have disastrous results.

Atrial Flutter and Fibrillation

Both of these arrhythmias are uncommon in children. Atrial flutter in a structurally normal heart is more commonly seen in infants than older children. There has been a rare association of atrial fibrillation with hyperthyroidism without any associated structural disease.[17] Both of these arrhythmias are more commonly seen in children with structurally abnormal atria, i.e. dilated atria from severe AV valve regurgitation, Ebstein's anomaly, s/p atrial partitioning surgery such as the Mustard, Senning, or Fontan procedures. Spontaneous conversions from atrial flutter to fibrillation or vice versa may occur.

Atrial flutter is described as a saw/tooth pattern of P waves on EKG, but this appearance depends upon the atrial rate and the ventricular response. In Figure 13, first tracing demonstrates atrial flutter with a rate of approximately 150 bpm; there is underlying first degree AV block. The second tracing has the typical saw tooth appearance of atrial flutter.

Atrial flutter can be difficult to diagnose because the flutter P waves may be hidden in the T waves. A sudden increase in vagal tone can slow conduction through the AV node, thereby making the flutter P waves more evident. Figure 14 is from a 5-year-old patient who was instructed to Valsalva (tall arrow marks onset of Valsalva maneuver); note the flutter P waves become evident (smaller consecutive arrows).

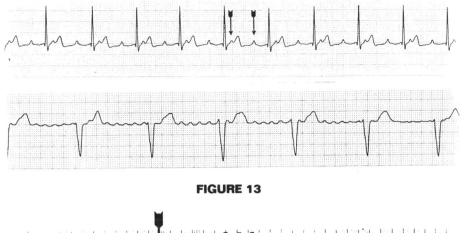

FIGURE 13

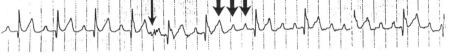

FIGURE 14

Adenosine can also help establish the diagnosis of atrial flutter by blocking AV nodal conduction, thereby transiently demonstrating the flutter P waves and a slower junctional escape rhythm. Typically, the atrial rate during flutter is >280 bpm with infant flutter rates as high as 450 bpm. The ventricular response may vary from 1:1 to multiple degrees of second degree block (i.e., 2:1, 3:1, 4:1, which describes how many P waves are associated with each QRS complex). Therefore, the R-R interval may be fixed or may vary depending upon the nature of conduction through the AV node. Atrial flutter is typically not a life-threatening arrhythmia and can be converted with oral medication. If the flutter has been long-standing (days or weeks) with rapid ventricular response, heart failure may occur. In this case synchronized DC cardioversion is indicated. After successful cardioversion, digoxin is given to prevent recurrence (see dosing table).

Atrial Fibrillation is classically described as causing an irregularly irregular EKG. No identifiable P waves are seen, but there is a coarse appearance to the baseline with irregularly spaced QRS complexes (Fig. 15).

Typically this is also not a life-threatening arrhythmia and may be converted with oral therapy. It may also spontaneously convert to sinus rhythm. If there is rapid AV conduction (as may been seen in patients with WPW syndrome), there may be hemodynamic compromise from rapid ventricular response; DC cardioversion is indicated in this circumstance. Atrial fibrillation is associated with sluggish or static flow through the atria, and therefore these patients are prone to thrombus formation. A cerebral embolus would be the likely explanation for a patient with neurologic symptoms and irregularly irregular pulse. Elective

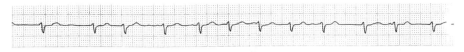

FIGURE 15

cardioversion in those who fail oral therapy should be preceded by echocardiography to rule out an atrial thrombus; several weeks of anticoagulation has been advocated prior to elective cardioversion to prevent embolic phenomenon. Oral conversion is usually with digoxin and/or propranolol.

Ventricular Tachycardia (VT)

This arrhythmia[8] is less common than SVT in the pediatric population. The adult EKG hallmarks for establishing the diagnosis are prolonged QRS duration and dissociation of P waves from QRS during tachycardia. These rules do not always hold true in pediatrics. The QRS duration is age dependent and relative prolongation may be missed if this is not kept in mind. Retrograde conduction is more commonly maintained in the young and may result in a 1:1 relationship between QRS and retrograde P waves. The etiology of VT includes the following:

Congenital heart disease, particularly unrepaired severe aortic stenosis and large VSDs (Eisenmenger syndrome). Postoperative VT is more commonly associated with surgeries requiring ventriculotomy or removal of ventricular muscle bundles (tetralogy of Fallot).

Structural heart disease: tumors, arrhythmogenic RV dysplasia (actually, a form of congenital heart disease but may not be macroscopic disease), dilated cardiomyopathy, hypertrophic cardiomyopathy.

Intrinsic heart or heart-lung disease: myocarditis, ischemia, long QT syndrome, pulmonary hypertension.

Metabolic: digitalis toxicity, theophylline, caffeine, amphetamines, cocaine, tricyclic antidepressants, phenothiazines, catecholamine infusions, hypokalemia, hyperkalemia, acidosis, hypoxia.

Nonsustained versus Sustained VT.   Nonsustained VT is defined as 3 or more consecutive beats up to 30 seconds duration.

Monomorphic VT.   (Fig. 16)

Treatment.   For patients with hemodynamic compromise, synchronized DC cardioversion is the treatment of choice; initially 1 joule/kg, which may be doubled if unsuccessful (the use of "synchronized" cardioversion is discussed under "Supraventricular Tachycardia"). Synchronized DC cardioversion should also be used if patients become hemodynamically unstable during drug infusions aimed at terminating VT. Hemodynamically stable sustained or recurrent nonsustained VT may be treated with the following infusions:

Lidocaine.   IV bolus loading dose over 1-2 minutes (1 mg/kg/dose); dose may be repeated once 5-10 minutes after the initial dose. This is followed by a continuous infusion of 10-50 μg/kg/min. Maximum dose 3-4.5 mg/kg/hour. Side effects include seizures, respiratory depression, hypotension/shock, arrhythmia, CNS symptoms (anxiety, euphoria, drowsiness). *Contraindicated in heart block.*

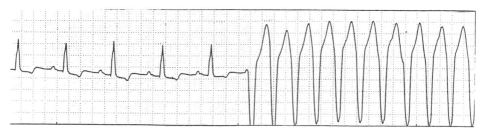

FIGURE 16

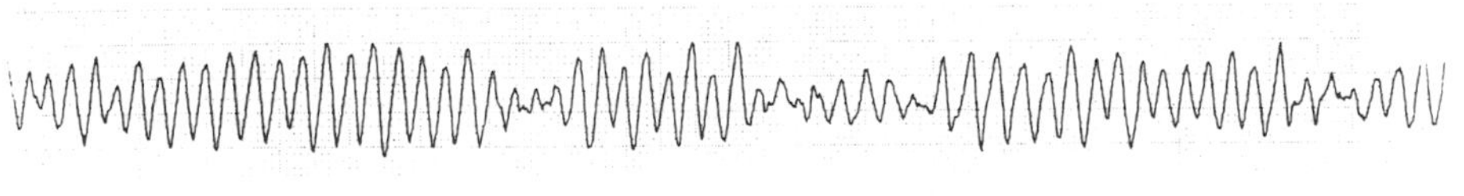

[ECG tracing]

FIGURE 17

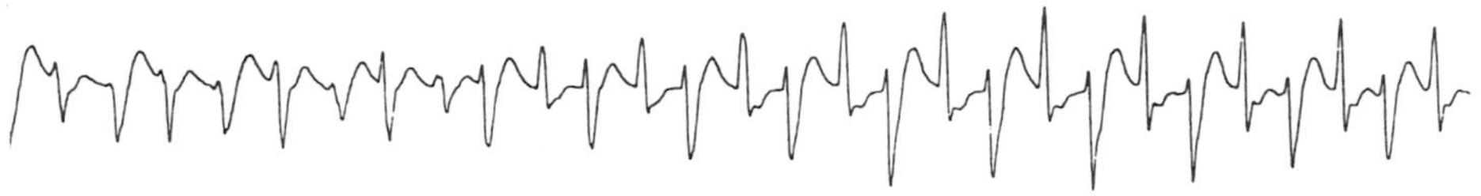

[ECG tracing]

FIGURE 18

Procainamide. IV bolus over 5 minutes (2–3 mg/kg/dose); may be repeated q 10–30 min prn (maximum 100 mg). This is followed by a continuous infusion of 20–80 μg/kg/min. Side effects include nausea, vomiting, rash, hypotension, arrhythmia, confusion or disorientation. *Contraindicated in complete heart block.*

Polymorphic VT.

Torsades de pointes. Usually associated with long QT syndrome. The QRS morphology gradually changes shape and appears to twist around the isoelectric line (Fig. 17).

Biodirectional VT. There is beat-to-beat alternation in QRS axis (Fig. 18). This is associated with digitalis toxicity, familial hyperkalemic paralysis, or catecholamine sensitivity.

Ventricular Fibrillation

Characterized by rapid, irregularly shaped complexes with hemodynamic compromise (Fig. 19). Treatment is unsynchronized cardioversion 2 joules/kg (synchronization may never result in discharge of energy as monitor may not be able to lock on to the rapid and irregular R waves).

Atrio-Ventricular Block

Varying degrees of AV block can be associated with multiple conditions:[6]

Structural Heart Disease. See discussion of congential AV block below.

Infectious Conditions. Viral or bacterial myocarditis, Lyme disease, Yersinia diarrheal illness, Chagas' disease, diphtheria, typhoid, Rocky Mountain spotted fever.

Inflammatory Conditions. Rheumatoid arthritis, Reiter's syndrome, Guillain-Barré.

Neurodegenerative Conditions and Muscular Dystrophies: Kearnes-Sayre syndrome.

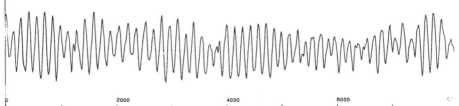

FIGURE 19

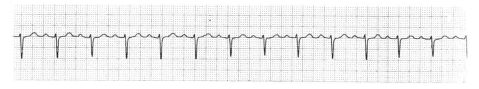

FIGURE 20

Infiltrative Disorders. Tuberous schlerosis, lymphoma, amyloidosis, sarcoidosis.

Trauma. Cardiac surgery, blunt chest trauma, penetrating chest trauma, radiation therapy.

Functional. Athlete's heart (high resting vagal tone), head trauma/cerebral edema.

Drugs. Tricyclic antidepressants, antiarrhythmics (digoxin in particular), clonidine.

Intermittent first- and second-degree AV block can be a normal variant in children, particularly in neonates and athletes; the etiology of this benign block is believed to be due to changes in autonomic tone. Persistent or high-grade second-degree block or complete (third-degree) block is always considered abnormal.

First-Degree AV Block

Defined as a fixed prolonged PR interval (Fig.20). Normal PR interval varies with age and heart rate. A PR > 0.20 sec is abnormal at any age. Neonatal PR is usually between 0.09 and 0.12 sec.

Second-Degree AV Block

Type I (Wenckebach block). Defined as progressive prolongation of PR interval with eventual nonconducted P wave (Fig.21).

Type II. Normal or lengthened PR interval but fixed in duration with occasional nonconducted P wave (Fig. 22).

Third-Degree AV Block

Congenital. Seen in 1 in 15,000–20,000 live births and may or may not be associated with structural heart disease. There is a definite association with

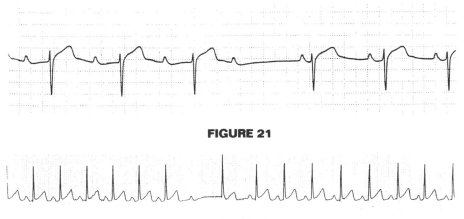

FIGURE 21

FIGURE 22

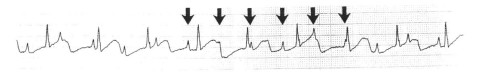

FIGURE 23

maternal connective tissue disease (most commonly systemic lupus erythematosus); maternal transfer of antibodies has been demonstrated, and these presumably cross-react with fetal cardiac conduction tissue at a critical stage in development. There is also an association with structural heart disease particularly L-transposition of the great arteries, left atrial isomerism, and AV septal defects.

Noncongenital. May result from a progression of first or second degree blocks.

Figure 23 demonstrates complete heart block. Note that the P waves "march through" the tracing.

Implantable Pacemakers

Electronic implantable pacemaker dysfunction can be life-threatening if the patient is pacemaker dependent. Pacing can be performed in the atrium, ventricle, or both. When the pacemaker generates an electrical impulse, the energy is delivered to the myocardium over a very brief period (0.1–1.0 milliseconds). This results in a vertical "spike" on surface EKG. If it is difficult to see the spike, the spike may be isoelectric; changing the lead (moving the EKG patches) may result in taller/deeper spikes. The spike should be immediately followed by a P wave if the atrium is being paced or QRS complex if the ventricle is being paced. A paced ventricular beat is generally a wide complex QRS since depolarization of the ventricle is occurring aberrantly from where the pacemaker wire is inserted and not in the normal fashion (the AV node and HIS bundles).

Figure 24 demonstrates normal pacemaker capture of a single lead ventricular pacemaker. Figure 25 demonstrates normal pacemaker capture of a double-lead or dual-chamber (atrial and ventricular) pacemaker.

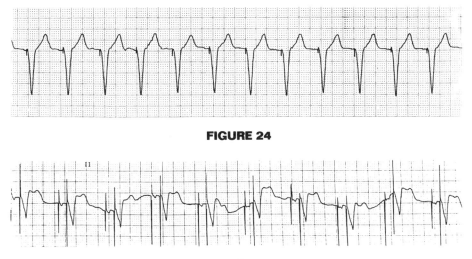

FIGURE 24

FIGURE 25

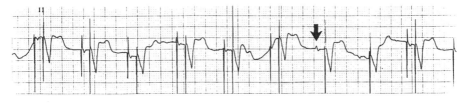

FIGURE 26

Not every heart beat may be generated by the electronic pacemaker; most pacemakers are programmed to sense intrinsic beats with subsequent inhibition of firing the electronically paced beat. Therefore the absence of pacing spikes does not mean the pacemaker is not functioning. Figure 26 shows a dual-chamber pacemaker with inhibition of pacemaker activity; the pacemaker "senses" the native electrical activity of the heart and therefore does not generate a pacemaker impulse (arrow marks the sensed P wave). However, if the patient is profoundly bradycardic it can be assumed that the pacemaker is not working or not capturing the myocardium.

Figure 27 demonstrates pacemaker dysfunction; the pacemaker is firing but not always capturing the myocardium. Note that the vertical pacing spikes are not always immediately followed by a QRS complex.

In pacemaker dysfunction, there is typically a slow ventricular escape rhythm which may be wide QRS morphology. Symptomatic patients should be started on intravenous chronotropic support such as isoproterenol or epinephrine.

X-rays will not cause pacemaker dysfunction. Intense magnetic fields such as those generated by MRI will adversely affect pacemakers (pacemakers are programmed/reprogrammed externally with electromagnetic signals). Cardioversion (DC) will often "reprogram" pacemakers into a default mode; the rate of firing may be different than that at which the patient or parent recalls it being programmed. Pacemakers are not a contraindication to DC cardioversion of life-threatening arrhythmias, but do not place the defibrillator puddle directly over the pacemaker. After cardioversion the pacemaker should be evaluated as soon as possible.

Ischemia

Electrocardiograms are often obtained to evaluate chest pain; ischemia in children is rare. It is associated with anomalous coronary arteries (the most common type is the left coronary artery arising from the main pulmonary artery); typically this presents in infancy with congestive heart failure. Marked ST-T wave changes in an infant should prompt investigation of this diagnosis. Note the ST elevation in this 4-month-old with anomalous left coronary artery (Fig 28).

Other considerations with ST-T wave changes include drug or toxin ingestion, pericarditis, myocarditis, and chest trauma.

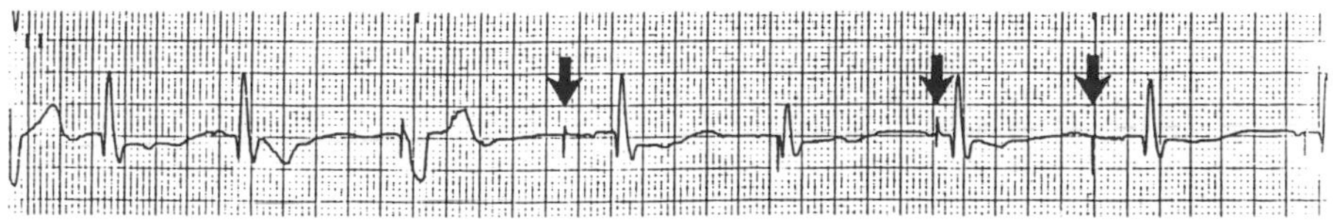

FIGURE 27

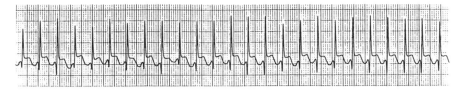

FIGURE 28

Endocarditis

Streptococcus viridans, *Streptococcus faecalis* (enterococcus), and *Staphylococcus aureus* are responsible for more than 90% of the cases. Empiric treatment is aimed at these common pathogens. Ideally blood cultures form two sites are obtained before initiating IV antibiotics. Penicillin G or oxacillin as well as gentamicin should be started after appropriate blood cultures are obtained.

REFERENCES

1. Barnea O, Austin EH, Richman B, Santamore WP: Balancing the circulation: Theoretic optimization of pulmonary/systemic flow ratio in hypoplastic left heart syndrome. J Am Coll Cardiol 24:1376, 1994.
2. Bove EL, Lupinetti FM: Tetralogy of Fallot. In Mavroudis C, Backer CL (eds): Pediatric Cardiac Surgery. St. Louis, Mosby, 1994.
3. de Leval M: Ventricular Septal Defect. In Stark J, de Leval M (eds): Surgery for Congenital Heart Defects, 2nd ed. Philadelphia, W.B. Saunders, 1994.
4. Deal BJ, Keane JF, Gillette PC, Garson A Jr: Wolff-Parkinson-White syndrome and supraventricular tachycardia during infancy: Management and follow-up. J Am Coll Cardiol 5:130, 1985.
5. Engle M: Postoperative Problems. In Adams F, Emmanouilides G, Riemenschneider T (eds): Heart Disease in Infants, Children, and Adolescents, 4th ed. Baltimore, Williams & Wilkins, 1989.
6. Fish F, Benson DW: Disorders of cardiac rhythm and conduction. In Emmanouilides G, et al (eds): Heart Disease in Infants, Children, and Adolescents, 5th ed. Baltimore, Williams & Wilkins, 1995.
7. Freedom RM, Benson LN: Hypoplastic left heart syndrome. In Emmanouilides G, et al (eds): Heart disease in Infants, Children, and Adolescents, 5th ed. Baltimore, Williams & Wilkins, 1995.
8. Garson A Jr: Ventricular arrhythmias. In Gillette PC, Garson A Jr (eds): Pediatric Arrhythmias: Electrophysiology and Pacing. Philadelphia, W.B. Saunders, 1990.
9. Haworth SG: Pulmonary vascular development. In Long WA (ed): Fetal and Neonatal Cardiology. Philadelphia, W.B. Saunders, 1990.
10. Helton JG, et al: Analysis of potential anatomic or physiologic determinants of outcome of palliative surgery for hypoplastic left heart syndrome. Circulation 74:70, 1986.
11. Jobes DR, Nicolson SC, Steven JM, et al: Carbon dioxide prevents pulmonary overcirculation in hypoplastic left heart syndrome. Ann Thorac Surg 54:150, 1992.
12. Kirklin JW, Barratt-Boyes BG (eds): Cardiac Surgery. New York, Churchill Livingstone, 1986, p 158.
13. Ko JK, Deal BJ, Strasburger JF, Benson DW: Supraventricular tachycardia mechanisms and their age distribution in pediatric patients. Am J Cardiol 69:1028, 1992.
14. Lees MH, King DH: Heart disease in the newborn. In Adams F, Emmanouilides G, Riemenschneider T (eds): Heart disease in Infants, Children, and Adolescents, 4th ed. Baltimore, Williams & Wilkins, 1989.
15. Lister G: Shock. In Emmanouilides G, et al (eds): Heart Disease in Infants, Children, and Adolescents, 5th ed. Baltimore, Williams & Wilkins, 1995.
16. Mehta AV, Sanchez GR, Sacks EJ: Ectopic automatic atrial tachycardia in children: Clinical characteristics, management and follow-up. J Am Coll Cardiol 11:379, 1988.
17. Perry LW, Jung W: Atrial fibrillation and hyperthyroidism in a 14-year old boy. J Pediatr 79:668, 1971.
18. Victoria BE: Cyanotic newborns. In Gessner IH, Victoria BE (eds): Pediatric Cardiology. Philadelphia, W.B. Saunders, 1993.

CHAPTER 9

Cardiopulmonary Resuscitation of Newborns During Transport

LUCKY JAIN, M.D.

With the regionalization of perinatal services and the introduction of newer modalities of treatment at tertiary care centers, the need for transport services with matching sophistication has increased. Although emphasis is rightly placed on transfer of mothers with the fetus in utero, tertiary care centers are often called for transport of sick neonates when unanticipated complications arise after the delivery, or when the mother is too unstable to be transferred. Since these patients are at risk for cardiopulmonary events during transport, personnel involved in transport should be highly skilled in all aspects of neonatal resuscitation.

Neonatal resuscitation, as performed in the delivery room has been the focus of several recent reviews.[2-5] An extensive textbook has been published jointly by the American Academy of Pediatrics and the American Heart Association on this subject.[6] The resuscitation procedure described in these publications is geared primarily for the delivery room. Effective application of this structured stepwise approach requires adequate personnel and equipment and prior knowledge of fetal jeopardy. Resuscitation of neonatal patients during transport usually requires some modification of this approach.[7] In this chapter we discuss salient features of neonatal resuscitation as it should be performed prior to and during transport.

BEING PREPARED

Adequate equipment and skilled personnel are essential for any transport. Before embarking on a transport, it is imperative that all equipment and medication stocks be checked. A checklist is useful for this purpose, and Table 1 shows the most commonly required items. Universal precautions should be taken during any resuscitation procedure. Gloves and other protective barriers should be worn when handling patients or contaminated equipment.[5]

Several studies have shown that hypothermia adversely affects the outcome of neonates and small infants.[8,9] This is particularly true for low-birthweight infants and asphyxiated infants who have difficulty tolerating cold environment and readily sustain cold injury.[8,9] Special precautions are necessary to prevent hypothermia during transport. The transport incubator should be prewarmed and have a fully charged battery pack. Wherever possible, the incubator should be plugged into an electrical outlet in the ambulance and in the transferring hospital, to prevent depletion of its battery. Gloves or bottles filled with warm water and warm blankets can be sources of additional heat.

TABLE 1.   Equipment for Neonatal Transports

Transport incubator	Laryngoscope blades, straight no. 0 and 1
Stethoscope	Umbilical catheters, 3.5F and 5F
Cardiotachometer with EKG or oscilloscope	Three-way stopcocks
Pulse oximeter	Sterile umbilical vessel catheterization tray
Suction with manometer	Syringes: 1 ml, 3 ml, 10 ml, 20 ml with needles
Bulb syringe	Feeding tubes
Oxygen source with flowmeter	Medications
Suction catheters, 5F, 6F, 8F and 10F	Epinephrine (1:10,000)
Resuscitation bag	Naloxone HCl (1 mg/ml or 0.4 mg/ml)
Face mask, newborn and premature sizes	Volume expander
Oral airways, newborn and premature sizes	Sodium bicarbonate (0.5 μg/ml)
Endotracheal tubes, sizes 2.5, 3.0, 3.5 and 4.0 mm	Dextrose solutions
Stylet (optional)	Lorazepam/phenobarbital
Laryngoscope (one spare)	Instant camera

Every effort should be made to ensure that the patient is as stable as possible prior to transport. This is sometimes a difficult decision when the condition of a sick infant or child is deteriorating. The transport team should be in close communication with the receiving team at the tertiary care center to decide on the best course of action. Special attention should be paid to the following questions:

1. Is the infant's temperature as close to thermoneutrality as possible?
2. Is the cardiac/respiratory status stable enough to withstand transport?
3. Is the blood glucose in the normal range?
4. Are all catheters/tubes in proper position and secure?

Vital signs should be monitored continuously during transport. These include heart rate, respiratory rate, blood pressure, oxygen saturation, and temperature. Several types of instruments are available for monitoring respirations and heart rate. We prefer instruments with a graphic display of cardiac rhythm and respirations rather than traditional apnea monitors. A pulse oximeter has become an essential component of neonatal and pediatric monitoring and should be used in all transports. In sick neonates who have an umbilical arterial catheter, a pressure transducer should be used to monitor blood pressure directly.

NEONATAL AIRWAY

A patent airway is a prerequisite for any successful resuscitation attempt. The patient should be placed supine or on his or her side with the neck in a neutral position. Overextension or flexion may produce airway obstruction and should be avoided. A blanket or towel (roughly 1 inch thick) placed under a neonate's shoulders may help maintain proper head position. For oral and nasal suctioning, a bulb suction device is usually adequate and is particularly useful during transports when appropriate wall suction may not be available. Deep or vigorous suctioning should be avoided and should be limited to 10 seconds at a time. Excessive stimulation of the oropharynx can produce reflex bradycardia.[10] When choanal atresia or micrognathia is suspected, an oral airway may be helpful. The airway should fit comfortably over the tongue, reaching the posterior pharynx with the flange just outside the lips.[6] Choosing the appropriate size is important because an airway that is too small may push the tongue backward and increase the obstruction, whereas one that is too large can lead to trauma (Fig. 1).

VENTILATION

As a general rule, any infant who requires prolonged ventilatory support should be intubated before transport. Such infants can then be ventilated either

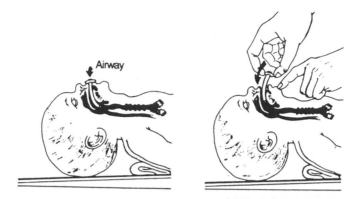

FIGURE 1. Selection and insertion of oral airway. (From American Academy of Pediatrics: Textbook of Neonatal Resuscitation. Elk Grove Village, IL, American Academy of Pediatrics, 1990; copyright American Heart Association.)

manually with a bag or with a transport ventilator. Signs of adequate ventilation include bilateral expansion of the lungs, as assessed by chest wall motion, and auscultation of breath sounds. A pressure manometer should be used whenever ventilating with a bag. Inability to inflate the lungs adequately during transport may be due to an obstructed airway or inadequate pressure. If a bag and mask are used for ventilation, care must be taken to ensure adequate seal between the face and the mask. All infants requiring prolonged positive pressure ventilation should have an orogastric tube placed, leaving it open to air to prevent gastric distention.

During air transports, special attention should be paid to the imbalance between the atmospheric pressure and the pressure of gases within the body (dysbarism). Infants with severe lung disease may experience hypoxia at high altitudes because of the reduction in the partial pressure of oxygen requiring an adjustment in the concentration of inspired oxygen.[11] Positive pressure ventilation is indicated for infants who have apnea, bradycardia (heart rate < 100 bpm) or persistent central cyanosis in spite of oxygen supplementation (Fig. 2). For infants who deteriorate during transport, initial attempts at ventilation should be made with bag and mask. For transports, we prefer to use the self-inflating bag because it can be used without an oxygen source. Ventilations should be performed at a rate of 40–60 times per minute. Because the tidal volume of newborn infants is small, infant-sized bags (volume 250 ml) with a pressure pop-off valve set at 35–40 cm should be used.

INTUBATION

As stated earlier, infants who require prolonged positive pressure ventilation ideally should have an endotracheal tube in place prior to transport. This prevents the need for emergency intubation en route and ensures proper positioning of the tube. Infants with diaphragmatic hernia should be ventilated only via an endotracheal tube. Radiologic confirmation of the tube position should be obtained before the transfer if possible. The tube should be adequately secured with tape to prevent accidental extubation in route. Displacement of the tube is a common cause for sudden deterioration in an infant's condition.[12] All transport teams should have at least one person skilled in emergency intubation. When reintubating an infant, a tube of appropriate size should be selected (Table 2) and attention paid to the vocal cord guide, a black line near the tip of most

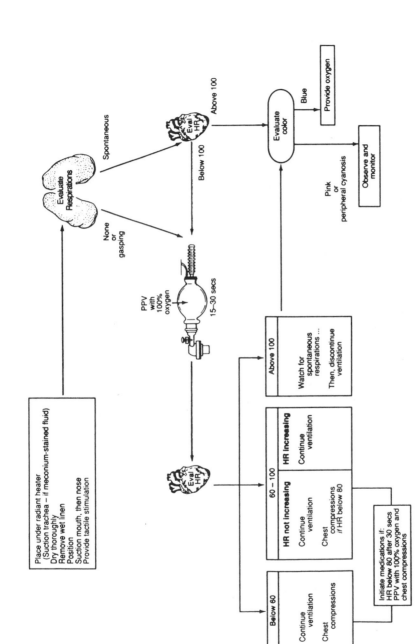

FIGURE 2. Overview of resuscitation in the delivery room. (From American Academy of Pediatrics: Textbook of Neonatal Resuscitation. Elk Grove Village, IL, American Academy of Pediatrics, 1990; copyright American Heart Association.)

TABLE 2. Endotracheal Intubation (Oral) for Newborns

Weight (g)	Endotracheal Tube Size (Internal diameter in mm)	Length to Corner of Mouth	Laryngoscope Blade Size
< 1250	2.5	7.5	0
1250–2000	3.0	8.0	0
> 2000	3.5	8.5	1

tubes. This guide should be positioned at the level of the cords to ensure that the tip is above the carina. A general guide to the proper depth of the endotracheal tube placement is a distance of 6 cm plus the infant's weight in kilograms.[5] After intubation, the position of the tube should be checked by:

1. Presence of symmetrical chest wall motion.
2. Presence of equal breath sounds, especially in the axillae, and absence of breath sounds over the stomach.
3. Presence of moisture in the tube during exhalation.
4. Absence of abdominal distention.
5. Improvement in the color, heart rate, and activity of the neonate.

When in doubt, tube position can also be confirmed by direct visualization of the larynx with a laryngoscope. Many centers prefer nasotracheal intubation over orotracheal because the tube is less likely to be dislodged in the former.

CHEST COMPRESSIONS

In the event of prolonged hypoxia due to respiratory insufficiency, bradycardia and cardiac arrest can supervene unless effective resuscitative measures are undertaken. Chest compressions are indicated if heart rate is less than 60 beats per minute or between 60 and 80 and not increasing despite adequate ventilatory efforts.[6] Figure 3 shows the two techniques commonly employed. Compressions with either of these methods are acceptable and should be accomplished in a smooth, nonjerky fashion. The two-thumb technique is preferable, especially when prolonged

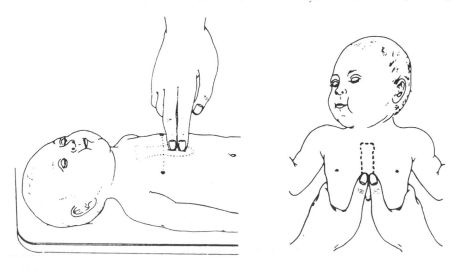

FIGURE 3. Position of fingers or thumbs during chest compressions. (From American Academy of Pediatrics: Textbook of Neonatal Resuscitation. Elk Grove Village, IL, American Academy of Pediatrics, 1990; copyright American Heart Association.)

chest compressions are required. The two thumbs are placed on the middle third of the sternum, with fingers encircling the chest and supporting the back. The pulse rate should be monitored periodically and compressions discontinued when the spontaneous heart rate reaches 80 beats per minute or greater. Compressions should always be accompanied by positive pressure ventilation with 100% oxygen. Since simultaneous delivery of chest compressions and positive pressure ventilations is likely to decrease the efficiency of ventilation, it is now recommended that chest compression be interposed with ventilations in a 3:1 ratio.[5] The rate of compressions combined with ventilations should be 120 per minute, which will result in provision of 90 compressions and 30 breaths each minute.

MEDICATIONS

Before transport, all sick newborns should have a secured site of vascular access. An umbilical venous catheter is ideal for such circumstances. A 3.5 or 5.0 French feeding tube or umbilical catheter with a single end-hole should be inserted into the vein until the tip of the catheter is just below the skin level and free flow of blood is obtained. Pushing the catheter in farther should be avoided because this may lodge the catheter tip in the liver, resulting in infusion of medications directly into the liver. When vascular access is not readily available, an endotracheal tube can be used to administer epinephrine during resuscitation. Consideration should be given to using higher doses of epinephrine (0.1–0.2 mg/kg) by the endotracheal route if the neonate does not respond to the standard dose.[5]

Medications are indicated if the heart rate continues to be less than 80 beats per minute despite adequate ventilation and chest compressions for 30 seconds. Medications most commonly used in resuscitation are shown in Table 3. Sodium bicarbonate should be used only in the presence of documented metabolic acidosis, and even then only sparingly. Recent evidence indicates that the alkali may correct extracellular metabolic acidosis, but only at the expense of transient aggravation of intracellular acidosis and a further decline in the contractile force of the heart.[13] Matten et al.[14] have shown that hyperosmolality resulting from the administration of sodium bicarbonate is an independent risk factor for death after successful resuscitation.

Albumin or normal saline comes in handy when volume expansion is necessary to combat shock resulting from acute blood loss. For infants with hypotension who fail to respond to volume expansion, inotropic support may be required. Dopamine is the most widely used agent for this purpose and has the primary effect of increasing cardiac contractibility, leading to an increase in cardiac output and blood pressure.[15] This is important, because prolonged hypoxia depresses myocardial contractility. Dopamine must be given as a continuous infusion via an infusion pump, and infants receiving the infusion need to have continuous monitoring of vital signs. Dopamine is used in the dose of 5–20 μg/kg per minute. The following formula can be used in preparing a dopamine solution[6]:

$$\frac{6 \times \text{infant's weight in kg} \times \text{desired dose } \mu\text{g/kg/min}}{\text{Desired amount of fluid ml/hr}} = \frac{\text{mg of dopamine}}{\text{per 100 ml of solution}}$$

Once the amount of dopamine to be added to each 100 ml solution has been calculated, the infusion pump can be adjusted to the desired infusion rate. Care should be taken to flush the tubing with the solution to clear the dead space. If necessary, the dose can be increased gradually up to 20 μg/kg/min of dopamine, beyond which it is unlikely to make any difference. If needed, either dobutamine or epinephrine can be used.

Hypoglycemia can be prevented by maintaining a constant infusion of glucose at 4–8 mg/kg/min during transport. Atropine and calcium have a limited role in resuscitation and should not be used.[16,17]

For infants in whom a ductus-dependent cardiac lesion is suspected, prostaglandin E, (PGE_1) infusion may be necessary.[18] Use of PGE_1 in transport should be limited to infants in whom definite diagnosis of cardiac condition warrants its use or when poor perfusion, acidosis, or profound cyanosis ($PO_2 < 25$ mmHg) are present.

Such infants often need to be intubated prior to the transport, since apnea is a known side effect of PGE_1 therapy. Also, an additional intravenous site may be necessary to combat hypotension which often occurs after PGE_1 infusion. Any patient whose condition deteriorates significantly after starting PGE_1 may have total anomalous pulmonary venous return with pulmonary venous obstruction; in this circumstance, PGE_1 infusion should be stopped.

SPECIAL CONSIDERATIONS

While the general principles of resuscitation during transport outlined in this chapter are applicable to most neonates, a few special situations are discussed here.

Preterm Infants

Since preterm infants are especially vulnerable to heat loss, every effort should be made to minimize such loss during transport. The transport isolette should be prewarmed. Plastic Saran wraps and warm bottles may be helpful. When delivering medications, care should be taken not to administer them too rapidly since sudden changes in vascular pressure and osmolarity can cause intraventricular hemorrhage. Many centers have standard guidelines for intubation of extremely low-birthweight infants. The decision to intubate any preterm infant prior to transport should be based on the condition of the infant and the level of expertise of the transport team.

Surgical Neonate

Infants with diaphragmatic hernia who have significant respiratory compromise should be intubated before transfer. Bag and mask ventilation should be avoided to prevent distention of the herniated viscus. A nasogastric tube should be inserted and kept open to air.

Infants with tracheoesophageal fistula should be transported prone with their heads elevated and a feeding tube in the esophageal pouch for suctioning.

Infants with meningomyelocele should also be transported in a prone position. A sterile dressing should be used to cover the defect.

Infants with omphalocele or gastroschisis should have the defect covered with gauze soaked in sterile warm saline and then with sterile plastic; plastic bags that enclose the lower half of the body as well as the defect are very useful. These infants are especially prone to heat and water loss. Undue pressure on or kinking of the exposed bowel should be avoided because this can cause necrosis of the already compromised tissue. The bowel should be decompressed with a nasogastric tube.

Congenital Heart Defects

Whenever possible, a chest radiograph, electrocardiogram, arterial blood gas study, and a history and physical examination should be used to arrive at a working

TABLE 3.   Medications for Neonatal Resuscitation

Medication	Concentration to Administer	Preparation	Dosage/Route	weight	Total Dose/Infant	total ml	Rate/Precautions
Epinephrine	1:10,000	1 ml	0.1–0.3 ml/kg IV or ET	1 kg 2 kg 3 kg 4 kg	**total ml** 0.1–0.3 ml 0.2–0.6 ml 0.3–0.9 ml 0.4–1.2 ml		Give rapidly
Volume expanders	Whole blood 5% albumin Normal saline Ringer's lactate	40 ml	10 ml/kg IV	1 kg 2 kg 3 kg 4 kg	**total ml** 10 ml 20 ml 30 ml 40 ml		Give over 5–10 min
Sodium bicarbonate	0.5 mEq/ml (4.2% solution)	20 ml or two 10-ml prefilled syringes	2 mEq/kg IV	1 kg 2 kg 3 kg 4 kg	**total dose** 2 mEq 4 mEq 6 mEq 8 mEq	**total ml** 4 ml 8 ml 12 ml 16 ml	Give *slowly*, over at least 2 min Give only if infant being effectively ventilated
Naloxone	0.4 mg/ml	1 ml	0.1 mg/kg (0.25 ml/kg) IV, ET, IM, SQ	1 kg 2 kg 3 kg 4 kg	**total dose** 0.1 mg 0.2 mg 0.3 mg 0.4 mg	**total ml** 0.25 ml 0.50 ml 0.75 ml 1.00 ml	Give rapidly IV, ET preferred IM, SQ acceptable
Naloxone	1.0 mg/ml	1 ml	0.1 mg/kg (0.1 ml/kg) IV, ET IM, SQ	1 kg 2 kg 3 kg 4 kg	**total dose** 0.1 mg 0.2 mg 0.3 mg 0.4 mg	**total ml** 0.1 ml 0.2 ml 0.3 ml 0.4 ml	
Dopamine	$\dfrac{6 \times \text{weight} \times \text{desired dose}}{(\text{kg}) \quad (\mu g/kg/min)}{\text{desired fluid (ml/hr)}}$ =	mg of dopamine per 100 ml of solution	Begin at 5 µg/kg/min (may increase to 20 µg/kg/min if necessary) IV	1 kg 2 kg 3 kg 4 kg	**total µg/min** 5–20 µg/min 10–40 µg/min 15–60 µg/min 20–80 µg/min		Give as a continuous infusion using an infusion pump Monitor HR and BP closely Seek consultation

$$\frac{6 \times \text{weight (kg)} \times \text{desired dose } (\mu g/kg/min)}{\text{desired fluid (ml/hr)}} = \text{mg of dopamine per 100 ml of solution}$$

IM = intramuscular; ET = endotracheal; IV = intravenous; SQ = subcutaneous.
From American Heart Association: Medications for neonatal resuscitation. In Textbook of Neonatal Resuscitation. Copyright American Heart Association, 1990; with permission.

diagnosis before the transport. If the cardiac defect suspected is a ductal dependent lesion, PGE_1 should be started at 0.05 mg/kg/min. This dose can be decreased to 0.01 mg/kg/min when an adequate effect has been achieved. When the diagnosis is not clear, PGE_1 should be reserved for sick infants with poor perfusion, acidosis or profound hypoxia. As discussed earlier, apnea, hypotension, and hypothermia are frequent complications of PGE_1 therapy and should be kept in mind.

Meconium Aspiration Syndrome

Infants with severe meconium aspiration syndrome (MAS) often have a component of pulmonary hypertension that makes their management somewhat difficult during transport. To minimize the risk of hypoxic pulmonary vasoconstriction, the oxygen tension should be maintained at the upper recommended levels. A sudden fall in oxygen tension during transport could be due to right-to-left shunting of blood secondary to pulmonary hypertension. It also could be due to air leak syndrome, since these infants are prone to air-trapping and hyperinflation. A portable transilluminator is very useful in this situation. A needle aspiration set should be kept ready during these transports. If a chest tube is placed, it can be vented into a flap valve (Heimlich valve) during the transport.

Seizures

Although unusual, seizures may present an unanticipated complication during transport. Infants with severe birth asphyxia are often affected. In managing an infant having seizures, priority should be given to maintaining patency of the airway and to adequacy of ventilation. Several anticonvulsant drugs are available for control of seizures. We prefer to use lorazepam (0.1 mg/kg) as the initial drug. Alternately, phenobarbital (15–20 mg/kg), or dilantin (15–20 mg/kg) can be used. Since hypoglycemia is a common cause of seizures in newborns, a Chem-Strip glucose level should always be obtained. If the glucose level is low, the patient should be given 2 ml/kg of 10% dextrose intravenously followed by a continuous infusion of 4–8 mg glucose/kg/min.

Ethical Dilemmas

Several new modalities of treatment have been introduced into neonatal-perinatal medicine in the last decade. Some interventions like extracorporeal membrane oxygenation and high-frequency ventilation are often used as last resorts and therefore require transfer of critically ill infants after conventional modes of treatment have failed. The transport team is thus sometimes faced with the dilemma of resuscitation and transport of a dying or seemingly nonviable infant. Infants with an invariably lethal diagnosis such as anencephaly need not be resuscitated, and there is no legal requirement for community hospitals to transfer such infants to tertiary care centers. Extremely premature infants and severely asphyxiated infants who are not resuscitated initially can be kept at the hospital of birth until they die.[20] In infants with cardiac standstill who do not respond to resuscitation in the delivery room, we have shown that survival is unlikely beyond 10 minutes of resuscitation (Fig. 4). The Child Abuse Amendment of 1984 and the Baby Doe regulations (1985), however, mandate that all medically indicated treatment should be provided to infants with life-threatening illness when such treatment is deemed to be effective in treating or correcting such conditions.[21,22] In situations where doubt exists about diagnosis or viability or when sudden deterioration occurs during transport, it is best to perform resuscitation and transport infants to the tertiary care center where a final decision can be made.

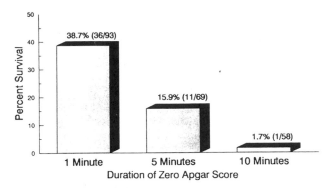

FIGURE 4. Survival among infants with persistent zero Apgar scores. (From Jain L, Ferre C, Vidyasagar D, et al: Cardiopulmonary resuscitation of apparently stillborn infants. J Pediatr 118:778–782, 1991, with permission.)

REFERENCES

1. American Academy of Pediatrics: Guidelines for Perinatal Care, 3rd ed. Evanston, IL, American Academy of Pediatrics, 1992.
2. Ballard RA: Resuscitation in the delivery room. In Avery ME, Taeusch HW (eds): Schaffer's Diseases of the Newborn, 6th ed. Philadelphia, W.B. Saunders, 1991.
3. David R: Neonatal resuscitation: Historical perspective and current practice. Clin Crit Care Med 13:1–20, 1988.
4. Sun SC: Resuscitation of newborns. Pediatr Rev 12:94, 1990.
5. Currents in Emergency Care, Vol. 3, No. 4, Winter 1992. American Heart Association/American Academy of Pediatrics: Neonatal Resuscitation. JAMA 268:2276–2281, 1992.
6. American Heart Association/American Academy of Pediatrics: Textbook of Neonatal Resuscitation, 1990.
7. Jain L, Vidyasagar D: Cardiopulmonary resuscitation of newborns. Its application to transport medicine. Pediatr Clin North Am 40:287–302, 1993.
8. Jolly H, Molyneux P, Newell DJ: A controlled study of the effect of temperature on premature babies. J Pediatr 60:889, 1962.
9. Miller JA Jr, Miller FS, Westin B: Hypothermia in the treatment of asphyxia neonatorum. Biol Neonat 6:148, 1964.
10. Cordero L Jr, Hon EH: Neonatal bradycardia following nasopharyngeal stimulation. J Pediatr 78:441, 1971.
11. Brink LW, Neuman B, Wynn J: Air Transport. Pediatr Clin North Am 40:439–456, 1993.
12. Little LA, Keonig JC, Newth CJL: Factors affecting accidental extubations in neonatal and pediatric intensive care patients. Crit Care Med 16:233, 1990.
13. Graf H, Leach W, Arieff AI: Evidence for detrimental effect of bicarbonate therapy in hypoxic lactic acidosis. Science 227:754, 1985.
14. Matten JA, Neil MH, Shubin H, et al: Cardiac arrest in the critically ill, II: Hyperosmolar states following cardiac arrest. Am J Med 56:162–168, 1974.
15. Bhatt MV, Nahata MC: Dopamine and dobutamine in pediatric therapy. Pharmacotherapy 9:303, 1989.
16. Adeni S, Shankararao R, Vidyasagar D: Does atropine have a role in neonatal cardiopulmonary resuscitation? Pediatr Res 27:27A, 1990.
17. Hughes WG, Ruedy JR: Should calcium be used in cardiac arrest? Am J Med 81:285, 1986.
18. Elliott RB, Starling MB, Neutze JM: Medical manipulation of the ductus arteriosus. Lancet 1:140, 1975.
19. Susan ED: Intra-transport stabilization and management of the pediatric patient. Pediatr Clin North Am 40:263–274, 1993.
20. Jain L, Ferre C, Vidyasagar D, et al: Cardiopulmonary resuscitation of apparently stillborn infants. J Pediatr 118:778–782, 1991.
21. Child Abuse and Neglect Prevention and Treatment Programs: Final Rule. 50 Federal Register 14, 878 (April 15, 1985) (45 CFR 1340).
22. Child Abuse Prevention and Treatment Act and Child Abuse Prevention and Treatment and Adoption Reform Act Amendments: Congressional Record-Senate (June 29, 1984). P. 58951.2.

CHAPTER 10

Pediatric Cardiopulmonary Resuscitation

DAVID G. JAIMOVICH, M.D.

Outcome studies have shown that the survival rate after cardiopulmonary arrest is in many cases below 15%. The incidence of pediatric cardiac arrest has risen with the increased length of survival of children with serious illnesses, including but not limited to immunodeficiency states, cardiac and pulmonary congenital disease, metabolic disorders, malignancy, and renal disorders. It is critical that health care professionals caring for children understand the pathophysiology of cardiopulmonary arrest and the various treatment modalities.

ETIOLOGY

Eisenberg et al.[1] reviewed the etiology of cardiopulmonary arrest in children and found that the most common presentation was associated with sudden infant death syndrome (SIDS), 32%. The second most common cause was drowning (22%), and most of the other causes were respiratory. Forty-five percent of the patients were less than one year of age. Therefore, it must be remembered that the majority of cardiac arrests on transport and out of hospital are due to respiratory causes or SIDS.

Cardiopulmonary resuscitation is divided into basic life support and advanced life support. The objective of basic life support is intended for external support of circulation and ventilation for a patient who has suffered a cardiopulmonary arrest. Performing CPR provides oxygen and nutrients to vital organs until normal circulation is restored. The approach to the critically ill or injured child should be:

1. To assess and to prioritize diagnosis and treatment.
2. To establish stability of the child's vital signs.
3. To establish the ABCs of the basic airway, breathing, and circulation.

Once unresponsiveness has been established, adequate ventilation and circulation should be assessed immediately. If ventilation is absent or inadequate, the airway should be opened and rescue breathing should begin. If the circulation is inadequate, cardiac massage, to establish artifical circulation, should be started.

RESUSCITATION OF THE PEDIATRIC PATIENT

Emergency medical services evolved to meet the needs of the pediatric patient in full cardiopulmonary arrest or impending arrest. Changes have included the training of lay people in basic life support, the establishment of advanced emergency medical services, development of prehospital care by paramedic services, and the development of air and ground pediatric transport teams.

Cardiopulmonary Assessment

The obvious signs of cardiopulmonary arrest include changes in skin color, loss of consciousness, apnea, and pulselessness. Emergency room evaluation may include electrocardiographic monitoring showing a terminal rhythm, such as asystole, ventricular fibrillation, electricomechanical dissociation, or a wide idioventricular rhythm. Basic life support will maintain oxygen delivery to both the myocardium and the central nervous system. Since mouth-to-mouth ventilation will deliver only an FiO_2 of 15–18% and closed compression will produce a cardiac output of 15–20% of normal; the rescue team must begin advanced life support as soon as possible to provide the necessary oxygen delivery to the myocardium, coronary blood flow, and cerebral perfusion pressure.

A rapid cardiopulmonary assessment is performed, which should be a physiologically oriented examination to establish the patient with an impending arrest, early signs and symptoms of respiratory failure or shock.

The rescuer must remember that the primary assessment should involve the airway, breathing, and circulation (ABCs).

Establishing the Airway

Regardless of the cause of the patient's cardiopulmonary embarrassment, the first priority in resuscitation is the airway. The patency of the airway must be determined by the adequacy of ventilation and should be divided into (1) self-maintaining, (2) maintainable by simple maneuvers, (3) unmaintainable without intubation.

Many cardiac arrests may be prevented by opening the airway and restoring breathing. The goal of opening the airway of an unconscious patient is aimed at relieving the obstruction, which is usually caused by the natural structures of the airway: the tongue and the palatopharyngeal tissues. The simple manipulation of the mandible forward will tilt the tongue away from the back of the throat and will clear the airway. If the patient is semiconscious and there is some tone to the muscles of the jaw, simple tilting of the head back will cause the mandible to move forward and thereby open the airway. If the patient needs active physical support of the mandible, the head tilt and chin lift (Fig. 1) will open the airway by moving the structures forward. In pediatrics, as opposed to adults, the rescuer must be careful not to overextend the head, especially in the infant, since this may result in airway obstruction by compression of the soft tissue of the infant's trachea. If the patient has a suspected head injury, the rescuer must consider this condition, and the jaw thrust (Fig. 2) should be performed without a head tilt, thereby not extending the neck, with the head carefully supported without turning or extending it. These maneuvers also include suctioning and positive pressure ventilation via bag-valve-mask device. The patient must be assessed after each maneuver before undertaking further intervention. If simple maneuvers fail to provide a self-sustaining stable airway, a rapid oral intubation should be performed by the most skilled person on the scene.

Breathing

By modulation of the respiratory rate and the tidal volume, chemoreceptors in the respiratory center stimulate the respiratory drive to maintain a PaO_2 of 80 mmHg, $PaCO_2$ of approximately 40 mmHg, and an approximate pH of 7.40.

3. Schleien CL: Cardiopulmonary resuscitation. In Nichols DG, Yaster M, Lappe DG, Buck JR (eds): The Golden Hour Handbook of Advanced Pediatric Life Support. St. Louis, Mosby, 1991.
4. Hornchen U, Schuttler J, Stoeckel H, et al: Endobronchial instillation of epinephrine during cardiopulmonary resuscitaiton. Crit Care Med 15:1037, 1987.
5. Roberts J, Greenberg M, Knaub M: Comparison of the pharmacological effects of epinephrine administered by the intravenous and endotracheal routes. J Am Coll Emerg Physicians 7:260, 1978.
6. Roberts J, Greenberg M, Knaub M: Blood levels following intravenous and endotracheal epinephrine adminstration. J Am Coll Emerg Physicians 8:53, 1979.
7. Greenberg MI, Roberts JR, Baskin SI: Use of endotracheally administered epinephrine in a pediatric patient, Am J Dis Child 135:767, 1981.
8. Melker R, Cavallaro D, Krischer J: A pediatric gastric tube airway. Crit Care Med 9:426, 1981.
9. Pilcher DB, DeMeules JE: Esophageal perforation following use of esophageal airway. Chest 69:377, 1976.
10. Pollack MW, Fields AI, Ruttimann UE: Sequential cardiopulmonary variables of infants and children in septic shock. Crit Care Med 12(7):554, 1984.
11. Gillette PC, Garson A: Pediatric Cardiac Dysrhythmias. New York, Grune & Stratton, 1981.
12. Dhingia R, Amat-y-Leon F, Wyndham C: Electrophysiologic effects of atropine on human sinus node and atrium. Am J Med 38:492, 1976.
13. Gilman AG, Rall TW, Nies AS, Taylor P: Goodman and Gilman's The Pharmacological Basis of Therapeutics, 8th ed. New York, McGraw-Hill, 1990.
14. Scheinman MM, Thorburn D, Abbott JA: Use of atropine in patients with acute myocardial infarction and sinus bradycardia. Circulation 52:627, 1975.
15. Haynes RE, Chinn TL, Copass MK, Cobb LA: Comparison of bretylium tosylate and lidocaine in management of out-of-hospital ventricular fibrillation: A randomized clinical trial. Am J Cardiol 48:353, 1981.
16. Bernstein JG, Koch-Weser J: Effectiveness of bretylium tosylate against refractive ventricular arrhythmias. Circulation 45:1024, 1972.
17. Markis JE, Koch-Weser J: Characteristics and mechanisms of inotropic and chronotropic actions of bretylium tosylate. J Pharmacol Exp Ther 178:94, 1971.
18. Koch-Weser J: Drug therapy—bretylium. N Engl J Med 300:473, 1979.
19. Katz AM, Reuter M: Cellular calcium and cardiac cell death. Am J Cardiol 44:188, 1979.
20. White BC, Winegar CD, Wilson RF, et al: Possible role of calcium blockers in cerebral resuscitation: A review of the literature and synthesis for future studies. Crit Care Med 11:202, 1983.
21. Heining MPD, Band DM Linton RAF: Choice of calcium salt: A comparison of the effects of calcium chloride and gluconate on plasma ionized calcium. Anaesthesia 39:276, 1986.
22. Stacpoole PW: Lactic acidosis: The case against bicarbonate therapy. Ann Intern Med 105:276, 1986.
23. Gueri AD, Chandra N, Johnson E, et al: Failure of sodium bicarbonate to improve resuscitation from ventricular fibrillation in dogs. Circulation 74:IV75, 1986.
24. Graf H, Leach W, Arieff AI: Evidence for a detrimental effect of bicarbonate therapy in hypoxic lactic acidosis. Science 227:754, 1985.
25. Cingolani HE, Mattiazi AR, Blesa ES: Contractility in isolated mammalian heart muscle after acid-base changes. Circ Res 26:269, 1970.
26. Pannier JL, Leusen I: Contraction characteristics of papillary muscle during changes in acid-base composition of the bathing fluid. Arch Int Physiol Biochem 76:624, 1968.
27. Steinhart CR, Permutt S, Gurtner GH, Traystman RJ: Beta-adrenergic activity and cardiovascular response to severe respiratory acidosis. Am J Physiol 244:H46, 1983.
28. Orlowski JP: Cardiopulmonary resuscitation in children. Pediatr Clin North Am 27:495, 1980.
29. Wood WB, Maley ES Jr, Woodbury RA: The effects of CO_2 induced respiratory acidosis on the depressor and pressor components of the dog's blood pressure to epinephrine. J Pharmacol Exp Ther 139:238, 1963.
30. Martinez LR, Holland S, Fitzgerald J, Kountz S: PH homeostasis during cardiopulmonary resuscitation in critically ill patients. Resuscitation 7:109, 1979.
31. Bishop RL, Weisfeld ML: Sodium bicarbonate administration during cardiac arrest: Effect of arterial pH, PCO_2, and osmolality. JAMA 235:506, 1976.
32. Grundler W, Weil MH, Rachow EC: Arteriovenous carbon dioxide and pH gradients during cardiac arrest. Circulation 77:234, 1988.
33. Weil MH, Rackow EC, Trevino R, et al: Differences in acid-base state between venous and arterial blood during cardiopulmonary resuscitation. N Engl J Med 315:153, 1986.
34. Desmukh HG, Gudipati CV, Weil MH, et al: Myocardial respiratory acidosis during CPR. Crit Care Med 14:433, 1986.

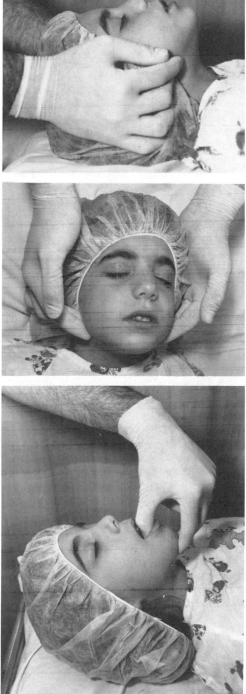

FIGURE 1, *A, B.* The head tilt-chin lift provides active physical support to the mandible and moves structures forward, clearing the airway.

FIGURE 2. The "jaw thrust" manipulates the mandible forward and lifts the tongue forward, thereby clearing the airway.

The assessment of a patient's ventilation and oxygenation is performed by the rise in the chest, inspiratory breath sounds, respiratory effort, and mucous membrane and skin color.

Once apnea has been established in the infant, the rescuer makes a tight seal covering the infant's mouth and nose, thereby providing an air-tight seal to deliver a breath. In the older child, the nose is pinched and the mouth of the patient is covered by the rescuer's mouth. Two slow breaths are delivered, once an air-tight seal has been established. Once the patient's chest rises, the rescuer may consider that an appropriate tidal volume is delivered. One breath should be administered at the end of every fifth chest compression. Patients who have a tracheostomy in place should have mouth-to-stoma or bag-valve-stoma artificial ventilation. If a leak exits through the mouth or nose, the rescuer should seal the mouth and nose with a hand.

During resuscitation and CPR, severe hypocarbia has been documented.[2] The rescue team should be acutely aware of preventing significant hypocarbia and alkalemia, since this may lead to a decreased ionized calcium level and precipitation of ventricular fibrillation.

In the pediatric patient gastric distension may occur during bag-valve-mask ventilation. This may interfere with ventilation by elevating the diaphragm and resulting in a decreased lung volume. As soon as the patient has been endotracheally intubated, a nasogastric or orogastric tube should be placed to relieve gastric distension.

Circulation

Perfusion is directly related to cardiac output, and both can be clinically assessed by evaluating the skin, central nervous system, extremities (**temperature, color, capillary refill**), urinary output, heart rate, and quality of the peripheral pulses. Hypotension can occur late in infants and children in shock or impending arrest; once this has occurred, it may be a very short time prior to a full cardiorespiratory arrest.

Once the airway has been adequately secured and breathing has been established, the pulse must be assessed. The absence of a pulse in the large arteries in an unconscious victim, without respirations, defines cardiac arrest. Owing to the infant's short neck, the carotid pulse is difficult to palpate. It is recommended that the *brachial* pulse be palpated in infants for the presence or absence of a cardiac arrest. This is located on the inside of the upper arm, midway between the elbow and shoulder. In older children and adults, while the head tilt is maintained, the carotid pulse may be palpated between the tracheal cartilage and the neck muscles.

This site is readily accessible to the rescuer who is performing artificial ventilation without the need to stop CPR. It is also appropriate to assess central circulation and not peripheral pulses such as the radial artery, which may no longer be palpable in a shock state.

External chest compression should be started when the pulse is absent or questionable. To perform external chest compression, the patient must be on a firm surface, in the supine position, and the head must not be above the level of the heart because of the effects of gravity.

The major difference in the technique of delivering chest compressions in the infant or younger child vs. the adult is the position of the heart in relationship to the rest of the chest. The recommended area of compression in these patients is one finger width below the intersection of the intermammary line and the sternum.

Two techniques may be performed for external chest compressions in the infant: one places two or three fingers on the sternum, and circles the chest of the infant forming a rigid surface on the back and using the thumbs to deliver compressions. Approximately 20% of the anteroposterior width of the infant's chest (half to one inch) should be compressed to deliver adequate cardiac output. If the child is too large for the three-finger or the encircling methods, the heel of one hand should be used two finger widths above the bottom of the sternum.

Vascular Access

Establishment of an intravenous line for the administration of fluids and medications is one of the key aspects of successful CPR. If possible, central venous access is preferable over peripheral access to administer fluids and medications. In children less than five years of age, if, after 90 seconds of attempts, a peripheral intravenous line is not established, then an intraosseous needle should be placed for vascular access.[3] Unless the rescue team has personnel experienced in the placement of central venous lines, time should not be wasted in attempting this type of cannulation.

Possible approaches to the central circulation include the internal and external jugular veins, and the subclavian, femoral, and axillary veins (see chapter on Equipment and Techniques for detailed explanation of procedures).

All medications and resuscitative fluids, including blood, used during CPR may be administered via the intraosseous route. This is considered a temporary measure when other vascular sites are not available and while the patient is being resuscitated. The benefits far outweigh the risks of this procedure and, therefore, should not be considered a "last-ditch" effort, but it should be placed after approximately 90 seconds of attempts at peripheral venous access (see chapter on Equipment and Techniques for procedure).

When peripheral venous access is not available, and intraosseous lines are either unsuccessful or cannot be placed, such as in multiple trauma of the lower extremities, the endotracheal route should be considered for rapid delivery of certain drugs during CPR. Medications included are lidocaine, atropine, naloxone, and epinephrine. Studies have shown that the rate of absorption and physiologic effects of lidocaine, epinephrine, and atropine administered via the endotracheal route compare favorably with the intravenous route.[4-6]

Large volumes of fluid should be avoided when drugs are delivered endotracheally. The total volume of fluid delivered into the trachea should not exceed 10 ml in the adult or 5 ml in the infant or small child.

Oxygen Delivery

It is not uncommon for a pediatric patient to present with mottling, which must be recognized as a changing pattern in the capillary beds as they open and close. Physiologically, it is the combination of areas of good and poor perfusion. Good perfusion is regarded as pink skin color, with saturated hemoglobin; areas of poor perfusion are regarded as cyanosis with desaturated hemoglobin from either hypoxemia or increased extraction in a low-flow state. As the patient's perfusion deteriorates, so does mental status. The infant and small child may go from an alert state to a state of combativeness or nonrecognition of parents; a more profound state of low perfusion to the central nervous system is unresponsiveness to pain. Fluctuating levels of consciousness are common in pediatric patients presenting in early states of shock. Failure to respond to a venipuncture should not be construed as "a good baby." Poor oxygen delivery to the muscles and central nervous system account for a progressive depression of the muscle tone.

INITIATING LIFE SUPPORT

Respiratory Failure

Pediatric patients may have a variety of clinical presentations leading to respiratory failure. Usually, if respiratory failure is due to pulmonary or neuromuscular disease, the patient will be alert and anxious. There will be an increased respiratory effort with the use of accessory muscles, including intercostal, subcostal, and suprasternal retractions, and nasal flaring. When these patients present with late respiratory failure, hypoxemia and hypercarbia will result in poor muscle tone, depressed central nervous system, and loss of consciousness.

In early respiratory failure, it is not always necessary to immediately intubate the patient. A rapid assessment and placing the child in a position of comfort, to maintain the airway and maintain parental contact, is of primary importance. The goal should be to minimize the patient's state of anxiety, thereby minimizing interventions such as taking rectal temperatures, performance of oral examinations, venipunctures for standard laboratory testing, and radiographic procedures which may not be necessary. The patient should have a high flow FiO_2 device, which should be administered preferably by the parent, eliminating added anxiety. The patient should not be given any oral medications or fluid to minimize the risk of aspiration should endotracheal intubation be required later.

In late respiratory failure, the parent and child must be separated, thereby providing the treating team with complete access to the patient. Immediate preoxygenation with FiO_2 1.0 should begin by bag-valve-mask ventilation. The trachea should be *orally* intubated in an emergency situation; nasotracheal intubation may be performed once the patient is stabilized. The equipment necessary for emergency tracheal intubation should always be readily available and adequately stocked (Table 1).

All patients should be considered for *full-stomach* intubation, and, therefore, cricoid pressure should be administered during the intubation procedure. By palpating the cricoid cartilage and exerting downward pressure, the esophagus is occluded between the trachea and the bodies of the cervical vertebrae. Once the endotracheal tube is in place (if uncuffed), or the cuff is inflated, cricoid pressure is released and breath sounds should be heard in the lung fields bilaterally.

Esophageal obturator airway devices are recommended for use only in adult patients. The use of this device is contraindicated in pediatric patients due to complications such as esophageal rupture, gastric distension and regurgitation, obstruction of the trachea,[8] and esophageal lacerations.[9]

TABLE 1.   Intubation Equipment

Laryngoscope with functioning bulbs
Laryngoscope blades (curved and straight)
Endotracheal tubes (appropriate size for age);
    uncuffed tubes in children $<$ 8 yrs of age
Syringe for cuff inflation
Oral airways (appropriate size for age)
Stylet
Tonsil suction
Tape
Benzoin to secure the tape
Magill forceps for possible foreign body extraction

Circulatory Failure

Once the patient is in shock, failure of the cardiovascular system to perfuse the other organ systems ensues. Decreased oxygen delivery, glucose, and the accumulation of toxic waste products in the tissues are a result of a low cardiac output state. Pediatric patients will maintain a state of normotensive shock (near normal or normal blood pressure) despite a low cardiac output in the early phases of shock; this is due to an increase in the systemic vascular resistance. The transport team should not feel secure when normal blood pressure is seen in a state of early cardiovascular shock, since the patient will also present with tachycardia, varying levels of consciousness, and poor capillary refill. When hypotension occurs, this is a late and often premorbid sign. The mortality rate for septic shock with hypotension has been reported as high as 55%.[10]

Even though the interventions chosen to restore perfusion depend on the etiology and mechanisms responsible for the state of cardiovascular collapse, the treatment for all types of shock, initially, until etiology is established, is *fluids, fluids, fluids* in boluses of 10–20 ml/kg. These fluids may be safely administered to most patients, with the exception of patients in cardiogenic shock and premature infants with an increased risk of intraventricular hemorrhage. Once the etiology has been established, appropriate therapy, including more fluids and vasoactive substances, should be administered. Clinical assessment of the patient should be performed after each intervention and prior to the administration of a new medication or more fluids.

MEDICATIONS

Atropine

Atropine increases the sinus rate and shortens the atrioventricular (AV) node conduction time[11] by blocking the cholinergic stimulation of the muscarinic receptors of the heart.[12] Atropine has very little effect on myocardial perfusion pressure, systemic vascular resistance, or myocardial contractility.[13]

In pediatric patients atropine is indicated for symptomatic bradycardia (associated with hypotension, premature ventricular beats, or poor perfusion) or asystole, and as a temporizing measure for second- and third-degree heart block.[14]

The recommended dose is 0.02 mg/kg (minimum 0.10 mg), repeated every five minutes to a maximum of 1 mg in a child and 2 mg in an adolescent. The recommended adult dose of atropine is 0.5 mg IV every five minutes until the desired heart rate is obtained. For asystole, 1 mg IV is given and repeated in five minutes if asystole persists. The onset of action of atropine is within 30 seconds and its peak effect occurs between one and two minutes after the IV dose.

Atropine increases myocardial oxygen consumption and can lead to ventricular fibrillation and tachycardia; therefore, it should be used with caution or not at all in patients with myocardial infarction or ischemia. If patients have a tendency toward life-threatening bradycardia, atropine should be avoided if possible. Patients with a diagnosis of pulmonary or systemic outflow tract obstruction and idiopathic hypertrophic subaortic stenosis should not have atropine administered, since it may decrease ventricular filling and thereby lead to a state of low cardiac output.

Bretylium Tosylate

Bretylium is effective in the treatment of ventricular dysrhythmias and is indicated when lidocaine fails to maintain a sinus rhythm. Currently there are no published data on its use in pediatric patients. Bretylium's effectiveness in adults suggests that it should be considered as a second-line antiarrhythmic in infants and children.

Since bretylium produces norepinephrine release, the cardiovascular system is most commonly affected. Usually, there is a transient increase in blood pressure[16] and a slight increase in heart rate, with a positive inotropic effect.[17] There was a mild decrease in blood pressure noted in 50 to 75% of adult patients who received bretylium.[18] It is thought to be secondary to the adrenergic blocking effects of bretylium.

The dose for ventricular fibrillation is 5 mg/kg by rapid intravenous infusion followed by another attempt at defibrillation. If ventricular fibrillation persists, administer 10 mg/kg followed by another attempt at defibrillation. In refractory ventricular tachycardia, administer 5 mg/kg; if ineffective follow this by a 10 mg/kg dose. Bretylium may be repeated every 15 to 30 minutes up to a total dose of 30 mg/kg.

Calcium

The use of calcium during CPR has fallen out of favor due to studies which have shown that in the setting of ischemia-reperfusion injury, the administration of calcium may worsen postischemia hypoperfusion and increase the likelihood of developing intracellular cytotoxic events which may lead to cellular death.[19,20]

Currently, if a patient suffers a cardiopulmonary arrest due to hypocalcemia, hyperkalemia, hypermagnesemia, or an overdose of a calcium channel blocker, calcium should be administered as a chloride salt. The pediatric dose is 10–20 mg/kg or 0.1 ml/kg of the 10% solution. Calcium gluconate seems to be as effective as calcium chloride in raising ionized calcium concentrations during CPR.[21] The calcium gluconate dosage is 100–200 mg/kg with a maximum dose of 2 gm in pediatric patients.

Sodium Bicarbonate

Cardiorespiratory arrest produces both respiratory acidosis (increased CO_2 content of the blood) and metabolic acidosis (lactic acid production secondary to poor tissue perfusion). To improve and reverse respiratory acidosis, the patient must be adequately ventilated. This usually requires that the patient receive appropriate bag-valve-mask ventilation or endotracheal intubation and adequate ventilation. The treatment for metabolic acidosis is restoration of adequate circulation and occasionally the administration of a buffer such as sodium bicarbonate.

The use of sodium bicarbonate during CPR is now a very controversial issue because of the lack of evidence showing actual benefit from receiving bicarbonate during CPR and because of the potential side effects of this drug.[22-24]

Sodium bicarbonate is indicated for the correction of significant metabolic acidosis. This acidosis depresses myocardial function by prolonging diastolic depolarization, which then depresses spontaneous cardiac activity, decreases the electrical threshold of ventricular fibrillation, and diminishes the inotropic state of the myocardium and the cardiac responsiveness to catecholamines.[25-28] Systemic vascular resistance subsequently decreases, and the responsiveness of the peripheral vasculature to catecholamines is ablated.[29] Furthermore, pulmonary vascular resistance *increases* with a decreasing pH.

Once adequate ventilation has been established and an arterial blood gas has been obtained to determine pH and $PaCO_2$, the dose of bicarbonate can be calculated by using the following formula:

$$[0.3 \times \text{weight (kg)} \times \text{base deficit}] = \text{mEq bicarbonate}$$

This equation represents half of the dose correction based on a volume of distribution of 0.6 for bicarbonate. If blood gases are not available, the initial dose should be 0.5 to 1 mEq/kg during an ongoing arrest.[30] The rescuers must remember that ventilation must be first and foremost, and once that is adequately established, it is then appropriate to administer sodium bicarbonate if necessary.

Adverse effects of sodium bicarbonate administration must be considered since these are associated with a high mortality rate (Table 2). Metabolic alkalosis will impair the release of oxygen from hemogobin to tissues[31] by causing a left shift of the oxyhemoglobin dissociation curve. Hypernatremia and hyperosmolality may decrease organ perfusion by increasing interstitial edema in the microvascular beds. The paradoxical intracellular acidosis occurs owing to the rapid entry of carbon dioxide into the cell and the slow egress of hydrogen ions out of the cell. Systemic venous and coronary sinus blood develop a hypercapnic acidosis during cardiac arrest and CPS which is worsened by the administration of bicarbonate.[32,33] A marked decrease in myocardial contractility occurs following this event.[25,26,34]

Glucose

The administration of glucose during CPR should be restricted to patients with documented hypoglycemia, since there is a potentially detrimental effect of hyperglycemia on the brain during ischemia. This may be due to an increased production of lactic acid in the brain by anaerobic metabolism. It has been shown that in a hyperglycemic environment, brain lactate concentration continues to rise for the duration of the ischemic period.[35] Studies have suggested that higher admission glucose concentrations may be an endogenous response to severe stress and not the cause of the more severe brain injury.[36] Recently, Voll et al.[37] showed that administering low-dose insulin to hyperglycemic rats after global brain ischemia can improve neurologic outcome. The medical team must be cautious since there are not enough studies to determine if the benefit of a tight control of serum glucose following cardiac arrest outweighs the risk of iatrogenic hypoglycemia.

Oxygen

Patients suffering from low cardiac output states or cardiopulmonary arrest should receive FiO_2 of 1.0. If minute ventilation is maintained and hemoglobin concentration is adequate for age, oxygen will increase arterial oxygen tension, hemoglobin saturation, and arterial oxygen content of the tissues. If adequate oxygenation is maintained, there will be a lowering of the pulmonary vascular resistance and a decrease in the right ventricular stroke work index. Even though patients may have chronic lung disease, such as bronchopulmonary dysplasia or chronic obstructive pulmonary disease, 100% oxygen should not be withheld during cardiac arrest.

TABLE 2.   Adverse Effects of Sodium Bicarbonate

Hypercapnia
Hyperosmolality
Hypernatremia
Decreased myocardial contractility
Paradoxical intracellular acidosis
Left shift of the oxyhemoglobin dissociation curve

Lidocaine

Lidocaine decreases automaticity, increases the ventricular defibrillatory threshold, and slightly increases or has no effect on the ventricular diastolic threshold for depolarization. Even though the effective refractory period of the Purkinje fibers and ventricular muscle is increased, the action potential of these fibers is decreased. Conduction times through the AV node and the interventricular septum are unaffected by lidocaine. Due to these physiologic effects, lidocaine has its antiarrhythmic action on the heart.

Animal studies have shown that when lidocaine is given by rapid intravenous bolus, there is a transient decrease in stroke work, blood pressure, systemic vascular resistance,[38] and left ventricular contractility;[39] consequently, these patients will show a compensatory slight increase in heart rate. When the usual bolus is administered at a slower rate, there doesn't seem to be any change in cardiac output, heart rate, or blood pressure when given to patients with recent myocardial infarction.[40]

Although dysrhythmias are not common in the pediatric population, patients with congenital heart disease (pre- and postsurgical) may present with life-threatening arrhythmias. Lidocaine has been shown to be effective in terminating ventricular premature beats (VPBs) and ventricular tachycardia (VT) during general surgery and pre- or postcardiac surgery. Patients suffering digitalis intoxication and acute myocardial infarctions have shown a beneficial effect from lidocaine. Patients undergoing cardiac catheterization and suffering ventricular arrhythmias during the procedure have a beneficial effect from lidocaine. It is indicated after cardioversion for ventricular fibrillation, especially with recurrent ventricular fibrillation or tachycardia. Lidocaine has shown no beneficial effect in the treatment of atrial or atrioventricular junctional arrhythmias.

Patients with severe hepatic disease or congestive heart failure commonly present with lidocaine toxicity. This is thought to be due to decreased hepatic flow secondary to a decreased cardiac output, thereby decreasing lidocaine clearance. Owing to these metabolic effects, patients with abnormal hepatic and cardiac function should receive a bolus no greater than 0.75 ml/kg, followed by an infusion rate of 10-20 μg/kg/min. An IV bolus of 1-2 mg/kg and a simultaneous administration of a constant intravenous infusion at 20-80 μg/kg/min are recommended in patients with normal cardiac and hepatic function. Toxic effects of lidocaine generally involve the central nervous system (Table 3).

Treatment for seizures and psychosis, because of lidocaine toxicity, is best handled with a benzodiazepine or barbiturate. These effects appear to be infrequent and occur only when large doses are administered. These potential side effects should not prohibit the cautious use of lidocaine.

VENTRICULAR FIBRILLATION

Ventricular fibrillation (V-Fib) is a sustained burst of multiple, uncoordinated ventricular depolarizations and contractions which have no effective cardiac output or myocardial blood flow. Reentrant impulses generated within the

TABLE 3. Adverse Effects of Lidocaine

Seizures	Disorientation
Psychosis	Muscle twitching
Drowsiness	Agitation
Paresthesias	Respiratory arrest

TABLE 4.   Causes of Lower Threshold in Ventricular Fibrillation

Hypoxia	Hypothermia
Hypercapnia	Metabolic acidosis
Myocardial ischemia	Electrolyte disturbances

ventricles, with multiple shifting circuits, maintain the fibrillatory pattern. There are many metabolic disturbances which may lower the threshold for V-Fib (Table 4). This is an uncommon rhythm in pediatric cardiac arrests, since studies have shown that over 90% of pediatric patients present with an initial electrical disturbance of bradyarrhythmia progressing to asystole, without any evidence for ventricular ectopy.[41] However, the rescue team must not forget that it is more common to see ventricular arrhythmias in adolescents and patients with congenital heart disease.[41] Electrical countershock is the treatment of choice for V-Fib and ventricular tachycardia when the patient is comatose or is pulseless. When high-voltage electric shock, properly applied, is sent through the heart, it terminates V-Fib by simultaneously depolarizing and causing a sustained contraction of the entire myocardium. Spontaneous cardiac contractions will commence, assuming the myocardium is well oxygenated and normal acid/base balance exists. Modern defibrillators deliver only direct-current (DC) shocks. Animal studies have shown that the higher the energy level, the greater the amount of myocardial damage which can potentially exist.[42,43] In addition, postdefibrillation arrhythmias may increase with higher energy doses.[44] In the majority of adult cases, energy levels of 100–300 joules (J) are successful when shocks are delivered with minimal delay.

Defibrillators should be checked periodically for accuracy in the low-energy dosages used in pediatric patients. It is preferable to use one that indicates both stored and delivered energy (see chapter on Equipment and Techniques). In general, the largest paddle that achieves full contact with the chest wall is used; this is usually 4.5 cm in diameter for infants and 8 cm for children. An interface substance should be used to provide the lowest impedance possible and the best transthoracic energy delivery. Electrode cream, electrode paste, saline-soaked gauze pads, and prepackaged pads are all acceptable. Alcohol pads should be avoided owing to serious burns that may be produced. Care must be taken so that the interface substance from one paddle does not come in contact with the substance from the other paddle, creating a short circuit and insufficient energy delivery to the heart.

The paddles must be placed so that the heart is between them. If both paddles are placed on the anterior chest, one paddle should be placed to the right of the sternum at the second intercostal space and the other placed in the left midclavicular line at the level of the xiphoid. For patients with dextrocardia, the position of the paddles should be a mirror image of the above. It is recommended that basic life support be initiated first in a patient who has been in cardiac arrest for an undetermined period of time, and performed for at least two minutes before attempting defibrillation in order to improve oxygenation and acid/base balance. Furthermore, the incidence of V-Fib as the cause of arrest in children is very low.

In the first defibrillatory attempt, 2 J/kg (maximum 200 J) should be administered initially. If unsuccessful, double the energy, 4 J/kg (maximum 360 J), and repeat twice if necessary. If the second attempt at the higher dose is unsuccessful, epinephrine should be administered (0.01 mg/kg—1:10,000 conc.), and sodium bicarbonate if metabolic acidosis is documented or if the duration of cardiac arrest warrants its administration. Basic CPR should continue, and an assessment of oxygenation and acid/base status should be done before repeating or increasing the energy dose. If V-Fib recurs frequently, an antiarrhythmic such as lidocaine or bretylium should be considered.

If open chest defibrillation is to be performed, a dose of 5–20 J of delivered energy should be used, always beginning with the lowest energy level. Paddles are applied directly to the heart and should have a diameter of no greater than 4 cm for children and 2 cm for infants. The handles should be insulated to protect the rescuer, and the paddles should be applied with saline-soaked pads. One electrode is placed behind the left ventricle and the other is placed over the right ventricle on the anterior surface of the heart.

Tachydysrhythmias are generally very sensitive to electrical conversion. There are no recently published standards for synchronized cardioversion. A dose of 0.25–0.50 J/kg, and doubled if unsuccessful, is used to terminate the rapid arrhythmia. Only those tachydysrhythmias that cause hemodynamic instability or symptoms requiring emergent treatment should be cardioverted. If the patient is stable, there is time to do a 12-lead EKG at the referring hospital attempting to clarify the diagnosis. Then, the patient should be transported with continuous cardiopulmonary monitoring and frequent reassessment of the patient's vital signs.

ELECTROMECHANICAL DISSOCIATION

Excluding ventricular tachycardia and defibrillation, electromechanical dissociation (EMD) is defined as organized EKG activity without clinical evidence of myocardial contractions. The etiology of EMD is divided into a primary and a secondary cause (Table 5).

Medications used in the treatment of primary or cardiac EMD include atropine, epinephrine, calcium, and sodium bicarbonate. In noncardiac, or secondary EMD, the primary underlying disorder must be treated to achieve a successful outcome.

A fluid value of 20 ml/kg of crystalloid solution should be considered in a patient who does not respond to medical intervention and in whom the cause of EMD is unknown, since often these patients may suffer from intravascular volume depletion. The rescuers must also consider placing pleural and pericardial needles to decompress potential air in the thoracic cavities, if clinically indicated.

CARDIAC PACING

Emergency cardiac pacing is successful in resuscitation only if initiated immediately after the onset of the arrest. Owing to the obvious pediatric emergency limitations, transcutaneous cardiac pacing may be applied to infants and children who present with this clinical picture.

The American Heart Association Advanced Cardiac Support Guidelines recommend the initial use of external pacemakers in patients with symptomatic bradycardia and suggest the use also for patients in asystole.[45]

TABLE 5.   Etiologies of Electromechanical Dissociation

Primary	Secondary
Cardiac	Hypovolemia due to pericardial tamponade
Noncardiac	Tension pneumothorax
Depletion of myocardial energy stores	Pulmonary embolism

Transcutaneous cardiac pacing has become a popular method of noninvasive pacing of the ventricles for a relatively short period of time. There are no clinical studies on the efficacy of transcutaneous pacing in pediatric resuscitation.

Patients who would benefit from cardiac pacing include those whose primary problem is impulse formation or conduction with preserved myocardial function. Patients with sinus bradycardia or high-grade AV block and a slow ventricular response would have the most benefit, as long as they have a sufficient stroke volume to generate a pulse.

Transcutaneous pacing essentially uses two stimulating electrodes on the thorax: one is placed anteriorly at the left sternal border, and the other posteriorly just below the left scapula. There are small pediatric electrodes available for infants and children, and the adult size may be used on children over 15 kg.[46] The demand, or asynchronous, mode should be selected when the patient is connected to the pacemaker; the EKG leads should be connected to the pacemaker. The stimulus output is increased until electrical capture is seen on the cardiac monitor. After electrical capture is achieved, evidence of arterial pulses must be established. To minimize the skeletal muscle contractions, which can be painful, large electrodes should be used, a 40-msec pulse duration, and the smallest stimulus should be required for capture. Patients should be sedated or administered analgesia if they are awake.

OPEN-CHEST CARDIAC MASSAGE CPR

From a physiologic standpoint, open-chest CPR is superior to closed-chest CPR in generating an appropriate cardiac output and vital organ perfusion pressure. Closed-chest CPR has replaced open-chest CPR since the early 1960s.[47] Patients receiving open-chest CPR have higher coronary and cerebral perfusion pressures[48,49] due to a lack of elevation of intrathoracic, right atrial, or intracranial pressure.

Even though there are a number of clinical indications for the use of open-chest CPR, most health care personnel cannot easily perform this procedure and the incidence of survival is very low. This is usually indicated if the patient already has an existing open chest wound and has suffered a traumatic arrest.

COMPLICATIONS OF CARDIOPULMONARY RESUSCITATION

Many complications are suffered during CPR, including injuries to the neck, thorax, and abdomen. Patients may suffer from air and bone marrow emboli, they may aspirate gastric contents, have metabolic and electrolyte disturbances, and one must not forget complications secondary to misused or dysfunctional equipment.

The largest percentage of complications during CPR involve the thoracic cavity. Krischer et al. showed that up to one-third of patients had either rib fractures, sternal fractures, or anterior mediastinal injury.[50] In that same study, patients were also reported to have upper airway complications and abdominal visceral injuries.

Pulmonary edema seems to be a frequent complication of CPR.[50,51] The etiology is diverse and includes a number of factors (Table 6). Other complications that must be considered are cardiac contusion and laceration or rupture of a coronary vessel.

Trauma to the neck, including cartilage and tracheal tears, as well as esophageal disturbances, have been reported.[52,53]

TABLE 6.   Causes of Pulmonary Edema

Airway obstruction	Left ventricular failure
Aspiration	Neurogenic pulmonary edema
Increase in negative intrathoracic pressure	Capillary leakage syndrome
Overhydration	

Metabolic and electrolyte imbalances frequently occur during CPR because of large changes of intravascular volume, administration of many drugs that increase the load of certain electrolytes (e.g., sodium bicarbonate), and severe swings in serum pH. Hypokalemia is commonly reported as a postresuscitation abnormality;[54,55] this may be due to either a rapid shift of potassium into the intracellular compartment or an endogenous hormonal release of epinephrine, insulin, or other agents.

Rescuer-associated complications are most commonly due to the spread of infection from the patient to the medical team member. This includes the transmission of hepatitis B virus and the AIDS virus.[56,57] There may be exchange of blood and/or saliva between the victim and the rescuer during mouth-to-mouth resuscitation or while performing invasive procedures.

The American Heart Association has published a physicians' statement on the theoretical risk of infection and supports a greater risk for salivary or aerosol transmission of *Herpes simplex, Neisseria meningitidis,* tuberculosis, and other respiratory infections.[45] There have been **no** documented cases of transmission of hepatitis B virus or HIV infection during mouth-to-mouth resuscitation. Mechanical ventilation or barrier devices should be accessible to all health care providers to minimize the theoretical risk of transmitting these potentially devastating viruses.[57]

SUMMARY

Unless a specific order **Do Not Resuscitate** is on the medical record, or there has been communication with the physician familiar with the patient's medical history, the decision to undertake CPR should always be made. There are a number of concerns to take into consideration when deciding to forgo CPR: these include the patient's medical history, the potential quality of life, the legal rights of the patient, treatment options, risks and benefits of therapy, and prognosis. There are many factors which will help the physician determine the course of CPR; once CPR is initiated, however, the decision to terminate resuscitation is based on many of these factors, including age, duration of CPR, and the presenting cardiac rhythm. The medical team must remember that the absence of neurologic function *should not* be applied as a criterion to stop CPR, since this is an unreliable prognostic sign. The neurologic status should be determined only after cardiovascular function is reestablished.

The outcome of the patient who receives CPR is generally balanced by two factors: the severity of the underlying illness and the time to the response of the cardiorespiratory arrest. In order to enhance survival, we must further study and come to understand the pathophysiology of cardiac arrest and vital organ perfusion.

REFERENCES

1. Eisenberg M, Bergner L, Hallstrom A: Epidemiology of cardiac arrest and resuscitation in children. Ann Emreg Med 12:672, 1983.
2. Lee WR, Baillie HD, Clarke AD, et al: An experimental comparison in dogs of expired air and oxygen ventilation during external cardiac massage. Br J Anaesth 43:38, 1971.

35. Siesjo BK: Cerebral circulation and metabolism. Neurosurgery 60:883, 1984.
36. Longstreth WT, Diehr P, Cobb LA, et al: Neurologic outcome and blood glucose levels during out-of-hospital cardiopulmonary resuscitation. Neurology 36:1186, 1988.
37. Voll CL, Auer RN: The effect of post-ischemic blood glucose levels on ischemic brain damage in the rat. Ann Neurol 36:1186, 1988.
38. Constantino RT, Crockett SE, Vasko JS: Cardiovascular effects and dose response relationships of lidocaine. Circulation 36(Suppl II):89, 1967.
39. Austen WG, Moran JM: Cardiac and peripheral vascular effects of lidocaine and procainamide Am J Cardiol 16:701, 1965.
40. Jewitt DE, Kishow Y, Thomas M: Lidocaine in the management of arrhythmias after myocardial infarction. Circulation 37:965, 1968.
41. Walsh CK, Krongrad E: Terminal cardiac electrical activity in pediatric patients. Am J Cardiol 51:557, 1983.
42. Dahl CF, Ewy GA, Warner ED, Thomas ED: Myocardial necrosis from direct current counter-shock: Effect of paddle electrode size and time interval between discharges. Circulation 50:956, 1974.
43. DiCola VC, Freedman GS, Downing SE, Zaret BL: Myocardial uptake of technetium-99m stannous pyrophosphate following direct current transthoracic countershock. Circulation 54:980, 1976.
44. Peleska B: Cardiac arrhythmias following condenser discharges and their dependence upon strength of current and phase of cardiac cycle. Circ Res 13:21, 1963.
45. Standards and guidelines for cardiopulmonary resuscitation (CPR) and emergency cardiac care (ECC). JAMA 255:2905, 1986.
46. Beland MJ, Hesslein PS, Finlay CD, et al: Noninvasive transcutaneous cardiac pacing in children. PACE 10:1262, 1987.
47. Kouwenhoven WB, Ing DR, Jude JR, et al: Closed-chest cardiac massage. JAMA 173:94, 1960.
48. Bircher N, Safar P, Stewart R: A comparison of standard, "MAST"-augmented, and open-chest CPR in dogs: A preliminary investigation. Crit Care Med 8:147, 1980.
49. Weiser FM, Adler LN, Kuhn LA: Hemodynamic effects of closed and open-chest cardiac resuscitation in normal dogs and those with acute myocardial infarction. Am J Cardiol 10:555, 1962.
50. Krischer JP, Fine EG, Davis JH, Nagel E: Complications of cardiac resuscitation. Chest 92:287, 1987.
51. Dohi S: Post-cardiopulmonary resuscitation pulmonary edema. Crit Care Med 11:434, 1983.
52. Nagel EL, Fine EG, Krischer JP, David JH: Complications of CPR. Crit Care Med 9:424, 1981.
53. Powner DJ, Holcombe PA, Mello LA: Cardiopulmonary resuscitation–related injuries. Crit Care Med 12:54, 1984.
54. Daniell HW: Hypokalemia after resuscitation [editorial]. JAMA 250:1025, 1983.
55. Thompson RG, Cobb LA: Hypokalemia after resuscitation from out-of-hospital ventricular fibrillation. JAMA 248:2860, 1982.
56. JAMA: Infection control guidelines for CPR providers. JAMA 262:2732, 1989.
57. JAMA: Risk of infection during CPR training and rescue: Supplemental guidelines. JAMA 262:2714, 1989.

CHAPTER 11

Shock

M. MICHELE MOSS, M.D.

Acute hemodynamic instability is a common reason for pediatric patients to need emergent interhospital transport. Shock is an acute, life-threatening disorder characterized by a lack of tissue perfusion and therefore a lack of tissue oxygen delivery. Despite multiple etiologies, poor tissue perfusion has predictable signs and symptoms and requires the same stabilizing therapies whatever the cause. Often empiric therapy is required when an etiology cannot easily be determined.

Oxygen delivery to the tissues is defined as the product of cardiac output and the oxygen content of arterial blood. The arterial blood oxygen content is the sum of oxygen carried by hemoglobin and dissolved oxygen. Cardiac output is the product of the heart rate and stroke volume, which in turn is determined by the cardiac preload, afterload, and myocardial contractility. Therefore, oxygen delivery to the tissues is determined by multiple variables, alterations of which can result in shock with loss of tissue oxygenation and eventual tissue death. Alternatively, if a deficit in one of these variables exists, improving one or more of the other variables can overcome the deficiency and allow for tissue preservation.

ETIOLOGY

The etiologies of shock can be categorized according to pathophysiologic mechanism, as outlined in Table 1, although overlap occurs between categories.

Hypovolemic Shock

Hypovolemic shock occurs because of a lack of preload, or ventricular filling, leading to decreased stroke volume and cardiac output. The loss of preload may be due to hemorrhage, the loss of whole blood, or to extracorporeal losses, most commonly gastrointestinal or urinary fluid loss.

Hemorrhagic Shock

Acute loss of blood, whether arterial or venous, can result in shock. Blood loss not only decreases oxygen delivery by lowering preload and hence cardiac output, but also decreases the hemoglobin level. Trauma is the most common cause of hemorrhagic shock in pediatric patients. However, any violation of the vasculature, as with surgery, invasive procedures or gastrointestinal bleeding, can result in enough blood loss to cause shock. Losing as little as 15% of the total blood volume can result in tissue hypoperfusion with physical findings of tachycardia, delayed capillary refill, and change in sensorium. With more severe blood loss, the examination reveals increased tachycardia, worsened peripheral perfusion, and severe alterations in mental status including coma.[1]

In general, patients with hemorrhagic shock have a history consistent with trauma or violation of the vasculature. However, trauma can be occult, especially in children who have been abused. Significant occult blood loss can occur with gastrointestinal bleeding or with trauma, as in cephalhematoma, retroperitoneal bleeding, or hematoma around large bony fractures.

Nonhemorrhagic Shock

Gastrointestinal fluid loss, particularly diarrhea, is the most common cause for nonhemorrhagic hypovolemia in infants and children. Vomiting alone rarely causes hypovolemic shock but contributes significantly if diarrhea is also present. Urinary losses in such disorders as diabetes insipidus or diabetes mellitus or postobstructive uropathy also can result in severe hypovolemia. Physical findings include evidence of dehydration with poor skin turgor, sunken fontanelle, dry mucous membranes, and lack of tears.

Third space losses result from tissue damage that causes the endothelial cell junctions to become loose and to allow fluid to leak from the vascular space to the extravascular space, or "capillary leak." The injury may be due, for example, to sepsis, burns, or pancreatitis. Third space losses often accompany other forms of shock, especially septic shock, thereby complicating the clinical picture.

Cardiogenic Shock

Cardiogenic shock is a broad term that covers multiple mechanisms stemming from a primarily cardiac problem. The mechanism can be an intrinsic cardiac problem, such as decreased contractility due to inflammation, or can be extrinsic, such as tension pneumothorax from chest trauma.

Decreased Contractility

Inflammation, ischemia, and toxins can injure the myocardium, decreasing its contractile function enough to cause shock. In pediatric patients, inflammation of the myocardium due to viral myocarditis or rheumatic fever is the most common cause of primary myocardial failure. Ischemia can occur with diffuse hypoxic-ischemic injuries such as near-drowning or with congenital abnormalities of the coronary arteries. Toxins, such as anthracycline chemotherapeutic drugs or endotoxin, also cause decreased contractility.

The history is helpful in determining the etiology of the decreased contractility. A history of viral symptoms (upper respiratory symptoms or gastrointestinal symptoms) or documented strep throat indicates viral myocarditis or rheumatic carditis, respectively. Infants with anomalous coronary arteries often have a history of irritability or colic, presumably secondary to angina.

Arrhythmias

Drastic changes in heart rate, either fast or slow, can decrease cardiac output. Too rapid a heart rate does not allow the ventricles to fill adequately and hence to eject enough stroke volume. Too slow a heart rate will not provide enough output over time. The most common primary arrhythmia in pediatric patients is supraventricular tachycardia. Most pediatric patients tolerate this arrhythmia well with few symptoms, but if the tachycardia continues for a prolonged period, especially at rates greater that 280 bpm, signs and symptoms of poor perfusion will develop. Other atrial arrhythmias, such as atrial flutter and atrial fibrillation, also produce poor perfusion if the ventricular rate is very fast.

Bradycardias are most commonly associated with respiratory insufficiency and failure and rarely are the primary cause of shock. Complete heart block causes loss of perfusion if it occurs acutely. Congenital complete heart block usually is well tolerated because of a compensatory increase in stroke volume. The acute onset of complete heart block occurs in patients with congenital anomalies of the heart especially ventricular inversion[2] as well as in patients with viral myocarditis or with ingestion of such toxic drugs as digoxin or propranolol.[3]

Although the history may not be specific enough to determine an arrhythmia as the cause of the hypoperfusion, the heart rate on physical examination is. Extreme tachycardia or bradycardia suggests an arrhythmia and warrants further investigation with an electrocardiogram.

Anatomic Obstruction

Anatomic obstruction to left ventricular output as a cause of shock is unique to infants in the first couple of weeks of life. Certain congenital cardiac defects listed in Table 1 require patency of the ductus arteriosus to perfuse the body. When the ductus closes postnatally, the infant acutely loses perfusion. Because the closure of the ductus arteriosus is often sudden, the history reflects the sudden onset of poor feeding, pallor, and irritability. Occasionally, the family gives the history of tachypnea or poor feeding since birth.

The physical examination is helpful early in the development of shock but is less useful when the shock is profound. As the ductus arteriosus closes in patients with coarctation and interruption of the aortic arch, the pulses are stronger before the obstruction and weak or absent below it. Accordingly, the arterial blood pressure is normal or increased in the extremities above the obstruction and markedly diminished or absent below. Perfusion to the right arm almost always originates from the aorta proximal to the obstruction; therefore, the right arm has a normal pulse and blood pressure. However, as the

TABLE 1. Categories and Etiologies of Shock

Hypovolemic	**Cardiogenic** (*(cont.)*
Hemorrhagic	Anatomic obstruction
Trauma	Coarctation of the aorta
Surgical	Hypoplastic left heart syndrome
Gastrointestinal bleeding	Interruption of the aortic arch
Nonhemorrhagic	Critical aortic stenosis
Extracorporeal loss	External obstruction
Gastrointestinal losses—vomiting,	Cardiac tamponade—penetrating trauma,
diarrhea	trauma, postoperative cardiac surgery,
Urinary loss	pericarditis
Third spacing	Tension pneumothorax
Pancreatitis	
Peritonitis	**Distributive**
Burns	Anaphylaxis
Sepsis	Hymenoptera stings
Cardiogenic	Drugs
Decreased contractility	Neurogenic
Inflammation—myocarditis, rheumatic fever	Spinal trauma
Ischemia	Drug overdose
Toxins—drugs, endotoxin	Tricyclic antidepressants
Arrhythmias	Barbiturates
Tachycardia	Sepsis
Supraventricular tachycardia	Bacteria
Other atrial tachycardias	Viruses
Ventricular tachycardia	Fungi
Bradycardia	Rickettsiae
Complete heart block	Protozoa
	Chlamydiae

shock becomes more profound, the myocardial contractility fails and all the pulses become weak.

The presence of a heart murmur in these patients is helpful in sorting out the etiology of the shock; however, in many patients a murmur is not present. Often in patients with critical aortic stenosis or coarctation the flow of blood across the obstruction is not sufficient to cause a murmur. Patients with hypoplastic left heart syndrome have a murmur of tricuspid regurgitation—if a murmur is present at all.

External Obstruction

External obstruction to left ventricular output can be due to fluid or blood collections in the pericardium or air collections in the pleural space. Cardiac tamponade occurs in the setting of chest trauma, either penetrating or blunt, or pericarditis. Pericarditis in children may be viral or postviral, bacterial, collagen vascular, or idiopathic. Bacterial pericarditis with pus in the pericardial space notoriously causes tamponade, whereas the other etiologies may not. The rate at which fluid collects rather than its volume determines whether tamponade is a risk. Hence less than 20 ml of fluid or blood that acutely enters the pericardial space can cause tamponade. Whereas, many patients with slowly developing effusions may have more than 100 ml of fluid without any evidence of cardiac tamponade.

The history in a patient with cardiac tamponade usually is obvious if chest trauma is the cause; however, patients with pericarditis can have a vague history of a viral syndrome and chest pain. In bacterial infections the presence of tamponade may be masked by other symptoms or signs of localized infections or septic shock. The physical examination with cardiac tamponade reveals muffled heart sounds, tachycardia, and jugular venous distention. A pericardial friction rub can be present, especially in patients with pericarditis. However, if the pericardial fluid collection is large, then no friction rub can be heard. Examination of the blood pressure shows a narrow pulse pressure and pulsus paradoxus. Pulsus paradoxus is accentuation of the variability in systolic blood pressure with inspiration and expiration.[4] On inspiration, patients with cardiac tamponade have a fall in pressure more than 10 mmHg lower than expiration. This alteration in pressure is best determined by auscultation of the blood pressure, but often can be detected by palpating the variability in pulse quality.

Tension pneumothorax occurs in patients who have suffered chest trauma or who have needed positive pressure ventilation, either bag-valve-mask or mechanical. Usually, the arterial blood gases deteriorate as poor perfusion develops with a tension pneumothorax. The physical examination reveals differential breath sounds and, in older children, jugular venous distention.

Distributive Shock

Distributive shock is due to abnormal distribution of cardiac output causing tissue hypoperfusion rather than lowered cardiac output. In fact, many patients with distributive shock have normal or increased values for cardiac output. Vasodilatation identified by warm extremities and bounding pulses is one of the characteristics of the physical examination with distributive shock. This vasodilatation is also the pathophysiologic mechanism for the shock in that the afterload is markedly decreased. Preload falls also because of pooling of the intravascular volume in the peripheral circulation. The most common cause of distributive shock is sepsis, but other causes include anaphylaxis, drug ingestion, and spinal cord trauma.

Anaphylaxis

Anaphylaxis is a systemic immune response, mediated by IgE in a previously sensitized patient, that results in distributive shock. The clinical scenarios for anaphylaxis include Hymenoptera stings and medications, especially penicillins. Histamine and leukotrienes C_4 and D_4 are released, causing massive vasodilatation with hypotension and endothelial injury with capillary leak. Clinically these patients are hypotensive with warm extremities and bounding pulses.

Other Causes

Massive drug overdoses, particularly tricyclic antidepressants and barbiturates, can cause a clinical picture of distributive shock. The patients will be hypotensive and vasodilated. This picture is due to massive blocking of α-receptors in the vasculature causing the vasodilatation. Injury to the spinal cord also can result in loss of sympathetic tone and massive vasodilatation with shock, termed "spinal shock." This clinical entity is difficult to differentiate in the presence of other trauma that suggests hypovolemic shock as the etiology of the hemodynamic instability.

Septic Shock

Although septic shock has many features of distributive shock, elements of hypovolemic and cardiogenic shock also are present. Septic shock is the result of a diffuse inflammatory response involving multiple different cascades of vaso-active mediators. The inflammatory response in sepsis is triggered by an infectious agent or its toxin.[5] Most commonly the infectious agent is bacterial, but it also can be viral, fungal, rickettsial, protozoan, or chlamydial. The diffuse inflammatory response can also be activated in the absence of infection by such triggers as severe pancreatitis or malignant diseases, mimicking sepsis. The cytokines, tumor necrosis factor and interleukin-1, are the two most extensively studied mediators in sepsis.[6,7] Other groups of mediators playing a role include the complement cascade and metabolites of arachidonic acid called eiconosoids, which includes the leukotrienes, prostaglandins, and thromboxanes.[8,9]

Septic shock has elements of all the major categories of shock—hypovolemia, impairment of cardiac contractility, and massive vasodilatation. The loss of vascular tone, present in the arterioles, venules, and microcirculation, leads to volume loss into the peripheral circulation and decreased return of blood to the heart. Third spacing of fluid significantly contributes to the intravascular volume loss. The microcirculation is also impaired by the presence of microemboli, fibrin aggregates, and cellular debris, preventing efficient transfer of oxygen to the tissues.[9] Although initially cardiac output can be increased in septic shock, cardiac dysfunction is present early. The maintenance of cardiac output appears to be a function of heart rate rather than improved stroke volume. Both left and right ventricular function appear to be impaired.[10] Diastolic dysfunction is present early, followed by dilation of the ventricles and systolic dysfunction.

Each patient has a varying degree of each of these components and can develop other components, often at unpredictable times. Classically, septic shock is described as having a "warm" phase and a "cold" phase. The warm phase represents the period when vasodilatation is predominant. The patient appears "well-perfused," with bounding pulses and warm extremities. The cardiac output can be normal or elevated. However, the patient will still have evidence of poor organ function, often with oliguria, altered mental status, and metabolic acidosis. The cold phase classically represents the period when cardiac output actually fails with decreased contractility. The extremities are cool with poor pulses and perfusion. These "phases" do not occur predictably, and this categorization has largely been abandoned. However, it remains important to be able to recognize the varying clinical face of septic shock.

PHYSICAL FINDINGS

The physical examination of the patient in shock shows decreased tissue perfusion, the body's attempt to compensate, and the specific etiology of the shock. Insufficient tissue perfusion is most easily assessed by examination of the extremities. Decreased peripheral pulses, delayed capillary refill, and cool and pale skin are the hallmarks of poor peripheral perfusion. Alterations in mental status also occur early with decreased perfusion. Initially the changes in mental status can be subtle, such as irritability or listlessness in an infant or confusion in an older child; but these progress to combativeness, stupor, or coma. Decreased perfusion to other organs is more difficult to assess by physical examination but can be detected with observation or laboratory evaluation. Decreased or absent urine output, the result of decreased blood flow to the kidneys, is not always obvious on initial examination but becomes apparent over time.

Compensation for poor cardiac output and poor tissue perfusion centers around redistribution of output to vital areas. Blood is redirected to the central organs, brain, heart, and kidneys—away from the peripheral tissues, skin and muscle. The poor peripheral perfusion is a result of this redistribution. Blood also may be shunted away from the gut, resulting in poor gastric emptying and intestinal ileus.

Increased heart rate is the major compensatory mechanism for improving or maintaining cardiac output when the stroke volume is limited. So, in all types of shock, tachycardia is needed to help maintain cardiac output and therefore peripheral perfusion. In patients with hypovolemic shock, the resolution of tachycardia parallels the improvement of preload as volume resuscitation occurs. The tachycardia also reflects increased demands for cardiac output, as with fever, and therefore may not resolve with resuscitation in other forms of shock if increased demands persist. The tachycardia should never be treated primarily unless a true cardiac arrhythmia is documented.

Normal values for the arterial blood pressure are age- and weight-dependent.[11] A general rule of thumb for determining the normal systolic blood pressure in a child is as follows:

$$\text{Systolic pressure} = 80 + (\text{Age in years} \times 2)$$

Hypotension is defined as a change in systolic blood pressure greater than 20% lower than the normal systolic blood pressure for the patient's age. Hypotension accompanies shock as loss of compensatory mechanisms are lost. However, arterial blood pressure is not always a dependable parameter to follow for evaluation of the severity of shock in children. In many types of shock the blood pressure may remain normal despite severe shock. Patients with distributive shock due to loss of α-receptor stimulation are more likely to develop hypotension early because of their massive vasodilatation.

Physical findings suggesting specific etiologies of shock are listed in Table 2.

LABORATORY EVALUATION

Certain laboratory and radiographic evaluations must be made in any patient in shock in order to further assess tissue insult and to guide therapy. Arterial blood gases are measured in any patient who demonstrates hemodynamic

TABLE 2.   Characteristic Physical Findings for Specific Types of Shock

Trauma	Obvious sites of bleeding Extensive bruising Cephalhematoma Lower extremity angulation or fracture
Dehydration	Sunken fontanelle (if still open) Dry mucous membranes Poor skin turgor Loss of tears
Third-spacing	Distended abdomen Tender abdomen
Decreased contractility	S_3 gallop rhythm Holosystolic murmur of mitral insufficiency
Anatomic obstruction	Differential pulses or blood pressures Murmur

Septic shock	Evidence of infection
	    Meningitis—stiff neck, bulging fontanelle
	    Pneumonia—abnormal lung examination
	    Skin infection—bullae, erythema
	    Open wounds

Anaphylaxis	Hives Angioedema of face
Spinal trauma	Neck pain Loss of lower body sensory or motor functions

instability. Determination of the arterial PO_2 assesses the presence of hypoxemia, which may be present due to decreased perfusion of the lungs in addition to any concurrent lung pathology. Correcting this hypoxemia is a crucial part of therapy. Determination of pH and PCO_2 assesses the presence and severity of metabolic acidosis secondary to tissue hypoperfusion and the patient's ability to compensate for the acidosis by increasing ventilation. Retention of CO_2 in the presence of metabolic acidosis is ominous; as it suggests that the patient is unable to ventilate adequately and respiratory arrest may be imminent.

The complete blood count includes the white blood count, hemoglobin and hematocrit levels, and the platelet count. An increased white blood count indicates presence of infection or stress. The presence of neutropenia with a low total white count also implicates an infectious process. The hemoglobin level assesses the adequacy of the blood's ability to carry oxygen. Even if blood loss is not the cause of the shock, blood replacement on the basis of the hemoglobin level is important in therapy. A lowered platelet count is indicative of diffuse intravascular coagulopathy, which can be triggered by shock with tissue damage, most commonly septic shock. Other laboratory measurements that determine the presence of DIC include elevated PT, PTT, and fibrin degradation products and a low fibrinogen level. Review of the blood smear reveals multiple injured red cells such as helmet cells.

Blood chemistries are often abnormal, especially if the patient has had loss of extravascular volume or third spacing. Significant hypocalcemia is often present in patients with capillary leak syndromes such as sepsis. Measurement of liver enzymes as well as bilirubin is useful to determine liver involvement either in the initiating process or as a result of hypoperfusion. Cultures of blood, urine, and spinal fluid are necessary in patients with presumed sepsis, especially if the etiology of the sepsis is not known. Assessment of spinal fluid may have to wait until the patient is stable hemodynamically because positioning the patient for a spinal tap may worsen hemodynamic and respiratory compromise.

Radiographic studies also should be performed. The chest radiograph allows determination of the presence of cardiomegaly suggesting cardiogenic shock, evidence of pneumonia suggesting an infectious process, or pulmonary edema which has a myriad of causes. The chest radiograph also can confirm the presence of a tension pneumothorax. Computed tomography and other radiographs are indicated in trauma patients. If a cardiac etiology is suspected, an echocardiogram is imperative for diagnosis. Structural heart disease, pericardial fluid, evidence of cardiac tamponade, and left ventricular function are all determined by the echocardiogram.

MONITORING

Monitoring of patients with hemodynamic instability includes both acute, noninvasive monitoring, which can be instituted quickly, and invasive monitoring, which is generally more accurate but more time-consuming to get in place, especially in pediatric patients. During transport of the patient, noninvasive methods are used most commonly, but at times a combination of modalities is available.

Noninvasive Monitoring

The most important aspect of monitoring is frequent repetitive assessment of the physical examination. After each therapeutic intervention, such as delivery of a volume bolus or adjustment of the dose of the inotropic infusion, reassessment of the patient's perfusion is performed. A key part of that assessment is close monitoring of the vital signs.

A continuous readout ECG is placed to assess heart rate and determine the presence of arrhythmias. The ability to print out rhythm strips is useful if arrhythmias are present. Blood pressure is measured noninvasively by manometric, Doppler, or oscillatory methods. Oscillatory methods are most convenient because they can provide automated readings at timed intervals, often with hard copy printouts. But, in cases of severe shock, oscillatory methods often cannot detect the pulse and therefore do not work. So alternative manual methods must also be available. In shocky infants blood pressure should be measured in all extremities initially to determine the presence of coarctation. Pulse oximetry gives continuous readout of the hemoglobin oxygen saturation, an important variable in oxygen delivery. As with oscillatory blood pressure monitoring, pulse oximetry will not work when perfusion is severely impaired. As perfusion improves, the pulse oximeter will be able to detect an adequate pulse and produce an oximetry reading.

Noninvasive monitoring can be performed in most modes of transport, although vibration in helicopters may hamper these methods, especially oscillatory methods of blood pressure measurement. Therefore, en route, blood pressure may need to be performed manually in an unstable patient.

Invasive Monitoring

Invasive monitoring may be very simple, as with a Foley catheter, or more complex, as with a pulmonary arterial catheter. Many pediatric patients requiring emergent transport are not yet "instrumented" with invasive monitors because of acute instability and the time needed to place certain intravascular catheters in infants and small children. However, patients who have been instrumented may need transport to another facility for further therapy or evaluation, and therefore transport personnel should be familiar with use of these devices.

Intraarterial catheters are placed for continuous blood pressure measurement and for sampling of arterial blood—most commonly, for blood gas analysis. All patients in shock who remain hemodynamically unstable should have placement of an intraarterial catheter. The most common sites for cannulation are the radial, dorsalis pedis, posterior tibial, and femoral arteries. These arteries have in common good collateral circulation and easy accessibility. Intraarterial catheters may be placed by percutaneous or direct visualization technique. Complications of intraarterial catheters include exsanguination in the event the catheter or tubing becomes disconnected or loss of perfusion distal to the catheter. The catheter and tubing must be secured carefully prior to transport to avoid disconnection during movement of the patient or secondary to continued vibration or turbulence. Frequent assessment of perfusion distal to the site of arterial cannulation is imperative.

Central venous catheterization is performed for many reasons including monitoring of central venous pressure (CVP) as a measure of preload, to secure venous access for infusion of vasoactive drugs, and for intravascular volume resuscitation. Percutaneous or direct visualization techniques are used for catheter insertion. The femoral vein is a common site for catheter placement because of its accessibility and low risk for complications. The subclavian vein and internal jugular vein are also used, more commonly in older children. In infants, these veins are less easily accessible unless one has had frequent experience; therefore, they are used less often. Alternate sites where catheters may be placed by direct visualization are the basilic vein and the axillary vein.

The tip of the central venous catheter should be within the thorax for a true central venous pressure reading. However, in the absence of abdominal distention, accurate reflections of the CVP are obtained from a catheter placed in the inferior vena cava.[12] The most common complication of central venous cannulation is infection, either at the site of insertion or within the catheter itself. This complication occurs when the catheter has been in place for a period of time and is not a problem acutely. However, the catheter should be secured with an occlusive sterile dressing after the site has been cleansed in order to deter future infection.

Pulmonary arterial catheters (PAC), often called Swan-Ganz catheters after the developers of the catheter,[13] provide a variety of hemodynamic information. The catheter consists of two pressure monitoring ports located 5–10 cm apart; the distal lumen allows measurement of pulmonary arterial pressure and the proximal reflects CVP. The tip also houses a balloon, which allows the catheter, when placed in the pulmonary artery, to advance into the smaller pulmonary arteries and occlude the lumen. This enables the distal lumen pressure port to assess pulmonary capillary pressure, a reflection of left ventricular preload. A thermistor is present near the tip of the catheter, allowing for cardiac output measurement by thermodilution technique. Other information obtained with a PAC includes mixed venous oxygen saturation, a good reflection of the adequacy of tissue oxygenation.

A PAC essentially is never indicated before emergent transport, but rarely will already be in place when moving a previously instrumented patient. When transporting a patient with a PAC, continuous monitoring of the pulmonary arterial port and the central venous port is done. A pulmonary arterial tracing should always be present. The PAC can drift into the pulmonary capillary wedge position, risking a pulmonary infarct. The catheter should also be carefully secured with a sterile dressing to prevent infection. Arrhythmias can occur with a catheter present inside the heart; therefore, the ECG is monitored continuously.

If the tip of the catheter falls back into the right ventricle, ventricular arrhythmias, including PVCs and ventricular tachycardia, can result. If the catheter falls back while in transport and cannot easily be floated back into the pulmonary artery by inflating the balloon, then the catheter should be withdrawn until central venous pressure is transduced from the distal port.

A Foley catheter is inserted to monitor urine output in patients who remain hemodynamically compromised. In the absence of renal glomerular or tubular damage, urine output is a good reflection of renal blood flow, and, hence, cardiac output. A nasogastric tube is also inserted in these patients to prevent gastric distention. When blood flow to the gut is diminished, poor gastric emptying and an ileus occur, resulting in abdominal distention. This distention hinders respiration, impedes venous return to the heart, and causes discomfort. The nasogastric tube also allows assessment of gastric pH and volume of gastric secretions.

THERAPY

Treatment of shock involves improvement of oxygen delivery to the tissues and treating the underlying cause of the shock. Often the latter is empiric therapy until a definitive diagnosis can be made. Maximizing oxygen delivery focuses on optimizing the determinants of cardiac output as well as arterial oxygenation and hemoglobin concentrations.

Airway and Ventilation

In any unstable patient attention to the airway and adequacy of breathing is priority. Patients with stable airways and adequate ventilation still need supplemental oxygen to maximize the oxygen content of the blood. During the initial resuscitation, efforts should be made to keep the oxygen saturation at 100%, no matter the FIO_2 needed to accomplish that. After stabilization, adjustment of the FIO_2 can be done to prevent oxygen toxicity. Mechanical ventilation needs to be considered in all cases of severe shock to decrease the patient's oxygen utilization. Care is taken during intubation to avoid drugs that would further compromise the hemodynamic state.

Fluid Resuscitation

Optimizing ventricular filling, or preload, during stabilization of shock is paramount no matter the type of shock. In hypovolemic shock, volume resuscitation is the definitive therapy. For trauma patients, aggressive replacement of lost blood is crucial, although volume replacement with balanced salt solutions is the initial therapy. In patients with cardiogenic shock, increasing preload can improve cardiac output because the failing ventricle needs a higher preload. If the patient has had poor intake due to the illness, preload may not be adequate for best cardiac output. Patients with distributive shock also need massive amounts of fluids owing to the loss of vascular tone and the accompanying capillary leak. Despite development of edema, common in these patients, intravascular volume still must be increased to maintain cardiac output. In patients requiring large quantities of fluid, placement of a central venous catheter to monitor CVP is helpful. This allows determination of the "optimal" CVP, which provides the best oxygen delivery, determined at the bedside by improvement in perfusion, urine output, and clearance of metabolic acidosis.

Bolus Fluids

Initial volume expansion is performed with a balanced salt solution, either 0.9% saline ("normal saline") or Ringer's lactate solution. Both solutions are isotonic with blood. Dextrose-containing fluids are avoided for volume expansion to prevent hyperglycemia. The volume of fluid recommended is 20 ml/kg given rapidly in the vein or by intraosseous needle if venous access is delayed. Boluses of 20 ml/kg are repeated as necessary for stability. In trauma patients the amount and type of fluid for resuscitation can be given according to protocol based on the severity of shock and presumed amount of blood lost (Table 3). For patients with myocardial failure smaller boluses of 5-10 ml/kg given more slowly are indicated. Patients with distributive shock may need as much as 100 ml/kg fluid for stabilization. Other fluids used for volume expansion are colloidal fluids, 5% albumin, plasma protein concentrates, and fresh-frozen plasma. FFP is impractical in the initial resuscitative effort because it has to be thawed and therefore is not readily available. Although not consistently the case, many clinicians believe that less fluid is needed for massive volume resuscitation if colloid, rather than crystalloid, fluids are used.[14]

Transfusion

Optimizing the hemoglobin concentration helps maintain oxygen delivery in all shock states. Transfusion of packed RBCs to a hemoglobin level of 13–16 grams% maximizes the oxygen carrying capacity of the blood. Overtransfusion should be avoided because polycythemia actually decreases oxygen delivery by greatly increasing peripheral vascular resistance.[15]

Maintenance Fluids

Other considerations of fluid resuscitation include provision of necessary electrolytes and glucose. After the initial salt solutions are given, attention must be paid to providing maintenance amounts of sodium, potassium, calcium, and glucose. For patients with dehydration, replacement of deficits of sodium and water need to be calculated. This replacement is given over 24-48 hours, depending on the type of dehydration.[16] Calcium replacement is provided as bolus replacement or, with recalcitrant hypocalcemia, as a continuous infusion. Patients with severe blood loss need calcium replacement, as do those with capillary leak syndromes. Extreme hypocalcemia can be seen with capillary leak presumably secondary to loss of calcium, bound to albumin, as the albumin leaks out of the vasculature. Patients with shock most often are hyperglycemic as

TABLE 3. Volume Resuscitation in Trauma Patients

Estimated Blood Loss (%)	Initial Volume Resuscitation	Total Volume Resuscitation
15–25	20 ml/kg NS or RL	If improved, NS or RL at 5 ml/kg/hr for several hours
	If no response, repeat 20 ml/kg NS or RL	Then if stable, adjust IV rate downward towards maintenance rates
25–40	40 ml/kg NS or RL	If improved, NS or RL at 5 ml/kg/hr for several hours
	If no response, either 20–40 ml/kg NS or RL or 10–20 ml/kg PRBCs or surgery if indicated	If stable, adjust IV rate downward towards maintenance rates
		Consider transfusion of PRBCs based on clinical condition and hematocrit
>40	Push PRBCs or whole blood Push NS or RL Surgery	Replace with type specific blood

Adapted from Manual of Advanced Pediatric Life Support. American Academy of Pediatrics and American College of Emergency Physicians.

a response to stress, but small infants can develop hypoglycemia. Because of this risk, monitoring glucose frequently by bedside glucometer and providing supplemental glucose are important. Glucose in the concentration of 5% is provided unless hypoglycemia has been documented. Then a bolus of glucose, 2 ml/kg of $D_{10}W$, is given, followed by increasing the glucose concentration to 10% in the maintenance fluids.

Treatment of Acidosis

Metabolic acidosis is often present due to anaerobic metabolism in the tissues from lack of oxygen delivery. If acidosis is mild, the patient can compensate and maintain an adequate arterial pH by increasing ventilation. Also, improvement of oxygen delivery with fluid resuscitation or inotropic support can resolve a mild acidosis. However, if the acidosis is severe, treatment with a buffer to maintain arterial pH is needed. Metabolic acidosis in itself can decrease cardiac function and prevent improvement in contractility with inotropic agents.[17]

Sodium bicarbonate or tris(hydroxymethyl) aminomethane (THAM) provides additional buffering ability. If the patient is ventilating adequately, then sodium bicarbonate is the drug of choice. A dose of 1 mEq/kg can be given empirically. Alternatively, the dose can be given based on the base deficit calculated from the arterial blood gas as follows:

$$mEq \ NaHCO_3 = 0.3 \times weight \ (kg) \times base \ deficit$$

Complications of overdosage of sodium bicarbonate include hyperosmolality, hypernatremia, and metabolic alkalosis.

THAM also acts as a buffer with the advantage that ventilation does not need to be adequate for it to work. Therefore, it has usefulness in patients with pulmonary complications in addition to inadequate tissue perfusion. However, the volume needed for adequate buffering is quite large, limiting its usefulness in many pediatric situations. The dose given is the following:

$$mEq \ of \ THAM = 0.25 \times weight \ (kg) \times base \ deficit$$

Complications of metabolic alkalosis and hyperosmolality can also be seen with overdosage.

Inotropic Support

Short-acting vasoactive drugs that increase cardiac contractility or improve blood pressure are needed in hemodynamically unstable patients, especially those with cardiogenic shock and distributive shock (Table 4). Patients with hypovolemic shock who have not responded to volume expansion are also considered candidates for inotropic support. Most of these drugs are catecholamines having effects on the tissue receptors, alpha (α), beta$_1$ (β_1), beta$_2$ (β_2), and dopamine, in varying degrees. One drug, amrinone, represents a new class of inotropic drugs, the bipyridines.[18]

Dopamine

Dopamine stimulates dopamine, β, and α receptors depending on the dose. At low doses, 2-5 μg/kg/min, dopaminergic effects predominate, seen as vasodilatation of the renal and mesenteric blood supply. At doses of 5-10 μg/kg/min, β stimulation prevails, seen mostly as increased cardiac contractility. Increases in heart rate can be seen at these doses, but more commonly occur at higher doses.

TABLE 4.   Inotropic and Pressor Drugs

Drug	Dose	Effect	Adverse Effects
Dopamine	2.0–5.0 μg/kg/min	Dopamine receptors, renal and mesenteric vasodilation	Tachycardia, arrhythmias
	5.0–10 μg/kg/min	β_1—improved contractility, mild increase heart rate	
	10–20 μg/kg/min	$\beta_1 + \beta_2$ and α	
	> 20 μg/kg/min	α predominates, vaso-constriction	
Dobutamine	2.5–20 μg/kg/min	Predominantly β_1—increase contractility with mild increase heart rate; mild vasodilation	Arrhythmias and tachycardia at higher doses
Epinephrine	0.05–1.0 μg/kg/min	β_1 and β_2, some α at higher doses	Arrhythmias, tachycardia even at low doses, hyperglycemia, ketosis, increased myocardial oxygen demand
Norepinephrine	0.5–1.0 μg/kg/min	Predominantly α—profound vasoconstriction, increase contractility	Decreases perfusion to extremities, kidneys, liver, and other organs
Amrinone	Load: 0.75 μg/kg followed by infusion 5–10 μg/kg/min	Increases contractility; vasodilator	Thrombocytopenia, nausea

Adapted from Moss M: Syncope and hypotension. In Burg FD, Ingelfinger JR, Wald ER (eds): Gellis and Kagan's Current Pediatric Therapy, 14th ed. Philadelphia, W.B. Saunders, 1993.

Also at higher doses, the α effects begin to be apparent, and at doses greater than 20 μg/kg/min predominate. Although there remains continued increased contractility, vasoconstriction becomes apparent both clinically and by measurement of systemic vascular resistance. The starting dose of dopamine depends on what response is desired and the level of hemodynamic instability present. If improved renal blood flow—and hence urine output—is desired, then start at a dosage of 2 μg/kg/min. For poor perfusion or hypotension, begin with doses of 5–10 μg/kg/min. Because of its short half-life, the dose of dopamine can be changed rapidly by simply adjusting the infusion rate.

Dobutamine

In contrast to dopamine, dobutamine affects primarily the β_1 receptors located in the heart. Positive inotropic effects predominate, with little effect on heart rate or peripheral vascular tone. Dobutamine is most useful in patients with cardiogenic shock and poor contractility. For patients who are hypotensive due to distributive or hypovolemic shock, it has less usefulness. If the patient with distributive shock, especially septic shock, is felt to have poor contractility, then dobutamine can be of use. The starting dose is 5 μg/kg/min and is adjusted upward if necessary for improved results.

Epinephrine

Epinephrine is an endogenous hormone synthesized in the adrenal medulla. Blood levels vary over a wide range in critically ill children.[19] At low doses, epinephrine stimulates β_1 receptors, producing increased contractility. Heart rate is also increased, even at low doses, as is the risk of arrhythmias. At higher doses, β_2 receptors are stimulated, producing a fall in systemic vascular resistance.

When the dose is increased, α receptor stimulation is seen with systemic vascular resistance now increasing. Other clinical effects noted are hyperglycemia, ketogenesis, hypophosphatemia, and hypokalemia. Epinephrine is used as a continuous infusion in patients with severe shock and hypotension due to sepsis or myocardial failure. It is the drug of choice for anaphylaxis. Epinephrine should also be used after cardiac arrest with hypotension.

Norepinephrine

Norepinephrine demonstrates mostly α and β_1 receptor effects, predominately increased systemic vascular resistance (SVR) with some improvement in contractility. The increase in afterload produced by the rise in SVR can improve coronary perfusion. Blood flow to the liver, kidneys, and gut is decreased by norepinephrine in normal adults. Clinically this drug is most useful in patients with distributive shock who have hypotension on the basis of a fall in SVR.[20] Patients with septic shock who have been intravascularly volume resuscitated and have not improved with dopamine and possibly epinephrine are candidates for norepinephrine. Patients with drug overdoses or spinal trauma who have lost α receptor tone respond well to norepinephrine. The starting dose is .05 μg/kg/min and is adjusted as high as 1 μg/kg/min.

Amrinone

Amrinone is pharmacologically different from the catecholamine drugs discussed above. Its action occurs by inhibition of phosphodiesterase, causing positive inotropic effects as well as relaxation of vascular smooth muscle. Clinically amrinone appears most useful in patients with primary myocardial failure. Amrinone has a relatively long half-life for a vasoactive drug and is metabolized in the liver. The organ dysfunction related to many shock syndromes makes using this drug problematic. The dosage recommended is for a loading dose of 0.75 mg/kg, followed by an infusion of 5–10 μg/kg/min. This dose was based on data from adults, not infants or children. In a small reported study of children, the loading dose recommended was higher, 3–4 mg/kg in children and infants.[21] Many clinicians bypass the loading dose and start with a continuous infusion, realizing that peak effect may not be noted for several hours.

Specific Therapies

Besides improving tissue oxygen delivery, one must start specific therapy for the cause of the shock as soon as possible to reverse the situation. Often, however, this specific therapy must be started empirically while definitive tests are being performed.

Antibiotics

The use of antibiotics is the best example of the use of empiric therapy. The definitive diagnosis of bacterial infection as the cause of shock can take considerable time, especially since culture results may not be available for several days. Of course, in septic shock antibiotics must be started immediately upon suspicion of bacterial infection, not when culture results are available. After the patient stabilizes, and if the cultures show no evidence of bacterial infection, antibiotics can be discontinued. Often a decision is made to continue the empiric antibiotics for a full course because of inconclusive results or concern that, clinically, a bacterial infection was the inciting event, despite lack of positive culture results. Choice of empiric antibiotics is based on the age of the patient, predisposing conditions, and the associated source of infection. Infants less than one month of age are at risk from infections due to Group B Streptococcus and enteric gram-negative organisms. *Listeria monocytogenes* is a risk in patients up to three months old. Previous healthy older infants and children develop septic shock predominantly by *Streptococcus pneumoniae, Neisseria meningitidis,* and *Haemophilus influenzae,* although the incidence of the latter has decreased markedly since routine vaccination began. Infants and children with chronic conditions requiring in-dwelling instrumentation are predisposed to infections by staphylococcal and gram-negative organisms. Antibiotics appropriate for these infectious agents are necessary for appropriate empiric therapy.

Prostaglandin E$_1$

Infants felt to have obstruction to left heart outflow need infusions of Prostaglandin E$_1$ to restore patency of the ductus arteriosus (DA). An infant with left heart obstruction whose DA has closed cannot be stabilized until the vessel is opened, allowing blood flow to return to the body. The initial dose in a critically ill infant is 0.1 µg/kg/min. Often, if the DA is patent and the desire is to maintain its patency, a lower dose can be used. The side effects of PGE$_1$ include periodic breathing, apnea, hypotension secondary to vasodilatation, and irritability. Stabilization of the airway usually is necessary in these infants because of both the profound shock and the PGE$_1$. Volume infusions can reverse the hypotension from vasodilatation. PGE$_1$ also should be considered in infants less than 2 weeks old with shock of undetermined etiology—most commonly sepsis or left heart obstruction—until an echocardiogram can be performed to confirm the presence or absence of heart disease.

Vasodilators

In patients with decreased myocardial contractility, the compensatory increase in systemic vascular resistance can result in worsening of the cardiac output. Therefore, judicious adjustment of the systemic vascular resistance with vasodilating agents is often warranted—but only after inotropic drugs have been started and the blood pressure stabilized. Additionally, preload must be optimal before beginning a vasodilating agent. Starting these medications prior to adequate stabilization can result in severe hypotension. Intraarterial and, preferably, central venous monitoring should be in place. Nitroprusside is the initial drug of choice for vasodilatation. It works both on the arteriolar and venous circulations, causing a fall in systemic vascular resistance as well as a fall in preload. The starting dose is 0.5 µg/kg/min, increasing to a maximum of 10 µg/kg/min. Accumulation of toxic degradation products with build-up of cyanide has been reported, especially in patients with organ dysfunction and with total cumulative doses greater than 10 mg/kg. Other vasodilators used are phentolamine, an α-blocker, nitroglycerin and captopril, an ACE-inhibitor. Captopril is available in enteric form only. Enalaprilat is an intravenous ACE-inhibitor, but is given in bolus form, not as a constant infusion.

Pericardiocentesis

External cardiac obstruction, cardiac tamponade, or tension pneumothorax must be treated by drainage of the obstruction. Hemodynamic stability is not possible without relief of the obstruction. Tension pneumothorax can be emergently relieved by needle thoracentesis, followed by placement of a chest tube. The needle thoracentesis can acutely relieve the "tension" by draining off some of the air, but a tube must be inserted to prevent reaccumulation of air, blood, or other fluid. Cardiac tamponade also can be relieved by needle pericardiocentesis.

If blood or pus is the cause, a large-bore needle, 14- or 16-gauge, is needed to drain enough fluid to relieve the tension. Reaccumulation of fluid in pericarditis is prevented by a pericardial drainage tube, which can be placed percutaneously. In chest trauma patients with cardiac tamponade, surgical exploration is necessary. When pus from bacterial infection is the cause of the tamponade, surgical drainage with a pericardial window is the treatment of choice to drain the pus adequately and to prevent creation of constrictive pericarditis later.

Antihistamines

Patients with anaphylaxis, in addition to epinephrine and volume expansion to maintain cardiac output, need antihistamine and anti-inflammatory therapy. Diphenhydramine is given at a dose of 1-2 mg/kg intravenously and repeated as needed every 4-6 hours. Corticosteroids, either dexamethasone, 0.25-0.5 mg/kg intravenously, or methylprednisolone, 1-2 mg/kg intravenously, are also given, particularly if airway edema or bronchospasm is present. Beta-agonist bronchodilators also can be administered, if necessary, in addition to the epinephrine infusion if bronchospasm is problematic.

REFERENCES

1. Manual of Advanced Pediatric Life Support. American Academy of Pediatrics and American College of Emergency Physicians, 1989.
2. Mullins CE: Ventricular inversion. In Garson A, Bricker JT, McNamara DG (eds): The Science and Practice of Pediatric Cardiology. Philadelphia, Lea & Febiger, 1990.
3. Johnson JL, Lee LP: Complete atrioventricular heart block secondary to acute myocarditis requiring intracardiac pacing. J Pediatr 78:312-316, 1971.
4. Curtis EI, Reddy PS, Uretsky BF, et al: Pulsus paradoxus: Definition and relation to the severity of cardiac tamponade. Am Heart J 115(2):391, 1988.
5. Danner RL, Natanson C, et al: Microbial toxins: Role in the pathogenesis of septic shock and multiple organ failure. In Bihari DJ, Cerra FB (eds): New Horizons: Multiple Organ Failure. Fullerton, Society of Critical Care Medicine, 1989.
6. Michie HR, Manogue KR, et al: Detection of circulating tumor necrosis factor after endotoxin administration. N Engl J Med 318:1481, 1988.
7. Baracos V, Rodemann HP, et al: Stimulation of muscle degradation and prostaglandin E$_2$ release by leukocyte pyrogen (interleukin-1). N Engl J Med 308:553, 1983.
8. Zimmerman JJ: Sepsis/septic shock. In Fuhrman BP, Zimmerman JJ (eds): Pediatric Critical Care. St. Louis, Mosby, 1992.
9. Rackow EC, Astiz ME: Mechanisms and management of septic shock. Crit Care Clin 9(2):219, 1993.
10. Parker MM, Shelhamer JH, et al: Profound but reversible myocardial depression in patients in septic shock. Ann Intern Med 100:483, 1984.
11. Report of the Second Task Force on Blood Pressure Control in Children. Pediatrics 79:1, 1987.
12. Chait HI, Kuhn MA, Baum VC: Inferior vena caval pressure reliably predicts right atrial pressure in pediatric cardiac surgical patients. Crit Care Med 22(2):219, 1994.
13. Pollack MM, et al: Bedside pulmonary artery catheterization in pediatrics. J Pediatr 96:274, 1980.
14. Imm A, Carlson RW: Fluid resuscitation in circulatory shock. Crit Care Clin 9:(2):313, 1994.
15. Lister GL, Hellenbrand W, et al: Physiologic effects of increasing hemoglobin concentration in left-to-right shunting in infants with ventricular septal defects. N Engl J Med 306:502, 1982.
16. Parenteral fluid therapy: Deficit therapy. In Behrman RE, Kliegman RM (eds): Nelson Textbook of Pediatrics. Philadelphia, W.B. Saunders, 1992.
17. Perkin RM, Anas NG: Nonsurgical contractility manipulation of the failing circulation. Clin Crit Care Med 10:229, 1986.
18. Notterman DA: Pharmacology of the cardiovascular system. In Fuhrman BP, Zimmerman JJ (eds): Pediatric Critical Care. St Louis, Mosby, 1992.
19. Notterman DA, DeBruin W, Metakis L: Plasma catecholamine concentrations in critically ill children—evidence of early beta-adrenergic receptor desensitization. Pediatr Res 25:42A, 1989.
20. Desjars P, Pinaud M, et al: A reappraisal of norepinephrine therapy in human septic shock. Crit Care Med 15:2, 1987.
21. Lawless S, Burckart G, et al: Amrinone in neonates and infants after cardiac surgery. Crit Care Med 17:751, 1989.

CHAPTER 12

Airway Management

RICHARD BERENS, M.D.
SUSAN DAY, M.D.

The pediatric airway deserves special attention in this handbook of pediatric transport medicine. Knowledge of the anatomic development and normal physiology of the airway is the basis for understanding the pathophysiology and management of respiratory disease in the children under our care. We begin this journey as all good travelers do by understanding the "lay of the land."

INTRODUCTION TO THE AIRWAY

The anatomy of the airway (Fig. 1[1-5]) begins at the point of air entry through the nares or mouth. The air travels down the nasopharynx, past the turbinates,[1] the adenoidal tissue,[2] and the velopharyngeal sphincter, arriving at the oropharynx.[3] Air also flows orally from the lips past the teeth, the tongue, and the tonsillar tissue and meets the nasopharyngeal air at the oropharynx. Once through the oropharynx, the air is directed past the epiglottis,[4] the arytenoids, the false cords, the true cords, the subglottic space, and into the trachea.[5] Once in the trachea, the gas is moved through the bronchi and bronchioles into the alveoli, where gas exchange occurs.

The pediatric airway has some important characteristics that should be understood by the patient care providers on the transport team. We will describe the normal features followed by examples of congenital and acquired pathology.

The nasopharynx is the primary path of respiration in the infant. The nasopharynx may become obstructed from tissue edema, such as from a viral upper respiratory infection or tissue hypertrophy as seen with either adenoidal hypertrophy or nasopharyngeal polyps. The infant may also have congenital choanal stenosis or atresia. These anomalies may present with apnea and cyanosis at rest, relieved only by crying. As the child matures, the nasopharyngeal diameter enlarges and obligate nasal breathing changes to a more balanced oronasal distribution.

The oropharynx of the infant differs from that of the adult. The tongue may appear to be enlarged if the mandible is small, as in Pierre Robin syndrome. The tongue, soft palate, and epiglottis function so that the infant is capable of eating and breathing without aspirating. Tonsillar tissue enlarges during upper respiratory infections, resulting in sonorous or stertorous breathing, especially while sleeping. The oropharynx may become obstructed from thickening of the retropharyngeal space secondary to cellulitis or an abscess.

The epiglottis normally has an elongated flexible consistency during childhood, as opposed to the rigid cartilaginous structure of the adult. The increased

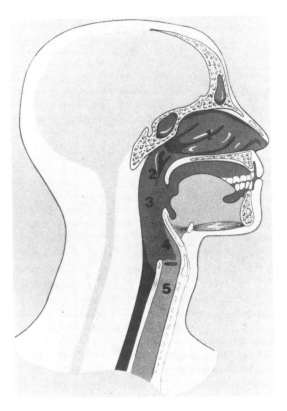

FIGURE 1. Normal anatomy of the pediatric airway. (From Roberts JT: Fundamentals of Tracheal Intubation. New York, Grune and Stratton, 1983, with permission.)

flexibility may respond to the negative inspiratory pressure of the normal respiratory effort by folding into the glottic opening, causing a high-pitched stridorous noise during inspiration. This condition, laryngomalacia, is a very common cause of stridor in the infant.[8,16] The epiglottis can be the site of infection from *Haemophilus influenzae* type B bacteria. This condition presents with fever, drooling, muffled voice, toxic appearance, and sometimes stridor. With the onset of immunizations against *H. influenzae*, the incidence of epiglottitis has dropped dramatically.[11]

The glottis of the child is positioned more caphalad, at the levels of C2–C4. By adulthood the maturation process elongates the head and neck structures, resulting in a migration of the glottis to C4–C6. The relatively short distance from the teeth to the glottis may be the reason that it is easy to overshoot the glottis during attempts at intubating children.

The narrowest part of the airway in children is the subglottic area, as opposed to the glottis in adults. The subglottic space of the infant, already narrowed at this stage of development, may be the site of edema from viruses, allergies, or trauma. The syndrome of croup, or laryngotracheobronchitis, consists of subglottic edema leading to a harsh seal-like barky cough and inspiratory stridor. The trachea and bronchial tree take on the cartilaginous consistency of the arytenoids and epiglottis. The trachea consists of a series of horseshoe-shaped cartilaginous rings with a soft membranous area posteriorly. The cricoid ring is a continuous circle of cartilage and the narrowest part of the trachea. The tracheal rings may be soft, responding to normal tidal breathing by partial occlusion and subsequent stridorous breath sounds (tracheomalacia). Congenital

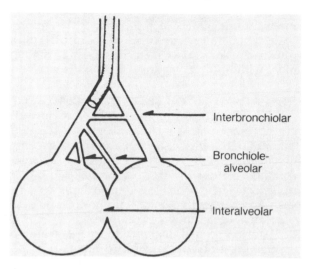

FIGURE 2. Collateral ventilation of the lung. (From Rogers M: Textbook of Pediatric Intensive Care, 2nd ed. Baltimore, Williams and Wilkins, 1992, with permission.)

Interbronchiolar

Bronchiole-alveolar

Interalveolar

vascular rings that encircle the trachea lead to maldevelopment of the cartilaginous structures, causing an isolated area of collapse that may persist for months to years after surgical repair of the vascular ring. Another congenital anomaly that may require emergent airway management is tracheoesophageal fistula.

The pulmonary parenchyma has a dynamic development from birth to adolescence. The total number of alveoli increases from 30 million to 300 million within the first eight years of life, a growth rate equal to one alveolar unit per second. Differential ventilation occurs with the development of pores of Kohn and channels of Lambert allowing for alveolus-to-alveolus and bronchiole-to-alveolus ventilation, respectively (Fig. 2). This process maintains functional residual capacity by preventing absorption atelectasis of alveoli in which the end bronchus is plugged with mucus.

With this brief description of the development of normal anatomy and some of the more common airway problems, we will now discuss the specific airway procedures and situations that may present themselves on transport of the critically ill or injured pediatric patient.

INDICATIONS FOR ENDOTRACHEAL INTUBATION

Indications for endotracheal intubation are listed in Table 1 and can be divided into these broad categories: failure of gas exchange; airway obstruction; airway protection; hemodynamic instability; and airway access for therapeutic

TABLE 1.   Indications for Endotracheal Intubation

Failure of gas exchange	Airway protection
Hypoxemia: $PaO_2 < 60$ with $FiO_2 \geq 0.6$ without	Loss of airway reflexes: gag, cough
cyanotic heart disease	Gastric lavage
Hypercapnia: $PaCO_2 > 50$, acute and unresponsive	Glasgow coma score < 9
to other airway maneuvers or medications	Hemodynamic instability
Apnea	CPR
Chest wall dysfunction: neuromuscular disease,	Shock
flail chest	Airway access for therapeutic interventions
Upper airway obstruction	Emergency drug administration
Viral or bacterial infection	Pulmonary toilet
Anaphylaxis	Hyperventilation: increased intracranial pressure,
Foreign body	metabolic acidosis, pulmonary hypertension

interventions. Often in the transport situation it is prudent to intubate the patient's trachea electively before definitive criteria have been reached. Thus, the transport team can avoid emergent airway management in an unstable environment with minimal resources at their disposal.

PREPARATION FOR ENDOTRACHEAL INTUBATION

The first responsibility of a care provider is assessment of the airway. The objective assessment includes reviewing the patient's clinical course, physical examination, pulse oximetry, and blood gas analysis. Respiratory failure, cardiovascular failure, and central nervous system decompensation are the most common reasons for assisting ventilation and intubating the trachea prior to transport. These patients tend to be the sickest, so we will review first the cardiovascular changes that occur with positive pressure ventilation before we discuss placement of the endotracheal tube.

During normal tidal breathing, we create negative intrapleural pressure by contracting the diaphragm, intercostal muscles, and accessory muscles. The sicker the patient, whether from extrinsic obstruction of the airway or intrinsic pulmonary disease, the more negative pressure the patient generates to provide air movement and gas exchange. As negative intrapleural pressure develops, blood flow increases to the right ventricle, and with expansion of the lungs, the pulmonary vessels are compressed, filling the left ventricle. Thus, adequate cardiac output is preserved. Initiation of positive pressure alone utilizing a Mapleson device with continuous positive airway pressure (CPAP) may decrease venous return, causing significant hypotension in the hypovolemic patient. One must take care to evaluate fluid status before initiating any positive pressure manipulations.

The changes in carbon dioxide provide differential changes in the systemic and pulmonary vascular beds. Hypercarbia is a systemic vasoconstrictor, secondary to catecholamine release and intrinsic firing of peripheral autonomic nerves. The pulmonary bed responds with vasoconstriction, which increases right heart work and compromises the patient with acute right heart failure. Hypocapnia lowers the systemic and pulmonary vascular resistances. The cardiovascular responses to endotracheal intubation are profound. One sees an increase in both heart rate and blood pressure equal to other stressful situations. In those patients presenting with poor cardiovascular status—e.g., end-stage cardiomyopathy or atherosclerotic heart disease—the hemodynamic response to intubation may precipitate a myocardial infarction.

The process of intubating the trachea begins with adequate preparation. SOAP is a mnemonic device that is extremely useful for setting up equipment before intubation (Fig. 3).

"S" stands for suction. This is first and should NEVER be forgotten, because of the risk of vomiting and aspiration. The suction catheter should be the large-bore plastic type with multiple distal openings commonly referred to as a Yankauer. Two varieties are used in pediatrics, neonatal and regular, of which the smaller is useful only in premature babies. The suction pressure should always be at the highest level during intubation, approximately –200 mmHg.

"O" stands for oxygen. The patient in need of intubation will need supplemental oxygen, and appropriate oxygen sources should be identified prior to airway control and intubation. The patient's response to oxygen can be monitored noninvasively using a pulse oximeter.

"A" stands for airway equipment. The simplest of these is the patient's own unobstructed self-initiated airway control. Other adjuncts include nasopharyngeal

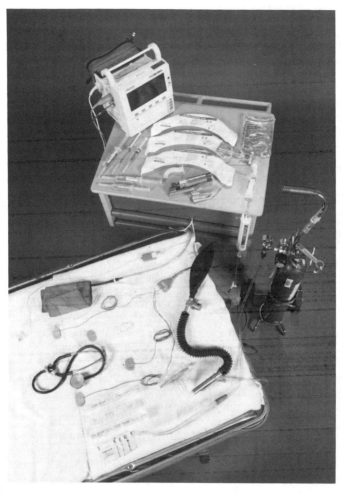

FIGURE 3. Airway adjuncts, intubation equipment, medications and monitoring equipment utilized for the routine endotracheal intubation.

airways, oropharyngeal airways, positive pressure devices with mask, endotracheal tubes and stylets, laryngoscopes, tracheostomy tubes, and cricothyrotomy kits. The preparation of this equipment will depend on the likelihood of need and your skill and experience. Remember, committing yourself to providing an artificial airway obligates you to have an alternative plan in case your first plan fails.

"P" has multiple meanings—personnel, positive pressure, and pharmacy. Airway management is not a task for one person. Once management is initiated, the adequacy of ventilation, oxygenation, and perfusion needs to be assessed. This may necessitate drawing blood gases, changing oximeter probes, and evaluating frequent vital signs and capillary refill. The caregivers may need to be replaced frequently, especially for the patient requiring high levels of respiratory and cardiovascular support.

Positive pressure devices are varied. The simplest is the caregiver's mouth and lungs. This option is undesirable for obvious reasons, yet is still an option nonetheless. Because of concerns about infectious diseases, we highly discourage the use of mouth-to-mouth, tube, or tracheostomy without some interposed one-way valve and/or filter. The other positive pressure devices are divided into hand-held devices and mechanical ventilators. We will limit our discussion to the hand-held devices: the Mapleson devices and the self-inflating devices.

The Mapleson devices most commonly used are of the D type. These consist of a universal adapter for attachment to the mask or endotracheal tube, a fresh gas inlet, a pop-off valve, and a conduit for exhaled gases leading to a collapsible neoprene or latex bag. The device can be used for both spontaneous and controlled ventilation. The closer the fresh gas flow to the endotracheal tube, the smaller the dead space with less rebreathing of carbon dioxide. The pop-off device is variable, allowing for changing levels of CPAP in the spontaneously breathing patient and peak inspiratory pressure (PIP) and positive end-expiratory pressure (PEEP) in the patient needing controlled ventilation. The device requires a minimum gas flow of twice the minute ventilation in order to prevent rebreathing of exhaled gases. This may limit its use in large patients with a high minute ventilation. These devices require continuous gas flow and cannot be used if continuous flow stops. For patients with extremely stiff lungs, these devices may fail as the compliance of the delivery bag may be better than that of the lungs, causing aneurysmal bulging of the delivery bag instead of lung expansion.

The self-inflating devices consist of a single unit that has a universal adapter to connect to the endotracheal tube or mask, a fixed, high-pressure pop-off valve, and a one-way valve that connects directly to the self-inflating reservoir bag. These are useful in the patient with normal pulmonary compliance in whom controlled ventilation is required. The devices require no fresh gas flow to function, as the self-inflating bag uses its own elastic properties to expand. This device should be with every intubated patient in case of fresh gas flow failure. The patient is protected against rebreathing inspired gases by the one-way valve, making this the device of choice in the large patient with a high minute ventilation exceeding 7.5 liters per minute of flow. This is based on the maximum limit of 15 lpm of most conventional oxygen flow meters. These devices produce forward flow of fresh gas only when the reservoir bag is squeezed. Therefore, their use is limited in the spontaneously breathing patient unless the care provider assists each breath. They may become useless in patients with poor pulmonary compliance, as the fixed high pressure limit of the pop-off valve may be reached before the patient's lungs are inflated.

One must ensure that all equipment is working properly before starting the management of the airway, especially when the caregiver begins to take over the work of breathing, either pharmacologically or mechanically.

PHARMACOLOGY OF AIRWAY MANAGEMENT

One prepares for intubation by assembling all the necessary equipment and personnel, positioning the patient in a fashion that will enhance visualization of the glottis, and proceeding with appropriate pharmacologic measures to enhance safe placement of the endotracheal tube. Each patient has his or her individual needs and no cookbook approach can be used. We will discuss the different pharmacologic agents in the order in which they are usually given (Table 2).

OXYGEN (O$_2$)

The first drug given to the patient prior to intubation should be oxygen. The delivery of O$_2$ should occur for three minutes of normal tidal ventilation, or for three vital capacity breaths. This is done to eliminate the nitrogen from the

TABLE 2. Medications to Facilitate Endotracheal Intubation

Medication	Dose	Onset	Effects
Anticholinergic agents			
Atropine	0.01–0.04 mg/kg (minimum 0.1 mg)	30–90 sec	Tachycardia, dry mouth, CNS toxicity
Glycopyrrolate	0.005–0.02 mg/kg	1 min	Tachycardia, dry mouth, no CNS effects
Sedative and hypnotic agents			
Diazepam	0.5–1.0 mg/kg	Immediate	Sedation, amnesia, anticonvulsant, hemodynamic stability in well-hydrated patient. Hypotension with narcotics. Thrombophlebitis
Midazolam	0.2–0.3 mg/kg	2–3 min	Same as diazepam. Less thrombophlebitis
Thiopental	3–5 mg/kg	30 sec	Anesthesia. Apnea, hypotension, tachycardia, reduction of ICP
Ketamine	1–2 mg/kg	30–60 sec	Dissociative anesthesia, minimal amnesia, analgesia. Hypertension, cardiovascular stimulation, emergence delirium. Sialorrhea. Preservation of airway reflexes, bronchodilation. Increased ICP
Morphine	0.05–0.1 mg/kg	1–2 min	Analgesia. Hypotension, bradycardia: worse with hypovolemia. Respiratory depression
Fentanyl	2–5 μg/kg	5–6 min	Analgesia. Fewer cardiovascular effects than morphine. Rigid chest or seizures with rapid injection
Meperidine	0.5–1.0 mg/kg	< 5 min	Analgesia
Etomidate	0.3 mg/kg	30–60 sec	Minimal cardiovascular effects. Adrenocortical suppression.
Neuromuscular blocking agents			
Succinylcholine	1–2 mg/kg	30–60 sec	Depolarization. Tachycardia or bradycardia; rise in serum K$^+$; increase in muscle tone, and intraocular, intracranial, and intragastric pressure
Vecuronium	0.1–0.3 mg/kg	60–90 sec (higher dose)	Nondepolarizing
Atracurium	0.4–0.5 mg/kg	2–3 min	Nondepolarizing. Hypotension, tachycardia
Pancuronium	0.08–0.1 mg/kg	3–5 min	Nondepolarizing, longer acting. Tachycardia

CNS = central nervous system; ICP = intracranial pressure.

alveoli. Functional residual capacity (FRC) is the volume of gas in the lungs at end expiration. This gas consists of 100% O_2 if pretreatment with O_2 is effective. The extra oxygen in the lungs at FRC allows time to perform the intubation before arterial desaturation occurs. This is especially important in the young child, who has a lower FRC and higher O_2 consumption per minute than the older child or adult. Additional factors that may heighten one's suspicion of low FRC are obesity, supine position, previous sedative agents, pneumonic or atelectatic pulmonary changes, or congestive heart failure. Concerns about O_2 toxicity should be deferred until after safe placement of the endotracheal tube and evidence that adequate tissue oxygenation has been achieved.

VAGOLYTIC AGENTS

Atropine

The next agent generally given could be a vagolytic agent to prevent bradycardia from vagal stimulation during laryngoscopy. This agent usually is atropine at a dose of 10–40 μg/kg, the onset of this drug is 30–90 seconds after intravenous administration. A minimal dose of 0.1 mg is recommended to prevent paradoxical bradycardia.[14] This dose also provides a beneficial side effect of drying salivary secretions, though the onset of this effect takes longer than 60–90 seconds. The tachycardia seen after administration may be detrimental to patients with myocardial ischemia of any etiology. It has a tertiary structure, allowing rapid transfer across the blood-brain barrier, making psychosis a potential side effect.

Glycopyrrolate

Glycopyrrolate is a competitive inhibitor of acetylcholine at the muscarinic receptors. It is a poorly soluble, synthetic quaternary ammonium compound. Because of its quarternary form it crosses the blood-brain barrier poorly. It has a less rapid onset than atropine and a more rapid clearance, with an elimination half-life of 1.25 hours. Compared to atropine it is a more potent drying agent, causes less tachycardia, and causes minimal drowsiness and mydriasis.

INDUCTION AGENTS

The induction agents are the next drugs of choice. The most commonly used agents include benzodiazepines, barbiturates, narcotics, and a variety of other drugs.

Benzodiazepines

Benzodiazepines provide a smooth hemodynamic induction compared with barbiturates. These agents have multiple central effects based on their propensity for mimicking naturally occurring central nervous system depressant substances, e.g., GABA (gamma-amino-butyric acid) and glycine. These responses include GABA's sedative and anticonvulsant effect, and glycine's antianxiety and muscle relaxant effect. The specific pharmacokinetics of each agent are discussed below.

Diazepam (Valium) is a viscid liquid dissolved in propylene glycol. Intramuscular and intravenous administration is painful, and may result in thrombophlebitis. The drug is metabolized by the liver, with an elimination half-life of 21–37 hours. The principal metabolite, desmethyldiazepam, has an elimination half-life of 48–96 hours and is only slightly less potent than the parent compound. The usual induction dose is 0.5–1.0 mg/kg. The well-hydrated patient tends to have a hemodynamically stable induction with diazepam compared with barbiturates; however, unexplained hypotension may occur. Overdoses of diazepam are unlikely to cause serious sequelae if cardiac and pulmonary systems are supported and other depressant medications are not used.

Midazolam (Versed) is the water-soluble equivalent to diazepam. It causes little pain with injection, and there is no thrombophlebitis. The elimination half-life is 1–4 hours. There is a rapid redistribution phase causing seemingly rapid recovery from a single intravenous dose. Midazolam is cleared primarily by the liver. It has anticonvulsant effects similar to diazepam, depresses ventilation, and causes little hemodynamic compromise in the well-hydrated patient. Significant hypotension, responsive to fluid administration, does occur when it is combined with narcotics. The induction dose of intravenous midazolam is 0.2–0.3 mg/kg, with onset of action in 2–3 minutes, approximately twice the induction time of pentothal. Both diazepam and midazolam display considerable antegrade amnesia for the events following their administration.

Barbiturates

The barbiturates are direct central nervous system depressants. The mechanism of action works directly on both presynaptic terminals and GABA-mediated postsynaptic terminals to provide an acute sleeplike state. The margin of safety of these agents is relatively small. Side effects include apnea and profound hypotension with compensatory tachycardia.

Thiopental has been the gold standard of intravenous induction agents since its introduction in 1934. It has a quick onset, with 3–5 mg/kg producing unconsciouness in 30 seconds. There is a rapid redistribution phase from vessel-rich tissue groups to vessel-poor and lipid tissue groups, providing a short recovery period of 3–5 minutes from the initial unconscious state. Its elimination half-life of approximately 12 hours is relatively long.[17] It is metabolized mostly by the liver, with a very small amount excreted by the kidneys. The clinical uses of thiopental include rapid onset of induction of anesthesia, and treatment of increased intracranial pressure. Once again, use of this agent in the hypovolemic patient should proceed with caution to prevent significant hypotension. Thiopental has no analgesic properties and in some studies has been shown to be hyperalgesic.

Narcotics

The narcotic medications are useful in treating pain and preventing hypertensive and tachycardic responses to noxious stimuli, including intubation. They work by binding to endogenous central opiate receptors, either in the brain or in the spinal cord. These agents achieve profound analgesia by increasing the threshold to pain. All opiate agonists cause some sedation, euphoria, nausea, urinary retention, decreased gastrointestinal tract motility, spasm of the sphincter of Oddi, and pruritus, generally around the mouth and nose. Despite the profound analgesia with narcotics, there is little amnestic effect. The incidence and degree of these side effects depend on the specific drug and the route of administration.

The narcotics fit into two classifications: naturally derived and synthetic. The naturally occurring opiates are morphine, codeine, and heroin. The synthetic agents are meperidine, fentanyl, sufentanil, alfentanil, and methadone. Morphine, fentanyl, and meperidine are the narcotics most commonly used in the transport environment. Their specific profiles and unique side effects are discussed below.

Morphine is the prototypical opiate agonist. It is better for dull aching pain than for sharp pain. It works best if given before the painful stimulus. The initial dose is 50–100 μg/kg, with a half-life of 2–3 hours. The cardiovascular side effects of hypotension and bradycardia occur most commonly in the volume-depleted patient or from rapid injection. These are initiated by a combination of histamine release, decrease in sympathetic tone, and increase in vagal tone. Secondary peak effects due to gastric sequestration occur with morphine and fentanyl.

Fentanyl is 10–100 times as potent as morphine. The initial intravenous dose may be 2–5 μg/kg, with initial onset time of 5–6 minutes. The elimination half-life is 3–6 hours. Because there is no histamine release, there is less hypotension than seen with morphine. The combination of fentanyl and a benzodiazepine has resulted in hypotension. A rapid bolus of fentanyl or other synthetic narcotics may cause a centrally induced rigid chest syndrome. The treatment of this condition is either with naloxone, a narcotic antagonist, or with neuromuscular relaxation. Rarely, seizures have been induced by rapid injection of fentanyl.

Meperidine is another synthetic narcotic, with one-tenth the potency of morphine. The initial dose is 0.5–1.0 mg/kg for an equianalgesic dose of meperidine. Normeperidine, a byproduct of meperidine metabolism, is half as potent an analgesic as meperidine. It has a half-life of 15–40 hours and is a central nervous system stimulant. The prolonged use of meperidine may lead to onset of seizures.

The use of narcotics during transport is common. One must be prepared to deal with the side effects of these medications. The most common serious side effects, hypotension and decreased minute ventilation, require immediate management. With adequate forethought and preparation, the duration and severity of the side effects can be minimized, allowing the patient to experience all the benefits of narcotic administration.

Ketamine

Ketamine is an induction agent from the phencyclidine drug classification. It causes a dissociative anesthetic state. The clinical effect is nonresponsiveness; the patient's eyes are usually open with a nystagmic gaze. Ketamine provides profound amnesia and analgesia, making it theoretically an ideal induction agent. At a dose of 1-2 mg/kg intravenously it has an onset time of 30-60 seconds, a rapid redistribution phase, and elimination half-life of 1-2 hours. It is metabolized by the liver, with a small percentage excreted unmetabolized by the urine. Unfortunately, it has side effects of hypertension, tachycardia, increase in intracranial pressure, and a high incidence of emergence delirium. With onset of anesthesia, the airway reflexes are maintained, as is spontaneous respiration. The drug does cause rather copious salivary secretions and may require pretreatment with an antisialogogue, such as glycopyrrolate. The cardiovascular stimulation seen with this drug makes it a favored agent in the acutely hypovolemic patient in need of sedation for airway support. Conversely, it is relatively contraindicated in those patients with preexisting cardiomyopathy or myocardial ischemic disease, as the hemodynamic consequences cause a higher myocardial work load without necessarily increasing oxygen supply. It is also contraindicated in patients with increased intracranial pressure. The emergence delirium may be prevented by pretreatment with a small dose of benzodiazepines.

Etomidate

Etomidate is an induction agent of the imidazole variety. It is dissolved in propylene glycol and is irritating to the veins. The induction after 0.3 mg/kg is rapid, 30-60 seconds, and it also has a rapid redistribution phase. It has less of a hangover effect than does thiopental. There is a higher incidence of myoclonic jerks after induction. The elimination half-life is 2-5 hours; the drug is metabolized by the liver and plasma esterases. It has minimal cardiovascular effects, making it very desirable for the patient with heart disease in whom rapid induction is desired. It may excite previous existing epileptic foci. There is evidence of adrenocortical suppression that resolves within six hours after a single bolus. This has restricted etomidate to use as a one-time induction agent.

NEUROMUSCULAR BLOCKING AGENTS

Neuromuscular blocking agents should be used during transport to facilitate placement of endotracheal tubes that cannot be placed without muscle relaxation. Unfortunately, these agents tend to be misunderstood and misused by caregivers, who use them only sporadically. These agents do not have any sedating or analgesic properties. It is quite possible to have a seemingly sedate and comfortable patient who is chemically restrained and distinctly aware of all the conversation, movement, noise, and pain associated with transporting a critically ill or injured patient.

The use of muscle relaxation for intubation must be planned thoroughly ahead of time, with all alternatives anticipated. The caregiver must be certain of an adequate airway and ventilation by either bag and mask ventilation or endotracheal intubation before eliminating the patient's own respiratory effort. Inability of the caregiver to ventilate after medications are given is common, and an alternative plan, whether that be more jaw thrust, repositioning the head, or surgical placement of an airway, depends on skill, experience, and expertise. Notice that an alternative plan does not include giving more medications at this point. Only the redistribution of the medications already given will allow the reinitiation of the patient's spontaneous ventilation.

DEPOLARIZING NEUROMUSCULAR BLOCKING AGENTS

Succinylcholine

To date, the only clinically useful depolarizing neuromuscular blocking agent is succinylcholine. A dose of 1–2 mg/kg has a rapid onset time of 30–60 seconds, with a relatively short duration of 3–5 minutes. This makes succinylcholine the drug of choice for those patients in whom the quickest neuromuscular blockade is desired. But this drug has multiple side effects that limit its desirability.

The hemodynamic side effects are by far the most common of succinylcholine administration and are related to the cholinergic actions at the ganglion. Therefore, based on the autonomic tone before drug administration, one may see either tachycardia or bradycardia.

The depolarizing property is effected by mimicking acetylcholine, opening ionic channels of Na^+ and K^+, and allowing initiation of muscle contractions. The metabolic result will be a mild rise in serum potassium of 0.5 to 1.0 mEq/L in the patient with normal neuromuscular junctions. Patients who have myopathies, an increase in the number of neuromuscular junctions, or compromised cellular integrity are at risk for a precipitous rise in serum potassium following succinylcholine administration and potential cardiac dysrhythmias. The increase in muscle tone that results from the succinylcholine-induced depolarization is a relatively brief event but may result in increased pressure at several sites. The tonic contracture from the extraocular muscles results in increased intraocular pressure, which may compromise those with an open globe injury. The contracture of the strap muscles of the neck may impede venous drainage of the cerebral vessels, causing a brief increase in the intracranial pressure, a rise that may be life-threatening in the severely head-injured patient with poor intracranial compliance. The contracture of the abdominal muscles may lead to an increase in intragastric pressure exceeding the lower esophageal pressure, resulting in passive reflux of stomach contents.

Other side effects associated with succinylcholine administration occur much less frequently. The skeletal muscle contracture may lead to sustained contracture in patients predisposed to malignant hyperthermia. The classic manifestation of this event is masseter spasm and inability to open the mouth; succinylcholine administration in this event worsens conditions for intubation. Unfortunately, this condition is rarely predictable, with the only treatment being time for metabolism of the succinylcholine already delivered. The muscle fasciculations from succinylcholine cause little myoglobinuria and myalgia. It is evident from this discussion that the availability of another agent with a rapid onset but without the multitude of side effects would greatly enhance safety.

Succinylcholine is contraindicated in those patients with Duchenne's muscular dystrophy and in patients with spinal cord injury of more than one week's duration. Outside of these instances it is still **the neuromuscular blocking agent of choice in the management of the emergency airway.**

NONDEPOLARIZING AGENTS

These agents cause neuromuscular blockade by blocking the effects of acetylcholine at the neuromuscular junction without allowing the ionic channels to open, thereby preventing muscular contraction. The blockade has a slower onset than succinylcholine and a longer duration of action. The cardiovascular side effects are related to sympathomimetic effects (pancuronium) and histamine release from the curare-like agents (atracurium, d-tubocurare, mivacurium). The drugs are cleared by a combination of renal and hepatic mechanisms.

Vecuronium

This drug is a medium-acting agent, with almost no hemodynamic consequences of its own. The intubating dose is 0.1–0.3 mg/kg. The onset time varies between 3–5 minutes for the low dose and 60–90 seconds for the higher dose. The trade-off for rapid onset is prolonged duration of action. The time to 25% recovery from a low dose is 25–30 minutes. The duration of block is longer in neonates than in adults,[12] and it is metabolized by the liver and excreted in the bile (80%) and urine (20%).

Atacurium

This is also a medium-action nondepolarizing agent. It has greater incidence of hypotension, with reflex tachycardia secondary to histamine release. The intubating dose is 0.4–0.5 mg/kg, with onset time of 2–3 minutes. The time to 25% recovery is 25–30 minutes. It is metabolized by Hoffman degradation and ester hydrolysis; both mechanisms are pH- and temperature-dependent. Therefore, it is not dependent on the liver or kidneys for excretion. Neonates tend to be more sensitive to the effects than are older children and to have a longer recovery.[4,5,6]

Pancuronium

This agent is a longer acting muscle relaxant whose major side effect is tachycardia. It is metabolized by both kidney and liver routes. The intubating dose of 0.08–0.1 mg/kg has an onset time of 3–5 minutes, with a 25% recovery time of 80–100 minutes. The excretion is 70–80% renal, and 15–20% from hepatic metabolism and biliary excretion.

THE ART OF INTUBATION

A well-planned intubation appears effortless in even the most stressful of situations. A poorly planned intubation is obvious to all, and involves more luck than skill if the end result is successful.

Orotracheal Intubation

Place yourself at the head of the bed with all your equipment. Remember the mnemonic SOAP. Identify your suction device, ensure that it is working, attach a Yankauer suction tip to the tubing and secure it near you, ready for use. Ensure adequate oxygen sources and functioning flowmeters, correct size mask, and Mapleson device and self-inflating bag. Have available all your airway devices: oropharyngeal and nasopharyngeal airways; laryngoscopes and functioning lighted blades; endotracheal tubes (including one half-size larger and one smaller than you predict will fit), with the appropriate size stylet in the first tube (Table 3). Make sure you have enough medications to manage the intubation and all the problems that may present themselves. This process can

TABLE 3. Guidelines for Laryngoscope Blade, ETT and Catheter Sizes

Age	Weight (kg)	Blade	ET Tube*	Suction (Fr)	NG Tube (Fr)
NB	3.5	1 (straight)	3.5	6–8	10
6 mo	7	1 (straight)	4.0	8	10
1 yr	10	2 (straight)	4..5	8	10
2 yr	12		4.5	8–10	10–12
3 yr	14		5.0	10	12
4 yr	16		5.0	10	12
5 yr	18	2 (straight or curved)	5.5	10	12
6 yr	21		5.5	10	12
7 yr	24		6.0	10	12
8 yr	27	2–3 (straight	6.0	10–12	14
9 yr	28	or curved)	6.5	12	14
10yr	30		7.0	12	14

* ETT sizes are approximate. One size larger or smaller may be needed.

take as little as 3-5 minutes if you have a well-devised plan. DO NOT RUSH. DO NOT proceed before you are ready unless an emergency dictates otherwise.

We will proceed at this point to discuss a normal sedated intubation without problems. Special circumstances surrounding problems with airways will be discussed later.

The patient should be monitored with EKG and pulse oximetry and placed in the sniffing position. A slight elevation under the occiput in patients over one year of age* will permit the straightest alignment of the glottic structures and maximal viewing area (Fig. 4). Preoxygenate the patient with 100% O_2 for 3-5 minutes before any intubation attempts. The intubation should be a two-person endeavor, one doing the procedure and an assistant available to do anything else. During preoxygenation, atropine or glycopyrrolate may be given to prevent reflex bradycardia from laryngoscopy. After oxygenation, titrate in the sedative medications. Continuously evaluate the airway and relieve any obstruction with appropriate maneuvers, such as a chin lift, jaw thrust, or placement of an oral airway. The gradual induction should allow you to take over the ventilatory work of the patient with manual bag-and-mask ventilation. By this process, you are assured that you can provide a mask airway when the patient becomes apneic. Once you demonstrate an ability to maintain the patient's airway, muscle relaxation and further sedation and analgesia can be given.

At this point the patient's cardiovascular status should be evaluated. Hypertension due to light anesthesia or hypercarbia should be alleviated with further sedation and increased ventilation. Conversely, the patient may become hypotensive secondary to previously given medications or following conversion from negative to positive pressure ventilation if dehydrated. The patient should be treated with isotonic fluid volume and pressor medications at this time. The stimulus of intubation causes a pressor response and may be beneficial in some of these instances to raise blood pressure. As long as an airway is maintained with a bag-and-mask device and the patient responds to your therapy, there is no reason to panic. This underscores the importance of having another person to help you.

---

* Patients under one year of age generally have a prominent occiput. Further occipital elevation may worsen intubating conditions.

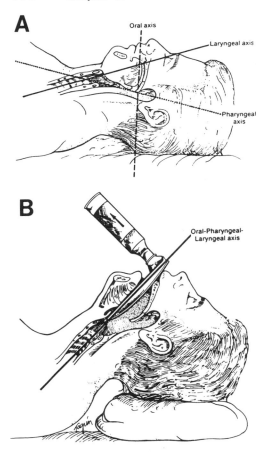

A

Oral axis

Laryngeal axis

Pharyngeal axis

B

Oral-Pharyngeal-Laryngeal axis

FIGURE 4. Axes of the airway in the neutral position (*A*) and with sniffing position (*B*). (From Wilkins R: MGH Textbook of Emergency Medicine. Baltimore, Williams and Wilkins, 1979, with permission.)

Once the patient is hemodynamically stable and fully relaxed, the act of placing the endotracheal tube can begin. Be aware of the risk of dental and soft tissue trauma from the laryngoscope blade. Place the blade gently into the right side of the mouth. Sweep the tongue to the left in order to keep it from blocking your view of the oropharyngeal and glottic structures. Begin to look immediately with placement of the blade. Slowly advance the blade along the contour of the tongue, identifying all structures as you pass them. The vallecula should be identified in all patients, if possible, and a decision made whether to place the blade into this structure or directly into the glottis to provide visualization of the cords. Proper technique with the laryngoscope handle generates the power of the lift from the shoulder with the wrist and elbow locked. This will prevent knocking the blade against the upper incisors. Figure 5 shows the proper force vectors to permit optimal visualization of the glottis.

Once the glottis is identified, gently pass the endotracheal tube through the cords into the trachea. Remember the number of lines at the cords or placement of the cuff for later documentation. Firmly hold the endotracheal tube with your right hand stabilized against the patient's face while the laryngoscope is gently removed. Breath sounds at the axillae and just beneath the clavicles should be evaluated bilaterally after placement. Vapor should be seen in the tube during exhalation. Ideally, one should have a small audible airleak around the endotracheal tube at 20–30 cm H_2O pressure, indicating minimal tracheal pressure at

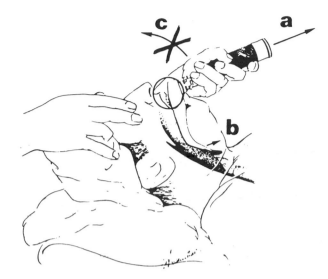

FIGURE 5. *A* and *B* show the proper force vectors for intubation, moving the tongue and soft tissues up and out, allowing full view of the glottic structures. *C* shows improper force vectors, using the teeth as a fulcrum. This motion may injure dental structures and cause the handle to move into the view of the glottis. (From Roberts JT: Fundamentals of Tracheal Intubation. New York, Grune and Stratton, 1983.)

the cricoid ring. Secure the endotracheal tube with adhesive tape to the upper and lower lips. In patients up to 8 years of age, the number of centimeters on the tube at the alveolar ridge or teeth should be equal to 11 plus the age in years. Pediatric endotracheal tubes usually have a circumferential dotted ring printed on the tube to indicate lip level for the average depth for age. Verify tube placement with a chest radiograph and ETCO$_2$ measurement if available. Send a blood gas to correlate with noninvasive monitors, if they are to be used for trending. Place a nasogastric or orogastric tube to keep the stomach decompressed.

Document the intubation procedure in the chart after completion. Documentation can be subdivided into pre-intubation, intubation and post-intubation categories. Pre-intubation should cover indications for the procedure. Then outline the intubation sequence, beginning with preoxygenation and medications followed by instruments used; record the laryngoscope blade and size, stylet and endotracheal tube size with or without cuff. Next use the "ABC" mnemonic: **A**traumatic or traumatic; **B**reath sounds equal or unequal; **C**ord structures visualized. The post-intubation documentation includes vital signs, blood gas analysis (if obtained), pulse oximetry, end-tidal CO$_2$ and chest radiograph. Any untoward events such as lost or broken teeth, vomiting, or aspiration during the procedure, should be clearly documented in a separate area marked "Complications." Having this documentation will be helpful to the child's caretakers in the ICU.

Nasotracheal Intubation

A nasotracheal tube can be placed fairly readily during direct laryngoscopy by those proficient in this skill. The benefits of this tube over an orally placed tube are its stability and our perception that children tolerate these tubes better. In an emergency, an orotracheal tube is sufficient. Nasotracheal placement is elective. The side effects include nose bleeds, nasopharyngeal incompetence, eustachian tube dysfunction, sinusitis, turbinate rupture, and nasal alae necrosis. This procedure is contraindicated in anyone suspected of having a basilar skull fracture. A blind nasal intubation in the pediatric patient is often unsuccessful owing to the accentuated anterocephalad location of the glottis in the child compared to the adult.

The safest way to start a nasotracheal intubation is to perform an orotracheal intubation as described above. Have an assistant hold the oral tube at the left corner of the mouth. Spraying a topical vasoconstricting agent, such as phenylephrine or Afrin, in the nasopharynx may decrease bleeding. Lubricate a second appropriate-size tube, without stylet. Direct the tube through a naris, perpendicular to the plane of the face, with firm but gentle pressure, until you feel it turn into the nasopharynx. With the laryngoscope blade in place, identify both the oral and nasal tubes. With Magill forceps, grasp the nasal tube near its tip, and advance it to a position close to the glottis. Ask an assistant to remove the oral tube and advance the nasal tube from above, while you guide it between the cords with the forceps. Slight flexion of the neck may help you advance the tube. Note the position of the lines on the tube with respect to the vocal cords.

SPECIAL TECHNIQUES

Rapid Sequence Induction

Any patient selected for rapid sequence intubation first must have a thorough airway evaluation. Any finding suggestive of a difficult intubation would be a relative contraindication. The technique is designed to provide an intubated airway within a minute, which requires a complete set-up before medications are given. The spontaneously breathing patient should be placed, head in the sniffing position, in a semi-sitting posture to prevent passive regurgitation from the stomach. A working wall suction capable of -200 mmHg with a large-bore, multiple-hole tip suction catheter attached should be at the head of the bed for easy access. The endotracheal tube should be of the appropriate size and a stylet in place with the tip of the stylet about 0.5 cm from the tip of the tube. The patient should be preoxygenated for 3–5 minutes, and cricoid pressure applied by a person dedicated to that role alone.

Cricoid pressure is a maneuver in which the circumferential laryngeal cricoid cartilage ring is pushed gently against the vertebral body of the spine, thereby occluding the esophagus. The intent of this maneuver is to prevent passive regurgitation of stomach contents into the pharynx.

Induction doses of both sedatives and neuromuscular blocking agents are pushed rapidly. No positive pressure breaths are given. The endotracheal tube is placed as soon as the patient is apneic and flaccid—about 60 seconds. Cricoid pressure should be held until proper endotracheal placement has been verified by auscultating the chest and abdomen. Placement also can be verified by exhaled CO_2, measured by capnography, and chest radiography.

If it is not possible to intubate the patient, gentle mask ventilation should be performed to keep the patient oxygenated during the apneic period. If both intubation and ventilation fail, a cricothyrotomy or tracheostomy is indicated. A new technique, the laryngeal mask airway, may be an appropriate adjunct before cricothyrotomy, but will not be discussed further here. An article by Pennant and co-workers[20] provides an excellent review of the technique and indications in pediatric patients.

Awake Intubation

The indication for an awake intubation is an anticipated inability to provide an airway once the patient has drug-induced apnea. Ideally, a complete explanation of the procedure and of the importance of doing this awake is provided. The "perfect" patient who would allow an intubation without some chemical preparation is very rare, especially in pediatrics. Another approach is to give sedative doses of medications and regional anesthesia, such as topical lidocaine to the oral mucosa. With each added medication, however, the line between awake and asleep is blurred, and the resultant effect is an induction halfway between one method and the other, while the benefits of both approaches are lost.

Cricothyrotomy

Inability to ventilate or oxygenate a patient is THE indication for performing a cricothyrotomy. The pediatric patient's anatomy makes this procedure considerably more difficult. However, no patient should be allowed to die for lack of an airway without this procedure being attempted. The equipment for cricothyrotomy can be obtained as a commercially-available kit or can be assembled from easily-obtainable materials: intravenous catheters, plastic syringes, oxygen, and tubing (Fig. 6).

The procedure must be done in a timely fashion. Remember, at this point there is nothing to lose. First, feel for the thyroid notch, or "Adam's apple." This becomes more pronounced after puberty, which is why it is sometimes harder to identify in prepubertal children. An 18-gauge catheter (Fig. 6A) on a syringe should be passed at a 45° angle through the cricothyroid membrane at the inferior pole of the thyroid cartilage. Suction should be applied to the catheter once the catheter is within the skin. Aspiration of air identifies the trachea. The angle of the syringe then should be lowered to 10–20° and advanced until the catheter is within the trachea, usually a few millimeters. Repeated aspiration of air verifies placement. If no air is aspirated, continue suction and pull back to the skin and repeat the first steps until air is aspirated. Advance the catheter into the trachea and remove the needle stylet.

Next, remove the plunger form a 5-ml syringe and attach the male end of the isolated barrel to the female end of the cricothyrotomy catheter. Take some simple oxygen tubing and cut a hole in the side of the tubing 3–4 inches from the end. Place the end of the oxygen tubing into the end of the barrel of the 5-ml syringe (Fig. 6B). Attach the oxygen tubing to a tank of oxygen or a wall source with 10 lpm of flow. Use one hand to stabilize the catheter at the neck and the other hand to regulate gas flow. With occlusion of the side hole (Fig. 6C) that you created, O_2 will flow into the trachea in a jet fashion. Release of your finger will allow exhalation if the only egress of air is through the 18-gauge cricothyrotomy catheter. This device is not designed to ventilate the patient, only to oxygenate. Once the patient is stabilized, further definitive airway maneuvers can be done.

SPECIAL AIRWAY PROBLEMS

Patients may present with disease processes that make the intubation procedure described above more risky than either a rapid sequence induction and intubation or awake intubation. There is always a risk/benefit assessment to be made when providing an airway for a critically injured child. The following scenarios will outline some of the risks associated with these situations.

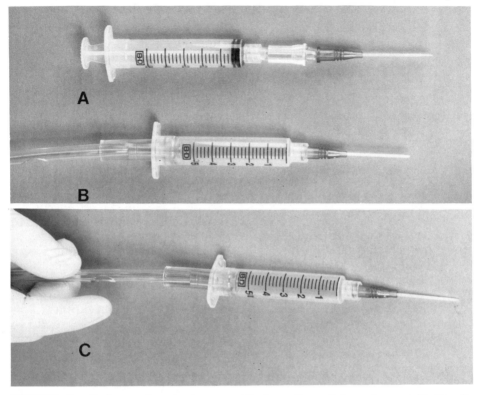

FIGURE 6. Equipment for cricothyrotomy. **A** shows the catheter-syringe combination for cricothyrotomy. **B** shows the catheter-syringe barrel with the oxygen tubing inserted. Note the side hole in the side of the oxygen tubing. **C** demonstrates use of the index finger to cover side hole to manipulate gas flow into and out of the catheter.

Full Stomach

Patients who present with trauma, acute onset of illness, upper gastrointestinal or pharyngeal bleeding, pregnancy, bowel obstruction, or intestinal ileus are assumed to have a full stomach. The risk is vomiting during endotracheal intubation. Once vomiting has occurred, the patient may aspirate both particulate matter and the acid contents of the stomach. The patient with intact cough and gag reflexes may be able to protect the airway during vomiting. The patient rendered unconscious for intubation depends on the skill of the intubator to prevent vomiting or passive regurgitation and aspiration. The choice to make is between an awake intubation or a rapid sequence induction and intubation as previously described. This latter approach may be used if the patient has no anatomic indicators of a difficult airway.

Facial Trauma

Facial trauma presents with many different scenarios. The involvement may be as simple as a controllable nose bleed or as complicated as crushed mid-facies with complete airway obstruction. Treatment obviously is dependent on the degree of injury and the severity of respiratory embarrassment. The factors responsible for airway embarrassment include the degree of active bleeding, soft tissue swelling, and loss of support of soft tissue secondary to facial fractures. With significant facial injury, one must also be suspicious of laryngeal and tracheal trauma, with resultant pneumothoraces and pneumomediastinum. Crepitus of the neck and chest, hoarseness, and differential breath sounds may help with diagnosing these problems.

Treatment of the airway requires a flexible approach to each individual. Minor trauma may require nothing more than close observation after a thorough exam. The patient with severe trauma and a compromised airway needs a premeditated plan with appropriate surgical support. Tracheostomy should be performed in the trauma patient with facial injuries and upper airway obstruction.[15] Instrumentation with nasotracheal and nasogastric tubes is contraindicated because of the likelihood of basilar skull fractures. One must remember that addition of any sedative medication may precipitate upper airway obstruction.

Suspected Cervical Spine Trauma

The management of the patient with suspected cervical spine (C-spine) trauma varies in the amount and type of mobility the caregiver is allowed without increasing the risk to the patient. One must be highly suspicious of C-spine injury in patients with head injury. The initial cardiorespiratory derangements—e.g., hypotension and respiratory embarrassment—may be caused directly by a C-spine injury. Special immobilization of the patient's C-spine will prevent any further injury that may result from flexion, extension or lateral rotation of the neck. The patient with spontaneous respiratory effort may benefit from supplemental O_2, since the depth of respiration may be diminished by loss of accessory muscle innervation. The patient may have minimal respiratory effort requiring prompt intubation. Instrumenting the airway in the C-spine–injured patient requires multiple assistants. For example, intubating the patient with a full stomach and possible C-spine injury would call for the intubator plus a person dedicated to midline immobilization of the C-spine and another dedicated to maintaining cricoid pressure. The patient may vomit spontaneously or during the intubation. The availability of suction devices and enough people to logroll the patient safely are essential to prevent aspiration. Direct laryngoscopy in a relaxed patient with orotracheal intubation is preferred, after administration of atropine, sedatives, and hypnotic agents.

Open Orbital Injury

Treatment of the child with an open globe injury has prompted much debate. These patients generally require a general anesthetic before any meaningful evaluation can take place. A rapid-sequence induction is commonly performed if the patient has a full stomach. The controversy lies in whether to use succinylcholine for muscle relaxation. One of the side effects of succinylcholine is a rise in intraocular pressure. The debate over the use of succinylcholine is split into two camps. Opponents claim the rise in intraocular pressure from this drug may promote loss of intraocular contents, thereby implicating this agent as a factor if loss of vision occurs. The proponents of succinylcholine cite it as the muscle relaxant of choice in the patient with a full stomach. The small increase in intraocular pressure from succinylcholine is far outweighed by the rise in intraocular pressure caused by the child's actions after the injury. These may include squinting from pain, active crying, and rubbing of the eye. The overall end-point of both groups is to provide a safe induction of general anesthesia in order to examine and subsequently treat an open globe injury. Studies exist to support either belief.[2,3,9,10,13,18]

Increased Intracranial Pressure

The management of the patient with isolated head injury revolves around the treatment of intracranial pressure already present and the prevention of any further elevation that may result from airway manipulation. The skull encloses three components: brain, blood, and water (CSF). Usually we are able to control only blood flow medically. This can be done with hyperventilation, which will cause central vasoconstriction. We can attempt to preserve cerebral autoregulation by maintaining the mean arterial BP between 50 and 150 mmHg. We also can prevent venous hypertension by allowing adequate jugular venous drainage with head position.

The pharmacology of intracranial pressure management deserves some discussion. One needs to provide medications that will cause some blunting of the hypertensive response to intubation. This may be provided by a number of medications used for induction. There is evidence to support that intravenous lidocaine, 1.5 mg/kg,[1] and fentanyl, 6 μg/kg,[7,19] given 3 minutes before intubation will blunt this hypertensive response. This should be followed with an induction medication that will decrease cerebral blood flow (CBF) and cerebral oxygen consumption ($CMRO_2$). Thiopental indeed decreases both; however, the CBF is decreased less than $CMRO_2$, providing a relatively luxuriant central nervous system perfusion.

The use of muscle relaxants adds some controversy to the management of the patient with intracranial pressure. Succinylcholine increases intracranial pressure. The use of a small amount of nondepolarizing muscle relaxant followed by succinylcholine may blunt this response. The use of succinylcholine in young pediatric patients may cause severe bradycardia and, therefore, should be preceded immediately by a dose of atropine. It is the drug of choice in patients with a full stomach because of its rapid onset of muscle relaxation. Nondepolarizing muscle relaxants such as vecuronium are not associated with elevations in intracranial pressure. There is, however, a longer onset to muscle relaxation and a more hazardous period of an unprotected airway.

The clinical management begins with proper head and bed positioning. This is followed by mild active hyperventilation with 100% FiO_2 to decrease the intracranial pressure. Care should be used to prevent insufflation of the stomach at this point. The patient should be presumed to have a full stomach, and cricoid pressure should be used during airway management. Lidocaine and fentanyl should be given, with cricoid pressure started as soon as management of the airway begins. The patient should be given sodium thiopental, 4-6 mg/kg, followed by vecuronium, 0.15 mg/kg. Hyperventilation should continue, with intubation attempted 60-90 seconds after the vecuronium is administered. The actual intubation should be kept to less than 15 seconds per attempt; longer times have been associated with increases in intracranial pressure.

COMPLICATIONS OF ENDOTRACHEAL INTUBATION

Invasive procedures are always associated with problems and side effects from the therapy itself. Endotracheal intubation is no different. Complications can occur during all facets of the procedure. The following are a few examples of these problems.

During the preparation of the patient, positioning becomes an important aspect of management. One must make sure that the patient is comfortably positioned and not lying on anything sharp. Maneuvering the head and neck to obtain optimal view of the glottic structures is a common procedure. Extra care should be taken in those patients with potential for cervical spine problems, e.g., trauma, Down syndrome, rheumatoid arthritis.

Medications are given during most intubations. All medications carry some systemic side effects that need to be considered. A rare side effect of atropine, for instance, is psychosis; its tertiary structure allows free penetration of the blood-brain barrier. The tachycardia from anticholinergic agents may compromise myocardial blood supply and oxygen demand, though this is not a serious threat in the previously healthy pediatric patient. Sedative medications commonly used to keep the intubated patient comfortable may lead to hypotension. The combination of benzodiazepines and narcotics[21] is a clear example of this.

The physical placement and presence of the endotracheal tube also have many side effects. The oropharynx and nasopharynx may sustain significant trauma during tube placement. Any movement of the tube causes trauma to the mucosal layer of the trachea. This may lead to stenosis or the formation of granulation tissue at the site of the injury. An endotracheal tube may fit too tightly, decreasing blood flow to the adjacent mucosal layer, leading to necrosis and stenosis of the trachea. The use of positive pressure and nonheated dry gas mixtures causes damage to mucosa and ciliary function. The secretions may dry out, leading to plugging of distal airways or the tube itself. The patient may develop hypothermia as the cool dry gases are warmed and humidified in the trachea. The tube may become dislodged, either into the pharynx or distally into a mainstem bronchus.

Positive pressure ventilation alone has adverse effects. The patient with hypovolemia or poor myocardial function may develop decreased cardiac output secondary to decreased venous return to the right heart. Excessive ventilation pressures may lead to barotrauma, resulting in subcutaneous emphysema, pneumothorax, pneumomediastinum, pneumopericardium, or pneumoperitoneum.

As one can see, the use of an endotracheal tube is not a benign undertaking. A comprehensive approach to the whole process will help prevent some of the side effects. Diligence in placement of the endotracheal tube will minimize trauma during placement. A full understanding of the desired medications and their side effects may prevent or shorten the adverse effects of these agents. The caretaker should monitor inflating pressures and use adequate positive pressure to promote physiologic gas exchange and to prevent barotrauma. Warmed and humidified gases will prevent the drying of secretions and heat loss that may occur with cool dry gases.

MONITORING DURING TRANSPORT

The extent of monitoring of the transported pediatric patient depends on the severity of illness and expected complications. The critical care transport team should be ready to provide all state-of-the-art monitoring but also be able to use basic skills of airway and cardiac assessment in order to adjust the care of the patient as the status changes.

The transport environment, whether in a ground ambulance or aircraft, is not predictably stable. Often the patient has just recently been intubated and stabilized. The airway and intravascular catheters must be secured and preserved. Adequate sedation with benzodiazepines and narcotics and, if necessary, muscle relaxation agents, are reasonable adjuncts to the patient's transport. A full understanding of the hemodynamic side effects should be understood before using these medications.

The heart rate, respiratory rate and temperature should be continuously monitored. The blood pressure should be assessed every 3-5 minutes during transport of critically ill patients. The patient's O_2 saturations should be monitored continuously. The end-tidal CO_2 monitor, if available, is an excellent monitor, not only for adequacy of ventilation but also of cardiac output in the compromised patient.

Acknowledgment.   The authors thank Dr. Nancy France for her help in reviewing this manuscript.

REFERENCES

1. Bedford R, Persing J, Poberskin L, Butler A: Lidocaine or thiopental for rapid control of intracranial hypertension. Anesth Analg 59:435, 1980.
2. Bowen D, McGrand J, Hamilton A: Intraocular pressures after suxamethonium and endotracheal intubation. Anesthesiology 33:518, 1978.
3. Bowen D, McGrand J, Palmer R: Intraocular pressures after suxamethonium and endotracheal intubation in patients pretreated with pancuronium. Br J Anaesth 48:1201, 1976.
4. Brandom B, Cook D, Woelfel S: Atracurium infusion requirements in children during halothane, isoflurane and narcotic anesthesia. Anesth Analg 64:471, 1985.
5. Brandom B, Rudd G, Cook D: Clinical pharmacology of atracurium in pediatric patients. Br J Anaesth 55:117, 1983.
6. Brandom B, Woelfel S, Cook D: Clinical pharmacology of atracurium in infants. Anesth Analg 63:309, 1984.
7. Carlsson C, Smith D, Keykhah M, et al: The effects of high dose fentanyl on cerebral circulation and metabolism in rats. Anesth 57:375, 1982.
8. Cotton R, Richardson M: Congenital laryngeal anomalies. Otolaryngol Clin North Am 14:203, 1981.
9. Cunliffe M: Neuromuscular blockade for rapid tracheal intubation in children: Comparison of succinylcholine and pancuronium. Can Anaesth Soc J 33:760, 1985.
10. Cunningham A, Barry P: Intraocular pressure—physiology and implications for anaesthetic management. Can Anaesth Soc J 33:195, 1986.
11. Eskola J, Kayhty H, Takala A, et al: A randomized prospective field trial of a conjugate vaccine in the protection of infants and young children against invasive Haemophilus influenzae type B. N Engl J Med 323:1381, 1990.
12. Fisher D, Castagnoli K, Miller R: Vecuronium kinetics and dynamics in anesthetized children and infants. Clin Pharmacol Ther 37:402, 1985.
13. France N, France T, Woodburn J: Succinylcholine alteration of the forced duction test. Opthalmology 87:1282, 1980.
14. Goodman L, Gilman A: The Pharmacologic Basis of Therapeutics, 8th ed. New York, Macmillan, 1990.
15. Handler S: Trauma to the larynx and upper airway. Int Anesthesiol Clin 26:39, 1988.
16. Holinger L: Etiology of stridor in the neonate, infant and child. Ann Otol 89:397, 1980.
17. Hudson R, Stanski D, Burch P: Pharmacokinetics of methohexital and thiopental in surgical patients. Anesthesiology 59:215, 1983.
18. Libonati M, Leahy J, Ellison N: The use of succinylcholine in open eye surgery. Anesthesiology 62:637, 1985.
19. Martin D, Rosenberg H, Aukburg S, et al: Low dose fentanyl blunts circulatory response to tracheal intubation. Anesth Analg 61: 680, 1982.
20. Pennant J, White P: The laryngeal mask airway. Anesthesiology 79(1):144, 1993.
21. Tomicheck R, Rosow C, Philbin D, et al: Diazepam-fentanyl interaction: Hemodynamic and hormonal effects in coronary artery surgery. Anesth Analg 62:881, 1983.

SUGGESTED READING

1. Gregory G: Pediatric Anesthesia, 2nd ed. New York, Churchill Livingstone, 1989.
2. Otherson H: The Pediatric Airway. Philadelphia, W.B. Saunders, 1991.
3. Rogers M: Textbook of Pediatric Intensive Care, 2nd ed. Baltimore, Williams & Wilkins, 1992.
4. Stoelting R: Pharmacology and Physiology in Anesthesia Practice, 2nd ed. Philadelphia: J.B. Lippincott, 1991.
5. Goodman L, Gilman A: The Pharmacologic Basis of Therapeutics, 8th ed. New York, Macmillan, 1990.
6. Roberts J: Fundamentals of Tracheal Intubation. New York, Gruen & Stratton, 1983.

CHAPTER 13

Respiratory Failure Management During Transport

STEVEN E. KRUG, M.D.

BACKGROUND/DEFINITION

Acute respiratory illnesses are quite common in infants and children. If not promptly recognized and properly treated, these illnesses can result in significant morbidity and mortality. Illnesses producing respiratory failure are the leading cause of cardiopulmonary arrest in children.[3,18] Respiratory failure is generally preceded by respiratory distress. In respiratory distress, respiratory performance still provides for adequate gas exchange through physiologic mechanisms that maximize the patient's pulmonary capacity; in respiratory failure, there is inadequate gas exchange, namely elimination of carbon dioxide and oxygenation of blood. Respiratory failure may arise from intrinsic lung or airway disease, from inadequate respiratory effort, or from the effect of associated organ system dysfunction.

MANAGEMENT IN THE FIELD

The outcome of the child suffering from an acute illness or injury frequently depends on the emergency care delivered prior to the arrival of the transport team during the prehospital and emergency department phases of care. Unfortunately, in many communities, the ability to consistently provide appropriate emergency medical services for children (EMSC) has been lacking.[8] Much has been written about perceived deficiencies in EMSC.[4,17,18] These deficiencies relate to inadequate personnel training and equipment and then are further magnified by a lack of ongoing clinical experience with pediatric critical illness among most emergency care providers.

These deficiencies in EMSC may result in either inaccurate or underassessment of illness severity (e.g., failing to recognize shock or respiratory failure) or an inability to meet the advanced life support needs of a child who has been appropriately assessed. Accurate patient assessment is a vital determinant of patient outcome for critically ill children. The recognition of prearrest states, such as respiratory distress or failure, combined with appropriate basic and advanced life support interventions, prevents illness progression to physiologic conditions that may not be remediable.[3,10] The well-documented and abysmal outcome for children suffering cardiopulmonary arrest dictates that successful resuscitative interventions must occur early in the progression to cardiopulmonary failure.[13,14,22,25]

The goal of prehospital care should be to meet the patient's basic life support needs and, in certain situations, the child's advanced life support needs. The prehospital assessment of the child in respiratory distress should focus on the ABCs. Unless contraindicated by a suspected diagnosis of critical partial upper airway obstruction (e.g., a child with epiglottitis), all children should have 100% oxygen administered as part of their care. All children should be transported to the hospital in a position of comfort, not forced into a position (e.g., supine) that adds to their respiratory distress by promoting additional airway obstruction or by limiting respiratory performance.

The extent of care provided to ill children in the field depends on the training and experience of the prehospital care providers and their traditional scope of practice. Depending on the training or certification level of the prehospital care providers (e.g., EMT vs. paramedic) and the limits of practice afforded by standing protocols or the on-line medical control officer, the scope of prehospital care for the child in acute respiratory failure can be fairly sophisticated, ranging from the provision of an aerosolized beta-agonist agent for acute bronchospasm to assisted ventilation and endotracheal intubation for the apneic patient.

CLINICAL PRESENTATIONS

As noted earlier, respiratory failure typically is preceded by a compensated state of respiratory distress. In distress, respiratory performance still provides adequate gas exchange through physiologic mechanisms that maximize ventilatory capacity and increase the work of breathing. Clinically, respiratory distress may be characterized by the work of breathing efforts, including the use of accessory respiratory muscles, inspiratory retractions, nasal flaring, grunting, diaphoresis, tachypnea, and tachycardia. Grunting is a particulary worrisome finding because it represents the patient's efforts to generate additional continuous positive airway pressure (CPAP). Because the range of normal vital signs varies from one age group to the next, the definition of tachycardia or tachypnea must be age-related (Table 1). In addition to findings of increased work of breathing, there may also be disease-specific symptoms that depend on the causative disorder (see Pathophysiology).

The clinical signs of respiratory failure result from end-organ dysfunction created by progressive tissue hypoxia and acidosis. These signs include altered level of consciousness (confusion, restlessness, lethargy); hypotonia; tachycardia; and weak pulses. Later and more ominous signs of respiratory failure include bradycardia; hypotension; cyanosis; and irregular respiration. These late signs of respiratory failure represent a premorbid event. In other words, although the time elapsed from the onset of respiratory illness to respiratory failure may be

TABLE 1. Normal Vital Signs

Age	Heart Rate		Respiratory Rate		Blood Pressure	
	Range	Mean	Range	Mean	Minimum	Maximum
Newborn	100–180	120	26–44	32	55/30	95/60
Infant < 1 yr	100–190	140	24–60	30	75/50	100/70
Toddler 1–3 yrs	100–180	130	20–32	26	90/55	130/85
Child 3–8 yrs	60–150	100	18–28	24	95/55	135/85
Child 8–12 yrs	50–100	80	14–24	18	95/60	140/90
Adolescent	50–100	75	12–20	16	95/60	140/90

From Krug SE: Cardiopulmonary arrest and resuscitation. In Reece RM (ed): Manual of Emergency Pediatrics. Philadelphia, W.B. Saunders, 1992, with permission.

fairly long, the progression from respiratory failure to cardiopulmonary arrest is fairly rapid.

PATHOPHYSIOLOGY

Acute respiratory failure can result from many different diseases (Table 2) and therefore may evolve through a variety of mechanisms. Primary respiratory failure is caused by a direct insult to (or a malfunction involving) the airway, lung parenchyma, or thorax. In secondary respiratory failure, respiratory dysfunction is due to the impact of a disease or disorder that has had a deleterious effect on another organ system (e.g., central nervous system, cardiovascular system).

Central Nervous System Disorders

The central nervous system (CNS) plays an important role in both the control and maintenance of normal respiration. Disorders affecting the CNS can impair respiratory performance via depression of respiratory drive or by suppression of protective airway reflexes. Children with a significant alteration in their mental status are at greater risk for airway compromise or hypoventilation. In the transport environment, one should assume the worst with such patients and entertain presumptive airway control (e.g, intubation) with assisted ventilation, even in children who on initial assessment have an intact airway and adequate ventilation.

Peripheral (and central) neuromuscular diseases can also affect respiratory performance by direct action on respiratory muscle function. A general assessment of respiratory muscle function should be included in the evaluation of the patient with respiratory disease. A subjective assessment can be performed at the bedside. The patient's ability to swallow, cough, and breathe deeply provide some insight into respiratory muscle function. Neuromuscular weakness frequently leads to the development of atelectasis.[16] Assisted ventilation should be considered for patients with impaired pharyngeal muscle function, significant atelectasis, or those with hypercapnia and/or hypoxemia.[9]

Upper Airway Disorders

Upper airway diseases impair respiratory performance through partial or complete airway obstruction. Partial obstruction of the airway produces turbulent airflow and a characteristic noise. Depending on the location of the obstructing lesion, the noise generated will present as stridor and/or wheezing. Disorders affecting the proximal airway may be acute or chronic. Chronic airway obstruction has also been linked to the development of pulmonary edema, pulmonary hypertension, and cor pulmonale.[24]

Stridor is a sound created by partial proximal airway obstruction most frequently located between the larynx and the thoracic inlet of the trachea. In this segment of the airway, the combination of negative intraluminal airway pressure and a positive atmospheric pressure cause a narrowing of the airway during inspiration. Any lesion affecting the lumen size in this portion of the airway will be accentuated during inspiration. Stridor is a sound created by turbulent airway flow, and may be loud or soft, high- or low-pitched, or harsh. Children with proximal airway obstruction may also have a "barky" cough.

Wheezing is a sound created by partial airway obstruction at the level of the intrathoracic conducting airways. In this portion of the airway, the combination of positive intrathoracic pressure and airway elastic tissue forces cause a narrowing of the airway during expiration. Turbulent airflow created by this

TABLE 2.   Causes of Acute Respiratory Failure in Children

Neurologic disease	Airway disorders (cont.)
Central nervous system	Lower airway
Status epilepticus	Reactive airways disease
Severe static encephalopathy	Foreign body aspiration
Acute meningoencephalitis	Cystic fibrosis
Brain abscess, hematoma, tumor	Bronchiectasis
Brain stem insult	Tracheobronchomalacia
CNS malformation	Bronchopulmonary dysplasia
Arnold-Chiari malformation	Alpha$_1$-antitrypsin deficiency
Drug intoxication	Hydrocarbon ingestion
General anesthesia	Congenital lobar emphysema
Spinal/anterior horn cell	
Transverse myelitis	Chest wall and mechanical disorders
Poliomyelitis	Diaphragmatic hernia
Polyradiculitis (Guillain-Barré)	Pneumo-, hemo-, or chylothorax
Werdnig-Hoffman syndrome	Kyphoscoliosis
Neuromuscular junction	
Myasthenia gravis	Lung parenchyma disorders
Botulism	Infectious pneumonias
Tetanus	Tuberculosis
Myopathy	Pertussis, parapertussis
Neuropathy	Cystic fibrosis
General anesthetics, drugs, poisons	Drug-induced pulmonary disease
	Vasculitis, collagen-vascular disease
Airway disorders	Pulmonary dysgenesis
Upper airway	Pulmonary edema
Acute epiglottitis	Near-drowning
Laryngotracheobronchitis (croup)	
Foreign body aspiration	Other diseases
Adenotonsillar hypertrophy	Cardiac disease
Retropharyngeal abscess	Anemia
Subglottic stenosis, web, hemangioma	Methemoglobinemia
Tracheomalacia	Carbon monoxide poisoning
Laryngomalacia	Cyanide poisoning
Congenital anomalies	Hypothermia, hyperthermia
Static encephalopathy	Sepsis
	Obstructive sleep apnea

From Baker MD, Ruddy RM: Pulmonary emergencies. In Fleisher GR, Ludwig S (eds): Textbook of Pediatric Emergency Medicine, 3rd ed. Baltimore, Williams & Wilkins, 1993, with permission.

relative narrowing presents as wheezing. Wheezing and stridor may sound the same and are therefore frequently confused. Further complicating the discrimination between stridor and wheezing is that each can be heard in the opposite phase of respiration (e.g., expiratory stridor and inspiratory wheezing) as the degree of partial airway obstruction advances.

Finally, there are diseases (e.g., croup) that can cause functional airway obstruction in both portions of the airway, producing both stridor and wheezing.

Lower Airway Disorders

Lower airway disorders are a very common cause of respiratory failure in all pediatric age groups. Respiratory failure from these diseases usually is mediated by a combination of bronchoconstriction, airway wall edema, and airway lumen obstruction by secretions. Reactive airway disease (asthma) is perhaps the commonest entity in this group of disorders. Although the musculature of distal airways is poorly developed in children under two years of age, reversible airway obstruction, or reactive airway disease, has been well documented in infants.[5] Bronchiolitis is the other common lower airway disorder affecting younger children. Unlike asthma, it tends to be seasonal in its occurrence, with respiratory syncytial virus as its principal pathogen.

Depending on the disease, any of these three mechanisms may predominate. The sum total of the three leads to a functional narrowing of the airway lumen and partial or complete airway obstruction. For lower tract airways, the obstruction first occurs in expiration, resulting in air trapping. As the obstruction progresses, the airway lumen then becomes obstructed during inspiration as well. This creates areas of poorly ventilated alveoli and resulting ventilation/ perfusion mismatching. Significant mismatching may be found even in patients with clinically mild illness.[23]

This mismatch of ventilation and perfusion manifests initially as arterial hypoxemia. It has been observed that children with apparently mild respiratory illness can indeed have clinically significant hypoxemia. It is this experience that has resulted in the recommendation that children presenting with respiratory illness to an acute care setting receive routine noninvasive (e.g., pulse oximetry) screening for hypoxemia.[12]

Compared to adults, children are especially prone to the effects of airway obstruction. The diameter of an infant's tracheal lumen is approximately one-third that of an adult-sized airway, and the infant bronchiole is one-half the size of its adult counterpart.[6] Pouseille's law (the resistance to airflow is related to the fourth power of the radius of the airway) dictates that even minimal changes in lumen size can have a profound impact on the resulting resistance to airflow. The impact of lower airway disease on respiratory performance in children is further magnified by the observation that lower airways make a greater contribution to total airway resistance in children than they do in adults.[5]

Children are at further risk for respiratory failure based on the anatomy and mechanics of the immature thorax. Young children have a soft, pliable rib cage, causing a higher compliance than seen in older children and adults. The horizontal positioning of the ribs to the sternum and diaphragm in infants also places them at a mechanical disadvantage. The infant diaphragm has been demonstrated to contain a greater percentage of fast-twitch muscle fibers, which are known to fatigue more easily. These features all add to the work of breathing in a patient with partial airway obstruction and make children more prone to the evolution of respiratory failure.[5]

Lung Parenchyma Diseases

The lung parenchyma disorders causing respiratory failure that are most frequently encountered in interhospital transport include infections, atelectasis, pulmonary edema, and, occasionally, adult-type respiratory distress syndrome (ARDS). While the causative mechanisms of these diseases are somewhat different, they all share a common final pathway, namely a mismatching of alveolar perfusion and ventilation.

Lower respiratory tract infections are exceedingly common in children, with a peak incidence in the first year of life. A significant percentage of infants with pneumonia will require hospitalization, with as many as 25% of those hospitalized requiring critical care.[21] The bacterial and viral pathogens responsible for pneumonia vary with age and time of year. Bacterial pathogens are an uncommon cause of critical illness in healthy hosts. While the development of rapid diagnostic technology has significantly improved management of these infections, integration of seasonal and age-related epidemiologic factors may assist in the selection of antimicrobial theory.

The signs or symptoms of lower tract infections can be fairly variable. In addition to nonspecific symptoms related to respiratory distress, there may be little else to direct the diagnosis toward pneumonia. Other findings may include irritability, vomiting, abdominal pain, or lethargy. Fever may or may not be present. Breath sounds may be asymmetric with crackles or rales appreciated on auscultation. Radiographic findings of an infiltrate, or an associated pleural effusion are frequently though not universally found.

Atelectasis is the most common lung parenchyma disorder encountered in an ICU setting.[21] Atelectasis may be the product of bronchial obstruction and/or direct parenchyma compression. Bronchial obstruction may be created by actual blockade of the bronchial lumen (e.g., foreign body, secretions) or by extra-bronchial compression (e.g., vascular ring, masses). In addition to evidence of increased work of breathing, the findings in patients with atelectasis include decreased breath sounds and dullness to percussion over the involved lung segment. Large areas of atelectasis may result in unilateral volume loss with shifting of the mediastinal structures on x-ray. This type of atelectasis is typically created by complete large airway (segmental bronchi or larger) obstruction. One important cause of such obstruction is endotracheal tube malposition.

While fairly uncommon in healthy pediatric populations, pulmonary edema is a common problem in critically ill children. It can be the result of any disorder that disrupts the forces governing the movement of fluid across the alveolar microvascular membrane (increased microvascular pressure, decreased interstitial tissue pressure, decreased plasma colloid osmotic pressure, increased interstitial osmotic pressure, increased vascular permeability, decreased lymphatic drainage). As most systemic diseases have some adverse impact on the lungs, the list of disorders that can create pulmonary edema is extensive. In addition to evidence of increased work of breathing, clinical findings in patients with pulmonary edema may include crackles on auscultation, wheezing, jugular venous distention, hepatomegaly, and pink-tinged, frothy sputum.

ARDS is a disease state characterized by diffuse alveolar disease or injury. The pathophysiology of this disorder, and its epidemiology in children, remain poorly understood. Its presentation can be fairly abrupt, as seen in children who have sustained blunt chest trauma or aspiration, or it can develop gradually, as might be seen in a child with sepsis. While ARDS is certainly not the most frequent cause of respiratory failure in children, it remains an important disorder because the overall mortality of this syndrome is nearly 60% in pediatric populations.[15]

The diagnosis of ARDS is based on the presence of characteristic clinical, radiographic, and physiologic findings. Patients with ARDS will demonstrate evidence of increased work of breathing with hypoxemia in spite of their increased minute ventilation. Hypoxemia that is refractory to maximal supplemental oxygen therapy and assisted ventilation is typical of severe ARDS. Interstitial lung markings are the radiographic finding early in the course of the illness, progressing to diffuse alveolar filling or a "white-out" pattern as the disease progresses.

Chest Wall and Mechanical Impairments

Mechanical impairments in the form of chest wall deformities or other structural barriers to ventilation can result in respiratory failure. These disorders act by reducing lung vital capacity. For certain acquired chest wall deformities (e.g., flail chest) and structural barriers (e.g., tension pneumothorax), the acute reduction in vital capacity can be severe enough to create respiratory failure. Children with congenital mechanical disorders (e.g., scoliosis) may poorly tolerate mild respiratory illnesses due to their limited ability to increase their respiratory performance.

Cardiac and Other Disorders

Respiratory performance is inexorably linked to the function of the cardiovascular system. Cardiac disease, if severe enough, can result in the development of secondary respiratory failure. Children with significant underlying chronic heart disease are also less tolerant of "ordinary" or mild respiratory illnesses. These children are therefore more prone to the development of "primary" respiratory failure. In addition to cardiac disease, severe anemia, acidemia, sepsis, heat illness, and certain toxins can cause respiratory failure.

PRETRANSPORT HOSPITAL MANAGEMENT

The phone call requesting the transport of an ill child provides an opportunity for the transport system to gather data regarding the patient's clinical status and, equally important, to provide advice to the referring team on how best to care for the patient pending the arrival of the transport team.[11] Although there may be significant limits to the scope of diagnostic or therapeutic interventions available to the patient, any direction that results in the improvement of care undoubtedly will have a positive impact on outcome.

The diagnosis of respiratory distress or respiratory failure can and should be made clinically at the time of the referred call. An objective physiologic evaluation with data to support that clinical suspicion should save precious time, assisting the arriving transport team to proceed directly to the critical therapeutic interventions required by the patient. As a general rule, all ill children, and certainly all those with respiratory distress, should be placed on continuous cardiorespiratory monitoring and given supplemental oxygen. The only exception would be the child with critical upper airway obstruction (e.g., epiglottitis, foreign body) who tolerates this poorly.

The assessment of the referring team should be directed to include a compete set of serial vital signs. An accurate description of the signs of increased work of breathing is also helpful. In terms of objective data, noninvasive pulse oximetry should be available at most emergency departments (although the correct-sized probe may not be). Of course, the data from pulse oximetry must be interpreted cautiously—a normal study does not rule out respiratory failure.

The gold standard diagnostic test is blood gas analysis, preferably from an arterial source. This provides a very objective assessment of pulmonary gas exchange, as well as a picture of the patient's acid-base status. Arterial blood sampling may be technically difficult in small children, and particularly in those who are not well. While the referring team should be encouraged to obtain these data, the stress of repeated painful or invasive procedures on an ill child should be considered when directing them to do so.

A chest x-ray also may be helpful in the assessment of an ill child with respiratory distress. A chest film may help to identify the cause or extent of the child's illness and can also help to evaluate certain invasive procedures (e.g., endotracheal intubation, central line placement). The referring team should be cautioned not to allow any lapse in the monitoring or care provided to a critically ill or injured child. Such a patient should never leave an acute care area to go to a radiology suite for an x-ray.

Advice regarding other diagnostic or therapeutic interventions depends on the clinical status of the patient, the suspected underlying disorder, the child's perceived needs, and the expertise or scope of care available at the referring facility. The transport program should be prepared to provide specific advice regarding pediatric resuscitation, including medication choices and dosing and tube or catheter sizes.

INTERHOSPITAL TRANSPORT MANAGEMENT

Upon the arrival of the transport team, the first priority should be a rapid cardiopulmonary assessment of the patient. The goal is to determine the patient's physiologic status and to provide necessary diagnostic and therapeutic interventions. The level of care provided should be equivalent to that received in a tertiary care pediatric critical care unit.

Recognizing that the transport vehicle and the period during which the patient is not in a hospital both represent a relatively unstable environment, the transport team must determine how to maximally stabilize the patient prior to departing the referring hospital. Most invasive procedures are more easily and successfully performed in the referring hospital, not in the helicopter or ambulance.[11]

Monitoring

As noted in the section on pretransport hospital management, it is important that a critically ill or injured child be continuously monitored. Making this rather difficult is the "background noise" generated during transport. The combination of vibration, electronic distortion, and background sound level challenges even the most technically advanced equipment. Recognizing this, the impetus for the transport team to maximally stabilize the patient prior to transport is even greater.

As a basic minimum, transported children should have continuous cardiopulmonary monitoring. In addition to a dynamic display of heart and respiratory rates, frequent or continous assessment of blood pressure should be done. As an adjunct or back-up to these monitors, continuous pulse oximetry also should be available for patients with critical illness. This can provide a very reliable assessment of the presence of hypoxemia.[19]

The concentration of delivered oxygen should be monitored at all times. Because children are particularly prone to heat loss, temperature monitoring of the pediatric patient is also essential. Finally, the evolving technology of noninvasive CO_2 (end-tidal, transcutaneous) measurement may allow confirmation of endotracheal tube placement and patency, the adequacy of assisted ventilation, or the presence of effective circulation.

All tubes and catheters should be checked for location and patency prior to departing the referring hospital. If the child is to be ventilated during transport, the patient should, if possible, be placed on the ventilator prior to leaving, with the adequacy of ventilation carefully assessed. Complications of assisted ventilation should be anticipated with replacement tubes and the necessary instruments kept readily available.

The specific goal for the transport management of respiratory failure is to relieve alveolar hypoventilation and tissue hypoxemia. Specific therapeutic modalities can be placed into one of three categories, those directed toward primary hypoxemia, the treatment of primary hypoventilation, and adjunctive therapies (Table 3).

TABLE 3. Management of Acute Respiratory Failure

Tissue hypoxemia	Alveolar hypoventilation (*cont.*)
Supplemental oxygen (titrate to color or oximetry)	Assisted ventilation with bag and mask
Assisted ventilation with bag and mask	Adequate tidal volume and pressure
Adequate tidal volume (10–15 ml/kg)	Increase expiratory time and/or rate
Positive end-expiratory pressure (PEEP)	Adjunctive therapy
Continuous positive airway pressure (CPAP)	IV fluid therapy to achieve normal vascular
Increase inspiratory time and/or rate	volume and tissue perfusion
Endotracheal intubation	Catecholamine/pressor therapy to assist
Treat the underlying cause	perfusion
Alveolar hypoventilation	Diuretic therapy for fluid overload or
Supplemental oxygen	pulmonary edema
Noninvasive and invasive airway support	Sedatives/analgesics
Chin lift or jaw thrust	Neuromuscular blockade
Suction	Antimicrobial therapy
Oral/nasal pharyngeal tube	Oral/nasal gastric tube insertion
Endotracheal intubation	Normothermia

From Baker MD, Ruddy RM: Pulmonary emergencies. In Fleisher GR, Ludwig S (eds): Textbook of Pediatric Emergency Medicine, 3rd ed. Baltimore, Williams & Wilkins, 1993, with permission.

Management of Primary Hypoxemia

Even in the absence of objective clinical evidence of hypoxemia (e.g., cyanosis or mental status changes), it should be assumed that children with signs of respiratory distress are suffering from hypoxemia. All such children should receive supplemental oxygen therapy. Oxygen therapy can be titrated against clinical signs (e.g., cyanosis) or by serial determinations of arterial oxygen content. Minimally acceptable PaO_2 levels are 60 torr in newborns and 70 torr in older children. If pulse oximetry is to be used to measure oxygen content, oxygen saturation should be maintained above 90%.

If supplemental oxygen therapy alone proves unsuccessful in reversing hypoxemia, respiratory care should be advanced to include assisted positive pressure ventilation. As a general rule, transport candidates who require assisted ventilation in order to maintain adequate oxygenation (or sufficient alveolar ventilation) should be intubated prior to transport. Assisted ventilation should deliver a sufficient tidal volume, generally 10–15 ml/kg, providing adequate chest expansion at an age-appropriate respiratory rate.

Depending on the underlying disorder, higher than normal pressures may be required to ventilate the patient. Increases in both the positive end-expiratory pressure (PEEP) and constant positive airway pressure (CPAP) may be needed for maximal end-expiratory lung volume and sufficient alveolar ventilation in children suffering from partial airway obstruction, atelectasis, diminished lung volume, or poor lung compliance. Increases in respiratory rate, inspiratory time, and tidal volume will also promote oxygenation. Finally, the diagnosis and specific treatment of an underlying disorder should assist efforts to oxygenate the patient.

Management of Primary Alveolar Hypoventilation

While supplemental oxygen therapy is a reasonable first intervention for a child with primary hypoventilation, it does not solve the underlying physiologic deficit. As a first step, a careful assessment of the patency and stability of the child's airway and the adequacy of the patient's ventilation should be performed. An obstructed or jeopardized airway should receive aggressive noninvasive (jaw thrust, chin lift, oral or nasal airway insertion, suction) and invasive (endotracheal intubation, surgical airway insertion) airway support.

While airway management may relieve hypoventilation due to upper airway obstruction, most children with primary hypoventilation suffer from lower airway or lung parenchyma diseases, or from disorders of respiratory control. These patients need assisted positive pressure ventilation with a bag and mask. As previously noted for children with primary hypoxemia requiring assisted ventilation, these children should also be intubated prior to transport.

Assisted ventilation should start at tidal volumes or pressures that provide sufficient chest expansion and gas exchange at an age-appropriate respiratory rate. If this fails to provide adequate alveolar ventilation, this assisted ventilation can be augmented through increases in respiratory rate, expiratory time, and tidal volume or pressure.

Adjunctive Therapy

Respiratory distress is frequently accompanied by disorders of other organ systems. Furthermore, children with nonacute or prolonged respiratory failure generally have developed multisystem organ failure. The optimal care of the child with respiratory distress or failure must therefore encompass evaluation and support of other key organ systems, such as the circulatory system.

Normal pulmonary function is highly dependent on the cardiovascular system, both for the delivery of blood to the lungs for alveolar/capillary gas exchange and for the delivery (and removal) of metabolic substrates (or byproducts) from tissues. Intravenous fluid therapy should be aimed at achieving normal vascular volume and perfusion pressures. In critically ill children, this may need to be augmented with catecholamines or pressors. While decreased vascular volume is certainly bad for ill children, so is fluid excess. Fluid therapy should be monitored carefully in these children. Iatrogenic fluid overload or pulmonary edema secondary to cardiovascular failure may require diuretic therapy.

Once it has been determined that a transport candidate will require assisted positive pressure ventilation with endotracheal intubation, serious consideration should be given to both sedative/analgesic therapy and neuromuscular blockade. Arguably, most patients are best intubated with the assistance of a rapid sequence induction technique. One can further argue that these patients should then remain paralyzed and sedated during the course of their transport. There are a number of perceived benefits from this practice, including decreasing the distressed patient's work of breathing and decreasing active or passive resistance of the patient during assisted ventilation.

If a pulmonary or related systemic infection is believed to be either the primary cause of respiratory failure or a significant accompanying factor, adjunctive therapy should include culturing the appropriate body fluids, and/or rapid immunoassay, and antimicrobial therapy. This may not have an immediate impact on respiratory function, but prompt intervention may help prevent continued deterioration and expedite long-term recovery. Additional therapeutic considerations in children with respiratory distress include maintenance of a neutral thermal environment. Hypothermia and hyperthermia have a profound and negative impact on metabolic function. Children with respiratory distress, or those who have received bag/mask ventilation, tend to have swallowed large amounts of air. An air-filled stomach can pose a problem for lung compliance, particularly if there is to be an air transport. As part of a general routine, all such children should have a nasal or orogastric tube in place.

MANAGEMENT OF POSSIBLE COMPLICATIONS

The provision of advanced life support for a child with respiratory failure exposes the patient to complications stemming from those interventions. The transport team must carefully assess and reassess the patient for these events, particularly during the transport. Any significant change in the patient's condition must be suspected as arising from such a complication until proved otherwise.

The first major category of complications are those related to the patient's airway—in particular, complications related to endotracheal intubation. Although it represents a tool to relieve airway obstruction or protect a jeopardized airway, the presence of an artifical airway places the patient at risk for acute airway obstruction or respiratory failure. This may be due to inadverent extubation, kinking or obstruction of the tube, or main stem bronchus (or esophageal) intubation.

The tube's position and patency should be carefully reaffirmed before departing the referring hospital, but Murphy's law and practical reality dictate that complications will occur during physical transfer of the patient (e.g., from stretcher to stretcher) or while the patient is being moved or transported. Any sudden change in the patient's condition should first be suspected as representing an airway problem. The transport team should always have a laryngoscope, an appropriate endotracheal tube and stylet, and a suction device with catheters immediately available.

The second category of complications are related to the provision of assisted positive pressure ventilation. While the long-term complicatons of oxygen toxicity and barotrauma may not be appreciated during the period of transport, excessive pressure or volume ventilation can result in a pneumothorax. The occurrence of this complication can be limited by careful monitoring of the tidal volume and ventilatory pressures used. The presence of free air in the thorax may be further exacerbated by the effects of high altitude or by the development of a tension pneumothorax. As noted for airway complications, these too are most likely to occur during the actual transport.

The suspicion of a pneumothorax should be raised prior to leaving the referring hospital. This is especially important if the patient is to be transported by air. If clinical suspicions warrant, a chest film should be obtained before departure. Finding a pneumothorax in an air transport patient should prompt the placement of a chest tube prior to departure. Of course, if time, the condition of the patient, or resources will not permit an x-ray, then a chest tube should be placed in the side(s) that are suspect.

Similarly, the diagnosis of a tension pneumothorax should be made clinically. In the scenario of a patient receiving assisted positive pressure ventilation who suffers an acute and severe cardiopulmonary decompensation, this diagnosis should be pursued after ensuring that the airway is intact and that equipment failure is not the cause. Even in the absence of clinical findings (e.g., decreased breath sounds) supporting the diagnosis, needle thoracostomy should be pursued on the suspect hemithorax, and on the contralateral hemithorax if the initial attempt is unsuccessful.

The third set of complications are related to equipment failure. The transport team must be prepared to maintain the patient's level of care in spite of the malfunction of key monitoring or therapeutic devices. It is always advisable to have some back-up power systems or equipment for cardiorespiratory monitoring. As an example, while not equivalent to a dynamic cardiac monitor, continuous pulse oximetry can provide adequate baseline monitoring data (pulse rate, O_2 saturation). If a mechanical ventilator is used to support a patient in respiratory failure, the team should be prepared to hand ventilate the patient if the ventilator fails, or if it is unable to support adequately the patient's needs.

REFERENCES

1. Baker MD, Ruddy RM: Pulmonary emergencies. In Fleisher GR, Ludwig S (eds): Textbook of Pediatric Emergency Medicine, 3rd ed. Baltimore, Williams & Wilkins, 1993.
2. Bushore M: Pediatric emergency care: Where do we go from here? A pediatrician's view. Pediatr Emerg Care 2:258, 1986.
3. Chameides L, Hazinksi MF (eds): Textbook of Pediatric Advanced Life Support, 2nd ed. American Heart Association, 1994, pp 2-1.
4. Committee on Pediatric Emergency Medicine: Emergency Medical Services for Children: The Role of the Primary Care Provider. Elk Grove Village, IL, American Academy of Pediatrics, 1992.
5. Eigen H, Gerberding KM: Lower airway disease. In Holbrook PR (ed): Textbook of Pediatric Critical Care. Philadelphia, W.B. Saunders, 1993.
6. Engel S: The Child's Lung: Developmental Anatomy, Physiology, and Pathology. London, Edward Arnold, 1947.
7. Haller JA: Towards a comprehensive emergency medical system for children. Pediatrics 86:120, 1990.
8. Institute of Medicine Committee on Pediatric Emergency Medical Services: Emergency Medical Services for Children. Washington, DC, National Academy Press, 1993.
9. Kanter RK: Neuromuscular disorders. In Holbrook PR (ed): Textbook of Pediatric Critical Care. Philadelphia, W.B. Saunders, 1993.
10. Krug SE: Cardiopulmonary arrest and resuscitation. In Reece RM (ed): Manual of Emergency Pediatrics. Philadelphia, W.B. Saunders, 1992.
11. Krug SE: Principles and philosophy of transport stabilization. In McCloskey KA, Orr RA (eds): Pediatric Transport Medicine. St. Louis, Mosby, 1995.
12. Maneker AJ, Petrack EM, Krug SE: The contribution of routine pulse oximetry to patient evaluation and management in a pediatric emergency department. Pediatrics 25:38, 1995.
13. O'Rourke PP: Outcome of children who are apneic and pulseless in the emergency room. Crit Care Med 15:667, 1986.
14. Rosenberg NM: Pediatric cardiopulmonary arrest in the emergency department. Am J Emerg Med 12:497, 1984.
15. Royall JA, Levin DL: Adult respiratory distress syndrome in pediatric patients. Clinical aspects, pathophysiology and pathology, and mechanisms of lung injury. J Pediatr 112:169, 1988.
16. Schmidt-Nowara WW, Altman AR: Atelectasis and neuromuscular respiratory failure. Chest 85:792, 1984.
17. Seidel JS: History of EMS for children. In Dieckmann RA (ed): Pediatric Emergency Care Systems: Planning and Management. Baltimore, Williams & Wilkins, 1992.
18. Seidel JS, Henderson DP (eds): Emergency Medical Services for Children: A Report to the Nation. Washington, DC, National Center for Education in Maternal and Child Health, 1991.
19. Silverman BK (ed): APLS: The Pediatric Emergency Medicine Course, 2nd ed. Elk Grove Village, IL, American Academy of Pediatrics, 1993, p 3.
20. Task Force on Interhospital Transport: Guidelines for Air and Ground Transport of Neonatal and Pediatric Patients. Elk Grove Village, IL, American Academy of Pediatrics, 1993.
21. Tilden SJ, Logan JJ: Lung parenchyma. In Holbrook PR (ed): Textbook of Pediatric Critical Care. Philadelphia, W.B. Saunders, 1993.
22. Torphy DE, Minter MG, Thompson BM: Cardiorespiratory arrest and resuscitation of children. Am J Dis Child 138:1099, 1984.
23. Wagner DP, Dantzker DR, Iacovoni VE, et al: Ventilation-perfusion inequality in asymptomatic asthma. Am Rev Respir Dis 118:511–524, 1978.
24. Weibley RE: Disorders of the proximal airway. In Holbrook PR (ed): Textbook of Pediatric Critical Care. Philadelphia, W.B. Saunders, 1993.
25. Zaritsky A: Cardiopulmonary resuscitation in children. Clin Chest Med 8:561, 1987.

Transport Issues in Neonates with Respiratory Problems

RAVI S. IYER, M.D.
DHARMAPURI VIDYASAGAR, M.D.

The transition from the uterine to extrauterine environment requires a series of complex physiologic changes affecting virtually every organ of the infant's system. This transition depends upon various factors involving pregnancy, labor, and delivery. The most obvious change at birth is the onset of breathing. Various stimuli, such as thermal, tactile, chemical, and neural reflexes, play a role in establishing respiration. Any compromise in utero, during, or soon after delivery may affect this phenomenon.

Respiratory problems are the most common reason for a neonate to be transported to the regional perinatal center. These problems are different in babies who are preterm, term, or post-term. An accurate assessment of the gestational age is critical in determining the most probable diagnosis. A combination of maternal dates, prenatal ultrasound (fetal growth, biparietal diameter, femur length, crown-rump length), and newborn physical and neurologic characteristics can predict the gestational age with an accuracy of ± 2 weeks. This, along with the birth weight, help in assessing the potential or the occurrence, the seriousness of the respiratory problem, and mortality and morbidity secondary to the disease.

The decision to transfer a high-risk newborn is to be made according to specific criteria developed within each region and based on the needs of the infant and local resources. Infants 28–34 weeks' gestation without significant respiratory problems may be managed in the community hospital.

Preterm infants are most commonly referred for problems of respiratory insufficiency, respiratory distress syndrome (or hyaline membrane disease), and apnea. In the term and post-term infant, respiratory distress secondary to aspiration, pneumothorax, or respiratory failure due to perinatal asphyxia frequently require immediate referral. Congenital anomalies such as diaphragmatic hernia, airway obstruction (laryngomalacia, vocal cord paralysis), or chest cage anomalies also require specialized care at the perinatal center (Table 1).

On receiving the call at the perinatal center, it is important to obtain a brief summary of events. Of particular importance is the gestational age, birth weight, Apgar scores, age (in hours), symptoms and time of onset, clinical course, interventions (oxygen, intubation, and ventilation), blood gases, current respiratory support, any obvious congenital anomalies, chest x-ray, and maternal history (fever, prolonged rupture of membranes, chorioamnionitis, oligo- or

TABLE 1. Respiratory Problems Requiring Neonatal Transport

Respiratory distress syndrome	Congenital anomalies (*Cont.*)
Apnea of prematurity	Diaphragmatic hernia
Transient tachypnea of newborn	Severe eventration of diaphragm
Respiratory insufficiency	Laryngotracheomalacia
Air leak syndromes (pneumothorax,	Choanal atresia
pneumomediastinum)	Thoracic dystrophy
Meconium aspiration syndrome	Cystic hygroma
Perinatal asphyxia with respiratory failure	Vascular rings
Diaphragmatic paralysis	Tracheoesophageal fistula
Vocal cord paralysis	Pleural effusions (secondary to hydrops,
Congenital anomalies	chylothorax)
Trisomy 13, 18	Bacterial or viral pneumonia (e.g., group B
Pierre Robin syndrome	streptococci)

polyhydramnios). Consolidation of this information helps in arriving at the diagnosis and assessing the seriousness of the situation, as well as in preparing for the transport. Sometimes, the problem may be minor and potentially resolve over a short period of time. The perinatal center would then be consulted for recommendation on the management.

A standard information sheet may be distributed among the network hospitals. When the need for consultation or transport arises, this form can be filled out and faxed to the perinatal center followed by a phone call. This form helps in accurate documentation of the transport call by the centers and gives some time for the physician to analyze the data. It also helps in deciding the composition of the transport team and assigning priorities. The perinatal center physician may also recommend certain interventions (e.g., administration of surfactant) before the child's arrival.

MECHANICS OF ARRANGING A TRANSPORT

Equipment
Once it is decided to transport the baby, the transport equipment should be checked thoroughly for readiness. The list of equipment commonly needed for a neonatal transport is given in Table 2.

It should be emphasized that in preparing for the transport of a critically ill neonate, the neonatal intensive care unit of the perinatal center is being extended into the community hospital. It is important therefore to ensure that all equipment is functioning properly. For a baby with respiratory problems, the transport incubator with a ventilator and oxygen-delivery system is the central piece of equipment. The transport team members should be aware of the functioning of the respiratory equipment and deal with any trouble-shooting. Remember Murphy's law: "If something can go wrong, it will!"

The electronic equipment must be easily adaptable to the power supply in the transport vehicle. Most equipment needs a conversion device that converts the 12-V DC current to 100-V/60 Hz AC current. All these units must have adequate grounding in the transport vehicle.

Advances in biomedical technology have helped in miniaturizing much of the equipment. Most of the monitoring devices for heart rate (EKG), respiration, on-line blood pressure, and pulse oximetry are available as a single unit mounted on the transport incubator frame. Many of them take into account the vibrations, bumps, and electronic interference in a transport vehicle and give reliable readings.

TABLE 2. Equipment Needed for Transport

Electrical	**IV accessories** *(Cont.)*
Transport ventilator	Sterile water vials
Transport incubator	Normal saline (flush) vials
Oxygen analyzer	Heparin lock flush (10 U/ml)
Pulse oximeter	**Drugs**
Laryngoscope with blades (size 0 and 1)	5% albumin
Infusion pumps	Normal saline
Cardiorespiratory and blood pressure monitor	Ringer's lactate
Respiratory care	Dopamine vial
Endotracheal tubes (2.5, 3.0, 3.5, and 4.0 mm)	Morphine vial
Suction catheters (nos. 6 and 8)	Pancuronium/vecuronium vial
Chest tubes	Phenobarbital vial
Heimlich valve	Furosemide vial
Laryngoscope bulbs	Phytonadione ampule
Batteries	Epinephrine 1:10000
Oxygen cylinders	Atropine vial
Oxygen tubing	Calcium fluconate vial
Oxygen facemask (nos. 0, 1, and 2)	Sodium bicarbonate vial
Self-inflating bag	Naloxone ampule
Stethoscope	Midazolam ampule
Bulb syringe	Ampicillin vial
Monitoring accessories	Gentamicin vial
EKG monitor leads	Digoxin ampule
Pressure transducer	Prostaglandin E_1 (ped)
Lancets	Tolazoline vial
Capillary tubes	Isoproterenol ampule
Dextrostix/Accuchek strips	Lidocaine vial
Pulse oximeter probe	IV fluids (D5W, D10W, normal saline)
IV accessories	**Miscellaneous**
Alcohol swabs	Feeding tubes (nos. 5 and 8 Fr)
Povidone-iodine swabs	Suction catheters (6, 8, and 10 Fr)
Gauze pads (2 × 2, 4 × 4 in)	Umbilical arterial catheters (3.5 and 5 Fr)
Syringes (3, 5, 10, 20, and 30 ml)	Umbilical ligature
Angiocatheters (24, 22 gauge)	Silk suture, with needle (3.0)
Tape (½ and 1 in)	Blunt needle adapters (18, 19, and 20)
Scalp vein needles (25, 23, 22, and 21 gauge)	Diapers
Three-way stopcocks	Blankets
Needles (19, 20, 22, and 25 gauge)	Flash light
Infusion pump tubing	Admission and other consent forms, hospital
Blood culture bottles (aerobic, anaerobic)	area map, nursery visitor's guidelines

Oxygen for transport is available in a compressed gas cylinder. It is important to be familiar with the various capacities of the oxygen cylinders available and their expected duration of life at various flow rates (Table 3). If an oxygen blender indicates the FiO_2 is not available, a mixture of air and oxygen can be given and the FiO_2 calculated based on their flow rates (Table 4). However, many transport units now are supplied with an oxygen blender for more accurate oxygen delivery. Oxygen cylinders that can be carried with the incubator are usually type E. Some extra oxygen is used to drive the ventilator, thus emptying the oxygen cylinder earlier than anticipated with the flow rate. A margin should also be provided for problems during the ride, such as a traffic delay of acute events in the neonate necessitating a stop en route. Larger oxygen cylinders are available in ambulances and may be used during the transport. Switching from the transport incubator source to that in the ambulance must be easy and swift. Hence, connecting ends of the tubing must be compatible. Care should be taken to inform the ambulance crew of these special needs in advance.

The transport ventilator should be checked for proper functioning. The ventilator tubing must be set up and anchored at an appropriate place in the

TABLE 3.   Approximate Hours of Flow for Standard Oxygen Cylinders Supplying MVP-10 Time-Cycled at a Rate of 50/Minute*

Flow Rate (l/min)	Standard Cylinder and Capacity (hrs)			
	D-360	E-620	M-3450	H-6900
1.0	1.2	2.1	11.5	23.0
1.5	1.2	1.9	10.5	20.9
2.0	1.0	1.7	9.6	19.2
2.5	0.92	1.6	8.8	17.7
3.0	0.86	1.5	8.2	16.4
3.5	0.80	1.4	7.7	15.3
4.0	0.75	1.3	7.2	14.4
4.5	0.71	1.2	6.8	13.5
5.0	0.67	1.1	6.4	12.8
5.5	0.63	1.1	6.1	12.1
6.0	0.60	1.0	5.8	11.5
7.0	0.55	0.94	5.2	10.5
8.0	0.50	0.86	4.8	9.6
9.0	0.46	0.79	4.4	8.8
10.0	0.43	0.74	4.1	8.2
11.0	0.40	0.69	3.8	7.7
12.0	0.38	0.65	3.6	7.2

* These figures express the tank life in hours with a full tank capacity. The tank life is dependent on factors other than flow rate, including cycling rate (increased cycling rate causes decreased tank life), use of positive end-expiratory pressure and continuous positive airway pressure, and capacity of the tank at the time of usage (e.g., if the tank were half full at the start of ventilation, these tank life figures would be reduced by 50%).

incubator. Some transport incubators have a connecting board, where tubing from the ventilator is attached to the outside of the incubator onto a bulkhead and those from the baby to the inside. This board prevents traction on the endotracheal tube due to the weight of the tubing and accidental extubation. However, care should be taken to monitor for disconnections at the board. Transport ventilators with rate and pressure alarms are available. In the absence of these, constant vigil should be maintained on the ventilator pressure gauge to check for cycling with the appropriate rate and pressure. A circuit should also be arranged for hand ventilation with a manometer in case of ventilator failure or acute events.

TABLE 4.   Effective FiO_2 Delivery from Various Combinations of Air and Oxygen Flow

Air Flow (l/min)	Oxygen Flow (l/min)								
	1	2	3	4	5	6	7	8	9
10	0.93	0.87	0.82	0.77	0.74	0.70	0.67	0.65	0.63
9	0.92	0.86	0.80	0.76	0.72	0.68	0.65	0.63	0.61
8	0.91	0.84	0.76	0.74	0.70	0.66	0.63	0.61	0.58
7	0.90	0.82	0.76	0.71	0.67	0.64	0.61	0.58	0.56
6	0.89	0.80	0.74	0.68	0.64	0.61	0.57	0.55	0.53
5	0.87	0.77	0.70	0.65	0.61	0.57	0.54	0.51	0.49
4	0.84	0.74	0.66	0.61	0.56	0.53	0.50	0.47	0.45
3	0.80	0.68	0.61	0.55	0.51	0.47	0.45	0.43	0.41
2	0.74	0.61	0.53	0.47	0.44	0.41	0.39	0.37	0.35
1	0.61	0.47	0.41	0.37	0.34	0.32	0.30	0.30	0.29

The pulse oximeter may be mounted separately or may be part of a combined monitoring system. Appropriate oximeter probes must be present in the equipment.

Although all electronic equipment would be hooked up to the transport vehicle's electrical source, they should have backup batteries to last the duration of transport in case the vehicular source fails. The oxygen source should be similarly self-sufficient.

TRANSPORT TEAM

The composition of the transport team is critical and depends on the nature and severity of the neonate's problem. It is important that the team personnel are adequately trained in care of the sick newborn. A sufficient volume of transports (> 300/year) merits organization of a separate team and roster. In other instances, the team may be formed by personnel on call in the neonatal unit.

When a physician accompanies the transport, he or she assumes responsibility and coordinates the efforts of team members. The need for a physician in the team depends on the seriousness of the problem in the neonate, availability of coverage in the neonatal intensive care unit (NICU) and policies laid down by the division. Currently, nurses are playing a greater role as transport team members. Some transport teams consist of nurse clinicians who are specially trained in neonatal problems and transport. Their training allows them to identify and treat respiratory distress, air leaks, and apnea with procedures including intubation and chest tube insertion. Respiratory therapists familiar with the needs of a neonate being ventilated form an important part of the team. Their expertise in managing the ventilator helps the physician concentrate on the other aspects of the critically ill neonate.

The transport team must function as a unit, with each member recognizing the other's capabilities and responsibility. When a physician is present, he or she assumes the role of team leader. In other instances, the senior transport nurse assumes that role. During transport, any major changes in the baby should be communicated to the base unit. The ambulance personnel assume the responsibility of the vehicle movement, route, and help in communication with the base hospital.

The behavior of the team members at the referral hospital needs special attention. The referral hospital team has worked hard to keep the baby stable and managed the situation as best as they could. They also are very concerned about the neonate and have been the first to impart the news of the baby's illness and need for transport to the parents. Hence, criticisms of management or a patronizing attitude on the part of the transport team should be avoided. Many things may be learned by the team on managing a sick baby when faced with limited resources. The referral hospital team is often eager to learn about other techniques of stabilization, procedures (e.g., endotracheal tube fixing), and new equipment. The transport team should take the opportunity to demonstrate these briefly during their visit. Such attitude of camaraderie will help in the rapport between the two hospitals.

STABILIZATION OF THE INFANT IN THE REFERRAL HOSPITAL

One of the major functions of the transport team in the referral hospital is to stabilize the baby before departure. Sometimes, the personnel at the referral hospital expect the transport team to "swoop and scoop." However, first the position of the endotracheal tube should be checked by clinical examination and, if necessary, x-ray. The positions of central lines should be looked at for

TABLE 5.   Endotracheal Tube (ETT) Size (Oral) for Newborns

Weight (gm)	ETT Size— ID (mm)	Length to Corner of Mouth (cm)	Laryngoscope Blade Size
< 1250	2.5	7.5	0
1250–2000	3.0	8.0	0
> 2000	3.5	8.5	1

appropriate positioning. The clinical course should be evaluated. If one was not done recently, a blood gas analysis should be done to assess the need for changes on the ventilator. Hypothermia, hypotension, hypoglycemia, and metabolic acidosis worsen the condition of a neonate with respiratory distress. Hence, these imbalances should be corrected before the baby leaves the referral hospital. The vital signs should help in deciding the need for vasopressors (dopamine, dobutamine) or volume infusion (albumin, normal saline). In cases of respiratory distress syndrome, surfactant may need to be administered. The trachea should be suctioned before departure. A "small" pneumothorax may worsen rapidly during transport; as it is more difficult to insert a chest tube in the narrow confines of an ambulance, due consideration should be given to performing this procedure at the referral hospital.

AIRWAY MANAGEMENT

Babies with severe respiratory disease need to be intubated and ventilated. If this procedure has not been done already, the transport team may need to do it. The size of the endotracheal tube should be selected according to infant's weight (Table 5). The tube should be adequately secured with tape to prevent accidental extubation en route (Fig. 1).

Most neonates do not need to be sedated for the purpose of intubation. However, some term infants remain vigorous and may need sedation and muscle relaxants during transport. Table 6 lists the drugs used for sedation. Most frequently used in neonates are morphine and fentanyl.

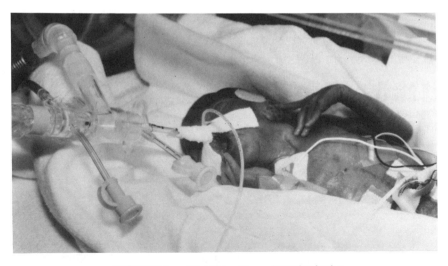

FIGURE 1.   Stabilizing the endotracheal tube.

TABLE 6. Sedatives Used in Airway Management in Neonates

Drug	Dose
Benzodiazepine	
Midazolam*	70–200 μg/kg/dose
Narcotics	
Morphine	50–100 μg/kg/dose
Fentanyl	1–4 μg/kg/dose

Care should be taken when using morphine in hypotensive neonates. Babies with meconium aspiration syndrome may be on high inspiratory pressures. When the baby breathes against the ventilator, intrathoracic pressure increases rapidly and may result in pneumothorax. Use of muscle relaxants helps prevent this to some extent (Table 7). Commonly used relaxants are pancuronium and vecuronium.

Accidental extubation en route is the most frequent respiratory complication. Recognition of this event during transport may be delayed because of various factors, such as poor lighting, absence of alarms, and poor accessibility. Reintubating a baby in the ambulance may be catastrophic considering the space limitations and movement of the vehicle. It may be necessary to pull over to the roadside and stop until the neonate is stable. In addition to securing the endotracheal tube properly and providing sedative medications and muscle relaxants, judicious use of physical restraints with sheets or Velcro straps helps in preventing these events. If the baby is agitated *despite adequate oxygenation*, additional doses of the sedative may be given en route.

A sudden deterioration in respiratory status may be due to a pneumothorax. Clinical examination and transillumination of the chest determine the location. Because it is difficult to insert a chest tube in the ambulance, a large-bore angiocatheter may be inserted and left in place until arrival to base unit. Though it is not as good as a chest tube, the procedure might save the infant's life and keep him or her stable during a short trip.

Severe hypotension may also present a similar picture, especially in term infants with persistent pulmonary hypertension and on hyperventilation. Volume supplementation with 20 ml/kg of 5% albumin may be given. Maintenance of temperature during transport is important. The transport incubator temperature should be set within the thermoneutral range for the baby's weight. Failure of power source can result in hypothermia. Use of prewarmed blankets or warm water beds should be considered. The baby should continue to receive appropriate intravenous fluids to prevent hypoglycemia (particularly babies at risk, such as those who are preterm or small-for-gestational age, or with diabetes mellitus, hypoxia, or sepsis) or dehydration. If there are any changes in the baby's condition en route, the Perinatal center NICU should be updated. Most ambulances have a portable cellular telephone, and constant communication should be maintained during transport.

TABLE 7. Drugs Used as Muscle Relaxants in Neonates

Drug	Dose
Pancuronium	40–150 μg/kg/dose
Vecuronium	30–150 μg/kg/dose

MANAGEMENT OF PARENTAL ANXIETY

The team leader should take time to talk with the baby's mother, explaining her infant's respiratory problem, the need for transport to another hospital, and the treatment planned. Parents are very anxious about their baby's medical condition, transfer to a new hospital, and the need to get to know and interact with a new group of caregivers. Time should be spent with them in allaying as much of this anxiety as possible. It would be helpful to write down the names of physicians and nurses who may be involved in the baby's care at the perinatal center. A brief explanation should be given as to why the baby is being transferred and what course of action will be taken at the parinatal center. Consents for admission and immediately possible procedures, such as catheter insertion or blood transfusion, could be explained and obtained at this time. The possibility of transporting the baby back to the referral hospital as soon as he or she is stable should also be discussed. Parents should be given a map showing the exact location of the base hospital, location of the NICU, and a telephone number to call. Before departure, the mother should have an opportunity to see and touch her baby. This act goes a long way in the mother's dealing with the separation from her infant. Space constraints and state laws may not permit parents or their relatives to travel in the ambulance with the baby, but the parents should be called soon after reaching the base hospital with an update on their baby's condition.

Before leaving the referral hospital, the transport team should call the perinatal center NICU regarding the baby's condition, ventilator set-up, and required intravenous lines or medications.

SPECIFIC PROBLEMS

Respiratory Distress Syndrome

Respiratory distress syndrome (RDS) is the commonest respiratory problem in premature infants. It results from inadequate surfactant production by type II alveolar epithelium. The major role of surfactant is to decrease surface tension and prevent the collapse of alveoli. Surfactant is a mixture of phospholipids and various proteins. At 35 weeks' gestation, the lecithin-sphingomyelin ratio is 2:1, which indicates adequate pulmonary maturity. However, factors such as diabetes, acute asphyxia, and maternal hemorrhage and acidosis can retard the production of surfactant, whereas chronic hypertension, placental insufficiency, antenatal steroids, prolonged rupture of the membranes, and drug abuse (e.g., heroin) result in accelerated pulmonary maturity. The primary effect of inadequate surfactant is alveolar atelectasis (Fig. 2). This condition results in hypoxia, hypercarbia, and acidosis leading to decreased pulmonary perfusion; a right to left shunt occurs in the lungs. Alveolar capillary damage due to hypoxia and poor perfusion results in capillary leak and edema formation. It also interferes in surfactant production. Surfactant may also be inactivated by the edema fluid containing plasma proteins. Low pH and hypoxia may cause pulmonary vasoconstriction, further decreasing pulmonary blood flow. It may also cause cardiac dysfunction and hypotension. The increased work of breathing causes further hypoxia and respiratory failure ensues.

Management

The use of antenatal steroids has decreased the incidence of RDS considerably. Even in those infants who go on to develop RDS, the disease is less severe. Surfactant replacement is the key to treatment of RDS. Respiratory support,

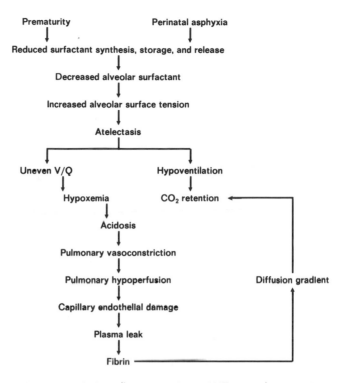

FIGURE 2. Pathophysiology of respiratory distress syndrome. V/Q = ventilation/perfusion.

oxygenation, acid-base balance, thermoregulation, and adequate tissue perfusion are major supportive measures. Babies with respiratory distress, grunting, and chest retractions should be intubated in the delivery room. The goal of adequate oxygenation is to maintain PaO_2 between 60–90 mmHg. If a chest x-ray shows reticulogranular pattern, airbronchogram, or bilateral haziness, it confirms the presence of RDS (Fig. 3).

Surfactant must be given via the endotracheal tube as early as possible. Though several types of surfactant are available, only Survanta (natural, bovine lung extract) and Exosurf (synthetic) are currently approved by the FDA. The endotracheal tube should not be suctioned for 2 hours after surfactant administration. Following this, oxygenation improves and care should be taken to wean the FiO_2 to prevent hyperoxia. As the pulmonary compliance improves, the ventilatory pressures (positive inspiratory pressure [PIP] and positive end-expiratory pressure [PEEP]) must be decreased appropriately to prevent air leaks (e.g., pneumothorax). Further doses of surfactant may be needed depending on the severity of RDS and response to initial dose. If the baby continues to require an $FiO_2 > 0.4$ despite adequate ventilation, further doses (up to four doses) may be given. Rarely, a baby with RDS may fail to respond to surfactant.

The ventilatory strategy is to oxygenate well without resulting in hyperoxia and with minimal barotrauma. Some very low birth weight infants do not have RDS and may need respiratory support only. PEEP is a valuable tool in babies with RDS; it may be maintained between 3–5 cm H_2O, though the optimal PEEP for each baby may vary. PaO_2 may be maintained between 60–90 mmHg by changing FiO_2 or other ventilatory parameters, such as PIP, PEEP, or respiratory rate.

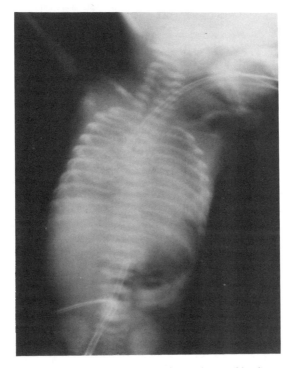

FIGURE 3.   X-ray showing diffuse haziness and granularity of hyaline membrane disease.

Maintenance of blood pressure appropriate for gestational age is important for adequate tissue perfusion. Vasopressors such as dopamine and dobutamine may be used early if necessary. If there has been blood loss, as in antepartum hemorrhage or from birth trauma, a packed cell transfusion must be given. Occasionally, 5% albumin or normal saline may be used, and this should be followed by adequate fluid therapy with 5% dextrose or 10% dextrose in water. Hypoglycemia must be treated with an intravenous bolus of 10% dextrose solution, 2 ml/kg, and an increase in dextrose infusion (> 6 mg/kg/min).

Mild metabolic acidosis is corrected with these measures. If it is not or if the acidosis is severe, sodium bicarbonate, 1–2 mEq/kg (0.5 mEq/ml) may be given slowly intravenously over 0.5 hour. Respiratory acidosis may be treated with changes in ventilation parameters. Care should be taken to rule out mechanical causes such as airway obstruction due to endotracheal tube or pneumothorax.

With extensive handling and initial procedures, hypothermia may result and should be prevented by using a radiant warmer, plastic wrap, or aluminum foil wrap. Placing the baby in an incubator is more useful in maintaining a neutral thermal environment. It is difficult to distinguish respiratory distress due to RDS from pneumonia. Hence, antibiotics (ampicillin and gentamicin) must be started after drawing blood for a complete blood count and blood culture. If the results are not suggestive of sepsis, antibiotics may be stopped.

Transport Issues in RDS

The transport team should evaluate the infant with RDS for the severity of symptoms. If they are mild, nasal continuous positive airway pressure (CPAP) may be adequate. However, as many of these babies deteriorate, it is better to intubate them electively in the community hospital rather than as an emergency in the ambulance during transport. The ambulance ride is stressful and would contribute to worsening of the clinical status. If the baby is already intubated, the following procedures are to be done:

1. Check endotracheal tube position by clinical examination and the most recent chest x-ray. Reposition if necessary.

2. Check for proper securement of the endotracheal tube, and retape if needed.

3. Evaluate clinical signs of adequate ventilation, such as color, chest movement, and breath sounds.

4. If chest movement is inappropriate, the inspiratory pressure may need to be changed.

5. Evaluate the most recent blood gas or obtain one if not done recently.

6. If RDS is confirmed, surfactant may be given before departure.

7. If surfactant is already given, the oxygenation and/or lung compliance may have improved. Appropriate weaning should be done on the ventilator, and if necessary, reevaluated with a blood gas.

8. All efforts should be made to have an arterial line (UAC or radial artery) in place for adequate monitoring of oxygenation and blood pressure.

9. The blood glucose, temperature, and blood pressure should be stabilized by appropriate measures.

10. Agitation and irritability may be due to hypoxia. If hypoxia is ruled out, a sedative-analgesic (e.g., morphine) may be used. If the baby is on high inspiratory pressures, consideration may be given to skeletal muscle paralysis also.

During transport, the major problems are endotracheal tube dislodgement and pneumothorax. The latter should be considered in a baby with acute deterioration. Transillumination is positive on the affect side. Aspiration of the pneumothorax should be done with a 25-gauge butterfly needle connected to a 20-ml syringe via a three-way stopcock. Chest tube insertion can be very difficult in the limited space of an ambulance. Alternatively, a 24-gauge angiocatheter may be used for aspiration. Small changes in oxygen saturation may be overcome by increasing the FiO_2.

Meconium Aspiration Syndrome

Meconium-stained amniotic fluid may be seen in 10–15% of deliveries. The passage of meconium may be physiologic or due to hypoxia. It occurs mostly in post-term and small-for-gestational-age infants.

Aspiration of the meconium by the neonate may occur either in utero or intrapartum. Amniotic fluid with thick meconium is more likely to cause problems. The pathophysiology is outlined in Figure 4. Post-term and small-for-gestational-age fetuses should be monitored adequately for occurrence of asphyxia. A critical step toward preventing intrapartum aspiration is suctioning of the mouth and pharynx by the obstetrician soon after delivery of the head at the perineum. Subsequently, the pediatrician should suction the trachea, especially if meconium is thick. There is an increased mortality and morbidity in infants born from pregnancies with meconium-stained amniotic fluid.

Symptoms of respiratory distress may occur soon after or within the first few hours after birth. They may be mild, with only tachypnea and borderline oxygen saturation. Cyanosis may not be seen until significant hypoxia occurs in view of the high oxygen affinity of fetal hemoglobin. Worsening tachypnea, grunting,

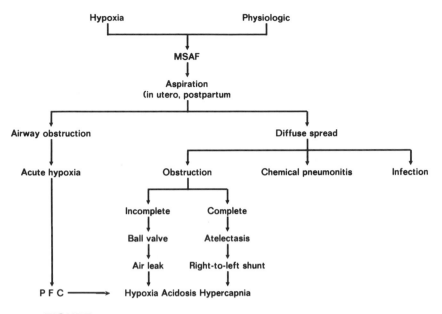

FIGURE 4.   Pathophysiology of meconium aspiration syndrome.

and chest retractions may occur. The chest may look hyperinflated. A chest x-ray shows irregular, patchy densities on one or both sides interspersed with areas of hyperaeration. Pneumothorax or pneumomediastinum may also be seen and may be the cause of a sudden deterioration in clinical status. Many times, the severity of chest x-ray findings may not correlate with the clinical status. Rapidly worsening oxygenation may also indicate the presence of persistent pulmonary hypertension (PPHN). This diagnosis should be suspected when there is persistent hypoxemia or acidosis despite ventilation with 100% oxygen. The following criteria can be used to confirm the diagnosis:

1. A difference in PaO_2 of 15 mmHg (or a difference of 10% on pulse oximeter) between preductal and postductal arterial blood samples. However, this difference may not be seen in a large right-to-left shunt across the foramen ovale.

2. A two-dimensional echocardiogram showing normal cardiac anatomy and prolongation of systolic time intervals (M-mode), indicating systemic/suprasystemic pulmonary artery pressure or a right-to-left shunt across the patent ductus arteriosus.

Management

Prevention of meconium aspiration is an ideal goal but not achievable many times. Adequate fetal monitoring, amnioinfusion, and timely delivery all help toward this goal. Suctioning of the mouth and pharynx on delivery at the perineum by the obstetrician and of the trachea soon after birth by the pediatrician minimizes intrapartum aspiration. Despite this, a significant number of babies aspirate meconium in utero and become symptomatic.

Adequate oxygenation will decrease pulmonary vasoconstriction and thus PPHN. Respiratory failure and hypoxia should be treated with mechanical ventilation with 100% oxygen. Hyperventilation to keep a pH 7.5–7.55 is the most common mode of ventilation. High mean airway pressures may need to be used to achieve adequate oxygenation. Hypotension worsens when there is increased intrathoracic pressure and decreased venous return. Vasopressors (dopamine, dobutamine) will be needed to keep systemic blood pressures more than the pulmonary blood pressures. This helps decrease the right-to-left shunting seen in PPHN.

Correction of metabolic acidosis with sodium bicarbonate will also help decreasing pulmonary vascular resistance. A continuous infusion of sodium bicarbonate may be considered to increase the pH. Hyperkalemia and hypocalcemia (secondary to alkalosis) need to be monitored closely. Antibiotics need to be considered if there is a question of pneumonia in the differential diagnosis. Tolazoline may be tried in severe PPHN. However, its use is limited by the severe systemic hypotension it causes. Surfactant has been tried with limited success. Use of high PEEP in conventional ventilation increases the risk of pneumothorax. Pulmonary barotrauma may result in air leak syndromes. Prompt intervention for pneumothorax with a chest tube is critical in these very sick infants. Inhaled nitric oxide has been shown to selectively decrease pulmonary vascular resistance with dramatic improvement. There has been a report on its use during transport from the referral hospital. Extracorporeal membrane oxygenation (ECMO) needs to be considered if the following criteria are met, although some infants respond to high-frequency ventilation without ECMO.

1. Alveolar–arterial PO_2 difference ($AaDO_2$) > 608 for 8 hours
2. $AaDO_2 > 604$ for 4 hours when PIP is > 38 cm
3. Oxygenation index (mean airway pressure $\times$ $FiO_2/PaO_2 \times 100$) > 40 for 4 hours
4. Barotrauma
5. Cardiac support
6. Acute deterioration

Transport Issues

Babies with meconium aspiration syndrome are usually very ill and have a potential for dramatic deterioration. They are known to have periods of good oxygenation and hypoxia without any change in ventilatory settings ("flip-flop" phenomenon). Hence, great care must be taken to stabilize these infants before departure:

1. Check the baby's respiratory status—clinical, chest x-ray, and arterial blood gases—and ventilatory setting.
2. An arterial line is crucial to monitor the blood pressure and PaO_2.
3. If ventilatory changes are necessary, repeat arterial blood gases in 0.5 hour.
4. If the baby has a pneumothorax, a chest tube should be in place before departure. The chest tube should be checked for adequate drainage.
5. A Heimlich valve (Fig. 6) is a one-way valve that can be used to drain a pneumothorax during transport. Its simple design, small size, and light weight make it ideal for transport.
6. Metabolic acidosis needs to be corrected promptly with injection of sodium bicarbonate, 1–2 mEq/kg as a slow bolus. It may also be used as an infusion to help maintain a high pH.
7. Evaluate a recent report of electrolytes and correct any abnormalities. Watch particularly for serum potassium and calcium values, which may be low in the presence of high pH.
8. Check the transport bed for adequate oxygen source. Also ensure that the ventilator in the bed is capable of delivering the high PIP by changing the pop-off valve settings if necessary. As soon as the baby is in the ambulance, consider a quick switch to the ambulance's oxygen source, as these are of a larger capacity.

9. If the baby is hypotensive, he or she may need a bolus infusion of normal saline or 5% albumin, 20 ml/kg. The baby may also need to be on vasopressors before departure.

10. Other measures, such as checking position of endotracheal tube and securing it properly, should be done.

11. Many of these babies are vigorous and "fight" the ventilator. The baby may be sedated using morphine or midazolam.

During transport, the commonest problem is ventilator malfunction. Be prepared to ventilate the baby with the hand-bag while correcting the problem. Running out of oxygen is also a major issue, as a high gas flow is needed to run the transport ventilator while the baby is on high PIP. Leaks or tears may occur in the hand-ventilatory bag (especially the anesthesia type). A spare one should be available in the transport kit. Vigorous babies may accidentally extubate themselves. A good physical restraint system using Velcro straps may be beneficial. A pneumothorax may occur at any time, and a chest tube will need to be inserted and connected to a Heimlich valve. The transport monitor should preferably be capable of monitoring the arterial blood pressure. If there is any drop in blood pressure, a fluid bolus needs to be given promptly. The endotracheal tube may get plugged with meconium or mucus.

Air Leak Syndromes

Pneumothorax, pneumomediastinum, pneumopericardium, and pulmonary interstitial emphysema are the common air leak syndromes seen in the NICU. Most often, these are associated with positive pressure ventilation. Occasionally, an infant may develop spontaneous pneumothorax and deteriorate rapidly. Disease processes such as meconium aspiration syndrome, diaphragmatic hernia, or hypoplastic lungs commonly predispose to air leak syndromes.

The accumulation of air in these spaces may be mild, requiring minimal or no direct intervention, to severe, needing immediate attention. Symptoms of respiratory distress such as tachypnea, grunting, and chest retractions due to the underlying primary condition may worsen rapidly, or there may not be any improvement despite adequate respiratory support. The chest on the affected side may be bulging. On the right side, the liver may be pushed down. Under these circumstances, a pneumothorax should be considered, and transillumination of the chest or a chest x-ray done. The x-ray will show air in the pleural space with a collapsed lung margin and shift of mediastinum to the opposite side (Fig. 5). If the lung is noncompliant, collapse may be minimal and pneumothorax difficult to detect. However, a small pneumothorax may increase and need intervention. If a tension penumothorax is seen, prompt relief with needle aspiration followed by a chest tube is needed.

Pneumomediastinum is usually mild and rarely requires any intervention. It is best seen on a lateral film of the chest as accumulation of air behind the sternum or elevating the lobes of thymus creating the "sail" sign. Pneumopericardium may cause cardiac tamponade and requires immediate drainage. Pulmonary interstitial emphysema usually manifests as worsening respiratory distress with gradually increasing PCO_2. Subsequent deterioration may be rapid. It is more common in very immature infants on a ventilator.

Transport Issues

Pneumothorax (unilateral or bilateral) without any underlying lung pathology has a better prognosis than when it complicates a respiratory disease.

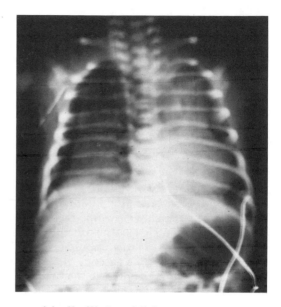

FIGURE 5. Chest x-ray showing pneumothorax.

In the latter instance, the baby is more critically ill. In addition to management of the underlying respiratory disease, care should be taken to assess the degree of pneumothorax. Even mild ones may worsen during transport due to the vibrations and bumps of the ride, resulting in erratic ventilatory pressures. Hence, it is advisable to drain the pneumothorax adequately and preferably keep a chest tube in place before departure. Check for proper drainage through the water seal and also with a chest x-ray to assess the degree of resolution of the pneumothorax.

During transport, underwater seal systems are bulky and difficult to manage in an ambulance. The pleural drainage may depend on a continuous suction being applied to the system. Moreover, the chest tube and its connections may move and get dislodged with the movement or vibrations of the ambulance. A Heimlich valve is light weight and small and allows air to drain one way (Fig. 6). Though it may not drain all the air in the pleural cavity, it serves well for a transport. Management of pulmonary interstitial emphysema should include using minimal ventilatory pressures to maintain sufficient oxygenation.

Diaphragmatic Hernia

A defect in the diaphragm due to failure of closure of the pleuroperitoneal canal during the eighth week of fetal life results in herniation of the bowel into

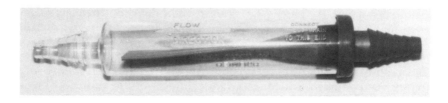

FIGURE 6. Heimlich valve.

the thoracic cavity. This in turn produces severe pulmonary hypoplasia and bowel obstruction. The size of herniation depends on the size of the defect. The defect commonly occurs at the left posterolateral lumbocostal triangle, on the left side in 85% of cases. The pulmonary hypoplasia results in a decreased number of pulmonary arterioles per unit area. This increases the vascular resistance. The clinical manifestations range from progressive respiratory distress with persistent pulmonary hypertension in severe cases to an asymptomatic infant in the milder hernias. Long-term outcome depends on the time of onset and severity of symptoms, gestational age, and postnatal management. Though variable, in those babies who present early in life, a survival rate of 40–60% is reported.

Management

The diagnosis of diaphragmatic hernia can be made with a prenatal ultrasound. After birth, the infant presents with progressive respiratory distress, scaphoid abdomen, and asymmetric breath sounds. A chest x-ray shows intestinal loops in the thoracic cavity with shift of the mediastinum to the opposite side (Fig. 7). An orogastric tube should be placed immediately to provide continuous suction, which prevents gaseous distention of the stomach and bowel. Endotracheal intubation is essential soon after the diagnosis is suspected. Bag and mask ventilation should be avoided to prevent intestinal distention. Appropriate positioning of the endotracheal tube is crucial to prevent selectivity in ventilating the hypoplastic lung. The underlying severe lung disease presents as persistent pulmonary hypertension. Hyperventilation with high ventilator rates and mean airway pressures may be tried with or without alkali therapy. Air leaks, particularly pneumothorax, are common and can cause a sudden deterioration in clinical status. Immediate placement of chest tubes is necessary. Hypotension is a common problem in these neonates, and volume infusion and vasopressors may be needed. ECMO can stabilize the baby for surgery. High-frequency ventilation, ECMO, and inhaled nitric oxide have also been found to be useful. The goal is surgical correction at the earliest.

Transport Issues

Optimal ventilatory management is crucial until the defect is surgically corrected. The respiratory therapist is a crucial part of the team and allows other team members to concentrate on other aspects of the baby's illness instead of the ventilator. The transport team should ensure proper position of the endotracheal tube, as confirmed by an x-ray. A recent arterial blood gas should be available, and ventilator settings may need to be adjusted to maintain good oxygenation. Maintenance of adequate perfusion is critical. The baby may need fluid bolus prior to departure and also vasopressors. Careful evaluation for the presence of a pneumothorax should be done. If one is found, placement of chest tubes should be strongly considered. The orogastric tube should be of large bore (8 Fr) and kept open for continuous drainage.

Before departure, the base NICU should be updated on the baby's status so that they are appropriately prepared to receive the baby. The pediatric surgeon should be appraised of the transport and estimated time of arrival so that there is an opportunity to evaluate the baby soon after arrival.

During transport, many of these babies are on maximal ventilatory support. Depending on the transit time, the oxygen cylinders on the transport incubator may soon run out. It may be better to switch to the larger cylinders from the ambulance source. Adequate functioning of the ventilator should be monitored closely. Ideally, the monitor should have a pressure transducer to record arterial

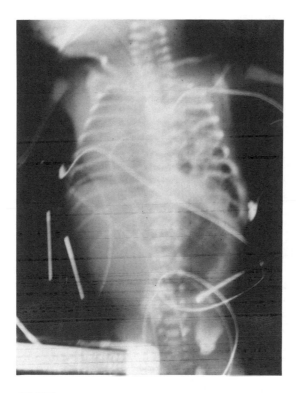

FIGURE 7.   Chest x-ray showing left diaphragmatic hernia.

pressure, as acute hypotension may occur during transport. A pneumothorax may be precipitated by the sudden jolts of a group ambulance, resulting in inappropriate intrathoracic pressures. Sedation of the baby and skeletal muscle relaxants must be considered.

Respiratory Depression

In apnea of prematurity and perinatal asphyxia, there is ineffective or no breathing depending on the severity of the problem. In both conditions, the central control of respiration is defective. In premature babies, respiratory stimulants such as aminophylline or caffeine may be tried. If apneas are significant enough to cause hypoxia, the baby needs ventilatory support until he or she is mature enough. Respiratory depression in perinatal asphyxia may be transient or may indicate a severe damage to the nervous system. Until a decision is made on the reversibility of the lesion, the respiratory failure has to be supported. In both diseases, the lungs are essentially normal. Hence, a minimal support in terms of inspiratory pressures or ventilatory rates is needed.

Transport Issues

These babies are generally stable when their respiration is supported. However, an asphyxiated infant may have symptoms related to brain injury (e.g., seizures). This needs to be controlled effectively with anticonvulsants before leaving the referral hospital. It is useful to know the number and severity of seizures so as to be prepared for one during transport. Diazepam or midazolam may be used for immediate control and phenobarbital for long-term use. In some babies, phenytoin may have to be added. Some babies with perinatal asphyxia may have respiratory distress and PPHN. Under these circumstances, the management is similar to that described in meconium aspiration syndrome with respect to PPHN.

Obstructive Lesions

Unilateral vocal cord paralysis may cause stridor with crying. It is usually secondary to excessive traction on the head during a breech or forceps delivery. Injury to the recurrent laryngeal branch is more common on the left side. Bilateral paralysis causes more severe respiratory symptoms. It is usually secondary to hypoxia or brainstem hemorrhage. These babies may have severe stridor, chest retractions, and aphonia. Immediate intubation and subsequently tracheostomy is necessary in many babies. Follow-up examination of vocal cords must be done. If improvement in their movement is observed, extubation may be tried. Most babies with unilateral paralysis recover over 4-6 weeks. Prognosis in bilateral paralysis depends on the severity of asphyxial injury.

Pierre Robin syndrome is a disorder of early hypoplasia of the mandible with resultant micrognathia, glossoptosis, and cleft palate. Presenting symptoms depend on the severity of posterior airway obstruction. In severe cases, an oral airway has to be inserted immediately. The baby can also be positioned prone and head down. The mandible develops with time and, hence, the airway and nutrition should be maintained until then.

Laryngotracheomalacia may be mild enough to cause inspiratory stridor only during drying or severe enough to cause obstruction during regular breathing. Under these circumstances, the baby may need to be intubated or a tracheostomy done for long-term care until the trachea improves.

In choanal atresia the neonate presents with respiratory distress and cyanosis at rest, with some improvement during crying because of mouth breathing. Placing an oral airway can produce dramatic improvement until corrective surgery is done.

Cystic hygroma or vascular rings may be severe enough to cause respiratory obstruction. Intubation may be difficult in babies with large hygromas, as also in Pierre Robin syndrome. Respiratory support is needed until surgical correction is done.

Babies with thoracic dystrophy present a management dilemma depending on whether the condition is lethal or not. Many of these babies need prolonged respiratory support, and they may die due to respiratory failure secondary to the restrictive disease.

Transport Issues

The common problem in management of these conditions is respiratory obstruction. Intubation may be easy, as in laryngotracheomalacia. If may be extremely difficult in some babies with Pierre Robin syndrome or a large cystic hygroma when the upper airway is displaced. During transport of such babies, the endotracheal tube should be secured well and babies sedated for the duration of transport. Intubating them during transport can turn out to be a disaster.

Other Disorders

Transient tachypnea of the newborn is secondary to delayed clearing of lung fluid. It is usually a self-limited disease and resolves over 48-72 hours. Oxygen may need to be given by hood or nasal cannula. Occasionally, it is severe enough to require ventilatory support.

Diaphragmatic paralysis is usually unilateral and secondary to phrenic nerve injury in upper brachial plexus palsy. Infants present with a wide range of respiratory symptoms from asymptomatic to severe respiratory distress. A chest x-ray shows an elevated diaphragm. Diagnosis may be confirmed by ultrasound or fluoroscopic examination for the movement of the diaphragm. Respiratory support may be needed in some infants for 4–6 weeks. If no improvement occurs at this time, plication may need to be considered.

Eventration of the diaphragm is a congenital weakness of a part of the diaphragm and may present with similar symptoms. It is more common on the left side with the liver being pulled up. Pneumonia may supervene due to atelectasis of the lung on the affected side. A chest x-ray shows an elevated diaphragm with paradoxical movement on fluoroscopy or ultrasound. Surgical plication at the earliest will relieve the symptoms.

Tracheoesophageal fistula may be of different types. In type 2 (85% of cases), when there is esophageal atresia (a blind pouch) and a fistula between the lower end of the trachea and the stomach or esophagus, the risk of aspiration is high. This may occur more commonly from inadequate drainage of secretions in the esophageal pouch. Aspiration pneumonia is a common reason for worsening respiratory status and need for support.

Bacterial pneumonia, particularly that due to group B streptococci, can present with severe symptoms with or without PPHN. In addition to antibiotics, PPHN must be managed with appropriate ventilatory strategy, which may include hyperventilation.

Transport Issues

Many of these infants may not need ventilatory support but may need oxygen. If pneumonia has supervened, antibiotics have to be given. During transport, the major issue is that of ventilatory support. The problems and issues have been addressed already in previous sections. In babies with tracheoesophageal fistula with esophageal atresia, care should be taken to adequately drain the esophageal pouch with a large-bore tube on continuous suction and head-up position to prevent aspiration. Babies with bacterial pneumonia and PPHN are very ill and need to be managed during transport as discussed for meconium aspiration syndrome and PPHN.

AIR TRANSPORT

Transport of newborn babies by helicopter or fixed-wing aircraft is increasingly used in areas where distance between the referral hospital and base NICU is large or when time is crucial. Air transport provides state-of-the-art neonatal services to remote areas. However, a change in altitude changes the barometric pressure in unpressurized aircraft. The sum of partial pressures of individual gases in the atmosphere defines the barometric pressure. Therefore, the partial pressure of oxygen (21% of atmosphere) decreases with increasing altitude (Table 8).

Hence, for the same FiO_2, this decrease in alveolar PO_2 with increasing altitude in turn decreases arterial PO_2. The hypoxia may increase the pulmonary vascular resistance if appropriate adjustments in FiO_2 are not made.

According to Boyle's law, at constant temperature, the volume of a gas varies inversely with the pressure. Therefore, the volume of gas within closed spaces, such as the thoracic cavity and intestines, changes with a change in barometric

TABLE 8.   Barometric Changes with Altitude

Altitude (ft)	Barometric Pressure (mmHg)
Sea level	0760
2,000	706
5,000	632
8,000	565
18,000	379

TABLE 9.   Gas Volume Changes with Altitude

Altitude (ft)	Atmosphere	Gas Volume
Sea level	1.00	1.00
5,000	0.83	1.20
8,000	0.77	1.33
10,000	0.50	2.00

pressure (Table 9). Air leak, such as pneumothorax, pneumomediastinum, or pneumopericardium, will expand and rapidly worsen the baby's condition. An endotracheal tube cuff may also expand and cause tracheal injury. However, in most neonates uncuffed endotracheal tubes are used.

Rapid descent can result in decompression of gases. If the baby is intubated, there is a risk of pneumothorax or air embolism occurring due to rapid reexpansion of respiratory gases. A slow ascent and descent is therefore recommended to reduce these problems.

Cabin pressurization minimizes some of these effects. Manipulation of the cabin pressure is within limits. Hence, the transport team must be aware of the barometric pressure within the aircraft in which they function. The change in PO_2 may also affect the transport team members and worsen fatigue or potentiate effect of some drugs, such as antihistamines or antivertigo agents.

REFERENCES

1. Bhende MS, Thompson AE, Orr RA: Utility of an end-tidal carbon dioxide detector during stabilization and transport of critically ill children. Pediatrics 89:1042-1044, 1992.
2. Donn SM, Faix RG, Gates MR: Neonatal transport. Curr Probl Pediatr 15(4):1-65, 1985.
3. Ferrara A, Harin A: Emergency Transfer of the High-Risk Neonate. St. Louis, Mosby, 1980.
4. Finsterwald W: Neonatal transport: Communication—the essential element. J Perinatol 8:358-360, 1988.
5. Jain L, Vidyasagar D: Cardiopulmonary resuscitation of newborns: Its application to transport medicine. Pediatr Clin North Am 40:287-301, 1993.
6. Johnson DE, Thompson TR: Resuscitation, stabilization and transport of the ill newborn infant. Minn Med (Apr):249-253, 1982.
7. Martin RJ, Fanaroff AA: The respiratory distress syndrome and its management. In Fanaroff AA, Martin RJ (eds): Neonatal-Perinatal Medicine: Disease of the Fetus and Infant, 5th ed. St. Louis, Mosby, 1992.
8. McDonald TB, Berkowitz RA: Airway management and sedation for pediatric transport. Pediatr Clin North Am 40:381-406, 1993.
9. Miller C: The physiologic effects of air transport on the neonate. Neonatal Netw 13(7):7-10, 1994.
10. Pettitt G, Bonnabel C, Bird C: Regionalization and transport in perinatal care. In Merenstein GB, Gardner SL (eds): Handbook of Neonatal Intensive Care. St. Louis, Mosby, 1989, pp 25-27.
11. Task Force on Interhospital Transport: Guidelines for Air and Ground Transport of Neonatal and Pediatric Patients. Elk Grove Village, IL, American Academy of Pediatrics, 1993.

CHAPTER 15

Transport Management of Acute Pediatric Asthma

ZEHAVA NOAH, M.D.
MARY GOMEZ, R.N., M.S.N.
STEVEN LESTRUD, M.D.

Asthma, or reactive airway disease, is a frequent cause for severe lower airway obstruction in infancy and childhood. Mortality continues to rise,[6] despite advances in the understanding of the pathophysiology of asthma and research focused on elucidating the best preventive measures and the development of appropriate treatment protocols.

Asthma affects 5–10% of children younger than 20 years.[17] Thus, it is the most common chronic illness in childhood. It is the leading cause of morbidity in childhood, with peak hospitalizations occurring in the fall months.[6] In children under 10 years, males were admitted twice as often as age-identical females.[19] Prevalence is higher in black children, despite a 40% overall increase in prevalence among white children in the United States.[23]

Asthma is frequently triggered by
- allergen exposure
- infections
- exercise
- emotional stress
- atmospheric causes such as weather, pollution, vapors.

Typical pathologic changes are bronchial smooth muscle spasm and hypertrophy, mucosal edema with influx of inflammatory cells, and mucus plugging with mucus gland hypertrophy.

Clinically, the patient presents with cough, dyspnea, wheezing, and respiratory distress. The chest radiograph may show hyperinflation, atelectasis, and peribronchial thickening.

Differential diagnoses may include
- bronchiolitis
- foreign body aspiration
- pneumonia
- pulmonary edema
- cystic fibrosis.

Status asthmaticus, the acute life-threatening manifestation of the disease, is characterized by airflow obstruction and bronchial hyperreactivity that does not respond to bronchodilators and may lead to respiratory failure (Table 1).

TABLE 1.   Clinical Indicators of Severe Asthma

Signs/Symptoms	Mild Phase	Moderate Phase	Severe Phase
Mental state	Age appropriate or at child's baseline	Agitated	Agitated, may be obtunded
Color	Pink in room air	Pink in oxygen	Cyanotic in oxygen
Chest expansion	Normal	Chest hyperinflation	Poor excursion, chest hyperinflation
Breath sounds	Present, wheezing/rales	Diminished, wheezing/rales	Markedly decreased
Respiratory rate	Tachypneic, 30% above the mean	Tachypneic, 30–50% above the mean	Tachypneic, over 50% above the mean, or may be slower due to fatigue
Retractions	None to mild intercostal retractions	Moderate intercostal retractions with tracheosternal retractions, use of sternocleidomastoid muscles	Severe intercostal retractions; tracheosternal retractions with nasal flaring during inspiration; retractions may decrease due to fatigue
Dyspnea	Uses complete sentences	Uses phrases, infant has difficulty sucking and feeding; cry is softer and shorter	1–2 Word dyspnea, infant stops feeding and sucking
Arterial blood gas			
pH	Alkalotic	Alkalotic	Acidotic
pO_2	WNL	Low	Low
pCO_2	< 35	< 40	> 40
Heart rate	Tachycardia	Tachycardia	Tachycardia
Blood pressure	Elevated, pulsus paradoxus < 10 mmHg	Elevated, pulsus paradoxus 10–20 mmHg	Pulsus paradoxus > 20 mmHg, dependent on hydration status
Oxygen saturation in room air	$> 95\%$	90–95%	$< 90\%$
Peak flow (for children 5 years old and older)	70–90% of predicted or personal best	50–70% of predicted or personal best	$< 50\%$ of predicted or personal best

Treatment and prevention of respiratory failure through oxygen administration, bronchodilators, and anti-inflammatory agents, and hemodynamic stability are the goals of therapy.

To transport a child safely during an acute exacerbation one has to be thoroughly familiar with the pathophysiology of the disease, its possible complications, and the level of care required during the different phases. Caregivers also must possess the skills and knowledge to deliver the necessary care for stabilization and transport.

INITIAL MANAGEMENT AND DECISION TO TRANSPORT

Care of the child in status asthmaticus requires simultaneous assessment and treatment. In the initial evaluation, the patients may be categorized as mild, moderate, or severe, as outlined in Table 1. Treatment and monitoring capabilities vary depending on whether care is at the pediatrician's office, a clinic, or a hospital Emergency Department (ED). Priorities of care, however, should follow the basic ABCs (airway, breathing, circulation) format prior to initiation of treatment (Table 2).

TABLE 2. Priorities and Equipment Needed for the Transport of the Acute Asthmatic Child

Priority	Assessment	Treatment Plan	Equipment Needed
A = Airway	Accommodate for position of comfort to facilitate aeration	Set up precautionary airway equipment	Face mask, nonrebreather; Intubation equipment: correct size endotracheal tube, stylet, laryngoscope, and blade; Appropriate bag and mask
B = Breathing	Assess respiratory rate, effort, color; Auscultate breath sounds	Give 100% O_2; Consider ABG; Check chest radiograph; Give preferred nebulized beta-agonist; Suction if needed; Have precautionary chest tubes and needle aspiration set-ups available	Oxygen delivery system, portable O_2 tank and O_2 tubing; Correct size chest tube and needle aspiration set-ups; Portable suction (battery operated and fully charged)
C = Circulation	Check heart rate, blood pressure, and O_2 saturation	Connect patient to cardiac monitor and pulse oximeter; Start IV with D5.2NS and 20 mEq KCL/L or D5.45NS and 20 mEq KCL/L at maintenance rates	Cardiac monitor; Pulse oximeter; End-tidal CO_2 monitor; Transcutaneous monitor, if available; Correct size IV catheters; Tubing, fluids, T-connector; Portable infusion pump
D = Drugs	Assess which medications have already been given; Assess if any drug allergies	Administer medications per protocol	Correct types and dosages of medications; Flush solutions, and syringes
E = Evaluate Evacuate Equipment	Continuously evaluate vital signs and overall status	Secure patient to stretcher; Secure tubings and equipment; Have equipment and IV easily visible during transport; Continuously monitor equipment function; Document patient findings	Equipment as listed above in A, B, C, D.

Patients presenting with a mild exacerbation may, after bronchodilators, need transfer from an office or clinic for worsening distress or because they are unresponsive to therapy. Moderate exacerbations will require transfer to an ED, if after appropriate bronchodilators and steroids, there is no marked improvement. For patients presenting in the severe phase and for high-risk patients, prompt transfer to a tertiary care center should be considered.

Transport of the child with severe asthma to the pediatric tertiary care center is indicated if stabilization cannot be achieved or continuing care cannot be delivered at the current setting—specifically, when the child's condition

- has been unresponsive to treatment
- exhibits increased respiratory distress and
- requires additional diagnostic and therapeutic modalities not available at the referral facility or
- the clinician requests transfer.

Since rapid deterioration can occur in status asthmaticus, preparation for transport should be made early. Consideration for transport based on the above parameters should include the length of time needed to access tertiary care.

TRANSPORT INFORMATION

The goals of transport are (1) safe, rapid transport; (2) the best possible stabilization of the patient's condition; and (3) minimizing stress and agitation. Once the decision for transport has been made, responsibility for care is a partnership between the referral hospital and the tertiary care facility. To initiate the transport process, exchange of information is essential. It should focus on the present state of the patient, whether improvement or deterioration has occurred, over what period of time, and the extent of services available in the referral facility. Data gathered on the phone will assist the transport team to anticipate the patient's needs. Preparation for transport arrangements should include such patient data as

- accurate description of the severity of respiratory distress
- fractional inspired oxygen (FiO_2) needed
- vital signs
- arterial blood gas (ABG) results
- brief history
- medications received at home
- medications administered at referral facility
- chest radiology results
- weight (for planning medication dosages)
- communication with parents
- parents' willingness to transport child.

Further information to facilitate transport logistics may include

- location of hospital
- optimal mode of transport (Appendix A)
- altitude concerns if applicable (Appendix B)
- landing facilities available (if necessary).

TRANSPORT PLANNING

Transport planning involves numerous details. It is recommended that team members utilize a checklist with each transport so that equipment and necessary notification calls are not forgotten. Planning the transport of the child in status asthmaticus may require the transport team to

- continue stabilization advice to the referral hospital
- premix medication drips
- organize, check, and secure equipment
- allocate a bed space and needed staff/equipment at the receiving institution
- designate contact/resource for referral hospital while team is en route
- ascertain estimated time of arrival (ETA) and inform necessary personnel.

Protocols guide many teams in the process of choosing medical management for the child with asthma, mode of transport (Appendix A), team composition, communication options, and equipment. Medical management of the child in status asthmaticus is described later in the chapter.

Team Composition

Factors that influence team composition include

- the child's severity of illness
- time and distance to the referring facility

- mode of transport
- experience of the team members
- need for advanced skill procedures such as possible intubation and chest tube insertion.

The child's condition may require skills not routinely available on advanced life support vehicles and may necessitate a pediatric speciality team. It is essential to focus on the skills the different members possess and match those skills to the situation. Thorough communication with the referral institution facilitates team composition selection.

Communication

Communication methods include the telephone, fax machine, cellular (mobile) phone, and dispatch radio systems. These systems are useful while the transport team is en route to the referral hospital. The team can ascertain if the patient's condition has changed. Regular contact will also reduce the amount of time spent discussing medical information at the referring institution and will allow the team to focus on direct patient care and stabilization. One should be cautious when utilizing communication systems that may cause electromagnetic interference (EMI) on flight instruments and medical equipment.

Equipment

The transport team should have well-charged equipment readily available. Transport equipment should comply with recommendations of durability, portability, and battery capability and should meet with all regulations for flight and electrical approval.[2] Prior to departure, transport members should confirm that the necessary equipment is ready and the appropriate people have been notified. Equipment and personnel should be properly secured into the vehicle.

EN ROUTE TO THE REFERRAL INSTITUTION

During the trip to the referring facility, the transport personnel should detail each team member's assignment. Team members also should calculate appropriate medication doses of anticipated asthma medications and emergency resuscitation and intubation drugs.

In addition, one must decide the size and type of equipment that may be needed, such as face masks and intravenous fluids. Equipment such as suction and oxygen systems should be set up and accessible. If medication drips are needed, one can prepare the solutions. Also, paperwork can be initiated to expedite the turnaround process. Finally, the transport personnel can contact the referring hospital to confirm the child's current status.

AT THE REFERRAL INSTITUTION

Upon arrival at the referral facility, the transport team should identify the staff members caring for the child. Brief introductions should facilitate the transfer process and create a congenial working environment. Patient assessment and current and proposed care plans must be reconciled, and tasks should be appropriately delegated to the transport team and referral hospital members to expedite stabilization and transfer.

Treatment protocols for transport of asthmatic patients vary but should include means to evaluate the degree of respiratory distress, initiate appropriate therapeutic measures, and apply monitoring for transport. After assuming care, simultaneous assessment and treatment are required following the ABC format in Table 2. This includes

- evaluation of the degree of respiratory distress
- evaluation of present status (vital signs and brief physical exam)
- obtainment of current medical history including previous ICU admissions, intubation, medications, allergies, precipitating events, and last oral intake
- consideration of pre- and post-bronchodilator peak flow measurements, unless in severe distress
- placement of the child in a position of comfort to facilitate aeration (may be on parent's lap).

Therapy will focus on the relief of bronchospasm and supportive care, which includes

- administration of supplemental oxygen per face mask
- assessment of hydration/initiation of fluid management
- assessment/treatment of underlying disease processes.

First-line therapy for an acute exacerbation is the application of beta-agonists, corticosteroids, methylxanthines, and consideration of anticholinergics.[9]

Beta-agonist receptor stimulation results in smooth muscle relaxation, with bronchodilation and vasodilation as well as tachycardia. Other frequent side effects include agitation, headache, tremors and hypokalemia. More specific beta-2 receptor agonists (albuterol and terbutaline) may result in less tachycardia.

Initial therapy for bronchospasm includes inhaled beta-agonist with oxygen, for patients not responding (those in status requiring transport), continuous beta-agonist nebulization is given. Subcutaneous administration of a beta-agonist (epinephrine or terbutaline) may be necessary with initial therapy if poor aeration limits nebulized drug delivery.

Intravenous bronchodilators are indicated for patients not clinically responding to nebulization therapy because of poor air exchange, elevated $PaCO_2$ (45 mmHg), or rising $PaCO_2$. Limiting factors are heart rates greater than 200–220 or 150% over baseline, chest pain, or dysrhythmias.[9]

BETA-AGONISTS
Albuterol
Nebulization: 0.1–0.2 mg/kg/dose to maximum 4 mg/dose in 5 ml normal saline every 15–20 min.
Continuous nebulization: 0.5 mg/kg/hr to maximum of 15 mg/dose/hr.
Terbutaline
Nebulization: 0.1–0.3 mg/kg/dose to maximum 3 mg/dose in 2.5 ml normal saline every 15–20 min.
SQ: 0.01 mg/kg/dose to maximum 0.3 mg/dose; repeat in 15–20 min for 3 doses.
IV: Load with 0.01 mg/kg over 10 min. Infuse 0.4 μg/kg/min initially, and increase as necessary by 0.2 μg/kg/min every 15–20 min. Maximum dose 6 μg/kg/min.
Epinephrine
SQ: 0.01 ml/kg/dose of 1:1000 to maximum of 0.3 ml/dose every 20 min up to 2 doses.
Isoproterenol
IV: 0.05 μg/kg/min increased by 0.05 μg/kg/min every 15 min as necessary for response to maximum 1 μg/kg/min.
Infusion should be through a second secure intravenous line.

CORTICOSTEROIDS
Methylprednisolone
IV: Load with 2 mg/kg; subsequent 1-2 mg/kg/dose every 6 hr.
Given early will up-regulate beta receptors and decrease inflammation and edema.

METHYLXANTHINES
Aminophylline may have a limited use in acute severe asthma; however, it is still widely used. Therapeutic levels between 10 and 15 μg/ml are associated with a lesser risk of toxicity and must be closely monitored. Aminophylline side effects include nausea, vomiting, tachycardia, dysrhythmias, and seizures. Blood levels may be increased and side effects more frequent in congestive heart failure, cor pulmonale, liver failure, and viral infections. The drug must be used cautiously.[9]

Aminophylline
Patients with no history of theophylline use:
Aminophylline bolus 6 mg/kg IV over 20 min; then run continuous drip.
Known theophylline level:
2 mg/kg IV bolus will increase serum level by 2 μg/ml.
Patients taking theophylline with unknown level:
Start continuous drip at appropriate rate while waiting for level.
Aminophylline drip rates:
6 weeks-6 months: 0.5 mg/kg/hr
6 months to 1 year: 0.6-0.7 mg/kg/hr
1 year to 9 years: 1 mg/kg/hr
9 to 16 years: 0.7 mg/kg/hr.

ANTICHOLINERGICS
Ipratropium
Metered dose inhaler only, two inhalations; repeat in 4-6 hr.
Atropine
Nebulization—0.03-0.05 mg/kg/dose over 10 min.
Additional pharmacologic agents may be used, but may not be feasible during transport. These include helium-oxygen mixtures, magnesium sulfate, and inhaled anesthetics.

Monitoring for transport provides a means for frequent assessment, evaluation of ongoing therapy, and detection of possible complications.
- place child on a cardiac monitor and pulse oximeter
- continue vital signs every 15 minutes
- consider arterial blood gases prior to departure
- obtain a chest radiograph
- continue pharmacologic therapy options (nebulizing treatments)
- evaluate the child's response to treatment
- copy chart, radiographs, and laboratory studies
- obtain repeat peak flow measurement, if feasible.

Indications for Intubation
Status asthmaticus occasionally will progress to respiratory failure despite maximal bronchodilator therapy. Indications for intubation and ventilation are based upon both clinical and laboratory data:

- exhaustion, poor respiratory effort
- absence of breath sounds and wheezing
- deteriorating mental status
- hypoxemia ($PaO_2 < 60$ mmHg in 60% FiO_2 or greater)
- hypercarbia ($PaCO_2 > 50$ mmHg or rising > 5 mmHg per hr)
- arrest, coma

Medications for Intubation

Endotracheal intubation may be poorly tolerated owing to hypoxemia, bronchospasm, and acidosis. Thus, personnel experienced in airway management should be utilized. Rapid-sequence induction may include atropine, ketamine, and succinylcholine with cricoid compression and oxygen supplementation. Conventional intubation may include atropine, analgesic/amnesic agents with a nondepolarizing neuromuscular blockade, with bag/mask ventilation and oxygen administration. Medications to be considered for intubation include:[9]

- **Atropine:** 0.01–0.02 mg/kg IV (0.1 mg minimum dose)
  maximum of 2 mg; anticholinergic reduces laryngospasm, bronchodilator
- Sedation/Analgesia*
  * Choose one of the following sedatives. Please note precautions prior to administration of any medication.
    Ketamine: 0.5–2.0 mg/kg IV; positive inotropy and bronchodilator
    Midazolam: 0.05–0.1 mg/kg IV; short-acting benzodiazepine
    Fentanyl: 1–2 μg/kg IV; less reported histamine release than with morphine
- Paralysis**
  ** Choose one of the following paralytics. Please note precautions prior to administration of any paralytics.
    Pancuronium: 0.1 mg/kg IV; longer acting, nondepolarizing muscle relaxant
    Vecuronium: 0.1 mg/kg IV; shorter acting, nondepolarizing muscle relaxant
    Succinylcholine: < 4 years 2 mg/kg IV; > 4 years 1 mg/kg IV; short-acting depolarizing muscle relaxant
    cholinergic effects not desirable
- **Lidocaine:** 1 mg/kg IV
  reduces laryngospasm and may blunt bronchospasm

Management of Ventilation

Strategies for ventilation should provide for adequate oxygenation and prevention of significant respiratory acidosis while avoiding barotrauma as bronchospasm resolves. To achieve these goals, the patient will require:

- oxygen supplementation
- paralysis and sedation
- continued bronchodilator therapy
- physiologic respiratory rate, tidal volumes 10–15 ml/kg
- short inspiratory time, maximal expiratory time
- low-level or no PEEP

Neuromuscular blockade and sedation are necessary to avoid hypoxia, bronchospasm, and barotrauma associated with resisting the ventilatory support. Low respiratory rates with a short inspiratory time allow maximal expiratory times, permitting proper emptying in air-trapped lungs. As a rule, positive end expiratory pressure (PEEP) is not necessary in lower airway obstruction as it may lead to overly distended alveoli and further cardiac and respiratory deterioration. For the duration of the transport, one should avoid severe acidosis; however, it is not always necessary to normalize $PaCO_2$. Elevated $PaCO_2$ (50–60 mmHg) may be tolerated if pH is within acceptable range and the patient is otherwise stable.

Potential Complications of Severe Asthma

Application of humidified oxygen, bronchodilators, and appropriate fluid management are adequate measures to treat most asthmatic exacerbations. The transport team, however, should attempt to anticipate acute complications and should be prepared to treat appropriately.

Hypoxia is common in asthmatic children upon presentation. Sudden worsening of hypoxia may be due to decreased air exchange, mucus plugging and atelectasis, developing pulmonary edema, and air leak. Administration of oxygen to keep saturations above 90% is done while evaluating the patient's air exchange and initiating more definitive treatment.

If patients develop **hypotension**, development of **pneumothorax** must be suspected with chest tube placement as necessary. Hypotension may result from **hypovolemia**, as many patients have had poor intake and have high intra-thoracic pressures impeding cardiac output, these patients will respond to intravenous fluid administration. Other causes for hypotension include dysrhythmias and tachycardia. **Dysrhythmias** and severe chest pain or other evidence of myocardial ischemia necessitate careful observation for worsening gas exchange while reducing beta-agonists or changing to more specific beta$_2$-agents.

Declining respiratory function may result in agitation or lethargy. **Agitation** not related to hypoxia or worsened air exchange may be due to therapy with beta-agonists or aminophylline and usually will respond to assurance. **Lethargy** is an ominous sign of respiratory failure, and intubation should be considered.

Complications of status asthmaticus may be due to the pharmacologic therapy. **Beta-agonists** contribute to tachycardia, agitation, hypokalemia, and hypoxia. **Isoproterenol**, in particular, has been associated with myocardial ischemia, tachycardia, and dysrhythmias. Patients with nausea and vomiting may have elevated **theophylline** levels. More serious side effects include gastrointestinal bleeding, dysrhythmias, tachycardia, and seizures. **Aminophylline and beta-agonist drips** must be carefully checked prior to transfer to insure they contain the appropriate concentrations to maintain therapeutic drug delivery.

PRIOR TO DEPARTURE

Before leaving the referral institution the transport team should notify the receiving facility of the

- child's condition
- care already given
- equipment and personnel needed
- estimated time of arrival.

Furthermore, the transport team should verify that the parents/legal guardians have the following information:

- a review of events
- prognosis
- plan of care
- informed consents
- directions to the tertiary care institution

- unit to which child will be admitted
- admitting physician responsible for care
- address the family's questions and concerns.

EN ROUTE BACK TO THE TERTIARY CARE FACILITY

Equipment should be well secured, visible to the team members, and audible if possible. Properly "packaging" the patient necessitates keeping the patient as comfortable as possible, keeping the child normothermic, and securing the child to the stretcher. Immediate access to intravenous sites, infusion pumps, and monitors is integral to evaluating the child's condition.

Potential for patient deterioration and equipment disconnects is high during the transition phases. Each patient movement between facilities and vehicles jeopardizes all connections and affects the child's response to the constant maneuvering. Emphasis is on continuous monitoring of the child and equipment. If the child's condition deteriorates, the receiving facility should be notified as soon as possible.

TRANSITION TO THE TERTIARY CARE FACILITY

In the pediatric intensive care unit, the transport team members assist in transition by monitoring vital signs, connecting equipment to hospital equipment, and giving the unit staff a thorough report.

Documentation of the transport should accurately reflect
- the child's condition upon arrival
- care that was rendered by the referral hospital
- care delivered by the transport team
- details of respiratory status
- times and doses of medications administered
- the child's response to treatments and the transport.

A phone call back to the referral hospital with an update of the child's condition is recommended. This allows for the transport team to offer their appreciation for assistance rendered during the transport. Furthermore, it offers the referral staff an opportunity to ask questions and confirm the child's safe arrival and current status.

CONCLUSION

Status asthmaticus is a frequent, life-threatening condition necessitating skilled transport to a pediatric referral center. Accurate assessment of the degree of respiratory distress; prompt application of bronchodilators, oxygen, and nonspecific therapy; clear concise communication between the referral center, transport team, and the pediatric ICU; and attention to details in monitoring will result in the safest, most efficient transport.

APPENDIX A

Effects of Mode of Transport on the Child with Severe Asthma

Mode of transport decisions may be critical to the safe transport of the child in severe respiratory distress. Each type of vehicle has advantages and disadvantages.[1,18] This will be briefly examined as pertinent to the child in status asthmaticus. Table 3 illustrates the overall advantages and disadvantages with each type of vehicle and implications for the transport of the child with severe asthma.

TABLE 3. Mode of Transport Considerations

Mode of Transport	Advantages	Disadvantages	Implications for the Child with Severe Asthma
Ground Ambulance	Provides door-to-door service; Can stop vehicle for emergency treatment; Can reroute to closest hospital; Easy to orient personnel to vehicle, thus can supplement with specialty teams; Multiple vehicles can be readily utilized for disaster situations/ multiple patients; In case of vehicle breakdown, alternate vehicle usually available; Few weather restrictions; Economical	Vulnerable to traffic delays; Cannot access remote areas; Potential for lengthy out of hospital transport times'; Repetitive acceleration/ deceleration; May not carry pediatric-sized equipment; Possibility of motion sickness	Potential spilling of nebulizer treatment; Parents may be able to ride along to reduce separation anxiety
Rotary-Wing (Helicopter)	Rapid transport times; Can access more remote areas; Flight crews typically have advanced medical skills; Sophisticated communication systems; Generally, smoother ride	Need for a helipad or adequate landing zone; Space and weight limitations; Noise and vibration; Restricted by severe weather; Expensive to operate; May need ambulance from helipad to hospital	Altitude concerns (see Table 4 for effects of altitude); Depending on aircraft, may be difficult to access patient
Fixed-Wing	Rapid transport times over long distances; Can usually accommodate more personnel; May be able to avoid inclement weather	Requires airport/runways facilities; Need for ground or helicopter transport to/from aircraft; Effects of altitude and possible need for pressurization; Expensive to operate; Difficult to divert to alternate facility if midair medical emergency arises	Altitude concerns

Ground ambulances provide readily available and economic services. Most ground ambulances allow for two or three team members in the back as a part of the team configuration in addition to the ambulance personnel. Factors such as ease of accessing patients at various locations and door-to-door service make surface ambulance systems the most popular mode of transport. A parent can ride in the vehicle if additional seat belts are available and not against team/ company policy. In pediatric cases, this may be advantageous in keeping a frightened child from becoming increasingly agitated. If the child deteriorates, the team can divert to the closest hospital or stop the ambulance in order to deliver additional care. Ground ambulances usually are able to continue services in most weather conditions. Transport, however, may be prolonged. Furthermore, precautions to avoid spilling nebulizer treatments should be employed.

Helicopter transport offers the benefit of a rapid response time and transit time back to the tertiary care facility. Another advantage is the helicopter's ability to access more remote locations. The primary drawback is the difficulty of chest auscultation owing to noise. Other disadvantages include the need for an adequate landing zone, space and weight limitations, and weather restrictions. In addition, the agitated or dyspneic asthmatic may require restraints if the patient

TABLE 4. Effects of Altitude on the Child with Severe Asthma

Gas Law	Effects of Altitude	Implications for the Asthmatic Child
Boyle's law	Increasing altitude and decreasing baro-metric pressure causes gas expansion in an enclosed space	Small air leaks may result in large pneumothoraces; Abdominal distention may aggravate respiratory distress
Dalton's law	Increasing altitude and decreasing baro-metric pressure causes less oxygen diffusion into bloodstream	Hypoxemia results in increased oxygen requirements
Henry's law	Increasing altitude and decreasing barometric pressure affects solubility of gases within a liquid	Rapid changes in altitude affect gas transfer between alveoli and blood resulting in decompression sickness: "chokes" and "bends"

stretcher configuration is near the pilot controls or may affect the safety of the medical crew.

Fixed-wing aircraft offer many options for long-distance transport. However, transport practitioners must understand the effects of flight physiology and how altitude can affect the severely asthmatic child. Cabin pressurization reduces the effects of altitude and can be useful in managing the asthmatic child during a fixed-wing flight. Since increased altitude equals a lower barometric pressure, controlling the cabin pressure will maintain the barometric pressure closer to sea level and thus reduce the possible risks of altitude.[1] Consequently, the importance of planning a flight is evident as one examines the physiologic effects and the possible dangers of placing a compromised patient at increased altitudes (see Appendix B and Table 4).

APPENDIX B

Effects of Altitude on the Child with Severe Asthma

Boyle's law states that an increase in altitude and the resulting decrease in barometric pressure cause gas expansion.[7] Its application to a patient situation is that enclosed areas such as the stomach can experience gas expansion or distention. This also applies to the pulmonary system. Since the child in status asthmaticus is at risk for pneumothoraces, a small air leak may increase at altitude, resulting in a devastating predicament. Pneumothoraces can be very difficult to diagnose in an asthmatic patient because the lungs do not collapse. It often presents itself as a lucidity over the diaphragm or as an extension to a pneumomediastinum. One must have a very high index of suspicion.

Dalton's law maintains that the increase in altitude and the decrease in barometric pressure result in less oxygen diffusion into the bloodstream. This leads to alveolar hypoxia and a need for additional O_2 during flight.

Henry's law addresses the solubility of gases within a liquid and the effects of altitude. The partial pressure of a gas and the solubility of the gas determine the amount of gas that will dissolve into a liquid. An example of this is decompression sickness (the bends). This can result from a loss of cabin pressurization.[7]

In addition, the level of humidity is decreased at higher altitudes and may impair mucus consistency and mobility. Its effect on the asthmatic child may lead to plugging of the airways. Temperature is decreased as altitude increases. One must monitor the patient's temperature.

REFERENCES

1. American Academy of Pediatrics: Task Force on Interhospital Transport. Guidelines for Air and Ground Transport of Neonatal and Pediatric Patients, 1993.
2. Air Medical Crew National Standard Curriculum, USDOT, National Highway Safety Administration, AAMS (formerly ASHBEAMS) and Samaritan Air Evac, 1988.
3. Aoki BY, McCloskey K: Evaluation, Stabilization, and Transport of the Critically Ill Child. St. Louis: Mosby, 1992.
4. Behrman RE: Asthma. In Nelson Textbook of Pediatrics. Philadelphia: W.B. Saunders, 1992.
5. Bhende MS, Thompson AE, Orr RA: Utility of end tidal carbon detector during stabilization and transport of critically ill children. Pediatrics 89:1042–1044, 1992.
6. Bloomberg GR, Strunk RC: Crisis in asthma care. Pediatr Clin North Am 39:1225–1241, 1992.
7. Blumen IJ, Abernethy MK, Dunne MJ: Flight physiology. Crit Care Clin 8:597–618, 1992.
8. Chernick V, Kendig EL: Disorders of the Respiratory Tract in Children. Philadelphia, W.B. Saunders, 1990.
9. Children's Formulary Handbook, 1st ed. Hudson, Ohio, Lexi-Comp, 1993.
10. Cox RG, Barker GA, Bohn DJ: Efficacy, results, and complications of mechanical ventilation in children with status asthmaticus. Pediatr Pulmonol 11:120–126, 1991.
11. Gomez M (unpublished): Transport Management of the Pediatric Patient with Asthma. Pediatric Transport Protocol, Children's Memorial Hospital. Chicago, 1993.
12. Guidelines for the Diagnosis and Management of Asthma: US Department of Health and Human Services, National Asthma Education Program Expert Panel Report, 1991.
13. Hathaway WE, et al: Current Pediatric Diagnosis and Treatment. Norwalk, CT, Appleton & Lange, 1993.
14. Jaimovich D, Kecskes SA: Management of reactive airway disease. Crit Care Clin 8:147–162, 1992.
15. McDonald TB, Berkowitz RA: Airway management and sedation for pediatric transport. Pediatr Clin North Am 40:381–406, 1993.
16. Provisional Committee on Quality Improvement, Practice Parameter: The office management of acute exacerbations of asthma in children. Pediatrics 93:119–126, 1994.
17. Rakel RE: Asthma in Children. Conn's Current Therapy. Philadelphia, W.B. Saunders, 1993.
18. Schneider C, Gomez MA, Lee R: Evaluation of ground ambulance, rotor-wing, and fixed-wing aircraft services. Crit Care Clin 8:533–564, 1992.
19. Skobeloff EM, et al: The influence of age and sex on asthma admissions. JAMA 268:3437, 1992.
20. Stein R, et al: Severe acute asthma in a pediatric intensive care unit: Six years' experience. Pediatrics 83:1023–1028, 1989.
21. Stempel DA, Redding GJ: Management of acute asthma. Pediatr Clin North Am 39:1311–1325, 1992.
22. Weiner C: Ventilatory management of respiratory failure in asthma. JAMA 269:2128–2131, 1993.
23. Weitzman M, et al: Recent trends in the prevalence and severity of childhood asthma. JAMA 268:2673–2677, 1992.

CHAPTER 16

Transport of Neonatal and Pediatric Patients Requiring Extracorporeal Life Support

DIANE OSTROWSKI, R.N.C., M.Ed.
DAVID G. JAIMOVICH, M.D.

Patients who present with acute reversible cardiac or respiratory failure refractory to conventional medical, ventilatory, or pharmacologic management may be candidates for extracorporeal membrane oxygenation (ECMO), whereby prolonged extracorporeal cardiopulmonary bypass via extrathoracic cannulation is performed. In these patients, ECMO provides for cardiopulmonary "rest," while avoiding deleterious "toxic" ventilation (high FiO_2 and high positive-pressure ventilation). The clinician must remember that ECMO is a supportive intervention and not a therapeutic one; therefore, it allows healing and resolution of reversible heart and lung pathology.[16]

HISTORICAL PERSPECTIVE

In 1965, the first successful trials of extracorporeal life support (ECLS) in children with oxygenation via pumpless arteriovenous flow through a bubble oxygenator was reported by Rashkind and associates. In these cases, extracorporeal circulation was necessary only for short periods of time (1–2 hours). Dorson et al., in 1969, and White et al., in 1971, reported the first attempts at the use of ECMO support in newborns with respiratory failure.[9,13] Efficacy was established with the use of prolonged ECLS and membrane oxygenation; unfortunately, the high incidence of intracranial hemorrhage precluded a successful outcome in these patients.

In 1972, Hill et al. reported the first successful use of prolonged ECLS in an adult with multiple trauma and respiratory failure.[17] Bartlett, Zapol, Hill, and Pyle and their coworkers reported separate clinical trials in the early 1970s in moribund adult patients with cardiac and respiratory insufficiency with variable success.[3,16,18,20,21]

In 1975, the National Institutes of Health (NIH) performed a multicenter, prospective, randomized study of ECMO in acute respiratory failure.[13,14] This study showed that although oxygenation uniformly improved with ECMO, survival was not prolonged and overall outcome was not improved significantly. Because of these results, studies on ECMO in adults with respiratory failure virtually stopped. The conclusions of the NIH study may have been misleading for several reasons: The cause of death in the majority of the control and ECMO-support patients was irreversible pulmonary disease manifested by postmortem findings of fibrosis and end-stage lung pathology.[10] Furthermore, the duration of the critical illness before entering the study may have been too long (9.6 days of ventilator therapy before receiving ECMO support), treating patients in both groups (conventional ventilation versus ECMO) with irreversible lung pathology regardless of the form of therapy. In addition, some of the ECMO patients continued to receive intensive ventilator therapy while on ECMO, not allowing for pulmonary "rest." This prolonged toxic ventilation may have contributed to the postmortem findings of pulmonary fibrosis and other irreversible lung pathology noted.[3,10,16,22]

Meanwhile, the efficacy of ECMO in reversible pulmonary disease was being demonstrated successfully in Europe by Gattinoni et al. in adult patients and in the United States by Bartlett et al. in neonates.[2,11,12]

For almost 25 years, ECMO has been applied in neonates (Fig. 1), children, and adults with cardiac and respiratory failure. The number of neonates treated with ECMO has increased exponentially, but the number of children and adults remains small in comparison. With the higher success rate in neonatal ECMO, selection and exclusion criteria were established by some ECMO centers.[5,6] Selection and exclusion criteria for pediatric and adult ECMO are poorly defined due to the difficulty in predicting morbidity and mortality in these patient populations.

PATIENT SELECTION

Neonatal Selection Criteria

Two types of criteria have been established from the cumulative experience of many ECMO centers. The first set, which is accepted by most ECMO centers, is designed to exclude neonates who are at high risk for serious complications associated with bypass. The second set of criteria is based on predictors of mortality in an attempt to determine, in a prospective fashion, which infants will likely fail conventional therapy.

Exclusion criteria include infants weighing < 2000 gm or with a gestational age of < 35 weeks (Table 1). The reasoning behind these limitations is due to Bartlett et al.'s findings, which showed that premature infants of < 35 weeks' gestation had an 89% incidence of spontaneous intracranial bleeding associated with systemic anticoagulation.[4] Once these criteria were established, later trials showed a reduction in the incidence of intracranial bleeding to < 10%.[4] Other exclusion criteria (Table 1) include the evidence of intracranial or systemic bleeding, since small brain parenchymal bleeding and greater than Grade 1 intraventricular hemorrhage may expand to catastrophic proportions. Also, continuous or uncontrolled bleeding from surgical wounds, chest tubes, lungs, or other sites is an obvious exclusion to this procedure.

Patients who have sustained > 7–10 days of "toxic" mechanical ventilation (high pressure, high FiO$_2$) should be excluded due to the potential for extensive barotrauma. Severe fatal congenital anomalies, including severe lung hypoplasia incompatible with long-term survival, are considered to be exclusion criteria. The presence of a severe congenital heart lesion is a relative contraindication, as ECMO may be used as a bridge to transplantation or to stabilize the patient prior to corrective surgery.

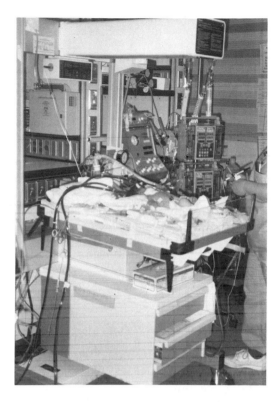

FIGURE 1.   Equipment for ECMO.

It is imperative that neonates who are identified as having severe respiratory failure be considered early enough for interhospital transport while the transfer would be tolerated, rather than to wait until the patient has met an extremely unstable clinical state; usually, the point for transfer is prior to the patient's meeting ECMO criteria. Each ECMO center has developed its own criteria based on some commonly held principles, including an estimated mortality of 80% or greater without ECMO therapy. Other frequently used criteria include an alveolar/arterial oxygen difference ($AaDO_2$) gradient > 600 mmHg for > 8-12 hours, which indicates the severity of the ventilation/perfusion mismatch in infants with persistent pulmonary hypertension, once standard therapeutic modalities have been exhausted. The general equation applied to measure the $AaDO_2$ gradient is as follows:

$$AaDO_2 = PAO_2 - PaO_2$$
$$PAO_2 = [FiO_2 (PB - PH_2O) - PaCO_2/0.8]$$

assuming a barometric pressure (PB) of 760 mmHg, partial pressure of water (PH_2O) of 46 mmHg, and a respiratory quotient of 0.8

TABLE 1.   Exclusion Criteria for Neonatal ECMO

Birth weight < 2000 gm or < 35 weeks' gestation
Evidence of Grade II intraventricular hemorrhage or systemic uncontrollable coagulopathy or bleeding
Mechanical ventilation with "toxic" parameters for > 7-10 days
Signs of irreversible or fatal congential anomalies

An oxygenation index (OI), which is based on arterial oxygenation and mean airway pressure (MAP), is computed according to the following formula[15]:

$$OI = \frac{(MAP \times FiO_2 \times 100)}{PaO_2}$$

which is applied to reflect the amount of ventilatory support being utilized to achieve any given PaO_2. An OI of ≥ 40 on *three of five* consecutive blood gas measurements obtained *30–60 minutes* apart within a *5-hour* period correlates with an 80% predicted mortality, whereas an OI ≥ 25 over the same time period correlates with a 50% predicted mortality.[4] A consistently supported recommendation is that transfer of patients with the clinical diagnosis of persistent pulmonary hypertension should take place after maximium medical therapy has been implemented and the OI is ≥ 25.

Peak inspiratory pressures ≥ 40 cm H_2O are highly predictive of eventual need for ECMO and may also be considered to be a criterion for transfer.

Patients who require ECMO present a tremendous challenge to the critical care transport team. The transport team should be extremely well versed in all of the transport issues, not only in extracorporeal cardiopulmonary support but also in the problems related to the pathophysiology of the disease, interhospital transport, and ground/flight safety. Communication is of utmost importance, and referring and receiving teams should discuss the patient's course, provide recommendations for treatment and management, and consider the stability (or lack thereof) to transfer the patient for ECMO.

It is recommended that the transport team for the infant or child requiring ECMO evaluation and possible implementation include a physician, pediatric critical care transport nurse, and pediatric respiratory therapist, if possible. The team must have extensive training in the care of the pre-ECMO patient, recognizing that these patients are extremely fragile and may respond adversely to even subtle changes such as noise, touch, or temperature. Obviously, significant physiologic changes, such as hypoxia, acidosis, or hypotension, will significantly adversely affect the patient. The transport team must discuss with the parents the severity of the situation and be honest about the potential for deterioration and perhaps even death during the transport.

Pediatric Selection Criteria

The pediatric patient poses a different challenge when potential ECMO support is required. These patients may suffer from a variety of pathologies including infection, trauma, and multiple organ system failure. Pediatric patients are usually on maximum support, including mechanical ventilation and high levels of positive end-expiratory pressure, inotropic support, and fluids to optimize cardiac output. Invasive cardiac monitoring (pulmonary artery catheter) is commonly instituted. These patients also have a high risk of barotrauma and air leaks.

In the past, pediatric patients with respiratory failure were supported with ECMO only after they had failed to respond to maximal conventional ventilator therapy and were in a moribund state. Criteria for intitiating ECMO are not as clear cut in pediatric patients as they are in neonates. The patient must have underlying reversible disease with a potentially lethal respiratory failure state. Variations of the neonatal entry criteria have been applied,[1] yet many of these criteria are not easily applicable to the pediatric patient.

Pediatric patients suffering from a number of insults, including sepsis, pulmonary hemorrhage, trauma, aspiration, and pulmonary infections which

TABLE 2.   Exclusion Criteria for Pediatric Patients Requiring ECMO

Prolonged "toxic" ventilatory support ($\geq$ 10 days)
Cardiac arrest
Active bleeding or coagulopathy
Significant irreversible neurologic injury
Terminal disease (e.g., underlying malignancy)

result in acute respiratory failure, may require extracorporeal lung support (ECLS). These patients present with multisystem organ failure, and as additional systems fail, the risk of mortality increases.

Although criteria for placing neonates on ECMO are uniform, pediatric criteria for initiating ECMO are not as clear. There have been many variations of neonatal criteria applied to pediatric patients,[1] although certain exclusion criteria (Table 2) transcend all age groups, including prolonged "toxic" ventilatory support ($\geq$ 10 days), cardiac arrest, active bleeding or coagulopathy, significant neurologic injury, or terminal disease. Patients who benefit most from ECMO are usually in the early acute phase of the disease, with < 6 days of mechanical ventilatory support.

TRANSPORT ISSUES

Transport of critically ill neonates and pediatric patients to a regional ECMO center is often associated with marked severe instability and, occasionally, cardiac arrest. Very often, these patients have existing or developing barotrauma, extremely noncompliant lungs, difficulty in maintaining adequate gas exchange, and often an unstable hemodynamic state. Due to this unstable clinical setting, ECMO transport teams have been organized in a few institutions. The ability to resuscitate, stabilize, and transport a patient on ECLS to a normal hospital setting requires extraordinary planning and coordination of experienced personnel.[8]

REFERENCES

1. Adolph V, Heaton J, Steiner R, et al: Extracorporeal membrane oxygenation for non-neonatal respiratory failure. J Pediatr Surg 26:326, 1991.
2. Bartlett RH, et al: Extracorporeal membrane oxygenation (ECMO) cardiopulmonary support in infancy. Trans ASAIO 22:80–93, 1976.
3. Bartlett RH, Gazzaniga AB, Fong SW, et al: Prolonged extracorporeal cardiopulmonary support in man. J Thorac Cardiovasc Surg 68:918–932, 1974.
4. Bartlett RH, Gazzaniga AB, Toomasian J: Extracorporeal membrane oxygenation (ECMO) in neonatal respiratory failure—100 cases. Ann Surg 204:236–245, 1986.
5. Bartlett RH, Roloff DW, Cornell RG, et al: Extracorporeal circulation in neonatal respiratory failure: A prospective randomized study. Pediatrics 76:479–487, 1985.
6. Beck R, Anderson KD, Pearson GD, et al: Criteria for extracorporeal membrane oxygenation in a population of infants with persistent pulmonary hypertension of the newborn. J Pediatr Surg 21:297–302, 1986.
7. Cornish JD, et al: Inflight use of extracorporeal membrane oxygenation for severe neonatal respiratory failure. Perfusion 1:281, 1986.
8. Cornish JD, Gerstmann DR, Begnaud MJ, et al: Inflight use of extracorporeal membrane oxygenation for severe neonatal respiratory failure. Perfusion 1:281, 1986.
9. Dorson W Jr, Baker E, Cohen ML, et al: A perfusion system for infants. Trans ASAIO 15:155–160, 1969.
10. Extracorporeal Support for Respiratory Insufficiency: A Collaborative Study. [Prepared in response to RFP-NHLI-73-20.] Bethesda, MD, National Institutes of Health, 1979.
11. Gattinoni L, Pesenti A, Mascheroni D, et al: Low-frequency positive-pressure ventilation with extracorporeal CO_2 removal in severe acute respiratory failure. JAMA 256:881–886, 1986.
12. Gattinoni L, Pessenti A, Pelizzola A, et al: Reversal of terminal acute respiratory failure by low frequency positive pressure ventilation with extracorporeal removal of CO_2 (LFPPV-ECCO$_2$R). Trans ASAIO 27:289–293, 1981.

13. Gille JP: World census of long term perfusion for respiratory support. Presented at the International Conference on Membrane Lung Technology and Prolonged Extracorporeal Perfusion, Copenhagen, Denmark, 1975.
14. Gille JP, Bagniewski AM: Ten years of use of extracorporeal membrane oxygenation (ECMO) in the treatment of acute respiratory insufficiency (ARI). Trans ASAIO 22:102-109, 1976.
15. Hallman M, Merritt A, Jarvenpaa A-L, et al: Exogenous human surfactant for treatment of severe respiratory distress syndrome: A randomized prospective clinical trial. J Pediatr 106:963-969, 1985.
16. Hill JD, DeLeval MR, Fallat RJ, et al: Acute respiratory insufficiency: Treatment with prolonged extracorporeal oxygenation. J Thorac Cardiovasc Surg 64:551-562, 1972.
17. Hill D, O'Brien TG, Murray JJ, et al: Extracorporeal oxygenation for acute post-traumatic respiratory failure (shock-lung syndrome): Use of the Bramson Membrane Lung. N Engl J Med 286:629-932, 1974.
18. Pyle RB, Helton WC, Johnson FW, et al: Clinical use of the membrane oxygenator. Arch Surg 110:966-970, 1975.
19. White JJ, Andrews HG, Risemberg H, et al: Prolonged respiratory support in newborn infants with a membrane oxygenator. Surgery 70:288-296, 1971.
20. Zapol W, Pontoppidan H, McCullough N, et al: Clinical membrane lung support for acute respiratory insufficiency. Trans ASAIO 18:629-636, 1972.
21. Zapol WM, Qvist J, Pontoppidan H, et al: Extracorporeal perfusion for acute respiratory failure: Recent experience with the spiral coil membrane lung. J Thorac Cardiovasc Surg 69:439-449, 1975.
22. Zapol WM, Snider MT, Hill JD, et al: Extracorporeal membrane oxygenation in severe acute respiratory failure: A randomized prospective study. JAMA 242:2193-2196, 1979.

CHAPTER 17

Neonatal Neurologic Problems

BETH ANN POPE, M.D.
MICHAEL J. PAINTER, M.D.

NEONATAL SEIZURES

Neonatal seizures may be difficult to recognize because of their subtle manifestations. The immature brain lacks complete myelin deposition, and electrical discharges usually remain localized to the hemisphere of origin. Many paroxysmal events are suspicious for seizures, and neurologic consultation often is obtained to differentiate normal neonatal movements from pathologic spells. A video electroencephalograph (EEG) may help distinguish abnormal neonatal movements from those of drug withdrawal, sleep activity, or clonus. An accurate diagnosis is essential for proper treatment.

Table 1 lists the possible etiologies of neonatal seizures. The most common cause of seizures in the infant is hypoxic ischemic encephalopathy, accounting for up to 65%.[2] Although the birth history may reveal the cause of the infant's seizures, the logistics of obtaining such information may be difficult. Efforts should be made to obtain detailed records of the labor and delivery before transport. Fetal asphyxia may be secondary to placental disease, maternal trauma or infection, or congenital syndromes. A careful physical examination including blood pressure, indirect fundoscopy, and skin examination may unveil certain clues regarding etiology.

The time of onset of the seizure activity helps one determine the etiology. Asphyxia, trauma, pyridoxine, and hypoglycemia are causes for seizures in the first 48 hours of life. Hypocalcemia, infection, and metabolic disease can cause seizures after the first 72 hours through the first week of life. After the history and careful physical examination, initial laboratory studies should include sodium, glucose, blood urea nitrogen, calcium, magnesium, bilirubin, blood gas (acid/base status), urinalysis, and toxicology. It is necessary to perform a lumbar puncture in the infant with seizures. Central nervous system infections account for 12–17% of neonatal seizures.[2] Table 2 shows key aspects of evaluation of an infant with seizures.

Neonatal head trauma can occur with precipitous delivery, prolonged labor, or difficult extraction. Intracranial hemorrhage is associated with seizures. Although subarachnoid hemorrhage usually is not of major clinical significance, it may be the etiology of clonic seizure activity. The cerebrospinal fluid (CSF) will contain blood when the lumbar puncture is performed as part of the initial

TABLE 1.   Possible Causes of Neonatal Seizures

Trauma	Drug withdrawal
Subdural hematoma	Barbiturate
Subarachnoid hemorrhage	Heroin
Intraparenchymal hemorrhage	Methadone
Cerebral contusion	Alcohol
Cortical vein thrombosis	Pyridoxine dependency
Asphyxia	Amino and organic acid disturbances
Watershed infarction	Maple syrup urine disease
Basal ganglia infarction	Nonketotic hyperglycinemia
Periventricular leukomalacia	Methylmalonic aciduria
Intraventricular hemorrhage	Propionic aciduria
Subarachnoid hemorrhage	Urea cycle abnormalities
Congenital anomalies (cerebral dysgenesis)	Kernicterus
Metabolic disorders	Toxins
Hypocalcemia	Local anesthetics
Hypoglycemia	Isoniazid
Electrolyte imbalance (hyper- and hyponatremia)	Familial seizures
Infections	Phakomatoses
Bacterial meningitis	Genetic syndrome with mental retardation
Cerebral abscess	Benign familial epilepsy
Herpes encephalitis	
Coxsackievirus meningoencephalitis	
Cytomegalovirus	
Rubella	
Toxoplasmosis	
Syphilis	

laboratory investigation. Subdural hemorrhage is more commonly related to birth trauma and manifested by focal seizures. Subarachnoid and subdural hemorrhage can be visualized with computed tomography (CT) of the head.

The most common and most treatable metabolic abnormalities that can result in seizures are hypoglycemia and hypocalcemia.[12] Hypoglycemia is seen with infection, metabolic defects including maple syrup urine disease, propionic acidemia and methylmalonic acidemia, and infants who are small for gestational age. Although infants of diabetic mothers frequently have low serum glucose, it rarely manifests as hypoglycemic seizures. Hypoglycemia is a whole blood glucose below 20 mg/dl in a preterm infant or 30 mg/dl in a full-term infant. In all infants after 72 hours of age, the whole blood glucose should be above 40 mg/dl.[12] Hypoglycemia is treated with a slow intravenous infusion of 10% dextrose, 2 ml/kg, followed by 6–10 mg/kg/min infusion until the underlying cause can be determined.

Hypocalcemia is defined as less than 8 mg/dl in a term infant and less than 7.5 mg/dl in a preterm infant. Early neonatal hypocalcemia seen in the first three

TABLE 2.   Laboratory Evaluation of Neonatal Convulsions

Immediate	If clinically indicated
Blood glucose	Urine for organic acids
Calcium	Serum for amino acids
Magnesium	Maternal and infant antibody titers against the following
Bicarbonate	Toxoplasmosis
Blood gas	Herpes simplex virus
Urea nitrogen	Cytomegalovirus
Toxicology screen	Rubella virus
Bilirubin	Syphilis
Lumbar puncture	Computed tomography scan

days of life is associated with premature infants, infants of diabetic mothers, DiGeorge syndrome, and birth asphyxia. Hypocalcemia occurring between 4 and 7 days is seen in high-phosphate feedings, maternal vitamin D deficiency, hypomagnesemia, and intestinal malabsorption. An electrocardiogram should be obtained in infants when hypocalcemia is suspected. Hypocalcemia lengthens the ST segment, and the Qo-Tc interval is increased. A Qo-Tc interval greater than 0.21 seconds in a preterm infant and 0.19 seconds in a term infant supports the diagnosis of low serum calcium.[12]

The major manifestations of neonatal hypocalcemia are jitteriness and seizures. The seizures usually are multifocal and migratory, and the infant is alert during the interictal period.[12] Treatment of infants with hypocalcemic seizures consists of an intravenous bolus of 10% calcium gluconate, 2 ml/kg, over 10 minutes. Any hypocalcemic infant not responding to this infusion must have a serum magnesium concentration measured. Hypocalcemia accompanying hypomagnesemia (serum concentration is less than 1 mEq/L) will respond to therapy only when the magnesium level is corrected. Hypomagnesemic neonates should be treated with 0.25 ml/kg of a 50% solution of magnesium sulfate given intramuscularly.

Pyridoxine dependency seizures occur shortly after birth, and multifocal clonic activity can progress rapidly to status epilepticus. Pyridoxine dependency is an autosomal recessive trait and is necessary for the synthesis of the inhibitory neurotransmitter, gamma-amino butyric acid (GABA). The seizures are recalcitrant to standard anticonvulsant therapy, responding only to pyridoxine. Following the intravenous administration of 100 mg of pyridoxine, the clonic activity ceases, and the EEG may normalize in less than 10 minutes.[6] The infant will require a lifetime dietary supplement of pyridoxine, ranging from 2–30 mg/kg/day.

Aminoacidopathies are an uncommon etiology of neonatal seizures. An underlying primary metabolic disorder should be suspected if the history shows poor feeding, a peculiar odor of the infant or urine, or if the initial laboratory data reveal acidosis or alkalosis. Analysis of the neonate's serum and urine confirms the diagnosis.

Once ventilation and perfusion are established, therapy should be initiated as listed in Table 3. Antiepileptic drugs should be used in the neonate in whom a specific metabolic abnormality has not been detected or in the presence of a structural defect in the central nervous system (CNS). Phenobarbital is the anticonvulsant most frequently used in the treatment of seizures in infants. A minimum loading dose of 20 mg/kg intravenously is required to achieve a therapeutic level. If seizures are refractory to a full 40 mg/kg dose of phenobarbital, phenytoin is used as an adjunctive agent. The loading dose of phenytoin is 20 mg/kg intravenously. The maintenance dose of phenobarbital and phenytoin is 3–5 mg/kg/day. Cardiac arrhythmia is the major toxicity of phenytoin. The drug must be administered slowly, not exceeding a rate of 1 mg/kg/min. If seizures persist, addition of a benzodiazepine is generally effective.

TABLE 3.   Acute Therapy of Neonatal Seizures

With hypoglycemia	Without hypoglycemia
Glucose, 10% solution: 2 ml/kg intravenously followed by a maintenance infusion	Pyridoxine: 100 mg intravenously
	Phenobarbital: 20 mg/kg intravenously, followed by an additional 5–20 mg/kg if necessary
	Phenytoin: 20 mg/kg intravenously

The etiology of the neonatal seizure will determine the duration of therapy. An acute, self-limited encephalopathy does not require prolonged anticonvulsant therapy, whereas cerebral dysgenesis, an abnormal neurologic exam, or atypical EEG pattern should be treated following discharge from the hospital.

SPINAL CORD INJURY

Despite a decrease in the incidence of spinal cord injury sustained during delivery, perinatal damage may be responsible for 11% of the cord injuries seen in the pediatric population.[16] Spinal cord lesions include epidural hemorrhages, meningeal lacerations, and trauma to the arteries, ligaments, musculature, and nerve roots. In the vast majority of infants, spinal cord injuries occur after vaginal delivery in the breech position, yet cases have been reported following cephalic delivery.

The infant spine is more deformable than the adult spine because of the elasticity of the interspinous ligaments, posterior joint capsule, and cartilaginous endplates.[16] This elasticity makes the infant spine more susceptible to hyperextension injury. The dura is the major supporting structure of the spinal cord. If a "pop" is heard during the delivery, it may signify the rupture of the dura mater and significant spinal cord injury.

In most breech deliveries, the mechanism of injury is traction, and the lesion usually is located in the lower cervical or upper thoracic cord. Along with hypotonia, the infant with a lower cervical injury may have diaphragmatic breathing and Horner syndrome. Lower thoracic lesions result in flaccid paralysis of the lower extremities and bowel and bladder dysfunction. Expulsion of urine following suprapubic pressure confirms bladder paralsyis. Lack of perceptible response to pain can help localize the level of injury.

Spinal cord injury from cephalic presentation usually is located in the upper to midcervical region. The uncinate processes are flat in the neonatal spine and are insufficient to withstand excessive torsional forces.[16] High cervical lesions may result in paralysis of the diaphragm and quadraplegia. A lesion above the fourth cervical vertebrae can be fatal unless respirations are supported.

Although the most common mechanism of spinal cord injury is traction, vascular compromise will result in cord ischemia. It is postulated that damage to the vertebral arteries by subluxation and dislocation can compromise the lumen of the arteries as they ascend through the foramina transversaria.[14] The consequent thrombosis may result in brainstem or upper cervical cord ischemia. Cord infarction is seen in newborns undergoing umbilical artery catheterization. The artery of Adamkiewicz is the major segmental artery to the thoracolumbar cord, arising between the levels of T10 and T12. If the catheter tip is placed in this region, embolization of the artery may occur, resulting in acute paraplegia.

Signs of spinal shock are flaccidity, loss of spontaneous movements, and absence of stretch reflexes. Such features may falsely be attributed to birth asphyxia or brain injury. The differential diagnoses of spinal cord injury at birth include myelodysplasia, infantile spinal muscular atrophy, and cerebral palsy. Bowel and bladder dysfunction and a sensory level to pinprick exam suggest a spinal cord injury.

Radiologic studies frequently are normal in infants with spinal cord injury.[16] Plain films may demonstrate subluxation, fracture, or anomalies, but the spinal cord can be ruptured by longitudinal distraction without disruption of the vertebral column. A normal myelogram or magnetic resonance image (MRI) does not exclude the diagnosis. Therefore, infants must be examined frequently for signs of spinal cord damage even if there is no radiographic evidence of injury.

The treatment of neonatal spinal cord injury has not been well established. A study performed by Bracken and coworkers concluded that treatment with methylprednisolone within the first 8 hours of injury is beneficial, but the study excluded children under the age of 13 years.[3] Prevention of neonatal spinal cord injury is the best approach.

BRACHIAL PLEXUS INJURY

Brachial plexus palsy is a well-known complication of both breech and cephalic delivery. While the majority of injuries are caused by traction of the plexus, injuries also occur from avulsion of the roots or transection of the nerves as they join to form the plexus. Injuries are more common on the right, perhaps because the left occiput anterior is the most frequent presentation. Stretch injuries have a good prognosis, whereas those due to avulsion may not recover function.

Erb palsy involves the upper segments of the brachial plexus, C5, and C6. The diagnosis is quickly suspected when the arm is held in the characteristic posture of adduction with internal rotation. This is due to paralysis of the deltoid and supra- and infraspinatus muscles. The elbow is extended and pronated because of weakness of the biceps and brachioradialis muscles. The biceps stretch reflex is absent, but the triceps reflex is spared. Wrist and hand movements should be preserved. A careful physical examination must be performed. Difficulty swallowing or sucking, intermittent stridor, or xiphoid retractions should alert the physician to possible hypoglossal nerve paralysis or recurrent laryngeal injury. Since 80–90% of phrenic nerve paralyses are associated with brachial plexus injury, a chest radiograph is warranted.[8]

Injury to the lower cord of the brachial plexus is termed Klumpke palsy. Injury to the C8 and T1 spinal nerve roots results in distal weakness, with flexion of the elbow, extension at the wrist, and hyperextension at the metacarpophalangeal joints. The tricep reflex is absent. Approximately one-third of cases are associated with Horner syndrome on the ipsilateral side.

In addition to the initial examination for long bone fractures, an electromyographic investigation performed at 6-week intervals is advantageous. It can distinguish the extent of the lesion and assess the recovery phase.[14] Favorable prognostic signs include early onset of recovery (2 weeks) and involvement of only the proximal upper extremity. By 12 months of age, 90% of the infants will have a normal neurologic exam.[8]

Therapy is aimed at preventing contractures. The arm should be immobilized against the abdomen to minimize swelling and/or hemorrhage and, beginning 7–10 days after the injury, passive range of motion exercises are recommended. The "Statue of Liberty" splint is no longer recommended because it reinforces the development of contractures. If an infant manifests signs of respiratory distress, mechanical ventilation should be instituted prior to transportation. Mortality associated with unilateral phrenic nerve palsy is as high as 15%, but in the remaining 85% recovery can be expected between 6–12 months.

INTRACRANIAL HEMORRHAGE

Subdural Hemorrhage

Improvement in obstetric technique has reduced the incidence of subdural hemorrhage. Tentorial subdural hemorrhage may occur in normal deliveries and remain undiagnosed with spontaneous recovery. Subdural bleeding results from rupture of the bridging veins overlying the cerebral hemispheres or dural sinus tears. Abnormal pressure on the skull from forceps, vacuum, or breech presentation may result in tearing of the tentorial attachments to the falx and petrous bones. Hemorrhage from a major tear of a dural sinus can extend into the posterior fossa, compress the cerebellum, and obstruct the fourth ventricle, and result in brainstem compression. Small tears or rupture of the bridging veins can result in subacute symptoms, presenting hours to days after delivery.

Clinical symptoms include irritability, weak or high-pitched cry, vomiting, and pallor. On examination, the infant is often hypotonic with a tense fontanel and may show an asymmetry of motor function. Seizures are frequent. Neonates should be monitored for early signs of brainstem compression: unequal pupils, bradycardia, irregular respiration, and oculomotor paralysis.

An infant with a molded head who, after a symptom-free interval, develops signs of intracranial hypertension should provoke the suspicion of tentorial tear and posterior fossa hemorrhage. CT is the technique of choice to verify subdural hemorrhage and should be obtained as quickly as possible. Although conservative management is advocated in the stable neonate,[18] surgical evacuation of the posterior fossa subdural bleed is necessary when brainstem signs occur. Subdural hemorrhage over the convexity of the cerebral hemisphere causing midline shift and transtentorial herniation is alleviated by tapping the subdural space. Repeated taps should not be performed if the infant is asymptomatic.

The prognosis of an infant with subdural hemorrhage depends on the degree of hemorrhage. Neonates with laceration of the falx or dural sinus often develop hydrocephalus and other sequelae. A more favorable outcome can be expected in infants with a convexity subdural hemorrhage.

Subarachnoid Hemorrhage

Subarachnoid hemorrhage in the newborn is unlike the dramatic arterial hemorrhage seen in adults. It originates from the vascular channels that are remnants of anastomoses of the leptomeningeal arteries or the bridging veins within the subarachnoid space.[17] It is thought to result from physiologic trauma or an hypoxic event during delivery.

Since the bleed is usually venous, clinical signs may be minimal or absent, and the hemorrhage is often self-limited. However, two additional clinical syndromes have been recognized.[17] Seizures can occur in an otherwise healthy infant interictally. The convulsions begin on the second day of life. In rare instances, neonates with large subarachnoid hemorrhages develop respiratory disturbances, brainstem dysfunction, and coma.

The diagnosis of symptomatic subarachonid hemorrhage is based primarily on CT findings. Other causes of blood in the subarachnoid space (hemorrhage associated with intraventricular or intracerebral bleeding) will be excluded by CT scan. A lumbar puncture should support the clinical suspicion with elevated red blood cells and protein, xanthochromia, and hypoglycorrhachia. Management is supportive, and hydrocephalus secondary to impaired cerebrospinal absorption occurs in some cases.

Intraventricular Hemorrhage in Term Infants

Although this lesion is more frequent in preterm infants, intraventricular hemorrhage (IVH) is detected by CT scan in full-term neonates. It may originate from the germinal matrix, the veins of the choroid plexus, or both. Perinatal asphyxia and trauma are often clinical correlates. Presentations are variable and consist of an altered level of consciousness, respiratory disturbances, seizures, and hemi- or quadraparesis. Posthemorrhagic hydrocephalus is common, and a ventriculoperitoneal shunt may be required. Diagnosis is made by ultrasound or CT scan. Management is similar to that of a preterm infant with IVH.

MYASTHENIA GRAVIS

Myasthenia gravis is a disorder of postsynaptic neuromuscular transmission and is included in the differential diagnosis of a hypotonic infant. Transient neonatal myasthenia occurs in approximately 21% of infants born to mothers with acquired myasthenia gravis.[15] Although the syndrome is believed to be due to the passive transfer of acetylcholine receptor (AChR) antibodies, the pathophysiology remains unclear, and the syndrome occurs in infants who are antibody-negative. Infants of mothers with acquired myasthenia gravis are at risk for developing transient neonatal myasthenia gravis.[15]

The majority of infants with transient myasthenia will develop symptoms within the first three days of life. Common clinical findings include shallow respiration, poor suck, hypotonia, and weak cry. Ptosis and ophthalmoplegia are less common. Mechanical respiration and gavage feedings are necessary in up to one-third of the patients.[15] Although some studies have correlated the severity of symptoms with the infant's antibody titers, others have not confirmed these findings.[15] Recovery is complete, and recurrence has not been reported.

Genetic defects causing myasthenia gravis in the neonate are uncommon. These infants are born to mothers without myasthenia gravis, and antibodies against the acetylcholine receptor protein are not detected. Several congenital syndromes are newly recognized; their diagnosis may require specialized techniques, such as microelectrode analysis of neuromuscular transmission or cytochemical studies.[5] The clinical features are similar to those of transient neonatal myasthenia, but long-term therapy may be necessary.

When the mother has myasthenia gravis, the diagnosis of transient neonatal myasthenia is not difficult. Besides detecting high serum titers of AChR antibody in the newborn, an anticholinesterase agent should be administered. A subcutaneous or intravenous injection of Tensilon, 0.15 mg/kg of body weight, should demonstrate a temporary reversal of an unequivocal neurologic deficit such as sucking or swallowing difficulties. Repetitive nerve stimulation is recommended in combination with the Tensilon injection, especially in infants born to mothers with acquired AChR antibody-negative myasthenia gravis.

Management of transient neonatal myasthenia gravis includes careful attention to airway maintenance, postural drainage, and nutritional status. Gavage feedings and mechanical ventilation are recommended in newborns with severe generalized weakness and respiratory distress. Nearly 20% of patients require only continuous surveillance and frequent small oral feedings.[15] The majority will require anticholinesterase medication. Neostigmine methylsulfate administered intramuscularly or subcutaneously (0.05 mg/kg) 20 minutes before feeding improves sucking and swallowing to allow adequate nutrition. Neostigmine also can be administered orally or through a nasal gastric tube (0.5 mg/kg) 30 minutes prior to feeding. The anticholinesterase medication is slowly discontinued when the patient is no longer symptomatic.

PERINATAL ASPHYXIA

Cerebral injury from hypoxemia is a major determinant of neurologic morbidity and mortality in neonates. Approximately 90% of the cases occur during the antenatal period.[9] Five principal mechanisms of asphyxia have been

TABLE 4.   Clinical Factors Associated with Hypoxic-Ischemic Injury

Maternal hypotension or hypertension	Umbilical cord compression
Maternal diabetes	Placental abruption, previa, or insufficiency
Maternal anemia	Altered fetal heart rate or acid-base disturbance
Maternal cardiopulmonary disease	Thick meconium
Preeclampsia	Infant cardiopulmonary disease
Intrauterine growth retardation	

described during the antepartum and intrapartum period: (1) interruption of umbilical circulation; (2) altered placental gas exchange; (3) inadequate maternal perfusion of the placenta; (4) decreased maternal oxygenation; and (5) failure of the infant to transition from fetal to neonatal cardiopulmonary circulation.[4] There are many etiologic factors in fetal asphyxia, as listed in Table 4. The clinical features of hypoxic-ischemic encephalopathy are nonspecific, however,

Neurologic signs and symptoms may be observed in the neonate with perinatal asphyxia. Whereas an intrapartum event may lead to neurologic signs hours to days later, infants that have sustained an hypoxic insult in utero may not be symptomatic in the neonatal period. A detailed examination will aid in the assessment of severity of hypoxic-ischemic encephalopathy. The spectrum is divided into three classes that have prognostic value.[9] Mild encephalopathy is characterized by jitteriness, uninhibited deep tendon reflexes, and hyperalertness and is not associated with long-term sequelae. Hypotonia, seizures, and lethargy are hallmarks of moderate encephalopathy, and if the symptoms persist for longer than 1 week, neurologic sequelae may exist in up to 40%.[9] Severe encephalopathy is associated with coma, seizures, brainstem dysfunction, and increased intracranial pressure. The majority of these infants will be affected with long-term sequelae such as microcephaly, mental retardation, spastic quadriplegia, and seizures.

Radiologic examination will help in the assessment of the extent of cerebral injury. CT scanning is the investigation of choice in the term newborn. Optimal timing of the scan is debated. It is often obtained during the initial evaluation of the asphyxiated infant, but the maximal extent of tissue damage visualized on CT is usually 2–4 days following the insult. Cranial ultrasound is beneficial in the premature infant to evaluate intraventricular hemorrhage and periventricular leukomalacia. An EEG recording also can aid in the evaluation of the asphyxiated newborn. Often it demonstrates a discontinuous pattern with marked slowing and reduced amplitude. If there is rapid resolution of the EEG abnormalities, however, the prognosis improves.[9]

Four major neuropathologic patterns of injury are summarized in Table 5. Distribution of the lesions reflects a combination of regional circulation and metabolic factors that change with the gestational age of the infant. The primary lesions seen on autopsy in term newborns are in the cortex and basal ganglia. In the premature infant, however, lesions generally occur in the germinal matrix and periventricular regions of the brain.

TABLE 5.   Neuropathologic Patterns of Hypoxic-Ischemic Injury

Pattern	Distribution
Selective neuronal necrosis	Hippocampus, cerebellum, brainstem
Staus marmoratus of the basal ganglia	Basal ganglia, thalamus
Parasagittal cerebral injury	Cerebral cortex, subcortical white matter
Focal and multifocal brain injury	Cerebral cortex

Efforts to resuscitate the infant should be directed toward adequate ventilation and perfusion, correction of accompanying metabolic acidosis, maintenance of normal blood pressure and glucose, and treatment of seizures. Antidiuretic hormone may be secreted inappropriately following a large cerebral insult, and fluid overload should be avoided. Serum osmolality and sodium concentration should be monitored to avoid the consequence of cerebral edema and seizures. Although seizures in the hypoxic-ischemic setting may be refractory to anticonvulsant therapy, treatment is recommended to reduce the incidence of apnea and hypertension. Handling should be minimized to reduce the incidence of hypoxemic episodes, especially in premature neonates.

REFERENCES

1. Alvord EC, et al: Neuropathologic observations in congenital phrenic nerve palsy. J Child Neurol 5:205, 1990.
2. Ballweg DD: Neonatal seizures: An overview. Neonatal Network 10:15, 1991.
3. Bracken MB, et al: Methylprednisolone or naloxone treatment after acute spinal cord injury: 1-year follow-up data. J Neurosurg 76:23, 1992.
4. Carter BS, et al: The definition of acute perinatal asphyxia. Clin Perinatol 20:287, 1993.
5. Engel AG: Congenital myasthenic syndromes. Neurol Clin 12:401, 1994.
6. Fenichel GM: Clinical Pediatric Neurology, 2nd ed. Philadelphia, W.B. Saunders, 1993, p 15.
7. Haenggeli CA, Lacourt G: Brachial plexus injury and hypoglossal paralysis. Pediatr Neurol 5:197, 1989.
8. Harris MC, Roth P: Neonatology. In Polin RA, Ditmar MF (eds): Pediatric Secrets. Philadelphia, Hanley & Belfus, 1989.
9. Hill A, Volpe JJ: Perinatal asphyxia: Clinical aspects. Clin Perinatol 16:435, 1989.
10. Huang CC, Shen YY: Tentorial subdural hemorrhage in term newborns: Ultrasonographic diagnosis and clinical correlates. Pediatr Neurol 7:171, 1991.
11. MacKinnon JA, et al: Spinal cord injury at birth: Diagnostic and prognostic data in twenty-two patients. J Pediatr 122:431, 1993.
12. Painter MJ, Bergman I, Crumrine P: Neonatal seizures. Pediatr Clin North Am 33:91, 1986.
13. Painter MJ, Gaus LM: Neonatal seizures: Diagnosis and treatment. J Child Neurol 6:101, 1991.
14. Painter MJ: Neurologic sequelae of birth. In Depp R, Eschenbach DA, Sciarra JJ (eds): Gynecology and Obstetrics. Philadelphia, Harper & Row, 1987.
15. Papazian O: Transient neonatal myasthenia gravis. J Child Neurol 7:135, 1992.
16. Rossitch E Jr, Oakes WJ: Perinatal spinal cord injury: Clinical, radiographic and pathologic features. Pediatr Neurosurg 18:149, 1992.
17. Volpe JJ: Neurology of the Newborn, 2nd ed. Philadelphia, W.B. Saunders, 1987, p 293.
18. von Gontard A, et al: Posterior fossa hemorrhage in the newborn—diagnosis and management. Pediatr Radiol 18:347, 1988.

CHAPTER 18

Transportation of the Child with Seizures

MARK G. GOETTING, M.D.
FERNANDO P. POLACK, M.D.

Seizures can be defined as pathologic paroxysmal electrical discharges in the cerebral cortex that produce any combination of the following: involuntary muscle movements or tone; abnormal sensory phenomena; altered mental status; and psychic alterations. When they produce simple stereotypic movements, usually jerking or posturing, they are termed *convulsions*. Seizures are significant in acute care medicine for several reasons. First, they are common. Second, they are frequently signs of an underlying structural, toxic, or metabolic insult to the brain that requires urgent attention. Third, the systemic effects of convulsions can create serious, even life-threatening complications. Fourth, prolonged seizures may directly impart, in extreme cases, permanent neurologic disability.

Seizures are one of the most common childhood emergencies and usually begin in the pre-hospital setting. Seizures often persist or recur following pre-hospital intervention and require a more vigorous pharmacologic approach in the emergency department. A small fraction of children will fail to respond to or will relapse following care in this setting. Thus, the child with seizures has an unpredictable course and can punctuate any transport with a convulsive crisis. A significant and stable portion of pediatric interhospital transports, about 20% performed by our institution and others,[1] is for the evaluation and therapy of the seizures and their underlying causes, as well as the treatment of non-neurologic, usually iatrogenic, complications. This chapter provides a review of the basic concepts necessary to the management of seizure emergencies, especially as they relate to the initial stabilization and transport of the child. Emphasis is placed on the child with prolonged or repetitive generalized convulsive seizures because their care is more difficult and the outcome more guarded.

CLASSIFICATION OF SEIZURES

Seizures are categorized by the cerebral site of origin and subsequent involvement, by whether they are symptomatic of a causative disorder or are idiopathic, by the manifested signs and symptoms, and by their frequency and duration. Epilepsy is a symptom complex that consists of recurrent, unprovoked seizures. In most children with epilepsy, the disease has no known cause. Proper classification of a seizure helps in the diagnosis of its cause, in selecting antiepileptic drugs (AEDs) and their dosage, and in prognostication. Careful observation and documentation of motor, behavioral, and autonomic events can have a dramatic influence on further care.

Site of Origin and Involvement

A *generalized* seizure, by definition, produces epileptiform discharges in all areas of the cerebral cortex as measured by electroencephalography. Clinically, consciousness is impaired and there may be bilateral motor manifestations. The common *tonic-clonic* convulsion is an example of a generalized seizure. Also, *absence*, formerly called petit mal, seizures are generalized. *Partial* (focal) seizures are restricted to a discrete region of the cortex. The areas involved may be small or may include an entire cerebral hemisphere. If consciousness is impaired, the seizure is called a *complex partial* seizure. Staring spells with automatisms such as lip smacking, previously termed psychomotor or temporal lobe seizures, are examples. It may be difficult to distinguish complex partial seizures from absence seizures without the aid of an electroencephalogram (EEG). If consciousness is preserved, these seizures are *simple partial* seizures. Clonic movements restricted to a single limb or side of the body fall into this category.

A generalized seizure may begin in one of two ways: simultaneously throughout the entire cortex or by spreading from a partial seizure. Those that involve the entire cortex from the onset are *primarily generalized* and frequently heritable. In *secondarily generalized* seizures the epileptogenic focus often consists of tissue injured from trauma, ischemia, or infection, or is the result of perturbed development. It is often impossible to separate primary from secondary generalized seizures because the spread from the epileptogenic focus in partial seizures can be extremely rapid, producing no observable localizing features in the convulsions. The distinction is frequently made only by electroencephalography. By contrast, some partial seizures begin by focal twitching of a limb and more gradually evolve into a secondarily generalized convulsion. Observation of asymmetries in a seizure, especially at its initiation, or behavioral manifestations are important in helping localize the brain abnormality and should be carefully noted.

Symptomatic Versus Idiopathic

Symptomatic seizures are those attributable to a known lesion, genetic condition, toxin, metabolic disturbance, or infection. Idiopathic seizures are without clear etiology. Although most children with epilepsy have idiopathic seizures, the majority of children transported with seizure-related emergencies have a diagnosable and treatable underlying cause, including febrile seizures. Even those known to have idiopathic epilepsy are subject to the same conditions that produce seizures in previously healthy children. Therefore, it is imperative to undertake a reasonable search for a cause in all patients with seizures.

Convulsive Versus Nonconvulsive

Convulsive seizures (*convulsions*) have obvious, usually dramatic motor involvement. Seizures without stereotypic and primitive motor involvement (clonic or tonic activity) are called *nonconvulsive*.[2-4] The outward manifestations of these seizures may consist solely of altered behavior, including staring, picking at clothes, mumbling, eyelid fluttering, or peculiar facial movements, or may resemble metabolic coma. Nonconvulsive seizures may follow convulsive seizures and often cause a prolonged apparent postictal period of depressed consciousness. The diagnosis is confirmed by EEG.

Frequency and Duration

Both seizure frequency and duration can vary immensely. For example, the frequency can be as low as once in a lifetime or can be nearly continuous. Likewise, duration can range from a myoclonic jerk of less than a second to nonconvulsive states that persist for days. Patient management is greatly influenced by these factors. For practical purposes, each patient can be placed in one of three categories: the single seizure, the seizure cluster, and the prolonged seizure.

A *single brief seizure* is most often important only as an indicator of brain dysfunction. Sometimes an unexpected seizure can produce a car accident or water submersion injury. Occasionally, medical complications from the seizure, such as aspiration or fractures, or iatrogenic problems from its treatment, require the patient to be cared for in an intensive care environment.

A *seizure cluster*, defined as three or more in the same day, indicates the likelihood of serious brain pathology and mandates hospital admission. Status epilepticus often follows if the patient is not treated properly. Systemic complications, such as neurogenic pulmonary edema, may occur. If the underlying cause cannot be immediately corrected, AEDs are required, but the risks involved in following the same intensive approach used for status epilepticus cannot be justified.

Status epilepticus can be defined as either a continuous seizure or a series of seizures (lasting 30 or more minutes) so frequent that consciousness is not recovered. This is a true medical emergency with potential for morbidity and mortality. In clinical practice seizures destined to meet the definition of status are stopped short whenever possible. Thus, it is appropriate to create a category called a *prolonged seizure*, one that lasts 10 or more minutes and is treated with great vigor in order to prevent it from becoming status.

Status epilepticus can have different presentations: repetitive or continuous generalized convulsive seizures with persistent depression of neurologic function; nonconvulsive seizures that produce a continuous or fluctuating confusional state; and repetitive or continuous partial seizures not associated with altered consciousness.

Refractory status epilepticus lasts longer than 60 minutes despite optimal therapy.

EPIDEMIOLOGY AND INCIDENCE

Over 4% of the American white middle class will have had a seizure by age 20 years.[6,7] The socioeconomically deprived have roughly double the likelihood. Epilepsy has no racial or gender preference. The rate of epilepsy in childhood is between 3 per thousand and 20 per thousand. More than half of epileptics had their first seizure during childhood. In the United States about 4 million persons have suffered at least one seizure, 2 million have suffered two or more seizures, and 200,000 suffer more than one seizure a month despite treatment.[5]

Although previous studies calculated the incidence of status epilepticus in the United States to be 50,000–60,000 cases each year,[8] these data could be a significant underestimation.[9] Approximately 12% of those with newly diagnosed epilepsy will present with a seizure lasting more than 30 minutes. About half of all cases of status epilepticus occur in children.[8] Those younger than 1 year have the highest incidence, and there is a gradual decline until early adulthood.[8] As many as 70% of those who become epileptic under 1 year of age will have at least one bout of status epilepticus during early childhood.[8]

TABLE 1.   Causes of Prolonged Seizures

	Admissions n = 148	Transports n = 36
Acute Symptomatic	39 (26%)	13 (36%)
CNS infection	12	3
Head trauma	10	4
Hyponatremia	6	3
Anoxic encephalopathy	5	2
Cerebrovascular disease	3	1
Hypocalcemia	1	0
Hypoglycemia	1	0
Toxic ingestion	1	0
Remote/Progressive Symptomatic	31 (21%)	10 (28%)
Without fever	20	6
With fever	11	4
Idiopathic	78 (53%)	13 (36%)
Without fever	41	6
With fever	37	7

ETIOLOGIES

The causes of prolonged seizures are myriad, and the distribution of etiologies varies with patient age and the community served. For example, febrile seizures almost always occur in children under 5 years.[10] Likewise, symptomatic hyponatremia and intracranial hemorrhage from child abuse mostly occur in the same age group. Hypoglycemic seizures occur more frequently in a malnourished community. Infectious and parainfectious causes may be seasonal and epidemic. The etiologies of consecutive cases admitted to our pediatric intensive care unit, including those we transported, are summarized in Table 1. Our experience seems similar to others.[8,9,11] Acute symptomatic patients had a newly diagnosed disorder that produced seizures. Remote/progressive patients had either a static or progressive neurologic disorder. Idiopathic patients had no known underlying neurologic problem other than seizures, including febrile convulsions. Many children in the latter two categories were chronically on AEDs, and about one-third were found to have subtherapeutic drug levels.

PATHOPHYSIOLOGY

A seizure is a temporary disturbance of the brain synaptic activity, an electrochemical event associated with an alteration in neural system function. Seizures can produce significant brain injury directly, although this would require hours of status epilepticus. More commonly, permanent neurologic disability is due to either the cause of status epilepticus or to complicating hypoxia, ischemia, or hypoglycemia. Prolonged seizures can have profound influences outside the nervous system. The metabolic strain convulsive status epilepticus imposes on the cardiovascular system, combined with reduced arterial oxygenation, metabolic and respiratory acidosis, hyperkalemia, reduced cardiac preload and increased afterload, and a hyperadrenergic state, place the patient in danger. Despite this, most children tolerate status epilepticus well when treated properly. However, the margin of safety may be small, especially in prolonged status epilepticus, and attention to detail is mandatory.

The physiologic perturbations from convulsive status epilepticus can be divided into two distinct phases.[12-14] The first phase is an uncompromised expression of the neurohumoral, motor, cardiovascular, and autonomic manifestations of the convulsion. Organ systems compensate and oblige to the excessive demands of the nervous system. The second phase is characterized by a subsequent decompensation and deterioration in organ system function, which may not begin simultaneously. Transition between phases 1 and 2 usually occurs between 30 and 60 minutes after the convulsion, but is highly variable.

Phase 1

Cerebral metabolism increases several fold, with a proportional increase in cerebral blood flow. Cerebral vascular engorgement produces elevated intracranial pressure. The hyperadrenergic state causes tachycardia, systemic and pulmonary arterial hypertension, increased cardiac output, pallor, perspiration, and mydriasis. Parasympathetic activity produces incontinence, hypersalivation, increased bronchial secretions, and vomiting. Airway reflexes are impaired and upper airway compromise is common from secretions, emesis, and pharyngeal collapse. Skeletal muscle contractions create hyperthermia, anaerobic metabolism with lactic acidosis, and impaired ventilation. Blood glucose and white blood cell levels increase in response to catecholamine release.

Phase 2

Cerebral metabolic demands persist, but oxygen and glucose delivery decline. Increasing hypoventilation, pulmonary aspiration, edema, and atelectasis, all contribute to arterial hypoxemia. Hypoglycemia results from depleted glucose stores and elevated insulin levels. Cerebral blood flow diminishes from depressed myocardial function, reduced preload, and arterial hypotension. Hyperkalemia, rhabdomyolysis, marked hyperpyrexia, worsening metabolic acidosis, and disseminated intravascular coagulopathy are frequently seen.[12-14]

PHARMACOTHERAPY

The ideal AED for seizure emergencies would be rapidly absorbed and effective from the intramuscular, intravenous, intraosseous, and rectal routes. It would not risk hemodynamic, respiratory, and neurologic depression. Finally, its duration of action would preclude seizure recurrence for at least 24 hours. No such ideal medication yet exists, but thoughtfully chosen combinations of existing AEDs provide satisfactory therapy without excessive risks and sedation for most patients.

Many medications have antiepileptic activity, leaving the clinician choices in the pharmacologic management of seizure emergencies. Mechanisms of antiepileptic action are complex and incompletely understood, but numerous animal and clinical studies have provided a sound basis for medication selection, its dosages and routes. Some drugs, such as lidocaine, isofluorane, and paraldehyde (although not currently available in the U.S.), have well documented efficacy in refractory status epilepticus. However, virtually all patients can be satisfactorily treated using a combination of benzodiazepines, barbiturates, and phenytoin. These medications are the most predictable, practical, and versatile. In short, they are the best and are all that one needs acutely.

The use of any AED appropriate for the emergency management of seizures risks hypotension, even cardiac arrest. In addition, most produce respiratory depression. Furthermore, phenytoin can cause vomiting and cardiac dysrhythmias, both of which may be life-threatening. Thus, pharmacologic intervention must be undertaken judiciously. Respiratory and hemodynamic monitoring can be challenging, but are essential in the management of the convulsing patient.

Airway management equipment and personnel with the skills to use it should be at hand. Vascular access is mandatory for those with sustained seizures, not only for AED delivery but as a portal for other emergency drugs and fluids.

Benzodiazepines

These lipophilic drugs have the most rapid onset of action compared to other AEDs and are effective in nearly all types of seizures.[15] Although benzodiazepines have been used clinically for status epilepticus at least 30 years, their mechanisms of action are complex and only recently are becoming understood.[16,17] They may both prevent the initiation and inhibit the spread of epileptiform discharges.[18] These medications are generally used as the initial agents to terminate seizures rapidly, and are usually followed by phenytoin or phenobarbital. Because of their rapid redistribution (alpha) phase, their anticonvulsant effect is relatively short-lived, especially diazepam and midazolam, making concomitant or immediately subsequent administration of a longer-acting drug desirable. Unlike barbiturates, they are not anesthetics, even in high doses.

Benzodiazepines are also effective in refractory status epilepticus by continuous infusion.[19-22] Initial experience suggests that they are highly effective and well-tolerated. Surprisingly, many children have been treated successfully without requiring mechanical ventilation.[20]

All benzodiazepines in clinical use for status epilepticus appear comparable in efficacy and will stop seizures in about 75% or more of patients in less than 10 minutes.[18,23-26] All are also known to cause hypotension and respiratory depression.[27-31] Three benzodiazepines, diazepam, lorazepam, and midazolam, each with its own advantages, will be discussed. When administered intravenously or intraosseously, the initial dose should be injected slowly, over a 10-minute period in those with cardiopulmonary instability, to minimize the risk of hypotension and apnea. If the seizure ceases before completing the injection, no more should be given; the function of the drug is only to rapidly halt the seizure.

Diazepam (Valium) has an extended serum half-life, but its clinical effectiveness ends within half an hour, thus making it inferior to lorazepam. Its diluent, propylene glycol, contributes to the problem of hypotension and can cause a burning sensation in peripheral veins. A major advantage of diazepam is its proven safety and efficacy by the rectal route, even when given in the home by parents and by prehospital providers.[26,32-34] Therapeutic serum levels are achieved within 2 or 3 minutes and peak levels within 10 minutes.[35] Respiratory failure is rare, presumably because of the more gradual absorption compared to the intravenous route.[26,36] The standard parenteral diazepam preparation, 5 mg/ml, is delivered about 5 cm into the rectum via a lubricated tuberculin syringe. The buttocks are then held closed to prevent leakage.

Lorazepam (Ativan) is more potent than diazepam but is also diluted in propylene glycol, increasing the risk of hypotension. However, it probably depresses respiratory drive the least, and its use may reduce the risk of respiratory arrest.[28-31] Because it can be an effective antiepileptic for 12 or more hours after a single dose, it is the benzodiazepine of choice when intravenous access is available. Occasional breakthrough seizures may occur, so it cannot be relied upon to provide seizure protection for this prolonged period.[37] Although it has been successfully used rectally, there is not yet enough experience to advocate this for routine clinical practice.[38,39]

Midazolam (Versed) is the newest drug of this class to be used as an AED. Its major advantage is its water solubility, which facilitates rapid absorption from the intramuscular route.[40] Initial clinical experience indicates that it is promptly effective and reasonably safe in the large majority of patients.[24,41,42] It probably has a slightly greater cardiovascular depressant effect than the other two benzodiazepines.[29] Recent reports document the efficacy of midazolam by continuous infusion for refractory generalized convulsive status epilepticus.[20,21]

With this understanding of these benzodiazepines, lorazepam is the drug of choice when intravenous or intraosseous access exists owing to its prolonged duration of action and reduced potential for respiratory arrest. Diazepam is better reserved for the rectal route and midazolam for the intramuscular route.[40]

Phenytoin

This major AED achieves peak anticonvulsant activity in 20–30 minutes following intravenous use and terminates convulsive status epilepticus in most patients, even when given as a sole agent. Its major advantages are that it can be given intravenously and that a loading dose usually provides a therapeutic serum level for a full day. It is minimally sedating and thus preserves the neurologic exam. Intraosseous administration should be avoided since subtherapeutic levels have been reported via this route. It is ineffective in absence and myoclonic seizures.

Rapid administration can result in hypotension, dysrhythmias, and vomiting; therefore, the loading dose should be given over 20 minutes, with electrocardiographic and blood pressure monitoring (Table 3). Also, phenytoin must be given with a saline solution because it precipitates in glucose-containing solutions. It is probably better to inject the medication into the port closest to the patient instead of mixing it into a burette of saline because the low pH of saline may produce precipitation.[43] The tubing must be flushed with saline before and after its administration; phenytoin is incompatible with many other drugs. The parenteral phenytoin preparation has a pH of 12 and contains propylene glycol. Extravasation can cause local irritation and necrosis at the injection site, so phenytoin should be administered into large veins when possible. Injection into the umbilical arteries may cause severe arterial spasm and ischemia of the legs. Intramuscular injection leads to muscle necrosis and poor absorption. Therefore, phenytoin should be given only intravenously.

Barbiturates

Phenobarbital is the most commonly used drug in this class in the treatment of seizure emergencies. Peak concentrations of phenobarbital occur in the brain within a few minutes, although the drug usually is not maximally effective for 30–60 minutes. Its duration of action following a loading dose ranges from 1–3 days. Its advantages include a long serum half-life and decades of experience with its use. Its disadvantages include respiratory, myocardial and neurologic depression. Cardiorespiratory compromise can be fatal.[44] Used alone, it is an alternative to the combined initial treatment with a benzodiazepine and phenytoin.[45] Simultaneous use of phenobarbital with a benzodiazepine may cause respiratory depression and hypotension.[18]

This drug, unlike phenytoin, is compatible with any usual intravenous fluid. The loading dose should be administered at a rate no greater than 1 mg/kg/min (maximum dose 30 mg/min) with electrocardiographic and blood pressure monitoring.

Pentobarbital, another barbiturate, often is used successfully for refractory status epilepticus. Its shorter half-life, about 20 hours, provides an advantage when discontinuing therapy, allowing earlier recovery from deep sedation. However, it produces marked cardiorespiratory and neurologic depression, and patients usually require mechanical ventilation, invasive hemodynamic monitoring, and, often, inotropic support when this drug is administered.

APPROACH TO THE SEIZING PATIENT

As with most emergencies, it is best to greet seizures with a plan. The many treatment options can create confusion and lead to serious mistakes. The following is a safe, simple, and effective approach for generalized convulsions. Other seizures do not demand the same urgency in treatment.

Almost all seizures last less than 5 minutes without treatment. Simple supportive care is all that is required in these cases. This includes the use of supplemental oxygen, discrete airway positioning and suctioning, lateral decubitus positioning when not contraindicated, and protecting the child from injury. Once these are accomplished, the clinician should prepare to treat the seizure pharmacologically if it continues beyond 10 minutes.

Prevention of Traumatic Complications

The convulsing patient needs to be protected from seizure-induced injury. The patient's head can be protected by placing padding or by keeping the rescuer's lap underneath it. Objects that can be dangerous to the patient should be removed from the area. The transport team should be alert to signs of trauma occurring prior to or during the seizure. Head injury, tongue biting, and fractures of the long bones and the spine can occur. The most common sites of injury are the skull, nose, mandible, spine at C5–6, clavicle, humerus, and tibia.[46]

Airway

The goal of emergency airway therapy is to anticipate and recognize respiratory problems and support or supplant those functions that are compromised or lost. Secretions, emesis, and pharyngeal hypotonia all contribute to airway compromise. Airway patency often can be restored by suctioning and positioning the head neutrally and performing a simple jaw lift maneuver or by placing the patient in the lateral decubitus position. Oral or nasal airways may be used to maintain airway patency but may produce vomiting. Gastric decompression should be considered to prevent emesis and secondary aspiration.

Oxygenation

Oxygen should always be administered because hypoxia often is unexpectedly severe in seizures. The brain is particularly susceptible to hypoxic injury because of its high metabolic demands. Also, pallor from the hyperadrenergic state may make cyanosis more difficult to detect. The patient should be immediately provided with oxygen by mask in the highest concentration available.

Ventilation

Assisted ventilation in a patient in respiratory failure must not await endotracheal intubation. Infants and children can be successfully ventilated by bag and mask, provided good positioning of the head, neck, and airway and a good seal around the mask are achieved. Often chest wall rigidity prevents effective bag-valve-mask ventilation and favors gastric distention. Therefore, great attention to ventilation technique is mandatory. One must be particularly cautious not to further impair central venous return and cardiac output with the application of positive pressure ventilation. If sufficient oxygenation cannot be achieved by bag-valve ventilation, endotracheal intubation is indicated.

Administration of an antiepileptic drug is a top priority because management of the airway and ventilation are substantially easier once the seizure has stopped. When intubation is required, short-acting barbiturates or neuromuscular blockers, or both, should be administered to stop the convulsion and avoid potential injury to the patient. A nondepolarizing neuromuscular blocker is preferred because of the risks of hyperkalemia and bradycardia associated with succinylcholine. Mivacurium is a good choice because of its short effective duration. It must be remembered that the termination of convulsive movements by muscular paralysis does not stop the seizure activity in the brain.

Cardiovascular Support

As cerebrovascular resistance falls and cerebral autoregulation is impaired, cerebral perfusion becomes dependent on systemic blood pressure.[12] Prolonged status epilepticus and AEDs can lead to hypotension and subsequent brain damage. A normal or slightly increased blood pressure should be maintained during a prolonged seizure and assured by frequent measurement. Also, continuous electrocardiographic monitoring is important because of the risk of dysrhythmias. An intravenous line should be established for fluid and glucose replacement and drug administration. When intravenous access cannot be established, an intraosseous line is an excellent route for fluids and medications, providing similar pharmacokinetic efficacy in most drugs,[47] phenytoin being the exception. Normal saline or lactated Ringer's solution are acceptable. With prolonged convulsions, fluid boluses may help prevent and treat hypotension. Dopamine is occasionally needed.

Initial Laboratory Assessment

All children with unexplained seizures should undergo certain emergent testing. This includes bedside serum glucose measurement and laboratory measurement of serum sodium, glucose, and ionized calcium. Those chronically receiving AEDs should have blood levels of the respective medications determined. Appropriate testing should be undertaken when poisoning is suspected (Table 2).

Additional testing often of value includes routine cerebrospinal fluid analysis and computed cranial tomography. Electroencephalography (EEG) may be useful to diagnose nonconvulsive status epilepticus and should be used liberally when the child does not emerge from postictal depression.[48]

Pharmacotherapy

Drug therapy should not be delayed beyond 10 minutes whenever possible. Further delay increases the chances of the patient being refractory to the first several drugs.[49,50] Nonetheless, drug treatment must be performed carefully to

TABLE 2.   Poisons that Can Cause Seizures

Anticholinergics	Carbon monoxide	Poisonous mushrooms	Organophosphates
Anticonvulsants	Cyanide	Lead	Phencyclidine
Antidepressants	Hypoglycemics	Lidocaine	Sympathomimetics
Camphor	Isoniazid	Nicotine	Theophylline

TABLE 3. Drug Therapy for Prolonged Seizures

Drug	Route	Dose (mg/kg)	Maximum Dose
Lorazepam	IV/IO	0.1	4 mg
Diazepam	IV/IO	0.3	10 mg
Diazepam	PR	0.5	20 mg
Midazolam	IM/IV/IO	0.1–0.2	5 mg
Phenytoin	IV	20	1500 mg
Phenobarbital	IV/IO	20	1500 mg

avoid complications. Ninety percent of patients with seizures lasting more than 10 minutes should respond to a well delineated seizure protocol. Dosages and routes are displayed on Table 3.

Therapy is begun with a benzodiazepine, the choice of which depends on drug accessibility and the delivery routes available. Intravenous and intraosseous routes provide greater control in medication administration, but treatment should not be unduly delayed in obtaining this vascular access. Care is necessary not to deliver these drugs faster than over 10 minutes intravenously or intraosseously because of the risks of apnea and hypotension. If the convulsion ceases before the infusion is complete, no more benzodiazepine should be given unless there is relapse.

Phenytoin should be given either simultaneously or immediately after the benzodiazepine. It should be administered over 20 minutes. If the seizure stops before its completion, the remaining drug can be given over 30–60 minutes.

If phenytoin fails, phenobarbital should follow immediately, also over 20 minutes. Because the risk of respiratory failure is high with the completion of the phenobarbital load, the infusion should be interrupted if the seizure stops before its completion.

REFRACTORY GENERALIZED CONVULSIVE STATUS EPILEPTICUS

Convulsions that continue after appropriate doses of a benzodiazepine, phenytoin, and phenobarbital are termed refractory and have a poorer prognosis. The recalcitrance of the seizures and the associated morbidity are usually due to the underlying condition. Our experience, and that of others, is that about 5–15% of those with status epilepticus are refractory to initial therapy.[51,52]

Treatment of the underlying cause is the best therapy. Pharmacotherapy is always successful in eradicating seizures provided the cardiovascular system of the patient can withstand the depressant effects. In addition, almost all patients will require mechanical ventilation. Therefore, it is prudent not to initiate the following therapy in transport.

Pentobarbital given intravenously will decrease blood pressure promptly, with recovery following within about 5 minutes.[53] Boluses of 5–15 mg/kg over 10 minutes may be repeated until the convulsions cease. Usually less than 20 mg/kg is needed.[54] Blood pressure monitoring should be continuous or nearly so, and the infusion should be interrupted whenever the age-appropriate blood pressure becomes unacceptably low. After completing the bolus, a continuous infusion of pentobarbital should begin at 3–5 mg/kg/hr. EEG monitoring is necessary as soon as possible to rule out nonconvulsive status epilepticus. Alternatively, a *loading dose of 30 mg/kg* followed by a continuous infusion with 5 mg/kg/hr provides reasonable assurance of arrest of seizure activity, but at the high risk of hypotension and decreased cardiac output.

More recently, midazolam has been used effectively in refractory status epilepticus.[20,21,55,56] This approach seems to produce less hypotension than pentobarbital and, in one series, to avoid the need for intubation. An intravenous loading dose of 0.15–0.2 mg/kg is followed by a continuous infusion of 1 μg/kg/min. Additional boluses of 0.1 mg/kg are given as needed with a concomitant increase in the drip by 12 μg/kg/min. With some exceptions, seizures are controlled with no more than 1 μg/kg/min and usually much less.

SEIZURE CLUSTERS

Children with serial seizures but with neurologic recovery do not require the intensive management of status epilepticus. These patients usually can be managed with treatment of their underlying disorder and rapid adjustment of their AEDs if they are on chronic therapy. If not, phenytoin 10 mg/kg IV once or 5 mg/kg every 2–3 hours for a total of 15 mg/kg generally will suffice.

SPECIAL CONDITIONS

While most patients can be effectively managed by the preceding protocol, exceptions exist. For example, when poisoning produces convulsions, decontamination and detoxification are essential. Antidotes, when available, may be the sole treatment.

The following are clinical conditions that warrant special discussion. They all are likely to be encountered, albeit infrequently in some cases, in a busy transport program.

Neonatal Seizures

Owing to immature myelination and other factors, seizures in newborns do not resemble those seen in older children. Seizures are frequently subtle and may be difficult to distinguish from nonepileptic manifestations of brain injury, such as posturing and brain stem release phenomena. Focal and multifocal tonic and clonic activity, especially if accompanied by altered vital signs such as tachycardia or apnea, suggests a true seizure (that is, one with an EEG correlate). Motor automatisms, such as pedaling, swimming, and stepping, likely are not seizures. The diagnosis of neonatal seizures often depends on EEG monitoring. When unavailable, it is reasonable to treat empirically.

The major causes of seizures in this age group are hypoxic-ischemic encephalopathy, meningitis, hypoglycemia, hypocalcemia, developmental defects, and intracranial hemorrhage. As with all children, treatment of the underlying disorder, when possible, is a high priority and may obviate AED use. The convulsing neonate may have the exceedingly rare condition of pyridoxine dependency, which responds promptly to intravenous pyridoxine, 50–100 mg/kg over 2 minutes. Thus, this intervention should be included for neonates with unexplained status epilepticus. Otherwise the choice, sequence and dosing of AEDs need not be altered for the neonate (Table 2).

Hyponatremia

Although it remains unclear whether it is the depressed serum sodium or chloride level which actually provokes seizures, hyponatremia is at least associated with refractory convulsions. In fact, the most common etiology of afebrile seizures in infancy is hyponatremia.[57] Usually there is a history of feeding large amounts of dilute formula, juices, or other hypotonic beverages. Occasionally infants take in enough water in swimming classes and bathing to produce convulsions.

Treatment of hyponatremic seizures with AEDs is often unsuccessful and may produce respiratory failure.[58] Infusion of 5 ml/kg of 3% saline over 5-10 minutes is more appropriate and typically will raise the serum sodium level by 3-5 mEq/L, almost always enough to promptly eliminate seizures. This treatment should be instituted empirically if the proper history is present. If later it is determined that the patient was normonatremic, no harm should result.

Hypoglycemia

Reduced blood glucose levels, usually less than 30 mg/dl, can produce seizures. Regardless of the cause of hypoglycemia, it must be corrected to eliminate seizures and prevent brain damage. Bedside glucose measurement provides this diagnosis within 2 minutes. Because seizures elevate stress hormone and catecholamine levels, which should increase blood glucose levels, a rapid reading of less than 100 mg/dl should prompt an immediate recheck. If confirmed, an infusion of glucose should follow while awaiting laboratory serum glucose measurement. Depending on the underlying cause of hypoglycemia, multiple 25% dextrose boluses (if intraosseous or a central line is available, otherwise, dilute to 12.5% for peripheral administration) and continuous infusions of up to 12.5% dextrose with coadministration of corticosteroids may be required to keep the serum glucose over 80 mg/dl. Frequent bedside glucose checks are needed to titrate therapy, sometimes as often as every 10 minutes. Correction of hypoglycemia may not immediately eliminate seizures even if caused by glucose deprivation, as restitution of cerebral glucose levels is not instantaneous.

Hypocalcemia

In neonates, birth asphyxia, other causes of circulatory shock, and maternal diabetes mellitus may produce severe hypocalcemia in the first week of life. Concomitant hypomagnesemia is not unusual and must also be treated in order to elevate the serum calcium levels. The high phosphate burden of "humanized" cow's milk-based formula will rarely cause status epilepticus in neonates in the second through fourth weeks of life.[59,60] Common causes of hypocalcemic seizures in children are phosphate poisoning, usually by sodium phosphate enemas,[61] and rickets. Parathyroid gland absence or dysfunction may also produce symptomatic hypocalcemia at any age.

Hypocalcemic seizures cannot always be discerned clinically from those of other etiologies, but there are certain observations that, when present, can so strongly suggest the diagnosis that AED use can be postponed until the diagnosis is ruled out by a normal serum ionized calcium level. For example, the neonate on a commercial formula who presents during the second through fourth week of life with escalating multifocal clonic and myoclonic activity and who remains alert during the jerking is likely hypocalcemic and, because of the alertness, is very unlikely to have a primary cerebral disease. Also, the infant who convulses for the first time shortly after the inappropriate administration of an adult-dosed enema should be treated with calcium unless there are mitigating conditions. Often, but not always, the QTc on the electrocardiogram will be prolonged beyond 0.460, rapidly confirming the diagnosis.[62]

One successful approach to the emergency correction of hypocalcemia is as follows. Calcium chloride, probably the most widely available salt, is infused during cardiac monitoring over about 5 minutes at a dose of 10 mg/kg. A continuous infusion of 10 mg/kg/hr is then begun. Frequent serum ionized calcium levels will indicate whether additional boluses and a higher infusion rate are necessary. Care must be taken to avoid extravasation of calcium as extensive tissue necrosis may result. The safest route is directly into the central venous compartment.

Status Myoclonicus following Cardiac Arrest

At least one-third of those who remain comatose following cardiopulmonary resuscitation develop seizures, usually within the first 12 hours. Status myoclonicus is unquestionably the most ominous postanoxic seizure disorder owing to its resistance to therapy and its almost uniform association with a fatal outcome.[63-66] Although its clinical appearance varies somewhat, by definition it persists at least 30 minutes and always involves rapid rhythmic or nearly rhythmic movements, usually every 1–10 seconds. Commonly it is multifocal and may be bilaterally synchronous or asynchronous. Sometimes it is restricted to a single body area, particularly a portion of the head or neck.

Controversy surrounds management of status myoclonicus. Some view this as an expression of the agonal brain that does not warrant intensive AED use.[64,65] Our experience supports this. Of 132 initial survivors of pediatric cardiac arrest, 43 developed status myoclonicus. All were refractory to phenobarbital and phenytoin, 20 mg/kg each. Only one child regained consciousness, a boy who suffered over 40 minutes' submersion in ice water. He received no additional AED and had pharmacologic neuromuscular blockade, yet made a full recovery. Among the others, many were poorly tolerant of even the initial AED administration because of a compromised cardiovascular system. Thus, if treatment of status myoclonicus is opted, it is very unlikely to improve outcome and may provoke cardiac arrest from iatrogenic hypotension.

Arterial Hypertension

Convulsions, especially status epilepticus, may cause ictal and postictal hypertension, thus raising the question of hypertensive encephalopathy as the cause of the seizures. Also, because elevated intracranial pressure may trigger arterial hypertension, an acute brain mass or hydrocephalus must be considered. Because status epilepticus is much more common than hypertensive encephalopathy in children, postictal hypertension is more likely to be attributable to the residual circulating catecholamines released during status epilepticus and should be ephemeral. However, a postictal blood pressure greater than four standard deviations above the age-defined mean strongly indicates hypertensive encephalopathy.[67] Focal postictal cortical deficits are compatible with a benign postictal state, hypertensive encephalopathy, and an acute brain lesion, and therefore do not help discriminate. Brain stem and cranial nerve deficits, however, are inconsistent with the former and usually mandate immediate neuroimaging.

PROGNOSIS

The prognosis of an infant or child with a seizure emergency is mostly determined by the cause of that seizure. Other influencing factors are the duration of the seizure, complicating effects of the seizure such as hypoglycemia, aspiration, hypotension and hypoxia, and unwanted effects of treatment, including cardiac arrest. Death during generalized convulsive status epilepticus in children is rare, when properly treated, and neurologic disability attributable solely to seizures also is rare.[5,8,11,57]

REFERENCES

1. Orr RA, Dimand RJ, Venkataraman ST, et al: Diazepam and intubation in emergency treatment of seizures in children. Ann Emerg Med 20:1009–1013, 1991.
2. De Negri M: Electrical status epilepticus in childhood: Neuropsychological impairment and therapeutic management. Dev Med Child Neurol 36:183–186, 1994.
3. Manning DJ, Rosenbloom L: Non-convulsive status epilepticus. Arch Dis Child 62:37–40, 1987.
4. Doose H: Nonconvulsive status epilepticus in childhood: Clinical aspects and classification. In Delgado-Escueta AV, Wasterlain CG, Treiman DM, Porter RJ (eds): Status Epilepticus. New York, Raven Press 1983, pp 83–92.
5. Hauser WA: Status epilepticus: Epidemiologic considerations. Neurology 40(Suppl 2):9–13, 1990.
6. Hauser WA, Nelson K: Epidemiology of epilepsy in children. Clev Clin J Med 56:S185, 1989.
7. Vining EPG: Psychosocial issues for children with epilepsy. Clev Clin J Med 56:S214, 1989.
8. DeLorenzo RJ, Towne AR, Pellock JM, Ko D: Status epilepticus in children, adults and the elderly. Epilepsia 33(Suppl 4):S15–S25, 1992.
9. Phillips SA, Shanahan RJ: Etiology and mortality of status epilepticus in children. A recent update. Arch Neurol 46:74–76, 1989.
10. Maytal J, Shinnar S: Febrile status epilepticus. Pediatrics 86:611–616, 1990.
11. Maytal J, Shinnar S, Moshe SL, Alvarez L: Low morbidity and mortality of status epilepticus in children. Pediatrics 83:323–331, 1989.
12. Lothman E: The biochemical basis and pathophysiology of status epilepticus. Neurology 40(Suppl 2):13–23, 1990.
13. Brown JK, Hussain IHMI: Status epilepticus. 1: Pathogenesis. Dev Med Child Neurol 33:3–17, 1991.
14. Shovron S: Tonic clonic status epilepticus. J Neurol Neurosurg Psychiatry 56:125–134, 1993.
15. Browne TR: The pharmacokinetics of agents used to treat status epilepticus. Neurology 40(Suppl 2):28–32, 1990.
16. Gastaut H, Naquet R, Poire R, et al: Treatment of status epilepticus with diazepam (Valium). Epilepsia 6:167–182, 1965.
17. Levine RL: Pharmacology of intravenous sedatives and opioids in critically ill patients. Crit Care Clin 10:709–731, 1994.
18. Treiman DM: The role of benzodiazepines in the management of status epilepticus. Neurology 40(Suppl 2):32–42, 1990.
19. Delgado-Escueta AV, Wasterlain C, Treiman DM, Porter RJ: Management of status epilepticus. N Engl N Med 306:1337–1340, 1982.
20. Rivera R, Segnini M, Baltodano A, Perez V: Midazolam in the treatment of status epilepticus in children. Crit Care Med 21:991–994, 1993.
21. Kumar A, Bleck TP: Intravenous midazolam for the treatment of refractory status epilepticus. Crit Care Med 20:483–488, 1992.
22. Labar DR, Ali A, Root J: High-dose intravenous lorazepam for the treatment of refractory status epilepticus. Neurology 44:1400–1403, 1994.
23. Galvin GM, Jelinek GA: Successful treatment of 75 patients in status epilepticus with intravenous midazolam. Emerg Med 4:11–12, 1992.
24. McDonagh TJ, Jelinek GA, Galvin GM: Intramuscular midazolam rapidly terminates seizures in children and adults. Emerg Med 4:77–81, 1992.
25. Giang DW, McBride MC: Lorazepam versus diazepam for the treatment of status epilepticus. Pediatr Neurol 4:358–361, 1988.
26. Dieckmann RA: Rectal diazepam for prehospital pediatric status epilepticus. Ann Emerg Med 23:216–214, 1994.
27. Treiman DM: Pharmacokinetics and clinical use of benzodiazepines in the management of status epilepticus. Epilepsia 30(Suppl 2):S4–S10, 1989.
28. Chiulli DA, Terndrup TE, Kanter RK: The influence of diazepam or lorazepam on the frequency of endotracheal intubation in childhood status epilepticus. J Emerg Med 9:13–17, 1991.
29. Reves JG, Glass PSA: Nonbarbiturate intravenous anesthetics. In Miller RD (ed): Anesthesia, 3rd ed. New York, Churchill Livingstone, 1990, p 246.
30. Lebowitz PW, Cote ME, Daniels AL, et al: Comparative cardiovascular effects of midazolam and thiopental in healthy patients. Anesth Analg 61:771–775, 1982.
31. Denaut M, Yernault JC, Coster AD, et al: Double-blind comparison of the respiratory effects of parenteral lorazepam and diazepam in patients with chronic obstructive lung disease. Curr Med Res Opin 2:611–615, 1975.
32. Knudsen FU: Rectal administration of diazepam in solution in the treatment of convulsions in infants and children. Arch Dis Child 54:855–857, 1979.

33. Hoppu K, Santavuori P: Diazepam rectal solution for home treatment of acute seizures in children. Acta Pediatr Scand 70:369-372, 1981.
34. Camfield CS, Camfield PR, Smith E, Dooley JM: Home use of rectal diazepam to prevent status epilepticus in children with convulsive disorders. J Child Neurol 4:125-126, 1989.
35. Dulac O, Aicardi J, Rey E, et al: Blood levels of diazepam after single rectal administration in infants and children. J Pediatr 93:1039-1041, 1978.
36. Seigler RS: The administration fo rectal diazepam for acute management of seizures. J Emerg Med 8:155-159, 1990.
37. Treiman DM, DeGiorgio CM, Ben-Menachem E, et al: Lorazepam vs phenytoin in the treatment of generalized convulsive status epilepticus: Report of an ongoing study [abstract]. Neurology 35(Suppl 1):284, 1985.
38. Dooley JM, Tibbles JAR, Rumney G, Dooley KC: Rectal lorazepam in the treatment of acute seizures in children. Ann Neurol 18:412-413, 1985.
39. Graves NM, Kriel RL, Jones-Saete C: Bioavailability of rectally administered lorazepam. Clin Neuropharmacol 10:555-559, 1987.
40. Raines A, Henderson TR, Swinyard EA, Dretchen KL: Comparison of midazolam and diazepam by the intramuscular route for the control of seizures in a mouse model of status epilepticus. Epilepsia 31:313-317, 1990.
41. Egli M, Albani C: Relief of status epilepticus after IM administration of the new short acting benzodiazepine midazolam [abstract]. Excerpta Medica 137:44, 1981.
42. Chamberlain JM, Altieri MA, Futterman C, et al: Intramuscular midazolam for the treatment of status epilepticus in children [abstract]. Pediatr Emerg Care 6:224, 1990.
43. Parke-Davis Company: Dilantin package insert, 1994.
44. Lombroso CT: Treatment of status epilepticus with diazepam. Neurology 16:629-634, 1966.
45. Shaner DM, McCurdy SA, Herring MO, Gabor AJ: Treatment of status epilepticus: A prospective comparison of diazepam and phenytoin versus phenobarbital and optional phenytoin. Neurology 38:202-207, 1988.
46. Finelli PF, Cardi JK: Seizures as a cause of fracture. Neurology 39:838-850, 1989.
47. Orlowski JP, Porembka DT, Gallagher JM, et al: Comparison of intraosseous, central intra-venous, and peripheral intravenous infusions of emergency drugs. Am J Dis Child 144:112-117, 1990.
48. Fagan KJ, Lee SI: Prolonged confusion following convulsions due to generalized nonconvulsive status epilepticus. Neurology 40:1689-1694, 1990.
49. Walton NY, Treiman DM: Response to status epilepticus induced by lithium and pilocarpine to treat with diazepam. Exp Neurol 101:267-275, 1988.
50. Treiman DM, Meyers PD, the DVA Status Epilepticus Cooperative Study Group: Utility of EEG pattern as a predictor of success in the treatment of generalized convulsive status epilepticus. Epilepsia 32(Suppl 3):93, 1991.
51. Bleck TP: Refractory status epilepticus. Neurology Chron 2;1-4, 1992.
52. Lowenstein DH, Alldredge BK: Status epilepticus in an urban public hospital in the 1980s. Neurology 43:483-488, 1993.
53. Swedlow DB, Schreiner MS: Management of Reye's syndrome. Crit Care Clin 1:285-311, 1985.
54. Orsorio I, Reed RC: Treatment of refractory generalized tonic-clonic status epilepticus with pentobarbital anesthesia after high-dose phenytoin. Epilepsia 30:464-471, 1989.
55. Bleck TP: Advances in the management of refractory status epilepticus. Crit Care Med 21:955-957, 1993.
56. Parent JM, Lowenstein DH: Treatment of refractory generalized status epilepticus with continuous infusion of midazolam. Neurology 44:1837-1840, 1994.
57. Dunn DW: Status epilepticus in children: Etiology, clinical features, and outcome. J Child Neurol 3:167-173, 1988.
58. Corneli HM, Gormley CJ, Baker RC: Hyponatremia and seizures presenting in the first two years of life. Pediatr Emerg Care 1:190, 1985.
59. Venkataraman PS, Tsang RC, Greer FR, et al: Late infantile tetany and secondary hyper-parathyroidism in infants fed humanized cow milk formula. Am J Dis Child 139:664-668, 1985.
60. Specker BL, Tsang RC, Ho ML, et al: Low serum calcium and high parathyroid hormone levels in neonates fed "humanized" cow's milk-based formula. Am J Dis Child 145:941-945, 1991.
61. Craig JC, Hodson EM, Martin HC: Phosphate enema poisoning in children. Med J Aust 160:347-351, 1994.
62. Goetting MG, Sowa B: Rapid diagnosis of hypocalcemic status epilepticus in infants [abstract]. Ann Neurol 24:317, 1988.
63. Krumholz A, Stern BJ, Weiss HD: Outcome from coma after cardiopulmonary resuscitation: Relation to seizures and myoclonus. Neurology 38:401-405, 1988.

64. Wijdicks EFM, Parisi JE, Sharbrough FW: Prognostic value of myoclonus status in comatose survivors of cardiac arrest. Ann Neurol 35:239–243, 1994.
65. Young GB, Gilbert JJ, Zochodne DW: The significance of myoclonic status epilepticus in postanoxic coma. Neurology 40:1843–1848, 1990.
66. Jumao-as A, Brenner RP: Myoclonic status epilepticus: A clinical and electrographic study. Neurology 40:1199–1202, 1990.
67. Proulx F, Lacroix J, Farrell CA, Gauthier M: Convulsions and hypertension in children: Differentiating cause from effect. Crit Car Med 21:1541–1546, 1993.

CHAPTER 19

Near-Drowning

DEBRA H. FISER, M.D.

BACKGROUND

Drowning may be defined as death secondary to submersion; near-drowning, on the other hand, implies that the victim has survived for some time following submersion, usually at least long enough to have gained hospital admission. Drowning is the cause of death for over 2000 American children each year; near-drowning is even more common, with over 7000 hospitalizations and over 30,000 emergency department (ED) visits per year for near-drowning events.[30]

The age groups at highest risk for death by drowning are children under the age of five years and between the ages of 15 and 19 years.[30] Owing to increased exposure and increased high-risk behaviors, males drown at a rate three to four times that of females.[24,30] Lower socioeconomic groups are also disproportionately affected.[7]

Geographically, southern and western states and Alaska in the US have the highest rates of drowning, peaking during summer months.[7] Natural bodies of water (e.g., lakes, rivers) are the site of most fatal submersions, especially for the adolescent age group, often related to a delay in locating the victim.[23] Preschoolers more often drown in residential swimming pools.[30] In contrast, infants under one year as well as older children with seizure disorders are at greatest risk for bathtub drowning.[23] Unfortunately, nearly one-fifth of submersions in children under five years of age have resulted from child abuse.[23]

Alcohol has been shown to play a contributing role in a large number of cases, particularly those which are boat-related.[2,22] In the home, swimming pool drownings frequently result from a brief lapse in adult supervision due to distraction by a telephone or doorbell.[23]

PATHOPHYSIOLOGY

Most pathology attributable to near-drowning is mediated by asphyxia.[1] However, hypothermia, aspiration, and associated injuries also are contributing factors.

Pathophysiology of the Drowning Episode

Unless the victim is unconscious at the time of submersion, a predictable sequence of events follows when the victim recognizes the trouble. Struggling occurs as the victim attempts to surface.[1] As a result of vigorous motor activity, the metabolic rate increases and body heat is lost to the surrounding water.[31] This cooling effect is particularly evident in children because of their large body surface-area to body-mass ratios. As the victim attempts to suppress the respiratory drive in order to avoid aspiration, he or she typically swallows a large amount of water. The resulting gastric distention enhances the risk of regurgitation so that, often, the victim aspirates both water and gastric contents, aggravating the pulmonary manifestations of near-drowning. Swallowed water, if not regurgitated or removed, is also absorbed from the gastrointestinal tract and may lead to free-water overload and hyponatremia. Alternatively, contact between the vocal cords and the water may produce laryngospasm.[1] As long as laryngospasm persists, the closed glottis protects the lungs from aspiration despite continued inspiratory stimulation. As a result 10–20% of all near-drowning events are "dry drownings," manifesting asphyxia but no evidence of aspiration. Loss of the respiratory drive or apnea with or without laryngospasm protects the victim from aspiration.

At times the victim loses consciousness under water. For example, swimmers who hyperventilate before submersion so that they can hold their breath longer may risk developing hypoxemia profound enough to produce loss of consciousness while swimming.[4] This occurs because, although it is not possible to willfully override the hypercarbic drive to breathe, it is possible to override the hypoxic drive to breathe, at least to the point of loss of consciousness when the PaO_2 plunges. In this situation, inspiratory effort would continue for a time and the presence or absence of associated laryngospasm would determine whether or not the victim aspirated water.

Pulmonary Pathophysiology

Torre and co-workers have described the scanning electron microscopic findings of the lung in drowning: dilation of the alveoli with stretching and even rupture of the septa; small lacerations of the epithelial lining of the alveoli, which at times reached the basal lamina and the capillary walls; and alterations of the surface of Type II alveolar cells.[28]

Although the presenting manifestations are indistinguishable clinically, the pathophysiology in the lung varies somewhat with the characteristics of the fluid aspirated.[9] Fresh water markedly disrupts the surfactant system, while salt water merely dilutes surfactant, but does not alter its surface tension properties. Owing to its hypertonicity, however, salt water pulls edema fluid into the alveoli from the vascular space. In either case, a picture of noncardiogenic pulmonary edema results. Within a few hours following aspiration, most patients exhibit fever and leukocytosis related to the pulmonary insult. These signs do not, however, imply that infection is present and should not alone be construed as indications for antibiotics.

Circulatory Pathophysiology

In contrast to the pulmonary pathology, Orlowski and co-workers demonstrated that the cardiovascular changes in near-drowning are not dependent on the tonicity of the fluid aspirated, but are the result of hypoxic-ischemic injury.[21] However, hypothermia plays an additive role in early hemodynamic instability and dysrhythmias.

Neurologic Pathophysiology

The neurologic manifestations are also primarily the result of the degree of hypoxic-ischemic encephalopathy. In addition, significant hypothermia may produce a clinical picture that resembles brain death, but may be reversible with rewarming. The protective effect of hypothermia is thought to be its lowering of metabolic rate and oxygen consumption by the brain. However, "miraculous" recoveries following prolonged submersion have only been reported following submersion in water that is not just cold, but icy.

Although the mammalian diving reflex has been credited with protection of the brain during cold water submersion of children, recent findings have called this assumption into question and seem to shift emphasis to hypothermia as the mechanism for enhanced survivability following cold water drowning in children.[10,12]

Other Pathophysiology

Other organ injury is related to ischemia far more than hypoxemia. The impact on the kidney may be acute tubular necrosis and associated renal failure. Transient hepatic enzyme elevations are common following ischemia of any etiology, but rarely are severe enough to impact outcome.

CLINICAL PRESENTATION

The clinical presentation of the near-drowning patient is most dependent on the duration of submersion and the time to return of effective respiration and circulation. Very brief submersions may produce only coughing or other mild respiratory symptoms or mild disorientation. At the other end of the spectrum, full cardiopulmonary arrest is common. If cardiopulmonary resuscitation (CPR) is successful, later findings may include acidosis, fulminant pulmonary edema and respiratory failure, hemodynamic instability, stupor, or coma.

Hypothermia is present in almost all cases of near-drowning, even in very warm weather, since the water temperature is invariably still lower than body temperature. In addition, the victim may present with signs and symptoms of an associated injury, such as cervical spine fracture from diving.

TREATMENT

Field Treatment

The field treatment of near-drowning begins with the safe rescue of the victim.[2,11] It is most important that the rescuer not endanger his or her own safety: drowning is very common among those attempting to rescue another victim. It is ideal to throw a life-line or flotation device to a victim if he or she is able to grasp it so that the rescuer does not have to enter the water. For swimming pool rescues, a shepherd's hook type device can be used to "fish" a victim from danger. However, if the victim is unconscious or cannot be located beneath the surface of the water, the rescuer should enter the water only after donning an appropriate flotation device.

Deep water resuscitation has been used successfully in some cases;[16,17] however, it should not delay removing the victim from the water for conventional resuscitation. In the process of securing the airway, rescuers should be cognizant of the potential for cervical spine injuries, especially in diving mishaps.[1] Rescue breathing should be instituted for patients with ineffectual or absent respiration. Techniques such as water drainage from the lung are not recommended; likewise, the Heimlich maneuver is recommended only in rare situations in which the airway is obstructed.[18] Bag-and-mask ventilation with supplemental O_2 and positive end expiratory pressure (PEEP) is the most effective means of restoring oxygenation, followed by endotracheal intubation.

After the airway is secured and effective ventilation has been instituted, stabilization of the circulation and establishment of vascular access can commence using usual advanced life support protocols. In infants and young children, placement of an intraosseous catheter is a viable alternative to placement of an intravenous catheter and may avoid unnecessary delay in transport.[8]

Field personnel should be alert to the potential for the near-drowning victim to become apneic, even if the patient is breathing spontaneously after being removed from the water. Later apnea is not uncommon; patients should be monitored carefully. Also, because of the large volume of water frequently swallowed during submersion, there is a great likelihood of vomiting, especially in association with assisted respiration.[16] Finally, drowning victims, even in hot summer months, typically become hypothermic. Removal of wet clothing and use of warm blankets en route to the ED may help to minimize this problem.

ED Treatment at Referring Hospital

All patients who have been near-drowning victims should be admitted for observation. Patients who have required CPR at the scene or in the ED, patients who have supplemental O_2 requirements exceeding 40%, and patients with any residual obtundation require admission to a tertiary-level pediatric ICU.

Priorities for stabilization prior to secondary transport begin with initial resuscitation per usual advanced life support guidelines with cervical spine precautions, if indicated. A nasogastric tube should be placed as soon as feasible after arrival to remove swallowed water.[1] Not only will this reduce the likelihood of vomiting, it will alleviate the gastric distention that may compromise ventilation in young infants.

Unfortunately, the prognosis for near-drowning victims requiring CPR in the ED is mostly dismal.[19] However, one aspect of resuscitation in the near-drowning victim that differs somewhat from other resuscitation settings is that of resuscitating the victim of near-drowning in icy water. A number of case reports exist documenting intact survival following prolonged submersion in icy water; therefore, more prolonged resuscitative efforts may be warranted in severely hypothermic cases (core temperature $< 33°C$) than would otherwise be appropriate for typical CPR.[3,14] Because hypothermia may contribute to refractory dysrhythmias, core rewarming should be instituted in the ED in addition to surface warming. Options include warmed intravenous fluids or lavage fluids, warmed inspired gases, and/or cardiopulmonary bypass.[15,20]

Pulmonary Management

The chest radiograph and a need for supplemental O_2 are the best prognostic indicators of pulmonary disease. However, it is a very rare patient with near-drowning who dies from late pulmonary complications. The vast majority of deaths in the hospital relate to global anoxic-ischemic injury.

Pulmonary management for the near-drowning victim is primarily supportive. Patients with O_2 requirements exceeding 0.40 to 0.50 are best managed with endotracheal intubation and PEEP. Only very rare cases fail to respond to conventional mechanical ventilation and require more heroic interventions such as oscillation or ECMO. Steroids have no role in the management of the patient with near-drowning and may worsen complications.[18] Likewise, prophylactic antibiotics are not routinely indicated except for victims who have been submerged in grossly contaminated water or other high-risk settings such as hot tubs.[18,29] Secondary infection, when present, usually does not occur until 48–72 hours after aspiration.

Circulatory Management

The circulatory support of the near-drowning patient centers on maintenance of adequate tissue perfusion and oxygenation to minimize secondary organ injury. The initial goal is restoration of normal sinus rhythm. Promotion of normal capillary refill occurs through judicious use of volume expansion with isotonic crystalloids and inotropic support as needed (dopamine if hypotensive or dobutamine if not). Evidence of adequacy of perfusion includes urine output exceeding 1-2 ml/kg/hr, spontaneous improvement in metabolic acidosis, and possibly improvement in level of consciousness. An indwelling bladder catheter should be placed as soon as possible to monitor urine output.

Free water should be limited somewhat in the patient with neurologic impairment. Typical initial maintenance fluids would be $D_5 1/2$ NS at 75-80% of usual maintenance rate.

Neurologic Management

The goal of neurologic management is the prevention of secondary or additional brain injury. Seizures are best treated initially with lorazepam (0.05 mg/kg IV) followed with an incremental loading dose of phenytoin (up to 15-20 mg/kg slow IV). Lorazepam may be repeated if needed for continued seizure activity. Other neurologic care is supportive using sedation for combativeness or agitation with or without neuromuscular blockade. Intracranial pressure monitoring and intensive control of intracranial pressure have not been shown to be associated with improved outcome following near-drowning.[5,25,26] Although most late deaths in near-drowning are secondary to cerebral edema and herniation, this edema reflects the severity of the anoxic injury occurring at the time of the submersion. No intervention after the fact has been shown to reverse this initial injury; however, additional injury may be preventable. CT scans on admission are indicated only if there is a question of associated intracranial injury secondary to blunt trauma (e.g., diving accident). Otherwise, the CT scan usually is normal initially and of no prognostic value.[27]

Other Management

While the resuscitation team is stabilizing the patient, it is important to remember to support the family. The incidence of adjustment problems in families following the near-drowning of a child is exceedingly high, with a very high divorce rate in subsequent months. Parents are racked with guilt and, not infrequently, blame themselves or their spouse for the event.[6] Professional help in defusing the situation is invaluable in the early stages as well as after hospitalization.

Intratransport Management

Patients should be as stable as possible before secondary transport to a tertiary care institution. The transport setting should not diminish the level of care provided to the child en route from that provided by the referring institution.[13] In fact, the level of care may improve with an experienced pediatric critical care transport team. The goals of the transport team are to maintain the stability of the airway, ventilation, and circulation en route, and to monitor for neurologic complications. Maintenance of thermal neutrality is also important.

Management of Possible Complications

Intratransport complications are best dealt with by anticipatory prevention. Maintenance of thermal neutrality poses an especially difficult problem on transport, especially in the near-drowning victim. Special care should be taken to avoid any unnecessary exposure to a cool environment.

Loss of an artificial airway en route is best prevented by careful tube taping, sedation, and neuromuscular blockade. Careful monitoring of pulse oximetry and/or color as well as chest excursion will alert the team to the possibility of a misplaced endotracheal tube without undue delay. Depending on the mode of transport (air or ground) and the degree of access to the patient airway, transport may have to be interrupted for tube replacement.

Another respiratory complication that may be encountered en route is pneumothorax. Pneumothorax is unusual in the near-drowning patient, but occasionally may develop as a result of resuscitation and become manifest only later during transport. Classic signs of pneumothorax include hypoxemia with unilateral decreased breath sounds and asymmetry of chest wall excursion. A small pneumothorax may be temporized with an increase in FiO_2 for a short transport; however, more significant hypoxemia or signs of tension require urgent needle thoracentesis for decompression followed by tube thoracostomy.

Noncardiogenic pulmonary edema may be manifest by voluminous pink- or red-tinged secretions welling forth in the endotracheal tube. It is important that transport personnel recognize these secretions as a sign of pulmonary edema, since the appropriate response is *not* frequent suctioning of the airway, but instead an increase in PEEP. Most of the secretions will disappear when the pressure is adjusted optimally; this may require some empiric increase in PEEP during transport.

Circulatory instability en route may require additional administration of normal saline or lactated Ringer's solution or adjustment of inotropic support.

The neurologic complications of near-drowning are quite common on transport and may include seizures, posturing, agitation, or herniation. Seizure management has already been discussed. Posturing and agitation are ideally treated with benzodiazepines, frequently with the addition of a muscle relaxant. We prefer short-acting agents such as midazolam and vecuronium so that we can assess the neurologic status more accurately at the time of arrival at the pediatric ICU. Herniation may occur in the most severely affected individuals and is usually suspected with absence of spontaneous movement or breathing and fixed, nonreactive pupils. Patients on cardiac and blood pressure monitors may exhibit a classic Cushing triad. The most appropriate acute response to this complication is manual hyperventilation. Mannitol may be administered (0.25 gm/kg IV); however, as previously discussed, it is uncertain whether empiric measures to control intracranial pressure following the anoxic event will affect outcome positively.

REFERENCES

1. Beyda DH: Pathophysiology of near-drowning and treatment of the child with a submersion incident. Crit Care Nurs Clin North Am 3:273, 1991.
2. Beyda DH: Prehospital care of the child with a submersion incident. Crit Care Nurs Clin North Am 3:281, 1991.
3. Biggart MJ, Bohn DJ: Effect of hypothermia and cardiac arrest on outcome of near-drowning accidents in children. J Pediatr 117:179, 1990.
4. Craig AB Jr: Causes of loss of consciousness during underwater swimming. J Appl Physiol 15:583, 1961.
5. Dean JM, McComb JG: Intracranial pressure monitoring in severe pediatric near-drowning. Neurosurgery 9:627, 1981.
6. Fandel I, Bancalari E: Near-drowning in children: Clinical aspects. Pediatrics 58:573, 1976.
7. Fiser DH: Current concepts: The intraosseous infusion technique. N Engl J Med 322:1579, 1990.

8. Fiser DH: Near-drowning. Pediatr Rev 14:148, 1993.
9. Giammona ST, Modell JH: Drowning by total immersion. Effects on pulmonary surfactant of distilled water, isotonic saline and sea water. Am J Dis Child 114:612, 1967.
10. Gooden BA: Why some people do not drown: Hypothermia versus the diving response. Med J Aust 157:629, 1992.
11. Haynes BE: Near-drowning: Rescuing victims effectively. Physician Sportsmed 19:31, 1991.
12. Hayward JS, Hay C, Matthews BR, Overweel CH, Radford DD: Temperature effect on the human dive response in relation to cold water near-drowning. J Appl Physiol 56:202, 1984.
13. Johnson CM, Gonyea MT: Transport of the critically ill child. Mayo Clin Proc 68:982, 1993.
14. Kram JA, Kizer KW: Submersion injury. Emerg Med Clin North Am 2:545, 1984.
15. Letsou GV, Kopf GS, Elefteriades JA, Carter JE, Baldwin JC, Hammond GL: Is cardiopulmonary bypass effective for treatment of hypothermic arrest due to drowning or exposure? Arch Surg 127:525, 1992.
16. Manolios N, Mackie I: Drowning and near-drowning on Australian beaches patrolled by life-savers: A 10-year study, 1973–1983. Med J Aust 148:165, 1988.
17. March NF, Matthews RC: New techniques in external cardia compressions: Aquatic cardiopulmonary resuscitation. JAMA 244:1229, 1980.
18. Modell JH: Drowning. N Engl J Med 328:253, 1993.
19. Nichter MA, Everett PB: Childhood near-drowning: Is cardiopulmonary resuscitation always indicated? Crit Care Med 17:993, 1989.
20. Norberg WJ, Agnew RF, Brunsvold R, Sivanna P, Browdie DA, Fisher D: Successful resuscitation of a cold water submersion victim with the use of cardiopulmonary bypass. Crit Car Med 20:1355, 1992.
21. Orlowski JP, Abulleil MM, Phillips JM: The hemodynamic and cardiovascular effects of near-drowning in hypotonic, isotonic, or hypertonic solutions. Ann Emerg Med 18:1044, 1989.
22. Pluckhahn VD: Alcohol and accidental drowning: A 25-year study. Med J Aust 141:22, 1984.
23. Quan L, Gore EJ, Wentz K, Allen J, Novack AH: Ten-year study of pediatric drownings and near-drownings in King County, Washington: Lessons in injury prevention. Pediatr 83:1035, 1989.
24. Rodgers GB: Factors contributing to child drownings and near-drownings in residential swimming pools. Human Factors 31:123, 1989.
25. Sarnaik AP, Preston G, Lieh-lai M, Eisenbrey AB: Intracranial pressure and cerebral perfusion pressure in near-drowning. Crit Care Med 13:224, 1985.
26. Sibbald WJ: Cerebral resuscitation therapy in pediatric near-drowning. J Pediatr 106:615, 1985.
27. Taylor SB, Quencer RM, Holzman BH, Naidich TP: Central nervous system anoxic-ischemic insult in children due to near-drowning. Radiology 156:641, 1985.
28. Torre C, Varetto L: Scanning electron microscope study of the lung in drowning. J Forens Sci 30:456, 1985.
29. Tron VA, Baldwin VJ, Pirie GE. Hot tub drownings. Pediatr 75:789, 1985.
30. Wintemute GJ: Childhood drowning and near-drowning in the United States. Am J Dis Child 144:663, 1990.
31. Young RSK, Zalneraitis EL, Dooling EC: Neurological outcome in cold water drowning. JAMA 244:1233, 1980.

CHAPTER 20

Endocrine and Metabolic Emergencies

PAUL L. MUELLER, M.D.
DAVID G. JAIMOVICH, M.D.

Although endocrine problems are relatively uncommon and the majority are treated with outpatient management, emergencies such as intractable hypoglycemia, hypocalcemia, or hyperkalemia may require transport to a tertiary care institution. An understanding of the differential diagnosis, pathophysiology, and treatment is necessary to identify the patient requiring transport and choose the correct diagnostic specimens, which in many situations are required before initial treatment. A discussion of the pathophysiology and differential diagnosis of endocrine conditions is included in this chapter.

HYPOGLYCEMIA

Hypoglycemia is defined statistically as a plasma glucose less than 30 mg/dl in small-for-gestational-age (SGA) or premature infants; less then 40 mg/dl in full-term infants in the first 3 days of life; and less than 50 mg/dl in full-term infants over 3 days of age.[1]

Pathophysiology

The various causes of hypoglycemia may be categorized as inadequate intake of glucose, defects in gluconeogenesis, or increased utilization of glucose[2,3] (Table 1).

In response to hypoglycemia, the body releases counter-regulatory hormones including glucagon, epinephrine, cortisol, and growth hormone in an attempt to raise the blood glucose concentration.[4,5] These hormones may cause symptoms of hyperglycemia that last for several hours. Although liver, muscle, and adipose tissue are usually considered the main targets of insulin action, insulin is also involved in metabolism within the central nervous system (CNS), although it is not required for glucose entry into the cells of the CNS. The neurologic complications appear to be proportional to the degree and duration of hypoglycemia. Normal levels for plasma glucose are derived from statistical data. The frequently quoted hypoglycemic threshold (30–40 mg/dl), above which the brain is protected from the effects of hypoglycemia, depends on many other metabolic conditions in the CNS.

Clinical Presentation

Symptoms are due to neuroglycopenia and adrenergic nervous system discharge.[6] Signs and symptoms in the newborn include twitching or seizures,

TABLE 1.   Etiology of Hypoglycemia in the Neonate and Child

Early neonatal hypoglycemia associated with physiologic stress	Decreased gluconeogenesis (cont.)
Asphyxia, toxemia, smaller twin, CNS hemorrhage, sepsis	Metabolic errors (cont.)
	Pyruvate carboxylase or phosphoenolpyruvate carboxykinase (PEPCK) deficiency (hepatomegaly, lactic acidosis)
Inadequate glucose intake	Fructose 1-6 diphosphatase deficiency (elevated lactate and alanine)
Starvation	Ethanol administration
Ketotic hypoglycemia (occurs after fasting, need to evaluate hormone deficiencies)	
	Increased utilization of glucose
Decreased gluconeogenesis	Hyperinsulinism
Hypopituitarism (deficiency of growth hormone, cortisol, thyroxine, or combinations)	Sudden withdrawal of intravenous glucose (infiltration of IV)
Metabolic errors (may be associated with acidosis)	Infant of diabetic mother
Galactosemia (reducing substances in urine after milk ingestion)	Small for gestational age infant
Aminoacidurias	Islet cell hyperplasia (nesidioblastosis)
Organic acidurias[8]	Erythroblastosis fetalis
MCAD deficiency	Beckwith syndrome
Carnitine deficiency	Islet cell adenoma (<2 months or >5 years of age)
Type 1 glycogen storage disease[4] (glucose-6-phosphate deficiency; hepatomegaly, lactic acidosis, hypoglycemia, abnormal response of glucose to glucagon or epinephrine)	Presenting sign of prediabetes (extremely rare in children)
	Excessive treatment with insulin
Fructose intolerance (reducing substance in urine after fruit is ingested)	Chronic seizures
	Insulin or oral hypoglycemics (sulfonureas)

limpness, lethargy, eye-rolling, high-pitched cry, apnea, irregular respirations, and possibly cyanosis. In the pediatric patient, seizures are a common sign of hypoglycemia. Symptoms in the child may include sweating, pallor, tachycardia, palpitations, anxiety, hunger, weakness, and possibly hypothermia.

The etiology of hypoglycemia in the neonate is given in Table 1. General systemic entities seen in critical care that may be associated with hypoglycemia include hepatic disease, renal disease, sepsis, total parenteral nutrition with inadequate glucose delivery, excessive insulin, oral hypoglycemic treatment, extensive thermal burns, starvation, or ethanol ingestion.[7]

Conditions in the differential diagnosis which may mimic hypoglycemia include anxiety, physiologic hyperinsulinism after glucose intake, pheochromocytoma, or the effect of medications, including theophylline, epinephrine, or Alupent.

Treatment

The initial treatment for significant hypoglycemia, regardless of its etiology, is first to immediately obtain a serum sample and then to administer a bolus of 0.2 gm/kg of glucose. This may be administered as a 25% dextrose solution if the patient has either central venous access or an intraosseous (IO) line in place. It is preferable to administer no greater than 12.5–15% dextrose into a peripheral intravenous line, because a higher concentration of dextrose may cause sclerosis in peripheral vessels. The initial bolus should be followed by intravenous fluids containing dextrose 10% (D10/W) and electrolytes.

In the neonate, errors of gluconeogenesis are managed by intravenous glucose at 10–15 mg/kg/min. Requirements over 15 mg/kg/min to prevent hypoglycemia indicate increased utilization of glucose due to hyperinsulinism.[9] If a patient has intravenous fluid administration at 150 ml/kg/day, D10/W provides approximately 10 mg/kg/min, and D15/W provides approximately 15 mg/kg/min.

Blood should be drawn for a STAT determination of glucose and lactate, and a serum sample sent for growth hormone, cortisol, and T_4 levels prior to treatment for hypoglycemia. The glucose and lactate must be done STAT, but the other specimens may be transported with the patient. Blood gases also should be obtained to determine the acid/base status. The presence of urinary ketones rules out hyperinsulinism. Metabolic acidosis suggests aminoaciduria or other errors of glucose metabolism. If acidosis is present, serum amino acids, urine amino acids, organic acids, and carnitine are obtained immediately, since in some cases they may change after treatment.

After adequate treatment with IV dextrose at 10–15 mg/kg/min, if the glucose again falls below 60 mg/dl, the diagnosis is likely to be hyperinsulinism. This may be treated with hydrocortisone (10 mg/kg/day) divided every six hours. This dose is decreased after two days to prevent peripheral edema or pulmonary edema, to 5 mg/kg/day (approximately 125 mg/m^2). When the blood glucose increases to 100–120 mg/dl, the dose may be reduced by 50% every one or two days.

Since cortisone takes 12–24 hours to raise the blood glucose, diazoxide may be administered for severe hypoglycemia (less than 40 mg/dl) due to hyperinsulinism.[10] Diazoxide is an anihypertensive that acutely inhibits insulin release from the pancreas. The initial dose is 5 mg/kg/day divided every six hours intravenously or orally with a maximal effect lasting up to four hours. If there is no increase in glucose by four hours, the subsequent dose is increased to 10 mg/kg/day divided into four equal doses. Again, if there is no response by four hours, the next dose may be increased to 15 mg/kg/day divided into four equal doses. The maximum recommended dose is 20 mg/kg/day in divided doses. Glucagon intramuscularly is indicated only for emergencies, e.g., when an intravenous line cannot be restarted. Somatostatin analogue (10–30 μg subcutaneously every 8 hours) also effectively inhibits the release of pancreatic insulin, although short-term rather than chronic use is recommended owing to gastrointestinal complications.[11]

Transport Management

After blood samples are drawn for laboratory diagnosis and an initial bolus of glucose is given, an intravenous line with D5/W or D10/W must be maintained to prevent a recurrence of the hypoglycemia during transport. A bedside glucose determination is monitored hourly or more frequently as needed. The glucose monitor will provide an immediate assessment of the glucose on a drop of blood. Visual reading of glucose strips may also be used to avoid long delays in waiting for a laboratory determination to be received. Anticonvulsant medications and intubation equipment must be available for use if the patient deteriorates and the airway must be secured.

Complications

Acute complications of hypoglycemia include seizures, coma, or aspiration and hypoxia secondary to an inability to maintain the airway. Late complications of hypoglycemia in the young child include possible learning disabilities or seizures. These are more common in children under 5 years of age presenting with blood glucose < 55 mg/dl.[12]

DIABETIC KETOACIDOSIS/HYPERGLYCEMIA

One of the most frequently encountered metabolic disorders in critical care is diabetic ketoacidosis (DKA). In spite of advances in the treatment of diabetes mellitus, DKA remains a significant source of morbidity and mortality in all age groups, with a reported mortality rate of 3–17%.[13]

Pathophysiology

The metabolic effects of insulin are as follows: (1) promotion of glucose transport across cell membranes and intracellular metabolism of glucose; (2) amino acid transport across cell membranes, protein synthesis, and growth; and (3) inhibition of lipoprotein, resulting in fat breakdown, weight loss, ketosis, and free fatty acids.[14] The average daily dose required to treat type I diabetes is 0.7 U/kg body weight in the prepubertal child, and 1–1.3 U/kg after puberty.

Hyperglycemia results from decreased utilization of glucose as a result of insulin deficiency in type I diabetes. In type II diabetes the cause is insulin resistance, although a relative insulin deficiency may coexist. Although the glucose production rate falls after several hours of hyperglycemia, decreased urinary excretion of glucose occurs secondary to hypovolemia and low glomerular filtration rate, contributing to the elevated concentration of glucose in the serum.

In addition to causing hyperglycemia, insulin deficiency and dehydration in DKA result in an overproduction of beta-hydroxybuterate, acetoacetate, acetone, and free fatty acids. In the presence of insulin deficiency, lipoprotein lipase is not inhibited, with resultant mobilization of free fatty acids, triglyceride, cholesterol and low-density lipoproteins. Free fatty acids further inhibit insulin action. Liver, muscle, and fat tissue convert from anabolic to catabolic metabolism with the release of both fatty acids and amino acids, which act as a substrate for liver gluconeogenesis and ketogenesis. In DKA, hyperglycemia causes an osmotic diuresis, producing intravascular dehydration. In this case tissue is hypoperfused, and anaerobic glycolysis produces lactic acidosis.

Factors precipitating DKA include lack of insulin, dietary excess, infection, trauma, or emotional stress. In addition to having underutilization of glucose secondary to insulin deficiency, patients in DKA may have elevated production of glucose secondary to cortisol, growth hormone, epinephrine, and norepinephrine release. Another response to volume depletion and hyperosmolality from osmotic diuresis in DKA is an elevation of vasopressin, plasma renin activity, and aldosterone concentrations. Because these hormones promote the retention of free water, patients may be at an increased risk of cerebral herniation if they are overhydrated.

Hyperchloremic acidosis is commonly seen in DKA owing in part to large amounts of chloride in intravenous fluid replacement. The most serious metabolic alteration in DKA is hypovolemia and associated hyperosmolality. The degree of hyperosmolality has been shown to correlate with the level of obtundation and electroencephalographic changes in patients with DKA.[15] As a result of hypovolemia, a decrease in glomerular filtration rate further slows the excretion of glucose, contributing to hyperglycemia.

In the differential diagnosis of hyperglycemia and ketosis, the transport team must be aware that treatment with prostaglandin E_1 infusion may produce hyperglycemia and ketosis. It is used to maintain a patent ductus arteriosus in patients suffering from ductus-dependent congenital cyanotic heart disease.

If the patient is not weighed on admission to the emergency department, body weight must be estimated from last known weight or from the child's apparent size. A child presenting in DKA may be safely estimated to have a water deficit of 10–15% of body weight.

Total body potassium deficiency is found in DKA due to osmotic diuresis and vomiting. Severe intracellular hypokalemia may result in cardiac arrhythmias or respiratory failure. After initial fluid resuscitation with a bolus of normal saline in 1-2 hours, potassium chloride is required at a rate of 30-40 mEq/L in the intravenous fluids to replace deficits and prevent further hypokalemia as a result of insulin administration. Despite depletion of total body stores, in some patients initial plasma levels of potassium may be high. In this case electrolytes are repeated in four hours and potassium in intravenous fluids is held until the serum potassium is normal.

Phosphate therapy is a controversial issue in the treatment of DKA. Patients may have depletion of total body phosphate stores and depressed levels of 2,3-diphosphoglycerate (2,3DPG). This fact prompted the use of potassium phosphate in treatment of DKA in an effort to increase oxygen-carrying capacity. However, recent clinical studies have not confirmed a clinical benefit from this treatment;[16] therefore, phosphate treatment is strongly recommended only if the serum phosphate is low.[17,18] An added benefit of using phosphate is to decrease the hyperchloremic acidosis produced by intravenous fluids. A combination of half potassium chloride and half potassium phosphate (typically 20 mEq chloride and 20 mEq phosphate/L) is provided in intravenous fluids.

Hyperchloremic acidosis is commonly seen in DKA owing in part to large amounts of chloride in intravenous fluid replacement. Severe acidosis in DKA may be life-threatening because of a negative inotropic effect on the myocardium. However, bicarbonate therapy remains controversial because of the risk of producing cerebral edema. Additional risks of unnecessary bicarbonate therapy include possible tissue hypoxia, paradoxical CNS acidosis, or further reduction of serum potassium or calcium levels. There is general agreement that bicarbonate is necessary in severe acidosis (pH <7.1) to prevent arrhythmia, confusion, stupor, or coma.[18] In cases of less severe acidosis, treatment with adequate fluids and insulin will improve the acidosis within 24 hours. It is preferable to administer bicarbonate by continuous infusion with a delivery concentration of 1 mEq/kg/hr. One to two mEq/kg may be safely administered over 1-2 hours before transport or en route. If more is given it is necessary to monitor the acid/base status on an hourly basis, which may be difficult during transport. When the acid/base status has improved (pH >7.20), the bicarbonate infusion is discontinued. In this situation adequate replacement of fluids and insulin will continue to reverse the acidotic state.

Clinical Presentation

The symptoms of DKA include polyuria and polyphagia. Polydipsia and weight loss are classic symptoms of insulin deficiency commonly present for 1-3 weeks. Fatigue, lethargy, hyperpnea, abdominal pain, and coma may result from ketoacidosis. Dehydration contributes to fever, weakness, and irritability in infants. Vaginal itching and candidiasis may be a presenting symptom. Hypoglycemia may be seen as an early sign in adults, but is rare in children.

The signs of DKA include dehydration manifested by dry buccal mucosa, tachycardia, weakness, and hypotension. Hyperpnea and a fruity odor on the breath are due to ketone production. Loss of subcutaneous tissue results from lipolysis. The diagnosis of DKA is made by the clinical signs and symptoms described above plus a confirming serum glucose above 140 mg/dl and ketonuria without another cause for ketones such as vomiting or dehydration.

In the differential diagnosis of DKA, one of the most common conditions to be considerd is viral gastritis, which may cause vomiting and small ketones but usually does not cause severe ketonuria or glucosuria. In diabetes insipidus, urine specific gravity is low (<1.010) with the absence of urinary ketones or glucose.

Stress, epinephrine, or steroids may produce hyperglycemia but usually not ketonuria. With fasting or dehydration, small ketones may be seen in the urine. In
Fanconi syndrome (renal tubular disease) proteinuria is found as well as glucosuria.

Treatment

Laboratory Tests

Initial laboratory examinations in patients with DKA include the following:
glucose; electrolytes; urine determination of ketones and glucose by dipstick in
the ER; venous pH or arterial blood gases; BUN; ketones; osmolality; calcium;
magnesium; and phosphate. In patients with possible cardiac or respiratory
compromise or severe dehydration, acidosis, or electrolyte abnormalities, electrolytes and pH may be required every 1-2 hours. However, routinely these studies
are obtained every four hours. A recent set of chemistries is desirable prior to
transport. Glucose is determined hourly either in the laboratory or at the bedside
by a glucose monitor. A lead II EKG strip should be monitored if patients have
severe acidosis or alterations of serum potassium or calcium. Accurate intake and
output (I&O) of fluids must be recorded. Patients presenting in shock require a
urinary bladder catheter to monitor output. Cultures of the blood, throat, or
urine are obtained in the emergency room if clinically indicated before antibiotic
therapy is given. A flow sheet is established to record the I&O, serum glucose,
electrolytes, pH, urine glucose, ketones, and insulin administration. The
patient's neurologic status should be assessed by the Glasgow coma score, at least
initially. The major cause of hyponatremia is total body sodium loss associated
with ketone diuresis. An additional apparent decrease in serum sodium is
produced by lipemia and glucosuria, which decrease the aqueous phase of the
blood. In hyperglycemia, the measured sodium is reduced 1.6 mEq/dl for every
100 mg/dl elevation of serum glucose above 200 mg/dl. In DKA, life-threatening
situations must be addressed promptly by the health care provider, as in any
critically ill patient. Management must be prioritized, with establishment of the
airway, breathing, and circulation (ABCs) given immediate attention.

Cerebral Edema

Altered sensorium in patients with DKA may be caused by either the
lethargy commonly associated with dehydration (intravascular volume depletion)
or by the much less common but more serious condition, cerebral edema,
beginning after treatment is instituted. Cerebral edema must be suspected
clinically if a patient develops rapidly changing lethargy, irritability, or altered
sensorium inappropriate for the degree of dehydration.[19,20] The index of
suspicion for cerebral edema is raised by a history of inappropriate large volumes
of fluid replacement in the first few hours (bolus with more than 40 ml/kg in
usual circumstances), the use of hypotonic saline (<0.45% NaCl), or with a rapid
drop (>100 mg/dl/hr) of glucose to below 250 mg/dl. If deteriorating Glasgow
coma scores or deepening coma are present, the patient may die.[19] Clinicians
appear to agree that euglycemia and rehydration should be performed cautiously
and in a controlled manner.[18] The transport team must be prudent when rehy-
drating the child with DKA. The situation is not analogous to treatment of a
patient with volume depletion due to blood loss because excessive or rapid
rehydration in a patient with DKA may contribute to the life-threatening
complication of cerebral edema.

If a child has fever in addition to shock, acidosis, and a clouded sensorium,
the differential diagnosis includes sepsis and meningoencephalitis. Physical

signs such as neck stiffening and irritability must be evaluated. In the patient who has severe cardiorespiratory compromise, a lumbar puncture may cause respiratory arrest by compromising the venous return to the heart or cerebral herniation if excess spinal fluid is withdrawn in the presence of cerebral edema. For these reasons antibiotics may be administered in the initial resuscitation and the lumbar puncture waived until the patient shows signs of cardiopulmonary stability. Antigenic evidence of the common bacterial infections and white blood cells in the CSF will allow a diagnosis of meningitis at a later hour.

In the patient with cerebral edema, mannitol (0.5–1 gm/kg IV) is given. If the child has progressive neurologic deterioration, is comatose, or has a Glasgow coma score <8, the patient should be intubated, both to prevent aspiration and to assist with hyperventilation in the treatment of cerebral edema. These patients benefit from a "pharmacologic cocktail" as an adjunct in endotracheal intubation. Barbiturates should be avoided because they may produce hypotension in an already hypovolemic and potentially hypotensive patient. To prevent cerebral compromise, the following drugs are given in rapid sequence for intubating the comatose child in DKA:

1. Atropine (0.02 mg/kg IV, minimum dose 0.1 mg)
2. Fentanyl (1–5 μg/kg IV) or lidocaine (1–2 mg/kg IV)
3. Pancuronium bromide (0.01 mg/kg IV defasciculating dose)
4. Succinylcholine (1 mg/kg IV)

Cardiac Dysrhythmias

Cardiac dysrhythmias are potentially life-threatening as a result of hyperkalemia, hypokalemia, or hypercalcemia in patients with DKA. Peaked T waves provide early evidence of intracellular hyperkalemia, and a lead II EKG strip provides a quick and reliable source for the diagnosis of this specific cardiac dysrhythmia. Therefore, patients in DKA should be placed on an EKG monitor throughout the transport if possible.

Pulmonary Edema or Aspiration

Patients in DKA may develop pulmonary edema diagnosed by increasing oxygen requirements and little or no radiographic changes. Possible causes of pulmonary edema include the following: low plasma oncotic pressure; increased pulmonary capillary permeability; myocardial failure; and a neurologic etiology. Infiltrates on a chest x-ray may suggest aspiration of gastric contents secondary to a decreased level of consciousness. To avoid prolonged acidosis and further tissue injury, adequate ventilation and oxygenation must be established and maintained.

Pretransport Treatment

Pretransport treatment of the patient with DKA begins with a thorough history of the signs and symptoms of DKA given above. Additionally the time of the last dose of insulin is recorded if the patient was previously on treatment. The presence of vomiting, fluid intake, viral illness or other infection, recent onset stress, overeating, or changes in exercise are noted.

The physical examination includes vital signs, mental status, weight, degree of dehydration, status of cardiopulmonary symptoms, and signs of infection. Cultures of blood, urine, and/or throat secretions if clinically indicated should be obtained before antibiotic therapy is started. A flowsheet is established for the I&O, serum glucose, electrolytes, urinary ketones, pH, and insulin administration. This flow sheet provides a continuous record for the health care providers from pretransport, during the transport, and after the transport care.

Zero to One Hour Management

An initial bolus of 20 ml/kg of 0.9% sodium chloride (NaCl) is given over 1 hour and repeated if necessary, determined by evidence of cardiovascular collapse by clinical criteria. Hypotonic fluids or repetitive unnecessary fluid boluses should be avoided to prevent the development of cerebral edema.[20] Vital signs, bedside glucose determinations, accurate I&O, and mental status (Glasgow coma score) should be obtained and recorded hourly. If hyperglycemia and ketosis have been documented, continuous intravenous infusion of regular insulin is established at a rate of 0.1 U/kg/hr (50 U reg insulin/250 ml 0.9% NaCl = 1 U/5 ml). An infusion rate of 0.1 U/kg/hr is necessary to improve the acidosis, resolve the ketosis, and slowly decrease the serum glucose by 50–100 mg/dl/hr. An initial bolus of intravenous insulin was standard treatment several years ago, but is no longer recommended because of resultant hypoglycemia. The serum glucose must be monitored hourly after insulin is given. When the glucose falls below 200–250 mg/dl, 5% dextrose should be added to the intravenous fluids while continuing with the insulin infusion. This is done to supply sufficient insulin to correct ketoacidosis and requires 12–36 hours of treatment. When the patient's serum glucose falls to less than 120–150 mg/dl, 10% dextrose is added to the intravenous fluids in order to continue the delivery of insulin at 0.1 U/kg/hr IV. On this treatment when the chemstrip falls below 100 mg/dl, usually in several hours, less insulin is then required. In that case D10 is continued but the insulin reduced to approximately 0.05 U/kg/hr. Usually the rapid decrease in glucose occurs only after many hours of treatment; rarely, it may occur suddenly if the patient has endogenous insulin release.

HYPEROSMOLAR HYPERGLYCEMIC NONKETOTIC COMA

Hyperosmolar hyperglycemic nonketotic coma (HHNC) occurs much more commonly in the elderly[21] than in the pediatric population.[22] It may mimic DKA by clinical manifestations including hyperglycemia, dehydration, hyperosmolality, and decreased sensorium, but in HHNC there is an absence of ketosis or acidosis. Causes of HHNC include infection, trauma, exogenous steroids, catecholamines, hyperalimentation, anticonvulsants (phenytoin), and thiazide diuretics. In adults the reported mortality is 40–60%.

Patients in HHNC frequently present in severe shock; fluid replacement is the primary basis of treatment. Isotonic fluids should be infused immediately (20 ml/kg) and repeated as needed to reverse the shock. Once shock has been reversed, intravenous fluids are changed to 0.45% NaCl + 20 mEq/L KCl (or as needed) without added glucose, at a rate of maintenance plus output (ongoing losses) to cautiously correct the hyperosmolar state. Insulin is administered at a much lower dose than in DKA because without acidosis the serum glucose levels may decrease precipitously. Continuous intravenous infusion of regular insulin is started at 0.03–0.05 U/kg/hr (one-third to one-half used in DKA). When the blood glucose falls below 250 mg/gl (which may occur during the transport), the insulin infusion rate must be decreased. If the glucose continues to fall, the administration of insulin should be discontinued.

ADRENAL INSUFFICIENCY/ADDISON'S DISEASE

In children adrenal failure may present as an acute life-threatening event such as shock or seizures.[23] On the other hand, adrenal insufficiency may present as a nonspecific state of malaise, weakness, weight loss, headache, or vomiting, where an adrenal etiology is not suspected, leading to a delay in diagnosis. It is unusual to make a primary diagnosis of adrenal insufficiency before transport.

However, the critically ill child with multiple organ failure is at risk of adrenal insufficiency, and glucocorticoids are frequently included in the emergency management prior to transport of these patients.

Pathophysiology

Glucocorticoids prevent hypotension; they exert a permissive action on catecholamines. Another major effect of glucocorticoids is to prevent hypoglycemia by increasing gluconeogenesis, decreasing glucose transport across the cell membrane, and decreasing the peripheral utilization of glucose.[24] Glucocorticoids counter the effect of insulin at several intracellular enzymatic sites of glucose utilization, which may explain their effectiveness in cases of hypoglycemia due to hyperinsulinism in the neonate. Aldosterone maintains the extracellular volume and electrolyte balance by promoting retention of sodium and water and excretion of potassium and hydrogen ions in the renal tubule by activation of the sodium-potassium ATPase pump. Because severe derangement of potassium or sodium may be life-threatening, it is evident that the transport team members must consider adrenal failure in the management of critically ill pediatric patients.

Hypothalamic corticotropin-releasing factor (CRF) stimulates the synthesis and release of pituitary adrenocorticotropic hormone (ACTH). Adrenal production of cortisone and aldosterone is induced by ACTH. Renin produced by the kidney stimulates the conversion of angiotensinogen to angiotensin-converting enzyme (ACE), which in turn converts angiotensin I to angiotensin II. Angiotensin II then promotes aldosterone secretion, which also is stimulated by potassium and ACTH. Aldosterone causes sodium retention and potassium excretion in the distal renal tubule.

Adrenal failure in the neonate may be caused by congenital virilizing adrenal hyperplasia (CVAH), an error in biosynthesis of cortisol and aldosterone.[25] Classically, salt-losing CVAH presents in the newborn at 7–10 days of age (1–3 weeks) as a critically ill infant in shock with vomiting, diarrhea, severely elevated serum potassium, and hyponatremia. The most common form is 21-hydroxylase deficiency; the female infant has ambiguous genitalia (female pseudohermaphrodite or virilized female) characterized by enlarged clitoris (phallus) and labial fusion. A rare autosomal recessive condition, CVAH has an incidence of 1:15,000. In 21-hydroxylase deficiency there is an elevated 17-hydroxyprogesterone (17-OHP), androstenedione (A), and testosterone (T), although one may not find a low serum cortisol in this condition. To treat the infant with CVAH in shock, fluids, sodium chloride, and glucose are required. Potassium must not be administered in the fluids since life-threatening hyperkalemia may result. At least half of the patients are salt losers requiring mineralocorticoid (9α-fluorocortisol) treatment.

The second most common form of CVAH is 11-hydroxylase deficiency, which occurs in approximately 10% of the cases and may present with hypertension in infancy or, more commonly, in later childhood. In this condition the hypertension is caused by elevated levels of deoxycorticosterone (DOC) or other adrenal steroids. It is diagnosed by an elevated ratio of DOC:aldosterone or elevated ratio of deoxycortisol:cortisol. It also produces an elevated 17-OHP and may be diagnosed on neonatal screening or identified by the physical appearance of virilization in the genitalia of the female newborn including labial fusion and possibly clitoromegaly (female pseudohermaphrodite). This diagnosis must be considered in the differential of hypertension and requires treatment with glucocorticoids.

A third form of adrenal hyperplasia, most often fatal although rare mild cases may survive, is 3 β-ol dehydrogenase deficiency. These patients may present with shock, elevated potassium, hyponatremia, and hypoglycemia. The male is undervirilized. This defect requires treatment as in the complete salt-dosing form of CVAH. Other defects in adrenal steroidogenesis that may produce life-threatening hypoglycemia, seizures, and shock in the critically ill child include adrenal lipoid hyperplasia, 20-22 desmolase deficiency, or adrenal hypoplasia. In these cases all of the adrenal steroids may be low, and the condition therefore would not be diagnosed by an elevated 17-OHP on the newborn state screen. Therefore, these forms of congenital adrenal failure must be considered in the emergency management of hypoglycemia and shock in the critically ill infant.

Clinical Manifestations

Adrenal failure may present with symptoms of glucocorticoid and/or mineralocorticoid deficiency. Common manifestations of adrenal insufficiency are listed in Table 2. Adrenal failure should be suspected in the patient with cardiovascular collapse that is unresponsive to fluids and inotropic support. Arrhythmias secondary to hyperkalemia may not respond to resuscitative efforts. Additional life-threatening complications of adrenal insufficiency may include profound hypoglycemia, which may cause seizures, aspiration, hypoxia due to airway compromise, severe metabolic acidosis, intractable seizures and encephalopathy, and death.[24]

Adrenal insufficiency (Table 3) must be considered in the differential diagnosis of a patient with suspected congenital heart disease or septic shock. Confirmation of the diagnosis of adrenal insufficiency requires obtaining a serum cortisol before starting steroid treatment in the critically ill patient. Cortisol data can be obtained on only a few drops of serum. Without the pretreatment specimen, the diagnosis may be masked by aggressive therapeutic intervention.

Adrenal insufficiency may cause a variety of clinical manifestations. Sudden death has been reported.[24] Patients may have psychosis, confusion, or apathy due to glucocorticoid deficiency. Abdominal pain, nausea, vomiting, and diarrhea are also commonly found.

The clinician must consider CVAH in the differential diagnosis of pyloric stenosis. The diagnosis of CVAH can be made by an earlier onset of vomiting and by hyponatremia, hyperkalemia, hypoglycemia, and metabolic acidosis. In contrast, the infant with pyloric stenosis is older (6–10 weeks) and has a normal serum sodium with metabolic alkalosis secondary to chloride loss from emesis.

Additionally, CVAH must be considered in the differential diagnosis of trauma, inborn errors of metabolism, sepsis, and congenital heart disease.

Treatment

It is important for the medical team to initiate fluid, electrolyte, and glucose replacement in cases of adrenal failure immediately after the patient arrives at the medical center in order to stabilize the hemodynamic and metabolic state.

Prior to treatment blood should be drawn for diagnostic tests, including cortisol, adrenocorticotropic hormone, serum electrolytes, and glucose, in addition to complete blood count and blood cultures.

TABLE 2. Signs of Adrenal Insufficiency

Hyperkalemia	Vomiting
Hyponatremia	Weight Loss
Hypoglycemia	Hypotension
Weakness	Hyperpigmentation

TABLE 3.   Etiology of Adrenal Failure

Congenital virilizing adrenal hyperplasia
Hemorrhage (Waterhouse-Friderichsen syndrome, meningococcemia)
Secondary to hypopituitarism (low adrenocorticotropic hormone)
Infection or infiltrative lesions of the adrenals (tuberculosis)
Resistance to adrenocorticotropic hormone (autosomal recessive inheritance)
Adrenal leukodystrophy
Congenital absence of the adrenals
Autoimmune Addison disease (in older children)
X-linked genetic forms
Associated with anticoagulant therapy
Withdrawal from prolonged (>1 month) administration of pharmacologic doses of glucocorticoids

In a critically ill child parenteral hydrocortisone in stress doses (75–100 mg/m^2) should be administered. Because cortisone has approximately 1/200 mineralocorticoid activity, these stress doses will provide some degree of aldosterone activity. However, in the newborn with CVAH, much larger doses of mineralocorticoid (9α-fluorocortisol, 0.1–0.2 mg daily) may be required; potassium is contraindicated. Dexamethasone, in doses commonly used, has little mineralocorticoid activity; glucose and normal saline are required in the intravenous fluids. The preferable intravenous solution is D10W/0.9% NaCl at 1.5 × maintenance. This will stabilize a patient's electrolytes and allow the serum 17-OHP to be obtained before administration of cortisone.

After transport and stabilization of the patient's condition, therapy is continued with glucocorticoids, mineralocorticoids, and additional sodium replacement as indicated after evaluation by a pediatric endocrinologist. The dose of cortisone required by patients is 10–15 mg/m^2 administered twice daily, in contrast to patients with CVAH requiring suppression of their pituitary ACTH, with 15–30 mg/m^2 cortisone administered every 8–12 hours. Patients with CVAH often require added sodium on a daily basis in addition to 9α-fluorocortisol.

THYROID DISEASES

Hyperthyroidism

Hyperthyroidism may present in the emergency setting with signs of hypertension, tachycardia, or headache.[26] Thyroid storm is a rare metabolic complication of hyperthyroidism and shock, often resulting in multisystem failure. This condition has a high mortality and requires aggressive treatment.[27]

Pathophysiology

Hyperthyroidism (Graves' disease) is an autoimmune disorder in which thyroid-stimulating immunoglobulin stimulates the thyroid gland to produce thyroxine.

Thyrotrophic-releasing hormone (TRH) is produced in the hypothalamus and travels down the pituitary stalk to stimulate the production and release of thyroid-stimulating hormone (TSH) in the anterior pituitary. Circulating TSH stimulates the thyroid gland to produce thyroxine (T$_4$) and triiodothyronine (T$_3$). T$_4$ is converted to T$_3$, which is the active form. The thyroid enlarges in the face of increased TSH production or environmental iodide deficiency. The action of thyroid hormone has a wide range of effects, maintaining heart rate, blood pressure, and metabolism in various tissues of the body. The normal range of T$_4$

in the neonate is 7–20 μg/dl, in contrast to a normal range of approximately 5–12 μg/dl in the older child. A surge of TSH occurs on the first day of life. Therefore, values obtained at this time should be interpreted with caution and repeated. In the sick infant, reverse T_3, which is inactive, is produced. Over 99% of T_3 and T_4 is protein-bound. Free T_4 is a more physiologic test than total T_4 and should be obtained whenever possible. The level of free thyroid hormone is not dependent on the concentration of thyroid-binding globulin in the serum. Normally, there is feedback inhibition of TSH production by circulating thyroid hormones.

Thyroid hormone causes an increase in chronotropic and inotropic effects without a concomitant increase in oxygen consumption. Thyroxine increases adrenergic receptor sites in myocardial cells. The hemodynamic and myocardial stimulation effects of T_4 can be reversed by beta-adrenergic blockade. Thyroid hormone is necessary for many metabolic activities, including growth, gonadal function, pituitary growth hormone secretion, and normal hypoxic and hypercapnic drives.

Clinical Presentation

Clinical signs of hyperthyroidism are due to hypermetabolism from excessive autonomic activity. Symptoms include tachycadia, nervousness, increased pulse pressure, increased appetite, proptosis, tremors, weight loss, and heat intolerance. Less frequently, dysrhythmias, psychosis, congestive heart failure, shock, coma, and seizures may be present.

Patients in thyroid storm present with confusion, lethargy, weakness, diaphoresis, cutaneous flushing, fever, and extreme tachycardia. Nausea, vomiting, hepatomegaly, and jaundice may be present in severe cases. If the patients are not treated promptly, symptoms may progress to extreme hyperpyrexia and coma. An altered mental status and tachycardia are present out of proportion to the fever. Thyroid storm must be considered in the differential diagnosis of the following conditions: anticholinergic poisoning; transfusion reactions; malignant hyperthermia; adrenal crisis; sepsis; anxiety, and drug ingestions. In some laboratories, a T_4 determination may be available in a few hours. If this is not the case, the transport team and the medical team at the referring institution must make a clinical diagnosis based on the history, signs, and symptoms. Emergency treatment may be required before the confirming laboratory tests of thyroid function are available. Of course, it is important to obtain the diagnostic specimens before treatment begins.

Pretransport Management of Thyroid Storm

Patients in thyrotoxic crisis with major organ system dysfunction need to be stabilized and to achieve a euthyroid state as soon as possible.[27] As with all life-threatening illnesses, the airway, breathing, and circulation (ABCs) must be given first attention; supplemental oxygen should be provided. Most children will maintain intact airway reflexes and not require endotracheal intubation. Vascular access should be secured with two large-bore intravenous catheters and hypovolemia corrected rapidly with 20 ml/kg of crystalloid solution. This may be administered as often as necessary to treat the hypovolemia. Serum glucose should be determined immediately at the bedside, to detect hypoglycemia, and dextrose included in the maintenance intravenous solution. Nonaspirin antipyretics should be administered for fever, because aspirin displaces thyroid hormone and may increase free thyroxine levels. External cooling methods also should be applied when necessary. If the patient has severe tachycardia prior to transport, propranolol (0.01 mg/kg) may be administered by slow intravenous push every 10 minutes until the patient's hemodynamic state has improved or until a total of 5 mg has been administered. Propranolol must be administered cautiously in patients with a history of severe reactive airway disease since beta-blockers may exacerbate an underlying respiratory condition. In order to limit continued release of T_4, propylthiouracil (PTU) (200 mg every 4 hours by naso-gastric tube) is administered. Also Lugol's solution of potassium iodide (5 drops every 8 hours) or sodium iodide (NaI; 250 mg/day over 24 hours with IV fluids) may be used. Stress doses of steroids used to treat hypotension (dexamethasone, 0.1 mg/kg) also inhibit the peripheral conversion of T_4 to T_3, as does propranolol (10-20 mg every 8 hours). If patients suffer symptomatic bradycardia secondary to beta-blocker administration, atropine and isoproterenol should be administered.

Neonatal thyrotoxicosis presents with goiter, crying, irritability, tachycardia, jitteriness, or diarrhea. The newborn with Graves' disease may become progressively more symptomatic during the first day, as propranolol or methimazole transferred from the placenta is cleared from the circulation. In the neonate, hyperthyroidism is treated with PTU with the dose adjusted for the child's weight and with propranolol if significant tachycardia is present.

The medical team must consider neonatal hyperthyroidism in the differential diagnosis of the following conditions: congenital and acquired infections; congenital heart disease; or drug withdrawal in the infant of a drug-abusing mother.

Chronic treatment of hyperthyroidism in children is more often undertaken by medication (PTU or methimazole). However, in the patient in whom this is not effective because of noncompliance, allergy to the medication, or some other reason, alternative treatments include surgery or radioactive iodine (RAI). RAI is an acceptable form of treatment, although it must not be used in patients who may be pregnant. Surgery must be done after the hyperthyroidism is adequately suppressed with iodides or propylthiouracil. An experienced thyroid surgeon is needed to prevent possible iatrogenic hypoparathyroidism or laryngeal nerve paralysis.

Clinical Presentation of Hypothyroidism

Neonatal hypothyroidism requires prompt consultation with a pediatric endocrinologist and treatment with T_4 to prevent mental retardation,[28] although it does not usually require emergency transport. Signs of hypothyroidism in the infant are given in Table 4.

Myxedema is seen most frequently in adults.[27] Patients present in a hypometabolic state with hypothermia, constipation, sluggishness, and bradycardia. More severe signs are coma, congestive heart failure, tachycardia, and pericardial effusion. Myxedema may be precipitated in the patient with hypothyroidism by a variety of metabolic stress conditions, such as anesthesia, surgery, severe cold exposure, intracerebral or gastrointestinal bleeding, and the use of sedatives or narcotics. The skin is characteristically cool, coarse, dry, thick, or doughy with a yellow or orange tint (carotenemia). Periorbital edema and dry brittle hair also may be present. Upper airway obstruction leading to respiratory compromise may be caused by macroglossia.

TABLE 4.   Signs of Hypothyroidism in Infancy

Large fontanelle	Distended abdomen
Macroglossia	Hypotonia
Hoarse cry	Lethargy
Prolonged neonatal jaundice	Feeding problems
Umbilical hernia	Hypothermia

If a pericardial effusion is present, patients will have muffled heart sounds, decreased intensity of the point of maximal impulse, and cardiomegaly. Rarely, they may have pericardial tamponade. Other clinical manifestations include an ileus or pseudoobstruction with decreased bowel sounds and abdominal distention.

Treatment of Patients with Myxedema

Treatment of patients with myxedema must address the life-threatening emergencies, metabolic complications, and infection. Establishment of the ABCs is primary. Severe hypothermia is best treated with passive rather than active rewarming. Active rewarming may cause rapid peripheral vasodilatation and worsen preexisting shock. Because inappropriate antidiuretic hormone secretion (SIADH) may be present, fluid restriction is indicated for hyponatremia. The patient with a serum sodium below 120 mEq/L is at risk for seizures, although the seizures are caused more by a rapid decrease in sodium than at a threshold of steady-state concentration. First priority is given to immediate correction of the hypoglycemia, hyponatremia, and hypoxia. Subsequently, if seizures occur and are not controlled by correction of serum Na, they may require treatment with a standard anticonvulsant. Identification of infections may be difficult in patients with myxedema because classic signs of fever, sweating, or leukocytosis may be absent.[27]

For myxedema, emergency intubation and assisted ventilation must be provided if patients have hypercapnia, hypoxia, or decreased airway reflexes. Aggressive fluid and inotropic support should be instituted if hypotension is present. Dopamine is the preferred inotropic agent in order to maintain renal and coronary blood flow. Because patients with myxedema may have Addison's disease in addition to the hypothyroidism, stress doses of glucocorticoids (100 mg/m^2/day) in four divided doses should be administered with the initial management after obtaining a serum cortisol and ACTH. An increased incidence of hypothyroidism is present with other autoimmune disorders, multiple endocrinopathies, Down syndrome, or diabetes mellitus.

The presumptive diagnosis and initial treatment of hypothyroidism must be based on a clinical judgment, since laboratory confirmation is not available on an emergency basis in most institutions. These patients may require emergency treatment to prevent mortality.

PHEOCHROMOCYTOMA OR ENDOCRINE HYPERTENSION

In children with severe unexplained hypertension, hypertensive encephalopathy, or cardiac failure, a diagnosis of pheochromocytoma should be considered. This is a rare tumor that secretes catecholamines.

Pathophysiology

Children with pheochromocytoma secrete primarily norepinephrine and epinephrine. The peak incidence is between 9 and 12 years of age, and the malignancy rate is 2–10%. The tumor is usually located within the adrenal medulla, but may be found elsewhere in the body.[29] The diagnosis is based on elevated plasma catecholamines or an elevated 24-hour urine catecholamine, metanephrine, or vanilmandelic acid (VMA). In preparation before surgery, phenoxybenzamine (Dibenzyline) is used for 10–14 days and, in some cases, propranolol. If surgery is not possible or effective, the condition may be treated medically by blocking cathecholamine synthesis with alpha-methyl tyrosine. Tyrosine is converted in neurons to L-Dopa, dopamine, norepinephrine, and epinephrine.

Clinical Presentation

Children usually present with sustained rather than intermittent symptoms of hypertension, headaches, sweating, nausea, vomiting, visual disturbance, and weight loss. Polydipsia, abdominal pain, tachycardia, and tremors also may be present. These patients have volume depletion, polycythemia, and an elevated hematocrit.

Pheochromocytoma must be considered in the differential diagnosis of other conditions, including the following: diabetes; hyperthyroidism; heart disease; polycystic renal disease; renal vascular hypertension; MEN syndromes II and III; and neurofibromatosis.

In the patient with severe hypertension, other endocrine causes that must be considered include the following: hyperthyroidism; Cushing syndrome; primary hyperaldosteronism; 11-beta hydroxylase deficiency (adrenal hyperplasia); use of anabolic steroids; glucocorticoids; or hypercalcemia.

Treatment

The transport team must be prepared to treat uncontrolled hypertension with sodium nitroprusside infusion at a low dose (0.25–1.0 μg/kg/min), with continuous cardiac and hemodynamic monitoring. If the patient develops tachydysrhythmias, lidocaine (1–2 mg/kg IV bolus in a continuous infusion at 20–80 μg/kg/min) is the treatment of choice. If control is not achieved, then intravenous propranolol (0.01–0.1 mg/kg IV slowly; maximum of 1 mg per dose) or esmolol (0.3–0.5 mg/kg over 5 minutes and an infusion of 0.025–0.1 mg/kg/min titrated to desired effect) should be considered. If the patient develops hypotension, a fluid bolus (20 ml/kg) should be administered as necessary.

The goal is to achieve a decrease in systemic pressure of no greater than 20–40 mmHg in the acute treatment of chronic hypertension and pheochromocytoma. The purpose of this is to prevent low perfusion pressure, since with chronic hypertension there is an upward shift in the lower limit of the autoregulatory curve, especially for cerebral blood flow.[30]

Treatment is then directed to control the hypertension for approximately 10 days with Dibenzyline and, if needed, propranolol in preparation for surgery.

HYPOCALCEMIA AND HYPOPARATHYROIDISM

Hypocalcemia is a common cause of seizures and tetany in the critically ill patient. In addition to maintaining central nervous system homeostasis, calcium is extremely important for modulation of heart rate changes and myocardial contractility.

The treatment team must be aware of the difference between total and ionized calcium. Because calcium is bound to albumin and other serum proteins, the total serum calcium level depends on the serum concentration of proteins. Measurement of ionized calcium rather than total serum calcium should be employed whenever possible because it is more meaningful physiologically.

Physiology

Calcium is necessary for central nervous system homeostasis, for myocardial contractility, and for regulation of heart rate. Intracellular calcium modulates many metabolic processes through activation of cyclic adenosine monophosphate (cAMP), a second messenger for many hormones.

The serum concentration of calcium is maintained by the renal resorption of calcium, linked to the excretion of phosphate, by the gastrointestinal absorption of calcium, and by resorption from bone, all under the control of calcitriol. Calcitonin may rapidly lower the serum calcium by promoting deposition in bone tissue.

Vitamin D (D) is formed from cholesterol by the action of ultraviolet light and 25-hydroxylation in the liver. It is subsequently 1-hydroxylated in the renal tubule to 1,25 dihydroxy D under the influence of parathyroid hormone (PTH). PTH also directly promotes renal phosphate excretion. In illness or malnutrition, the inactive form 24,25 (OH) to D is produced. Low serum calcium or phosphate levels stimulate 1-hydroxylation in the kidney.

Clinical Presentation

It is not uncommon for critically ill patients to have mild hypocalcemia without clinical manifestations.[31] Neuromuscular and cardiovascular signs are listed in Table 5. Irritability, twitching, hyperreflexia, muscle spasms, tetany, or seizures are common signs of hypocalcemia. Chvostek's sign is a lower facial spasm induced by tapping over the facial nerve. Other pathologic states induced by hypocalcemia may include bradycardia and hypotension due to decreased contraction of smooth muscle in the vasculature. Ineffective digitalization, prolonged curarization, urinary retention, papilledema, or infantile apnea also may be seen. Laryngospasm may be recognized by stridor, a crowing sound.

Common causes of hypocalcemia include deficiency of vitamin D, decreased intake of calcium, sudden release of calcitonin, or hypoparathyroidism (Table 6). More than one clinical condition may be causing hypocalcemia in the critically ill patient.[33] Patients presenting with hyperventilation-induced respiratory alkalosis may have tetany on the basis of a decreased ionized calcium.

Rapid infusion of concentrated albumin solutions, citrated blood, bicarbonate, or the use of phosphate enema solutions can transiently lower the ionized calcium level;[34] calcium binding to albumin is modulated by pH. Alkalosis increases calcium binding to proteins; acidosis decreases calcium binding.

In the neonate, hypocalcemia may present with seizures, jitteriness, apnea, prolonged QT interval, or myocardial dysfunction. Early neonatal hypocalcemia may be associated with prematurity, asphyxia, or prolonged labor or may be seen in infants of mothers with insulin-dependent diabetes (IDM). In later-onset neonatal hypocalcemia, occurring after one week of age, the etiology may be decreased intake of formula, transient hypoparathyroidism, exaggerated release of intracellular phosphate from cell destruction, increased phosphate content of cow's milk, calcitonin release precipitated by stress or asphyxia, bicarbonate or citrate administration, or renal resistance to vitamin D.

TABLE 5.   Clinical Features of Hypocalcemia

Neuromuscular	Cardiovascular	Respiratory
Increased neuronal irritability	Hypotension	Laryngeal spasm
Tetany	Bradycardia	Bronchospasm
Chvostek or Trousseau signs	Asystole	
Hyperreflexia	Dysrhythmia	
Paresthesia	Impaired cardiac contractility	
Weakness	EKG abnormalities	
Seizures	QT and ST prolongation	
Muscle spasms	Decreased catecholamine response	
	Decreased digitalis response	

Adapted from Jaimovich D: Endocrine and metabolic disorders. In McKloskey K, Orr R (eds): Textbook of Neonatal and Pediatric Transport Medicine. Philadelphia, Mosby, 1995.

TABLE 6. Etiology of Hypocalcemia

Parathyroid Hormone Insufficiency	Calcitriol Insufficiency	Losses
Idiopathic hypoparathyroidism	Vitamin D deficiency	Hyperphosphatemia
Autoimmune	(inadequte intake)	Citrate infusion
DiGeorge syndrome	Malabsorption of vitamin D	Tumor lysis syndrome
Acquired	Lack of sunlight	Toxic shock syndrome
Surgery (s/p thyroidectomy)	Advanced hepatic disease	Diffuse muscle necrosis
Trauma	Hypoparathyroidism	Drug toxicity
Sepsis	Pseudohypoparathyroidism	Ethylene glycol
Burns	Advanced renal disease	Sodium sulfate
Hypomagnesemia	Nephrotic syndrome	EDTA
Drugs	Vitamin D dependency	Sodium fluoride
Adrenergic blockers	(renal resistance)	Bone sequestration
Cimetidine		Cisplatin
Aminoglycosides		Mithramycin
		Calcitonin (stress or thyroid tumor)

Hypocalcemia in IDM may be caused by prematurity, asphyxia, limited calcium or vitamin D transfer from the mother, increased phosphate intake with cow's milk formula, decreased renal ability to excrete phosphate, elevated serum citrate levels after exchange blood transfusion, administration of furosemide, or decreased calcium levels due to hypoproteinemia.[35]

Rickets of prematurity affects 30% of premature infants.[36] Diagnostic findings include x-ray evidence of osteomalacia or osteoporosis, with a normal serum calcium, phosphorus, and alkaline phosphatase. Risk factors for this condition may include low-birthweight infants (less than 1000 gm) causing deficient body stores of calcium and phosphorus, chronically ill premature infants, total parenteral nutrition with inadequate mineral supplementation, human milk without added vitamin or mineral supplements, bronchopulmonary dysplasia, fluid restriction, decreased intake of formula, or treatment with furosemide, causing urinary losses of calcium and phosphorus.

Treatment

In the patient with seizures, tetany, or other signs of hypocalcemia, the transport team should obtain a serum sample for calcium levels (preferably ionized), magnesium, phosphate, PTH, and calcitriol for specific diagnostic testing. The patient with a serum calcium <7 mg/dl (ionized <2.8 mg/dl), neuromuscular signs, or cardiovascular collapse should have prompt treatment. In patients with hyperphosphatemia, the preferred method of treatment is to lower the serum phosphate to allow an improvement of hypocalcemia.[37] If patients have clinically significant hypomagnesemia (less than 1 mg/dl) treatment with magnesium should be undertaken.[38] In some cases, correction of the magnesium deficiency may correct the hypocalcemia.

If the patient is symptomatic, administration of calcium is a medical emergency. Intravenous calcium chloride (20–30 mg/kg/dose in a 10% solution) should be infused slowly; rapid administration may result in life-threatening arrhythmias, bradycardia, and asystole. The patient must be on a cardiac monitor and resuscitative drugs (atropine) kept readily available. Calcium chloride or other calcium salts should be diluted in dextrose water or normal saline prior to administration. A large-bore vein, central venous line, or IO line should be used, if possible, as extreme care must be taken if a peripheral intravenous line is used to avoid extravasation. Calcium is very irritating to tissues; extravasation may cause sclerosis and sloughing of skin from tissue damage.

HYPERCALCEMIA

Hypercalcemia is infrequently encountered in critically ill pediatric patients. Patients with a calcium level over 13 mg/dl may present with malaise, anorexia, polyuria, lethargy, and failure to thrive. Dehydration may be associated with deteriorating renal function if the hypercalcemia is severe (>14–15 mg/dl). Hyperparathyroidism is rare in children. A large number of medications or metabolic abnormalities may be associated with hypercalcemia in children,[35] including: (1) hyperparathyroidism; (2) immobilization; (3) thiazide diuretics; (4) excessive vitamin D intake; (5) benign familial hypocalciuric hypercalcemia; (6) idiopathic infantile hypercalcemia (William syndrome); and (7) renal tubular defects.

Hypercalcemia must be considered in the differential diagnosis of hypertension. Approximately 20% of children with hypercalcemia have elevated blood pressure. Serum calcium concentrations of 13–15 mg/dl may cause nausea and malaise, but are generally not life-threatening.

Volume expansion with isotonic saline at twice maintenance volume is the first measure in the therapeutic regimen of hypercalcemia. This corrects water and sodium depletion, expanding intracellular volume and, thereby, diluting extracellular fluid calcium and increasing excretion of calcium in the urine. Normal saline solution (10–20 ml/kg/hr) is followed by a loop diuretic such as furosemide (1 mg/kg/dose, 1–4 times daily) to produce a brisk excretion of calcium in the urine. In most cases, these treatments will be effective in the emergency correction of hypercalcemia in childhood. If patients with severe hypercalcemia also have hypokalemia or hypomagnesemia, replacement of potassium or magnesium should be undertaken to prevent worsening of those conditions by volume expansion.

Patients with immobilization, especially if accompanied by decreased renal function or dehydration, may have a sudden increase in serum calcium level. This is treated with restoration of fluid volume on an acute basis, with glucocorticoids (hydrocortisone, 10 mg/kg/day) to decrease the gastrointestinal absorption of calcium after several days, and with rapid weight-bearing and mobilization to prevent ongoing resorption of calcium from the bone.

The therapeutic interventions must be considered only temporizing measures and a primary diagnosis pursued to institute a specific treatment for the underlying cause of hypercalcemia.

PHOSPHATE

In the critically ill child, phosphate metabolism is essential for many biologic functions, including the oxygen-carrying capacity of hemoglobin and diaphragmatic and cardiac muscle function. In the child, the normal range of serum phosphate concentration is 4.0–7.1 mg/dl, although serum phosphate concentration is not reliable as a guide to total body phosphate stores, since the majority of phosphate is intracellular.

Pathophysiology

Several metabolic effects of phosphate may be of critical importance in acutely ill children. Phosphate is essential in the composition of 2,3DPG, which is necessary for modulation of oxygen hemoglobin dissociation and provision of oxygenation in tissues.[16] Phosphate is a constituent of nucleic acids, nucleic proteins, and cell membrane phospholipids and is necessary for cell membrane integrity. It plays an integral part in both neurologic function and in skeletal muscle, diaphragmatic, and cardiac muscle function. Severe hypophosphatemia, therefore, may clinically compromise the critically ill patient. Hyperphosphatemia leads to hypocalcemia and associated symptoms, such as seizures. Phosphate concentrations >10 mg/dl may be associated with an ionized calcium <1.5 mEq/L. The clinical signs of hypocalcemia in this case may include prolonged QT intervals, tetany, or seizures.

The serum phosphate concentration is altered by various physiologic events, including acid-base regulation of transcellular shifts of phosphate, dietary intake, renal losses, carbohydrate or fat ingestion, and the effects of exercise.

Hypophosphatemia may result from reduced intake, increased excretion, or shifts from extracellular to intracellular fluid spaces.

Clinical entities associated with hypophosphatemia include diabetic ketoacidosis, metabolic acidosis, heavy metal poisoning, hypocalcemia, paint or glue sniffing, renal tubular disorders, or Reye syndrome. Correction of a low cardiac output by saline infusion and/or inotropic agents may result in increased urine losses of phosphate due to an increased glomerular filtration rate. Hypophosphatemia may be due to increased losses in chronic gastrointestinal dysfunction, including emesis, diarrhea, or malabsorption associated with malnutrition.

The clinical complications which may result from low serum phosphate include phagocytosis, increased platelet and red blood cell destruction from rhabdomyolysis, liver failure, muscualr weakness, respiratory failure, sinus node dysfunction, or depressed myocardial function.

Treatment

Even in the presence of complications, the treatment of hypophosphatemia is undertaken with a slow infusion over 4-12 hours rather than at a rapid rate. Ideally, treatment begins at the referring institution or during transport. Only severe hypophosphatemia (<1 mg/dl) requires emergency intravenous treatment. If the serum phosphate level is between 0.5 and 1 mg/dl, diaphragmatic contractility may be depressed, with resultant respiratory distress or failure. Suggested treatment is 0.1-0.4 mEq/kg of phosphate, administered over a 4-12-hour intravenous rate.

If the patient presents with a serum phosphorus concentration below 0.5 mg/dl, more aggressive treatment should be administered with 0.2-0.9 mEq/kg phosphate over a 4-12-hour rate. The patient must be cautiously monitored by both clinical and laboratory criteria because acute treatment with phosphate may result in hypocalcemia, hypomagnesemia, hyperphosphatemia, hypotension, and acute renal failure. Treatment should begin at a dose in the lower recommended range, especially in the presence of hypocalcemia or renal failure. If the patient has severe hypocalcemia, phosphorus replacement should not be undertaken until the serum calcium has been corrected.

Clinical Presentation of Hyperphosphatemia

Hyperphosphatemia may be a diagnostic sign of hypoparathyroidism, or it may be due to inadequate excretion, excessive intake, or shifts from the extracellular to the intracellular fluid space. Inadequate excretion due to a decrease in glomerular filtration rate may be seen in patients with severe volume depletion, renal failure, or myocardial failure. Excessive intake may be seen in the child on high doses of vitamin D, with phosphate enemas, or with oral phosphate supplementation. Other causes of hyperphosphatemia include cytotoxic therapy and tumor lysis syndrome in the treatment of acute lymphoblastic leukemia[39] and Burkitt lymphoma.[40] In lactic acidosis and hypoperfusion secondary to shock, hyperphosphatemia may be seen due to shifts from intracellular to extracellular fluid space.[41] Spurious hyperphosphatemia due to lysis of red blood cells may result from blood-drawing. Iatrogenic hyperphosphatemia may result from excessive intravenous phosphorus replacement,[42] or oral or rectal phosphate-containing solutions prescribed as laxatives.[43]

Treatment

Restitution of the plasma volume with normal saline (20 ml/kg) may partially treat the hyperphosphatemia. If patients have symptomatic hypocalcemia, calcium chloride (10% solution), 20–30 mg/kg/dose IV slowly, should be administered. Antacid solutions containing aluminum hydroxide (1 mg/kg) may be administered by a nasogastric tube in an effort to bind phosphate; however, this process may take many hours.

HYPOMAGNESEMIA

Magnesium is an intracellular cation that is important as a cofactor for ATP in many enzymatic processes. Hypomagnesemia is suspected if a child has signs of hypocalcemia that do not respond to treatment with calcium. In this clinical situation, the hypomagnesemia may cause decreased PTH release; the low magnesium must be treated before serum calcium returns to normal. The normal range of total plasma magnesium concentration is 1.6–2.8 mg/dl, the majority of which is protein-bound. The patient with hypomagnesemia may require treatment if the serum level is <1 mg/dl.

Pathophysiology

A major portion of the plasma magnesium (65–85%) is bound to proteins. The extracellular magnesium, however, accounts for only 1% of the total body content, the majority of which is bound to tissues (bone 50%, muscle 25%, and other soft tissues).

Magnesium plays a role as a cofactor for ATP in the activation of many intracellular enzymes; it is essential for cell membrane functions, for mitochondrial function, and for the synthesis of both protein and DNA. The serum level of magnesium is controlled by PTH and calcitonin in a manner similar manner to that of calcium; stress due to asphyxia may cause calcitonin release and neonatal hypocalcemia. Hyperphosphatemia associated with cow's milk ingestion may contribute to hypomagnesemia in the neonate. In some cases of hypocalcemia, if the magnesium is low, it must be corrected before the calcium will return to normal.

EKG manifestations include increased PR and QT intervals, flat broad T waves and ST depression, and ventricular tachydysrhythmias.[32]

Clinical Presentation

The signs of hypomagnesemia are similar to those of hypocalcemia, including muscle twitching, seizures, severe confusion, and possible respiratory paralysis. Hypomagnesemia may present with neuromuscular or behavioral manifestations, including muscle fasiculations, cramps, paresthesias, spasticity, convulsions, delirium, hyperirritability, and tetany. In the neonate hypomagnesemia may cause a similar clinical presentation, with jitteriness, hyperalertness, weakness, and poor feeding. Skeletal and respiratory smooth muscle weakness has been reported.[44]

Up to 50% of critically ill adult patients are reported to have hypomagnesemia, especially patients with decreased renal function.[45]

The etiology of hypomagnesemia may be decreased magnesium intake, increased losses of magnesium in the gastrointestinal tract or renal system, or alterations in the distribution of magnesium. A decreased intake of magnesium is thought to be operative in cases of the infant of the diabetic mother, short bowel syndrome, or other causes of malabsorption, such as laxative abuse. Magnesium losses may occur in the infant receiving repeated transfusions with citrated blood, with malabsorption, renal acidosis, renal failure, or diabetic ketoacidosis. Drug-induced magnesium losses may occur with furosemide, thiazide diuretics, ethacrynic acid, digoxin,[46] aminoglycosides, mannitol, or calcium.

Pre- or postoperative patients with congenital heart disease on digoxin may be at risk for hypomagnesemia or digoxin-induced dysrhythmias.[47]

Treatment

In hypomagnesemia renal function must be assessed to evaluate the primary cause of magnesium loss. The transport team or emergency medicine physician must consider treatment in the patient with a critically low magnesium level (<1.0 mg/dl) or the symptomatic patient. Usually, magnesium replacement is performed over a period of 3-5 days. The treatment dose of magnesium sulfate is 25-50 mg/kg/dose (0.2-0.4 mEq/kg/dose) over 1-2 hours. Patients should be placed on a cardiorespiratory monitor and serial neurologic evaluations performed.

HYPERMAGNESEMIA

Hypermagnesemia may be present in the infant of a mother treated with magnesium sulfate for toxemia, or from magnesium administration in another manner. Hypermagnesemia may cause signs of muscular depression, central nervous system depression, or respiratory arrest. Hypotension may occur at a serum magnesium level >5 mg/dl; CNS depression may occur at approximately 7 mg/dl; and respiratory depression or coma at levels >15 mg/dl.

Treatment

Treatment for hypermagnesemia includes intravenous fluids, diuretics, or exchange transfusion.

HYPERNATREMIA AND DIABETES INSIPIDUS

Patients with diabetes insipidus (DI) have polyuria, polydipsia, and hypernatremia (sodium >150 mg/dl) due to an inability to conserve water[48]).

Pathophysiology

The clinician must suspect DI in the case of polyuria associated with a persistently low urine specific gravity (<1.010). The diagnosis is confirmed if the ratio of urine to serum osmolality is less than 1.4, especially if the urine osmolality is extremely low, below 200 mOsm/L. Three common causes of polyuria with a low urine osmolality are DI; nephrogenic DI (impaired renal response to antidiuretic hormone); and increased intake of free water. In the differential diagnosis, one would also consider diabetes mellitus, characterized by glucose and ketones in the urine; psychogenic water drinking, with hyponatremia rather than hypernatremia; enuresis, which occurs at night only; and urinary tract infection. In nephrogenic DI, there is no response to treatment with vasopressin.

Diabetes insipidus may be caused by hypothalamic or pituitary damage such as injuries causing cerebral ischemia, hypoxia, infections, or secondary to

TABLE 7. Etiology of Hypothalamic and Pituitary Lesions

Trauma	Other space-occupying lesions
Inflammation	Midline central nervous system developmental
Tumor (craniopharyngioma)	defects (absent corpus collosum)
Infiltrative disease (sarcoidosis, histiocytosis)	Hereditary diabetes insipidus
Infection (viral or bacterial meningitis, tuberculosis)	

a global insult.[48] The etiology of various hypothalamic or pituitary lesions is listed in Table 7.

Nephrogenic DI that does not respond to vasopressin with a decrease in urine output or increase in specific gravity may be caused by acute tubular necrosis, obstructive uropathy, pyelonephritis, polycystic kidney disease, sickle-cell anemia, protein starvation, and hypercalcemia.

In developed countries the most common causes of DI are head trauma or neurosurgery. Reports in children indicate that 10% of cases are caused by tumors, 37% are related to postsurgical intervention for intracranial tumors, and 3% related to nonsurgical trauma. Studies indicate that when DI accompanies global brain injury, it is associated with nearly 100% mortality in 1-5 days after the injury.[49]

Hereditary DI is a rare entity inherited in an autosomal dominant manner with incomplete penetration. In this condition, autopsy findings suggested a congenital defect in ADH synthesis. Histiocytosis X may cause DI, especially in cases with multisystem involvement. Septooptic dysplasia and other intracranial defects account for approximately 20% of cases of DI in children.

Treatment

As in all cases of critically ill patients with severe head injury, the ABCs should be achieved and maintained. Specifically, if volume losses are significant, these patients may enter a state of hemodynamic instability. For patients presenting in shock, 20 ml/kg of an isotonic solution, such as lactated Ringer's or isotonic saline, is indicated as often as necessary. Hypotonic saline must be avoided to prevent cerebral edema. Once shock is treated, care should be taken that full correction of the abnormality is done over an extended period. The transport team should have a recent set of electrolytes. Treatment is conservative rehydration with D5/0.45% NaCl at 1.5 × maintenance. A similar calculation is to give maintenance plus the deficit over 48 hours. This fluid restriction is sufficient treatment during the initial stabilization until the patient arrives at the tertiary care institution. If the transport team has established a diagnosis of DI, they may use vasopressin (0.03 U/kg subcutaneously) or DDAVP (10 μ intranasally or 1 μg intravenously) to decrease excessive urine output. Alternatively, they may prepare a vasopressin infusion (0.5-15 mU/kg/hr) to avoid the need for large volumes of fluids and accompanying risks of rapid shifts in electrolytes. The usual starting dose is 0.5 mU/kg/hr and, if no effect is seen in 30 minutes, the infusion is doubled and repeated every 30 minutes thereafter. It is rare that a patient will need more than 10 mU/kg/hr, with the average patient responding to 2-4 mU/kg/hr. The end-point is a decrease in urine output to less than 2 ml/kg/hr. The clinician must be aware of the vasoconstriction that may accompany vasopressin use in severe CNS injury. Excessively high rates of vasopressin infusion must be avoided. With excessive doses, complications include systemic vasoconstriction leading to tissue ischemia, profound lactic acidosis, and infarction of skin over extremities.

In the patient with suspected DI who has polyuria and dehydration, or after the end of a 7-hour water deprivation test, a trial of vasopressin may be given.

Urine is collected hourly for volume and specific gravity. An initial and final serum sodium and osmolality are obtained. A trial dose of aqueous vasopressin is given. A positive response to Pitressin confirms the diagnosis of central DI. This is found by an increase in specific gravity to >1.010 and by a decrease in the serum sodium and osmolality.

Alternatively, a trial of intranasal DDAVP once or twice daily may be given. The initial dose is 5–10 μg, increased as needed; the average dose is 10–20 μg (maximum = 40 μg) daily. The goal is to maintain the serum sodium between 130 and 150 mg/dl. Some patients may have an absent thirst mechanism and require regulation of the daily fluid intake at maintenance amounts.

Patients may be slow to respond to DDAVP. In this case, excessive amounts or frequent administration should be avoided because they may cause a prolonged period of subsequent hyponatremia, which is difficult to correct.

HYPONATREMIA AND SYNDROME OF INAPPROPRIATE ANTIDIURETIC HORMONE SECRETION

The syndrome of inappropriate antidiuretic hormone (SIADH) must be considered in the diagnosis of hyponatremia with decreased urine volume.[48]

Pathophysiology

Under normal conditions, a decrease in effective arterial blood volume or a rise in plasma osmolarity induces the release of antidiuretic hormone (ADH). However, in cases of postoperative brain surgery patients, and in meningitis or head trauma the excretion of ADH may be inappropriate. A diagnosis is one of excluding other causes of hyponatremia (Table 8), such as sodium loss in sweat, stool, renal dysfunction, or increased intake of free water. With the latter, urine volume is increased and urine specific gravity decreased.

Treatment

Treatment for SIADH begins in the referring institution or during transport. The treatment of choice is fluid restriction. Fluid restriction alone (one-fourth to two-thirds maintenance) usually will correct the problem. Patients with seizures, severe obtundation, or coma require 3% saline (0.5 mEq/ml) administered in an amount calculated to restore the serum sodium to 120–125 mEq/L according to the following formula:

$$(\text{Desired–actual Na}) \times 0.6 \times \text{kg} = \text{mEq of Na required}$$

Half of this amount can be infused over 5–10 minutes, and the remainder may be administered over 2–4 hours until the plasma sodium concentration has reached the desired level. If it is administered into a peripheral vessel, care should be

TABLE 8.   Etiology of Hyponatremia

Losses	Increased free water (cont.)
Gastrointestinal losses (diarrhea or fistula)	Water intoxication (increased urine volume, low specific gravity)
Renal losses (interstitial disease, renal tubular acidosis, diuretics)	Disorders of the osmostat (SIADH, hypothyroidism)
Third space (burns, peritonitis, pancreatitis)	Edema
Mineralocorticoid deficiency (adrenal failure)	Nephrosis
	Acute renal failure
Increased free water	Congestive heart failure
SIADH (decreased urine volume, increased specific gravity)	Hyperglycemia or mannitol therapy

taken to avoid extravasation, which may cause significant tissue injury. Preferably, it is administered into a large vessel, a central venous line, or an IO line.

If a child is hyponatremic and hypovolemic, blood volume must be restored. The intravenous fluids of choice in this case are normal saline or blood products, as clinically indicated.

After fluid restriction therapy is begun, an increase in urinary output should be seen within a relatively short time of 1–3 hours. When the transport team recognizes the diagnosis of hyponatremia, the clinician must decide if this is dilutional. If so, a possible clinical diagnosis of SIADH is suggested and therapy by fluid restriction is begun immediately.

HYPOKALEMIA

The serum potassium concentration is tightly regulated, and minor changes may lead to life-threatening arrhythmias. Potassium is the major intracellular cation, playing an important role in mitochondrial function, nerve conduction, and muscular contraction. Neuromuscular transmission is dependent on the ratio of intracelluar to extracellular potassium.

Pathophysiology

Hypokalemia may cause life-threatening arrhythmias; therefore, the treatment team must be aware of various causes of hypokalemia (Table 9).

Shifts between intracelluar and extracellular potassium may result from alterations in acid-base balance. Vomiting, a common sign in critically ill patients, may cause chloride and hydrogen ion loss, resulting in alkalemia. As a result, hydrogen ions move from intracellular to extracellular space and there is a concurrent efflux of potassium from extracellular to intracellular space, resulting in systemic hypokalemia. In addition, with metabolic acidosis, potassium is excreted by the kidney in exchange for hydrogen ions, which further contributes to hyperkalemia.

Other causes of metabolic alkalosis include chloride losses associated with diarrhea, sweating, cystic fibrosis, or diuretic administration.[50,51] These etiologies associated with chloride loss may be suspected if the urine chloride is low. On the other hand, if the urine chloride is high, the etiology of the metabolic alkalosis may be primarily potassium deficiency or Bartter's syndrome, a rare renal tubular disorder characterized by chloride wasting. In cystic fibrosis, hyponatremia and volume contraction cause hyperaldosteronism, resulting in loss of potassium and hydrogen ion, with resultant metabolic alkalosis.

Patients with periodic paralysis may experience profound muscle weakness associated with hypokalemia due to extracellular to intracellular shifts of potassium. In hypothermia, hypokalemia may be induced by potassium shifts to the intracellular space. Subsequent rewarming may then lead to an efflux of potassium into the intravascular space. Supplementation with potassium must be done cautiously to prevent hyperkalemia.

Cardiac patients must have serum potassium levels carefully monitored, especially if on diuretic or digitalis therapy; patients are at increased risk for arrhythmia

TABLE 9.   Etiology of Hypokalemia

Hyperaldosterone (elevated sodium)	Renal losses (diabetes, RTA, diuretics, carbenicillin,
Decreased intake of potassium (anorexia, starvation)	Bartter syndrome, Cushing syndrome)
Increased losses (vomiting, pyloric stenosis,	Alkalinization
gastric suctioning, diarrhea, laxative use,	Treatment with insulin
sweating, and cystic fibrosis)	Familial hypokalemic periodic paralysis

due to digitalis intoxication if hypokalemia or hypercalcemia is also present. Pediatric patients with congenital heart disease (CHD), postsurgical repair of CHD, or a history of atrial or ventricular dysrhythmias are at risk for hypokalemia-induced atrial or ventriculator ectopy, atrial tachycardia, atrial ventricular blocks, premature ventricular contractions, ventricular tachycardia, and fibrillation.

Clinical Presentation

One of the first manifestations of hypokalemia is muscle weakness, which in severe cases may progress to respiratory and generalized paralysis. Cramping, edema, and paresthesias may be seen. Muscle ischemia and rhabdomyolysis have been associated with hypokalemia.[52] Autonomic smooth muscle is affected by hypokalemia in cases of impaired gastric motility and paralytic ileus, producing nausea, vomiting, and constipation.

Treatment

If arrhythmias, muscle paralysis, or severe weakness is due to hypokalemia, the treatment of choice is rapid (over 1 hour) correction with intravenous potassium chloride. In DKA, potassium phosphate is recommended in addition to potassium chloride. The preferred route is a large peripheral central vein or IO line to diminish the risk of sclerosis in smaller vessels. Potassium should be mixed in solutions without dextrose, except in the case of DKA, since dextrose may stimulate endogenous insulin release with subsequent shift of potassium intracellularly. The maximum infusion rate is 0.5-1 mEq/kg/hour. During administration, the serum potassium must be monitored, since hyperkalemia may develop rapidly, especially in patients with acidemia, diabetes mellitus, or renal tubular acidosis. Medications that may prevent potassium from entering the cell and leading to hyperkalemia during treatment include nonsteroidal anti-inflammatory agents, angiotensin-converting enzyme inhibitors, or beta-blockers.

HYPERKALEMIA AND ALDOSTERONE DEFICIENCY

The serum potassium level is modulated by renal clearance. A potassium concentration >6 mEq/L in an unhemolyzed specimen on more than one occasion is significant and suggests possible aldosterone deficiency or congenital adrenal hyperplasia.

Hyperosmolality may produce cellular contraction, leading to potassium efflux from cells. A common cause of hyperkalemia in critical care is skeletal muscle injury due to motor vehicle accidents or catabolic states such as surgery, sepsis, or burns. Transient hyperkalemia may be caused by hemolysis. Renal disorders associated with urinary obstruction, sickle-cell nephropathy, lupus nephritis, and treatment with cyclosporine are much more common than adrenal insufficiency or Addison disease as a cause of hyperkalemia. One of the most common causes in the critical care setting is drug-induced hyperkalemia due to one of the following medications: nonsteroidal antiinflammatory agents; cyclo-sporine potassium-sparing diuretics; and angiotensin-converting enzyme inhibitors such as captopril or enalapril. It is important to evaluate possible iatrogenic causes such as oral potassium supplements or unmixed parenteral fluid additions as in potassium salts and penicillin, or other intravenous medications (Table 10).

Pathophysiology and Clinical Manifestations

Unless hyperkalemia is severe, it is usually asymptomatic. Alteration of the electrical conduction of the heartbeat forces prompt clinical attention because

TABLE 10. Etiology of Hyperkalemia

Hyperosmolarity (cellular contraction, efflux of potassium from cells)
Skeletal muscle injury (accident, surgery, sepsis, burns)
Hemolysis
Renal disease (urinary obstruction, lupus nephritis, sickle-cell nephropathy, cyclosporine)
Adrenal insufficiency (Addision disease, adrenal hyperplasia)
Drug-induced (nonsteroidal antiinflammatory agents, cyclosporine, potassium-sparing diuretics,
    angiotensin-converting enzyme inhibitors, e.g., captopril or enalapril)
Ingestion of oral potassium supplements
Potassium in penicillin or other intravenous medications

---

there is imminent danger of cardiac arrest or arrhythmia. A serum potassium concentration <6 mEq/L does not exhibit cardiotoxicity. With hyperkalemia, the initial change in the electrocardiogram is the appearance of tall peaked T-waves, especially in the precordial leads. If untreated, more serious EKG changes such as merging of the normal U and T waves may follow. The Q-T interval is normal or diminished in hyperkalemia. As intraventricular conduction becomes further delayed, the PR interval is prolonged, the P-wave amplitude decreases, and the QRS complexes widen into a sine wave pattern. This is ventricular flutter, which may progress to cardiac standstill. Concomitant electrolyte abnormalities such as hyponatremia, hypocalcemia, acidosis, or hypomagnesemia may exaggerate these electrocardiographic changes.

Pseudohyperkalemia is a condition of apparently high serum potassium by in vitro measurement and is due to elevated platelet ($>10^6$ platelets/mm^3) or white blood cell ($>50,000$/mm^3) counts. Although the serum potassium is not elevated, hyperkalemia may result from ischemic muscle distal to a tourniquet during blood drawing.

Management

Management of hyperkalemia in the pretransport or transport setting may be required before an exact cause is known. Methods of treatment include agents to reduce the effect of potassium directly on membrane potentials, to remove total body potassium, or to distribute potassium intracellularly. The initial treatment in cases of CVAH, adrenal failure, or aldosterone deficiency is hydration with normal saline (1.5 × maintenance) and the use of 9α-fluorocortisol.

If the serum potassium is greater than 7 mEq/L or if cardiac toxicity is present, identified by EKG changes showing loss of P waves or widening of the QRS complex, treatment with intravenous calcium is indicated to reduce membrane threshold potential and restore normal membrane excitability. Owing to the short duration of the potassium-lowering effect of calcium, it must be combined wiht therapy to lower the serum potassium level, such as insulin and dextrose, or with alkalinization.

If the serum potassium level is <7 mEq/dl, treatment may begin with measures to redistribute potassium intracellularly or promote excretion. Regular insulin (0.1 U/kg IV over 1 hour) promotes an intracellular shift of potassium. Unless the blood sugar is greater than 300 mg/dl, insulin is given with glucose (0.25 gm/kg IV) to prevent the development of hypoglycemia. Repeated infusions of insulin and glucose may be required.

Alkalinization using sodium bicarbonate also promotes cellular uptake of potassium. This is the treatment of choice in acidosis but is not limited to use in the acidotic patient. Bicarbonate is not recommended in cases of hypernatremia.

In conditions associated wiht hypocalcemia, such as uremic acidosis, calcium should also be administered to avoid hypokalemic tetany during the infusion of bicarbonate.

While the above therapy is undertaken, measures to remove potassium from the body should also begin promptly after the patient is stabilized. Unless end-stage renal therapy is present, loop diuretics such as furosemide should be administered to promote kaliuresis. These patients should be given adequate amounts of normal saline to avoid volume depletion.

Kayexalate may be administered if renal failure is severe, since potassium clearance by the colon can be augmented with this substance. This is a cation exchange resin that increases stool potassium in exchange for sodium. It can be given orally (1–2 gm/kg) with 20% sorbitol to avoid constipation. For a more rapid effect, or if ileus is present, a retention enema in a slurry of Kayexalate and sorbitol is preferable. The clinician should be cautious of sodium overload, which may occur if the patient has significantly compromised renal clearance.

REFERENCES

1. Conte FA, Grumbach MM: Endocrine disorders. In Grossman M, Dieckmann RA (eds): Pediatric Emergency Medicine. Philadelphia, J.B. Lippincott, 1991, pp 467–473.
2. Bacon GE, Spencer ML, Hopwood NJ, et al: A Practical Approach to Pediatric Endocrinology. Chicago, Yearbook, 1990.
3. Mueller PL, Varma SK: Endocrine disorders. In Manual of Pediatric Therapeutics. Boston, Little, Brown, 1974, pp 365–393.
4. Sperling MA: Hypoglycemia. In Behrman RE (ed): Nelson Textbook of Pediatrics. Philadelphia, W.B. Saunders, 1992, pp 409–419.
5. Cornblath M, Schwartz A: Hypoglycemia in the neonate. J Pediatr Endocrinol 6:113–115, 1993.
6. Fischer KF, Lees JA, Newman JH: Hypoglycemia in hospitalized patients: Causes and outcomes. N Engl J Med 315:1245–1250, 1986.
7. Malouf R, Brust JCM: Hypoglycemia: Causes, neurological manifestations, and outcome. Ann Neurol 17:421–430, 1985.
8. Yudkoff M: Metabolic emergencies (inborn errors of metabolism). In Fleisher GR, Ludwig S (eds): Textbook of Pediatric Emergency Medicine. Baltimore, Williams & Wilkins, 1993, pp 962–974.
9. Collins JE, Leonard JV, Teale D, et al: Hyperinsulinaemic hypoglycemia in small for dates babies. Arch Dis Child 65:1118–1120, 1990.
10. Grant DB, Dunger DB, Burns EC: Long-term treatment with diazoxide in childhood hyper-insulinism. Acta Endocrinol 279(Suppl):340–345.
11. Thornton PS, Alter CA, Levitt Katz LE, et al: Short and long-term use of octreotide in the treatment of congenital hyperinsulinsim. J Pediatr 123:637–643, 1993.
12. Ryan CM , Atchison J, Puczynski S, et al: Mild hypoglycemia associated with deterioration of mental efficiency in children with insulin-dependent diabetes mellitus. J Pediatr 32–38, 1990.
13. Holman RC, Herron CA, Sinnock P: Epidemiologic characteristics of mortality from diabetes with acidosis or coma, United States, 1970–78. Am J Public Health 73:1169–1173, 1983.
14. Karam J, Salber P, Forsham P: Pancreatic hormones and diabetes mellitus. In Greenspan F (ed): Basic and Clinical Endocrinology. Norwalk, CT, Appleton & Lange, 1991, pp 592–650.
15. Tsalikian E, Becker D, Crumrine P: Electroencephalographic changes in diabetic ketosis in children with newly and previously diagnosed insulin-dependent diabetes mellitus. J Pediatr 98:355, 1988.
16. Fisher JN, Kitabchi AE: A randomized study of phosphate therapy in the treatment of diabetic ketoacidosis. J Clin Endocrinol Metab 57:177–180, 1983.
17. Clerbaux T, Detry B, Reynaert M, et al: Reestimation of the effects of inorganic phosphates on the equilibrium between oxygen and hemoglobin. Intens Care Med 18:222–225, 1992.
18. Sperling MA: Diabetes mellitus. In Behrman RE (ed): Nelson Textbook of Pediatrics. Philadelphia, W.B. Saunders, 1992, pp 390–409.
19. Duck SC, Kohler E: Cerebral edema in diabetic ketoacidosis. J Pediatr 98:674, 1981.
20. Duck SC, Wyatt DT: Factors associated with brain herniation in the treatment of diabetic ketoacidosis. J Pediatr 113:10–14, 1988.
21. Cahill GF: Hyperglycemic hyperosmolar coma: A syndrome almost unique to the elderly. J Am Geriatr Soc 31:103–105, 1983.

22. Pildes RS: Neonatal hyperglycemia. J Pediatr 109:905, 1986.
23. Chin R: Adrenal crisis. Crit Care Clin 7:23, 1991.
24. Chin R, Cernow B: Corticosteroids. In Chernow B, Lake R (eds): The Pharmacologic Approach to the Critically Ill Patient. Baltimore, Williams & Wilkins, 1993, p 510.
25. Miller W: The adrenal cortex. In Rudolph AM (ed): Rudolph's Pediatrics. Norwalk, CT, Appleton and Lange, 1991, pp 1584–1613.
26. Fisher DA: The thyroid. In Rudolph AM (ed): Rudolph's Pediatrics. Norwalk, CT, Appleton and Lange, 1991, pp 1621–1644.
27. Menendez CE, Rivlin RS: Thyrotoxic crisis and myxedema coma. Med Clin North Am 57:1463–1470, 1973.
28. Klein AH, Meltzer S, Kenny FM: Improved prognosis in congenital hypothyroidism treated before age three months. J Pediatr 81:912–915, 1972.
29. Voorhees M: Disorders of the adrenal medulla; multiple endrocrine adenomatosis syndromes. In Kaplan S (ed): Clinical Pediatric and Adolescent Endocrinology. Philadelphia, W.B. Saunders, 1982, pp 207–210.
30. Reed G, Devous M: Cerebral blood flow autoregulation and hypertension. Am J Med Sci 289:37–44, 1985.
31. Zaloga GP: Calcium homeostasis in the critically ill patient. Magnesium 8:190, 1989.
32. Jaimovich D: Endocrine and metabolic disorders. In McKloskey K, Orr R (eds): Textbook of Neonatal and Pediatric Transport Medicine. Philadelphia, Mosby, 1995.
33. Arnaud C, Kolb F: The calcitropic hormones and metabolic bone disease. In Greenspan F (ed): Basic and Clinical Endocrinology. Norwalk, CT, Appleton & Lange, 1991, pp 247–322.
34. Chernow B, et al: Iatrogenic hyperphosphatemia: A metabolic consideration in critical care medicine. Crit Care Med 9:772–774, 1981.
35. Mimouni F, Tsang RC: Parathyroid and vitamin D related disorders. In Kaplan SA (ed): Clinical Pediatric Endocrinology. Philadelphia, W.B. Saunders, 1990, pp 427–453.
36. Koo WW, Sherman R, Succop P, et al: Serum vitamin D metabolites in very low birth weight infants with and without rickets and fractures. J Pediatr 114:1017–1022, 1989.
37. Zaloga GP: Phosphate disorders. In Zaloga GP (ed): Endocrine Emergencies, Problems in Critical Care. Philadelphia, J.B. Lippincott, 1990, pp 416–424.
38. Zaloga GP, Roberts JE: Magnesium disorders. In Zaloga GP (ed): Endocrine Emergencies, Problems in Critical Care. Philadelphia, J.B. Lippincott, 1990, pp 425–436.
39. Boles JM, Dutel JL, Briere J, et al: Acute renal failure caused by extreme hyperphosphatemia after chemotherapy of an acute lymphoblastic leukemia. Cancer 53:2425–2429, 1984.
40. Monballyu J, Zachee P, Verberchmoes R, et al: Transient acute renal failure due to tumor-lysis-induced severe phosphate load in a patient with Burkitt's lymphoma. Clin Nephrol 22:47–50, 1984.
41. Brautbar N, Kleeman CR: Hypophosphatemia and hyperphosphatemia: Clinical pathophysiologic aspect. In Clinical Disorders of Fluid and Electrolyte Metabolism, 4th ed. New York, McGraw Hill, 1987, pp 789–830.
42. Slatopolsky E, Rutherford WE, Rosenbaum R, et al: Hyperphosphatemia. Clin Nephrol 7:138–146, 1977.
43. Wason S, Tiller T, Cunha C: Severe hyperphosphatemia, hypocalcemia, acidosis, and shock in a 5-month-old child following the administration of an adult fleet enema. Ann Emerg Med 18:696–700, 1989.
44. Molloy DW, Dhingra S, Solven F, et al: Hypomagnesemia and respiratory muscle power. Am Rev Respir Dis 129:497–498, 1984.
45. Ryzen E, Wagers PW, Singer FR, et al: Magnesium deficiency in a medical ICU population. Crit Care Med 13:19–21, 1985.
46. Specter MJ, Schweizer E, Goldman RH: Studies on magnesium's mechanism of action in digitalis-induced arrhythmias. Circulation 52:1001–1005, 1975.
47. Martin BJ, McAlpine JK, Devine BL: Hypomagnesemia in elderly digitalized patients. Scott Med J 33:273–274, 1988.
48. Bode HH: Disorders of the posterior pituitary. In Kaplan SA (ed): Clinical Pediatric Endocrinology. Philadelphia, W.B. Saunders, 1990, pp 63–86.
49. Keren G, Barzilay Z, Schreiber M, et al: Diabetes insipidus indicating a dying brain. Crit Care Med 10:798, 1982.
50. Brewer ED: Disorders of the acid-base balance. Pediatr Clin North Am 37:429–447, 1990.
51. Finberg L: Water and electrolytes in pediatrics: Physiology, pathophysiology, and treatment. Philadelphia, W.B. Saunders, 1993.
52. Knochel JP, Schlein EM: On the mechanism of rhabdomyolysis in potassium depletion. J Clin Invest 51:1750–1758, 1972.

CHAPTER 21

Evaluation and Management of Renal Emergencies

KENNETH MILLER, M.D.
BARBARA ATKIN, RN, BSN, MBA

RENAL PHYSIOLOGY

The kidney is primarily responsible for maintaining salt and water balance in the body. Approximately 20–25% of the cardiac output is filtered through and by the kidney. The filtrate then flows down the tubular system, wherein both active and passive transport of salt and water occur. The filtrate (180 liters), which is formed daily, contains 25,000 mEq of sodium, 99% of which is reabsorbed by the kidneys.[1]

Body space distribution (body water) reaches mature adult proportions by two years of age. Water content in adults is approximately 70% of lean body mass (LBM). The above percentages also apply to infants older than 30 days of age. Intracellular fluid is approximately 45% LBM in the infant and 50% in children older than three years. Extracellular fluid volume is approximately 25% in infants and 20–23% in children over three years. Interstitial volume represents 22% of lean body mass from birth until 3 years, but only 15% in those over three years. Plasma volume is the same regardless of age, approximately 6%. The major cation in the extracellular fluid is sodium.[2]

Obligatory water losses fall into three essential categories; insensible water loss through evaporation (skin or respiratory tract), which equals 45 ml/100 calories (30 ml/100 calories through the skin, 15 ml/100 calories through the respiratory tract). The losses are mainly free water, except during times of high fever when there will also be obligatory losses of sodium, potassium, and chloride. Ventilatory losses can increase threefold with respiratory illnesses, and calories expended through the integument will increase by 13% for each 1° C rise over basal conditions. If body termperature decreases by 1.5 ° C, heat production (and evaporation loss) increases due to shivering.[3]

Obligatory loss of water through the urine is approximately 50 ml/100 calories; water losses through the urine are generally increased by any disorder that will affect concentrating ability such as diabetes insipidus, diabetes mellitus, or acute renal failure (polyuric state). As a rule, water loss through stool is small, roughly 5 ml/100 calories. Diarrhea, however, may increase water losses up to 30%. Vomiting not only increases losses, but also affects the child by the diminished intake.[3]

Abnormal water losses can occur via sequestration, such as secondary to mechanical bowel injury (ileus), where the fluid is transcellular, thus affecting the intravascular space. In addition, fluid shifts due to a decline in plasma volume, secondary to protein loss or due to a decline in protein production, will affect the oncotic pressure, and thus will shift fluid from the effective circulating volume.[3]

The kidney plays a role in the regulation of acid-base balance as well. Through glomerular filtration, sodium and potassium are provided as cations for the exchange of hydrogen ions in the tubular system. At the tubular level four mechanisms for the excretion of hydrogen ions exist: (1) carbonic anhydrase, which will lead to the formation of hydrogen ions and bicarbonate; (2) a tubular exchange mechanism involving sodium and potassium for hydrogen ions; (3) conversion of bicarbonate in the glomerular filtrate to carbon dioxide (CO_2) and water, which can decrease the net bicarbonate content in an acid urine to zero; and (4) the production of ammonia which will link the hydrogen ion to form ammonium. Finally, HPO_4 can act as a buffer, forming H_2PO_4. There are also other organic acids, and even creatinine, which can serve as buffers.[4,5]

The kidney is also responsible for the regulation of sodium, potassium, and chloride, involving renal hemodynamics, the renin angiotensin system (RAA), aldosterone, anti-diuretic hormone (ADH), and atrial natriuretic hormone.[6]

FLUID AND ELECTROLYTE DISORDERS

Many of the transport medical problems encountered in an acute setting will require fluid resuscitation. The choice of, and rate of administration of, such fluids may influence renal outcome and, indeed, patient outcome.

Although pulmonary, cardiac, endocrine, and GI disorders have been addressed in other chapters, several issues pertaining to fluid resuscitation are worth reiterating.

In the patient with asthma, an acute asthmatic attack will significantly increase insensible free water loss two- to three-fold, necessitating an adjustment in fluids. Salt requirements, however, would remain unchanged unless fever losses were present. In this situation, up to 45 mEq/L of sodium and 10 mEq/L of potassium may be lost through the skin. Conversely, in status asthmaticus, fluid requirements may need to be curtailed due to elevation of circulating ADH, which will lead to a more concentrated urine with decreased water excretion. Indeed, pulmonary edema may develop in the patient with status asthmaticus owing to a decrease in pleural pressure coupled with an increase in capillary presure and a decrease in oncotic pressure which may be associated with over-hydration. Thus, close monitoring of vital signs, urine output, skin and mucous membrane color, as well as skin turgor and consistency, is imperative.[7]

Fluid and electrolyte abnormalities are common in patients with cardiac disease, with or without congestive failure. Edema is often observed in such children, who are both salt- and water-overloaded. The kidney, however, senses a state of altered perfusion. This leads to the release of renin and subsequent production of angiotensin II and aldosterone; thus, salt retention will occur. In addition, ADH levels will be high, and water will accompany the salt retention. The causes of heart failure in children include myocarditis, arrhythmias, impaired coronary artery circulation, congenital heart disease with or without superimposed infection, or heart failure secondary to pulmonary or systemic hypertension. Hypoxia and acidosis may also accompany these conditions. Clearly, improvement in tissue oxygenation is essential in preventing the latter complications. Establishment of a brisk diuresis will help as well.[8] If hyponatremia is observed, it is most likely dilutional and related to excess water retention. Loop diuretics are the preferred first-line drugs because of the ability of these agents to increase free H_2O loss greater than salt loss. There are currently four such agents: furosemide, bumetanide, torsemide (not approved for children), and ethacrynic acid (which is the only one that lacks a sulfhydryl group and thus can be given to patients with a sulfa allergy). Chloride absorption is blocked at the ascending loop of Henle as is, in turn, sodium reabsorption. An initial dose of furosemide 1-2 mg/kg should be administered (1 mg of bumetanide = 20-40 mg of furosemide). If no response in 30 minutes, the dose may be doubled or consideration given to placing the child on a furosemide or bumetanide drip. A more sustained diuresis is often achieved with a continuous infusion, and the potential for ototoxicity is reduced. The initial starting dose of furosemide is 0.25 mg/kg/ hour with a maximum dose of 1 mg/kg/hour. Concomitant administration of an oral and/or IV thiazide diuretic often results in a synergistic response.

Contraction alkalosis accompanied by hypokalemia may be seen in patients on high-dose diuretics—e.g., the child with heart failure. The carbonic anhydrase inhibitor, acetazolamide (Diamox), and supplemental potassium may correct the abnormalities. Occasionally, a potassium-sparing diuretic, such as triamterene, amiloride, and/or aldactone may be required as well. Aldactone has a slow onset of action (24-48 hours). Its effects will, however, persist after it is discontinued, for two to four days.[9,10]

In diabetic ketoacidosis, one should appreciate that although these patients tend to become volume depleted rather quickly, they remain polyuric due to the osmotic gradient created by the hyperglycemia. A small percentage will even develop nonketotic hyperosmolar coma, which should be managed quite similarly to hypernatremic dehydration—i.e., slow restoration of normal osmolality with a low sodium, high potassium solution (provided urine output is excellent). Often, the serum sodium will appear low in the diabetic patient with ketoacidosis due to an elevated glucose. For every 100 mg/dl rise in glucose > 100 the serum sodium is lowered by 1.6 mEq/dl. In addition, hypophosphatemia can occur with diabetic ketoacidosis. Acid/base abnormalities do arise, but rapid correction of metabolic acidosis should be avoided to prevent cerebral edema and intracellular acidosis. If bicarbonate is given, it should be administered slowly and only if the pH is < 7.2 or if the serum bicarbonate level is < 12.

The transport team will often encounter an infant or young child in whom the hydration status is in question. A careful history regarding the cause of the underlying condition and its duration, concomitant disorders, and any medications administered during and prior to the illness is imperative. For example, in a child who appears to be dehydrated, the type of fluids administered prior to and during the hospitalization are important. In the hypernatremic dehydrated patient, one will often learn that the child was on milk products, i.e., high solute-containing solution. It is equally important to determine the number of times the child has voided as well as the volume of each voided specimen. Record admission weight and pre-illness weight. For the child who has had vomiting and diarrhea, it is important to try to record the number of episodes of emesis and diarrhea that have occurred. Record the character and color of the stool and perform a clinical assessment, including a vital sign determination, skin turgor (doughy in hypernatremic dehydration), moistness of the mucous membranes, and skin color. Neurologic assessment and observation for signs or symptoms of fluid overload (mottling, cyanosis, edema, heart failure, organomegaly, pallor, and/or rashes) should also be noted. The family and patient (when possible) should be queried regarding duration of fever and the average daily temperature.

PRERENAL AND RENAL FAILURE

In assessing adequacy of urine volume, remember that under normal physiologic conditions urine output is approximately 50 ml/24 hrs/100 cal, or 2 ml/1 hr/100 cal. In calculating appropriate minimum urine volume, one usually addresses the amount of urine necessary to excrete the obligatory renal solute load. An infant can vary urine solute concentration from 765 to 800 mOsm/L, after the first few weeks of life. This calculates to a urine volume of 31.8 ml/100 cal/24 hrs, or 1.3 ml/hr. The older child, from two months to two years, can concentrate up to 1000 to 1400 mOsm/L, or 24-25 ml/100 cal/24 hrs, or 1-1.25 ml/hr.[1-4]

When the dehydrated patient does not show significant clinical improvement or enhanced urine output after an initial fluid challenge of 10-20 ml/kg of a crystalloid solution (lactated Ringer's or normal saline) administered over 45 minutes and repeated one time, then the transport team is faced with a critical dilemma. Failure to respond may be due to inadequate expansion of the extracellular or intravascular compartments, or perhaps impairment of normal homeostatic mechanisms that maintain the integrity of the microvasculature, leading to capillary leak. Alternatively, myocardial dysfunction and/or parenchymal renal failure may account for failure to respond to volume expansion. If the patient's problem is related to capillary leak syndrome or inadequate expansion of the vascular space, blood pressure will remain low, the pulse rapid and weak, and the extremities cool with altered perfusion and decreased capillary refill, despite the fact that the patient may even have peripheral edema. One should judiciously continue to administer fluids, but perhaps substitute colloid for crystalloid. Clearly, in the patient who appears to be 15% dehydrated, colloid should be the first fluid administered either as 5% albumin or plasmanate.[13] Conversely, one may be faced with a child who responds, but with only a small volume of urine produced. It is then critical that the patient's electrolytes, urine specific gravity, and osmolality be measured. If enough urine exists, one could calculate the fractional excretion of sodium or renal failure index. In the prerenal state, the patient will have a low urine sodium ($<$ 20 mEq/L), a high specific gravity or osmolality, and a fractional excretion of sodium or renal failure index $<$ 1%. In this situation, administration of additional fluids is imperative. However, if urine sodium is high ($>$ 30 mEq/L) or the fractional excretion of sodium is $>$ 2.5 in the small infant or $>$ 3 in the older child, then renal failure is probably present.[14,15] Fluid administration should then be curtailed to insensible losses, plus extrarenal and renal losses. Insensible fluid losses would be administered as free water unless high fever existed. Correction for fever losses is imperative. For extrarenal losses, one could use D5W/0.45% normal saline, adding potassium only if urine output is at least 0.5 ml/kg/hr. In a patient who is managed correctly, weight loss will generally occur (between 0.2-1% of body weight). In stabilizing the child who appears dehydrated or in whom hydration status is unclear, a bladder catheter must be placed. This allows the clinician to determine if the patient has an outlet obstruction, determines if urine exists in the bladder, and provides a means to record output on a frequent basis. In addition, cultures should be sent if clinically appropriate. Clearly, if catheterization is accomplished without incident and there is no history of voiding dysfunction or other urinary problems, the likelihood of postrenal failure secondary to obstruction is remote. The only exception would be a

TABLE 1.   Complications of Renal Failure

Hyperkalemia	Seizures
Acidosis	Anemia
Hypocalcemia	Hypoglycemia
Hyperphosphatemia	Hypertension
Fluid overload	Rapidly rising BUN and creatinine

solitary obstructed kidney, which usually would be palpable on examination. In either event, if time permits, an ultrasound of the kidneys will determine if obstructive uropathy exists, and will show the size of the kidneys, indicating whether there is an acute or chronic process. Therefore, the transport team can prevent the patient with prerenal failure from progressing to renal failure if urine output is established with hydration, administration of low-dose dopamine (2–3 μg/kg/min), and/or the use of diuretic therapy after failure of appropriate fluid challenges and evaluation of the clinical status. The conversion of a patient from prerenal failure to polyuric renal failure is also of value, since the outcome of such patients is generally excellent.[16] In a polyuric state, adequate calories may be administered and provide all other necessary byproducts to support the patient. In summary, in the patient initially encountered by the transport team, early institution of adequate hydration is essential. Institution of low-dose dopamine at the onset may also be of value. Diuretic therapy should be reserved for situations in which adequate hydration has been established, but in which urine output greater than 1 ml/kg/hr has not occurred. If a patient has a poor urine response and one suspects renal failure, then all the potential complications of renal failure should be sought out (Table 1).

COMPLICATIONS OF RENAL FAILURE

Hyperkalemia is considered a potentially life-threatening complication of acute renal failure. It results from the shift in potassium from its normal intracellular location to the extracellular space. It is commonly encountered in patients with sepsis, rhabdomyolysis following trauma, or in the tumor lysis syndrome. It may also be seen with the hemolytic-uremic syndrome and/or acute glomerulonephritis. The concomitant presence of acidosis will further elevate potassium levels. Potentially life-threatening cardiac arrhythmias could develop from elevated potassium levels. The early signs of hyperkalemia by EKG are noted when the potassium levels are greater than 6.5. These include peaked T waves and prolongation of the PR interval. Widening of the QRS complex, loss of the P wave, and the eventual development of ventricular fibrillation can occur as potassium levels rise to 8 or greater. Intervention with agents to lower the potassium should be instituted when the potassium is $\geq$ 6. There are only two ways to truly lower total body potassium: one is with dialysis, of which hemodialysis is the only effective means of rapidly lowering potassium; the second is the use of the exchange resin sodium polystyrene sulfonate (kayexalate), which is generally administered when the potassium level is > 6. Using the resin, one exchanges sodium for potassium in the intestinal tract. This agent has a slow-onset of action, generally one to two hours, but its effects will last six to eight hours. As a rule, the potassium level is dropped by 1 mEq/L if we use a dose of 1 gm/kg of kayexalate. This agent is generally administered in either Sorbitol 20% or Sorbitol 70%, the latter given only orally. There is a pre-mixed solution 15 gm of kayexalate per 60 ml of 20% Sorbitol. The dose can be repeated every six to eight hours. Side effects include elevation of sodium levels and hypertension. When potassium levels are ≥ 7, administration of sodium bicarbonate 2–3 mEq/kg over 20–30 minutes with the concomitant administration of insulin and glucose (0.5 gm/kg glucose with insulin. 0.1 unit/kg over 30 minutes). Insulin is the most important pharmacologic agent promoting the shift of potassium intracellularly. The effect of the insulin/glucose cocktail in combination with sodium bicarbonate will last from two to eight hours. Sodium bicarbonate is most effective with severe acidemia. Hypernatremia, hypertension, and alterations in blood glucose are potential complications. Finally, the competitive antagonist calcium gluconate could be administered but only with continuous EKG monitoring if the potassium level is ≥ 8.0. The effects of calcium administration, although immediate, are gone as rapidly when the infusion is discontinued. Bradycardia and hypercalcemia are potential complications of calcium administration. The inhaled beta-adrenergic agent albuterol has also been used to treat hyperkalemia.[17,18]

Acidosis, which also accompanies renal failure, should be dealt with, but only if the pH is < 7.2 or if the serum bicarbonate level is ≤ 12. Acidosis should also be addressed if hyperkalemia is present or if maximum respiratory compensation is present, i.e., a $PaCO_2$ less than 25 torr. Correction to a pH of 7.25 or a bicarbonate level of 15 is adequate. The amount of bicarbonate to be given is calculated as 24 minus the observed bicarbonate × 0.5, which is the bicarbonate space times the patient's weight. Half of the calculated amount is generally given. Continuous infusion of bicarbonate and/or dialysis is necessary when intractable acidosis exists. Clearly, in such a situation, the patient will have arrived at the tertiary center. One should also calculate the anion gap (serum sodium minus the sum of chloride and bicarbonate). If greater than 15, one should search for causes of the increased gap, i.e., lactate, ethylene glycol, ethanol or methanol, aspirin intoxication, or diabetic acidosis.

Hyponatremia may also accompany renal failure. It is generally mild and is usually dilutional (excess water to salt retention). Edema will often be present. However, in the diuretic phase of acute tubular necrosis or in polyuric renal failure, the decline in serum sodium may be truly due to losses in the urine. Thus, urine and serum sodium must be obtained simultaneously. Sodium 3% is never given to such patients because of the risk of producing pulmonary edema. In addition, rapid correction of hyponatremia is not recommended.[19,20] In patients who have hyponatremic dehydration, slowly correct sodium at a rate of 0.5 mEq/hr in order to avoid the rare but serious complication of central pontine myelinosis.[21] Fortunately, hyponatremic dehydration, generally due to diarrheal illness, is rare (< 10% of cases).[22]

Hypocalcemia also occurs acutely in patients with renal failure of new onset, concomitantly with hyperphosphatemia. These changes are due to the inability of the renal tubule to excrete phosphorus as well as the inability of the renal tubule to produce the 1-alpha hydroxyvitamin D. The latter changes will result in altered calcium absorption from the intestinal tract and release of parathyroid hormone with subsequent leaching of calcium from the bones. Most children with hypocalcemia are asymptomatic. Rarely will tetany, seizures, or arrhythmias be seen; if they are, an infusion of calcium gluconate can be given. One should also be aware that correction of acidosis may worsen hypocalcemia,[17,23,24] since alkalinization of the blood will lead to binding of calcium to plasma proteins. Seizures in renal failure patients are generally due to hyponatremia (serum sodium < 110), hypoglycemia, and/or hypocalcemia.[17]

TABLE 2.   Causes of Renal Failure

Prerenal	Intrinsic Renal (Renal)	Postrenal
Decreased plasma volume	Congenital	Posterior urethral valves
Dehydration	Hypoplasia	Ureterovesical junction obstruction
Sepsis	Dysplasia	(bilateral)
Decreased renal perfusion	Vascular lesions	Ureteropelvic junction obstruction
Hypoxia	Renal artery thrombosis	(bilateral, solitary kidney)
Shock	Renal venous thrombosis	Urethral diverticulum
Heart failure	Ischemic injury	
	Shock	
	Hemorrhage	
	Sepsis	
	Interstitial nephrotoxic drugs	
	Antibiotics	
	Nonsteroidals	
	Uric Acid	

Hypertension may also be encountered in certain renal failure states, most commonly in acute glomerulonephritis and hemolytic uremic syndrome.[25]

Causes of renal failure in various age groups are shown in Table 2. In a neonate, the causes of renal failure can be divided into intrinsic or postrenal disorders. The latter are generally due to obstruction secondary to a congenital abnormality (bilateral uretero-pelvic junction obstruction, uretero-vesico junction obstruction, posterior urethral valves, or urethral diverticulum). A rare imperforate prepuce or a neurogenic bladder secondary to a meningomyelocele may lead to postrenal failure. In most instances, either a palpable mass or palpable bladder will be noted. A history of polyhydramnios may be obtained or there may be a history of an abnormal in-utero ultrasound. Pneumothorax without a clear-cut underlying etiology often indicates an underlying renal problem. The bladder, therefore, must be catheterized. Prompt attention also must be given to metabolic and electrolyte abnormalities.

Intrinsic causes of renal failure in the neonate include sepsis, dehydration, shock, and hemorrhage. Renal vein thrombosis, renal artery thrombosis, and renal failure secondary to nephrotoxic agents such as aminoglycosides and indomethacin can also be observed. On rare occasion, polycystic kidney disease or renal dysplasia may cause renal failure. Any of these disorders may initially present in the prerenal state. Thus, serum and urine chemistries must promptly be obtained. One or more fluid challenges with crystalloid (normal saline or lactated Ringer's solution) or colloid should be considered if volume depletion is suspected. Loop diuretics or dopamine in renal perfusion doses should be administered based on clinical and laboratory data.

Of the diarrheal diseases, hyponatremic diarrheal dehydration is rare. The majority of children with dehydration secondary to a diarrheal illness will have isotonic dehydration. Hypernatremic hydration, however, is associated with the highest incidence of complications (morbidity and mortality). Fortunately this illness occurs in only 10% of children. It is most commonly noted in colder climates and is usually related to the administration of high solute to solvent containing solution when a warm interior is increasing insensible losses. One should appreciate certain unique features of these children. Their skin tends to be doughy, leading one to underestimate the severity of the dehydration. However, the mucous membranes will appear dry. These children tend to lie still unless stimulated. They are then extremely irritable. Hypernatremic dehydration implies at least 10% dehydration by the time of arrival at the hospital.[26] If the patient is mottled or pale, dehydration may have approached 15%.

The serum sodium should be reduced at a rate no greater than 0.5 mEq sodium/hour if the sodium level is greater than 160. If seen at the time of transport and if fluid resuscitation is necessary, normal saline, lactated Ringer's, and/or 5% albumin should be given.[26,27] After urine output is established, then and only then would one switch hydration solutions to the generally more dilute solutions commonly administered. As a rule, correction of the dehydration in the hypernatremic patient is over 48–72 hours. The goal is to prevent seizures and intracranial hemorrhage. Concomitant electrolyte disorders include hypocalcemia and hypokalemia. Occasionally hyperglycemia and acidosis are present.

Severe crush injuries, heat stroke, or extensive electrical burns can produce rhabdomyolysis, which may also lead to renal failure by myoglobin becoming trapped in the renal tubules. Prompt institution of an alkaline solute diuresis will prevent acute renal failure since myoglobin goes into solution if the pH in the urine is > 6.5. Concomitant evaluation for associated electrolyte abnormalities, hypo- or hypercalcemia, hypokalemia or hyperkalemia, hyperuricemia, or hyperphosphatemia are important.[28]

HEMOLYTIC UREMIC SYNDROME

One of the more unique causes of acute renal failure in children is hemolytic uremic syndrome.[29,30] This condition is generally seen in outbreaks with a typical gastrointestinal prodrome (vomiting, diarrhea, often bloody) most commonly due to the verotoxin-producing *E. coli* 0157:H7. However, other agents can also produce this condition and on rare occasion, it may be seen in families without the typical prodromal illness. In addition. *S. pneumoniae* or other neuraminidase-producing organisms can produce an atypical hemolytic uremic syndrome.

The prognosis for familial type of hemolytic uremic syndrome not occurring during outbreaks or in those presenting with an atypical illness is generally poor, with end-stage renal disease developing. Prompt attention to electrolyte and acid-base disorders and concomitant complications such as hypertension or a rapidly rising BUN and creatinine is imperative. Early institution of dialysis is the key to management. Administration of packed red blood cells is instituted only if the hemoglobin is < 7. One should then use CMV-negative, washed or leukocyte poor, packed RBC's. Platelet administration is rarely, if ever, necessary in these children. Central nervous system complications and late GI complications, including stricture and perforation or ischemic bowel, can occur.

ACUTE GLOMERULONEPHRITIS

Acute glomerulonephritis can present with oliguric renal failure. Hypertension often complicates the course. Electrolyte problems, including hyponatremia, hyperkalemia, acidosis, hypocalcemia, and hyperphosphatemia are often present. Typically, such patients have an antecedent illness (viral or streptococcal) and a history of gross hematuria. They often will have gained excessive weight and have a decline in urine output and, depending on the degree of elevation of BUN and creatinine, may have alterations in their appetite and activity. Prompt recognition of these conditions and early institution of therapy for the various complications may prevent further difficulties and result in a shortened acute illness.[17]

HYPERTENSIVE EMERGENCIES

Hypertensive emergencies may also be encountered by the transport team and need to be adressed promptly and appropriately. Hypertensive emergency implies an immediate threat (within hours) to one or more vital organ systems (kidneys, heart, brain, or eyes). In such instances, evidence of target organ damage will often be present on exam. A history may be elicited of altered sensorium, visual disturbances, changes in patient's cardiopulmonary status, or urine output. Among the causes of hypertensive emergencies or hypertensive encephalopathy or accelerated (malignant) hypertension are acute glomerulonephritis, reflux nephropathy, renovascular hypertension, acute renal failure with fluid overload, pheochromocytoma, coarctation of the aorta, or hemolytic uremic syndrome.[25] Accelerated hypertension can also be observed in the renal transplant patient. Prompt therapy in an intensive care setting is necessary. Stabilization of the patient's hypertension prior to transport is essential. Although one wants to treat the hypertension and thus lower the pressure as promptly as possible, precipitous lowering of the blood pressure should be avoided to prevent alterations in cerebral blood flow, which could cause ischemic injury. Drugs of choice are generally those that allow minute-to-minute control. For transport purposes, labetalol or perhaps nicardipine may be the preferred choices.[25] Nitroprusside may be difficult to administer in a transport setting, but certainly would be considered a drug of choice in an ICU setting. The dosing ranges, mechanism of action, and adverse effect profile are shown in Table 3. An arterial line is generally considered essential for the administration of nitroprusside, but is not essential for the administration of labetalol or nicardipine.[25]

TABLE 3. Drugs Used in Hypertensive Emergencies or Urgencies

Preferred Drugs	Dose	Mechanism of Action	Onset of Action	Duration of Action	Adverse Effects and Disadvantages
First-line					
Nitroprusside	0.5–10 μg/kg/min IV	Direct arteriolar and venous vasodilator	Immediate	Only during infusion	Cyanide and thiocyanate toxicity, chest pain, headaches
Labetalol	0.5–3 mg/kg/h IV	α/β-Receptor blocker	Within minutes	Up to 24 hr after end of infusion	GI upset, headaches, scalp tingling, dizziness
Diazoxide	(1) 1–2 mg/kg/dose IV over 30 sec q10–15 min (2) 0.25–10.5 mg/kg/min IV (max 300 mg/kg/20 min)	Direct arteriolar vasodilator	Within minutes	Up to 24 hr	Hyperglycemia, hyperuricemia, salt and water retention, and acute hypotension
Phentolamine	0.1–0.2 mg/kg	α-Blocker (for pheochromocytoma)	Immediate	30–60 min	Tachycardia, abdominal pain, nausea, vomiting, hypotension
Nicardipine	0.1 μg/kg/min	Calcium channel blocker	Immediate	During infusion?	Flushing, tachycardia, headache

Table continued on following page.

TABLE 3. Drugs Used in Hypertensive Emergencies or Urgencies (*Continued*)

Preferred Drugs	Dose	Mechanism of Action	Onset of Action	Duration of Action	Adverse Effects and Disadvantages
Second-line					
Nifedipine	0.25–0.5 mg/kg/PO (max 20 mg) q4–6h	Calcium channel blocker	20–30 min	4–6 hr	Dizziness, facial flushing, paresthesias, headaches
Hydralazine*	(1) 0.1–0.5 mg/kg IV (max 25 mg) (2) 0.1 mg/kg bolus; then 1.5 mg/kg/ min (max 5 mg/ kg/min)	Direct arteriolar vasodilator	30 min	4–12 hr	Tachycardia, headaches, flushing, vomiting, hypotension
Propranolol	0.1–0.05 mg/kg IV over 1 hr (max 10 mg) q6–8h	β-Receptor antagonist	Immediate for heart rate	Up to 8 hr, 24 hr for blood pressure	Bradycardia, bronchospasm in predisposed individuals
Esmolol	100–300 µg/kg/min	β-Receptor antagonist	Immediate	Up to 8 min, 24 min for blood pressure	Bradycardia, bronchospasm in predisposed individuals
Furosemide	1–4 mg/kg IV 16–8h	Loop diuretic	5 min	2–3 hr	Electrolyte imbalance, hearing deficit, hyperglycemia
Captopril	Age < 6 mo; 0.05–0.5 mg/kg PO q8–12h Age > 6 mo; 0.3–2 mg/kg PO q8–12 h	ACE inhibitor	15 min	8–12 hr	Leukopenia (dysgeusia), rash, reversible renal failure
Enalaprilat	0.01–0.32 mgt/kg IV q6h	ACE inhibitor	20 min	6 hr	Leukopenia, reversible renal failure
Methyldopa	10 mg/kg/day IV or PO divided q6h	Centrally acting agent	20 min	6–8 hrs	Drowsiness, hemolytic anemia, hepatitis, depression

* Used initially for afterload reduction
Abbreviations: ACE = angiotensin converting enzyme; GI = gastrointestinal, IV = intravenous; min = minutes, mo = months; PO = oral; qxh = every x hours; qxmin = every x minutes; yr = years.

Urgent hypertension implies a potential risk of vital organ damage. Evidence of target organ damage may be absent or minimal. The blood pressure elevation may be significant but rarely produces symptoms. Generally, this is seen in postoperative patients who have undergone orthopedic, renal, or vascular procedures. Agents that can be used in such a situation often do not require close monitoring and include nifedipine, captopril, or IV enalapril. They have a slower onset of action (20–30 minutes). Nifedipine may cause more precipitous falls in pressure, and its duration of action is less predictable than those of the aforementioned agents. Dosing range, frequency of administration, and adverse effects are shown in Table 3.[25,31,32] If no reduction in blood pressure occurs within 30–60 minutes, the dose may be repeated or increased. On occasion, diuretics may be given (judiciously) to patients with significant hypertension. In the patient with a renal transplant, cyclosporin levels should be drawn since cyclosporin toxicity can cause hypertension and alter renal function. Renal artery stenosis must also be suspected in such patients. A renal scan can be ordered to look at perfusion of the kidney if time permits; BUN and creatinine should also be obtained. Acute rejection and/or renal artery stenosis could also account for the elevated pressures and the elevated BUN and creatinine.[25]

Thus, the management of patients with renal related problems is rather complex. A careful history and physical exam is imperative in order to recognize potentially life-threatening but correctable abnormalities.

REFERENCES

1. Corey HE, Spitzer A: Renal blood flow and glomerular filtration rate during development. In Edelmann CM Jr (ed): Pediatric Kidney Disease. Boston, Little Brown, 1992, pp 49–78.
2. Finberg L: Properties of water, ions, solutions and cells. In Finberg L, Kraveth RE, Fleischman AR (eds): Water and Electrolytes in Pediatrics. Philadelphia, W.B. Saunders, 1993, pp 2–10.
3. Finberg L: Water metabolism and regulation. In Finberg L, Kraveth, RE, Fleischman AR: Water and Electrolytes in Pediatrics. Philadelphia, W.B. Saunders, 1993, pp 17–21.
4. Hellerstein S: Renal physiology and renal regulation of water and electrolytes. In Finberg L, Kraveth RE, Fleischman AR (eds): Water and Electrolytes in Pediatrics. Philadelphia, W.G. Saunders, 1993, pp 50–67.
5. Schwartz GJ: Acid-base homeostasis. In Edelmann CM Jr (ed): Pediatric Kidney Disease. Boston, Little, Brown, 1992, pp 201–230.
6. Spitzer A, Aperia A: The renal transport of sodium and chloride. In Edelmann CM Jr (ed): pediatric Kidney Disease. Boston, Little, Brown, 1992, pp 93–126.
7. Kraveth RE: Asthma. In Finberg L, Kraveth AE, Fleischman AR (eds): Water and Electrolytes in Pediatrics. Philadelphia, W.B. Saunders, 1993, pp 235–239.
8. Kraveth RE: Heart failure. In Finberg L, Kraveth RE, Fleischman AR (ed): Water and Electrolytes in Pediatrics,. Philadelphia, W.B.Saunders, 1993, pp 215–220,
9. Barken RM, Rosen P: Congenital heart failure. In Barkin RM, Rosen P (eds): Emergency Pediatr. St. Louis, Mosby, 1994, pp 129–139.
10. Wells TG: The pharmacology and therapeutics of diuretics in the pediatric patient. Pediatr Clin North Am 37:463–504, 1990.
11. May JM, et al: Special problems of fluid and electrolyte metabolism in diabetic patients. In Chan JCM, Gill JR Jr (eds): Kidney Electrolyte Disorders. New York, Churchill Livingstone, 1990, pp 363–420.
12. Barkin RM, Rosen R: Dehydration. In Barkin RM, Rosen R (eds): Emergency Pediatrics. St. Louis, Mosby, 1994, pp 60–68.
13. Miller K: Personal communication.
14. Berns AS, Linas SL, Miller TR, et al: Urinary diagnostic indices in acute renal failure: Usefulness of diagnostic indices. Kidney Int 10:495, 1976.
15. Mathew OP, Jones AS, Jones E, et al: Neonatal renal failure: Usefulness of diagnostic indices. Pediatrics 65:57, 1980.
16. Anderson RJ, Lings SL, Berns AS, et al: Nonacute renal failure. N Engl J Med 96:1134–1138, 1977.
17. Long S, Gaudio KM, Siegel NJ: Non-dialytic treatment of acute renal failure. In Edelmann CM Jr (ed): Pediatric Kidney Disease. Boston, Little, Brown, 1992, pp 801–814.
18. Wesson DE: Disorders of potassium metabolism. In Greenberg A (ed): Primer on Kidney Diseases. Academic Press, 1994, pp 398–406.
19. Wesson DE: Hyperchloremic metabolic acidosis. In Adrogue HJ (ed): Acid Base and Electrolyte Disorders. New York, Churchill Livingstone, 1991, pp 97–116.
20. Battle DC: Metabolic Acidosis. In Greenberg A (ed): Primer on Kidney Diseases. Academic Press, 1994, pp 372–381.
21. Palevsky PM, Cox M: Disorders of sodium and water homeostasis. In Mandal AK, Jennette JC (eds): Diagnosis and Management of Renal Disease and Hypertension. Academic Press, 1994, pp 33–70.
22. Finberg L: Pathophysiology of hyponatremic states. In Finberg L, Kraveth SE, Hellerstein S (eds): Water and Electrolytes. Philadelphia, W.B. Saunders, 1993, pp 120–123.
23. Finberg L: Calcium, phosphorus and magnesium metabolism and regulation. In Finberg L, Kraveth SE, Hellerstein S (eds): Water and Electrolytes. Philadelphia, W.B. Saunders, 1993, pp 73–82.
24. Bushinsky DA: Homeostasis and disorders of calcium and phosphorus concentration. In Greenberg A (eds): Primer on Kidney Diseases. Academic Press, 1994, pp 406–413.

25. Miller K: Pharmacological management of hypertension in pediatric patients. Drugs 48:869–887, 1994.
26. Finberg L: Hypernatremic dehydration. In Finberg L, Kraveth SE, Hellerstein S (eds): Water and Electrolytes. Philadelphia, W.B. Saunders, 1993, pp 124–134.
27. Sterns RH, Narins RG: Hypernatremia and hyponatremia: Pathophysiology, diagnosis, and therapy. In Androgue HG (ed): Acid Base and Electrolyte Disorders. New York, Churchill Livingstone, 1991, pp 161–191.
28. Knochhel JP: Pigment nephropathy. In Greenberg A (eds): Primer on Kidney Diseases. Academic Press, 1994, pp 149–152.
29. Miller K, Kim Y: Hemolytic uremic syndrome. In Holliday M, Barratt TM, Vernier RL (eds): Pediatric Nephrology. Baltimore, Williams & Wilkins, 1987, pp 482–491.
30. Kaplan BS, Levin M, et al: The hemolytic uremic syndrome. In Edelmann CM Jr (ed): Pediatric Kidney Disease. Boston, Little, Brown, 1992, pp 1383–1398.
31. Farene M, Arbus GS: Management of hypertensive emergencies in children. Pediatr Emerg Care 5:51–55, 1989.
32. Dilmen U, Cagler MK, Senser A, et al: Nifedipine in hypertensive emergencies of children. Am J Dis Child 137:1162–1165, 1983.

CHAPTER 22

Poisoning, Ingestion, and Overdose

CURT M. STEINHART, M.D.
ANTHONY L. PEARSON-SHAVER, M.D.

Poisoning continues to be an important cause of morbidity for children in the United States. Of the 1,581,540 poison exposures reported by the 1989 Annual Report of the American Association of Poison Control Centers,[25] two-thirds occurred in children less than 13 years of age. Most accidentally poisoned children are toddlers.[25] Intentional poisonings due to substance abuse and suicide attempts remain a major problem among older children and adolescents. Transport teams must be familiar with symptom complexes associated with certain intoxications. In addition, transport team personnel should maintain a high index of suspicion for intoxications as the cause of conditions otherwise not explained.

HISTORY

The history is the single most important aspect in evaluating a poisoned patient. In several recent studies, history alone identified 85–90% of the toxic agents,[12,39] making extensive toxicologic screening unnecessary. A careful and detailed interview of caretakers or witnesses may be all that is needed for a clinical diagnosis. Questions to ask about poisoned patients include:

1. What toxic agents or medications were found near the patient?
2. What medications are in the home?
3. What approximate amount of the toxic agent was ingested?
4. How much of the agent was available before the ingestion?
5. How much of the agent remained after the ingestion?
6. When did the ingestion occur?
7. Were there characteristic odors at the scene of the ingestion?
8. Was the patient alert upon discovery?
9. Has the patient remained alert since the ingestion?
10. How has the patient behaved since the ingestion?
11. Does the patient have a history of substance abuse?

PHYSICAL FINDINGS

Central Nervous System Findings

Both trauma and poisoning often present with signs of central nervous system (CNS) depression. Therefore the possibility of trauma must be considered.

This is of particular concern in the unconscious adolescent patient. Evaluation of the cervical spine should be carried out. Patients poisoned by CNS depressants tend to present with consistent findings. Initially following the poisoning, cerebral function may be unaffected while vestibular and cerebellar functions become altered. This may result in nystagmus, ataxia, and/or dysarthria. Impaired consciousness may ensue later.

Central nervous system depressants may affect brainstem and somatic reflexes. Depression of oculocephalic (doll's eyes), oculovestibular (cold caloric response), and stetch reflexes may occur. If muscle tone is affected, patients may present with flaccidity. Pupillary light reflexes and ciliospinal reflexes tend to be resistant to most intoxicants and usually are preserved. CNS depressants cause symmetrical impairment of function, which may further assist in differentiating intoxication from trauma in which focal effects may be present.

Sometimes delirium and psychosis are features of poisoning and can provide clues to the toxic agent.[33] Delirium is a state of altered sensorium characterized by extreme motor and mental excitation, defective perception, impaired memory, and rapid succession of confused and unconnected ideas. Delirious patients are disoriented and confused and may have visual hallucinations. Delirium may be seen in anticholinergic poisoning.

Patients with psychosis have an intact sensorium. Psychosis is manifested by gross distortion or disorganization of a person's mental capacity, affective responses, capacity to recognize reality, and ability to communicate. Psychosis interferes with one's ability to cope with the demands of daily life. Psychotic patients may present with auditory hallucinations, illusions, and paranoia. Stimulants such as amphetamines and cocaine frequently cause psychosis.

Pupillary responses (Table 1) and gaze preferences can indicate the level of injury, which helps further differentiation between structural and toxic injury. Sluggish or absent pupillary responses indicate brainstem injury. Pupillary dilation can be caused by lesions in the midbrain or ipsilateral third nerve or by drugs such as atropine and scopolamine. Pupillary constriction can be caused by opioids and barbiturates as well as by lesions in the pons, medulla, spinal cord, and hypothalamus.

Respiratory Findings

Poisons can cause respiratory failure by central respiratory depression or respiratory muscle failure or both. Opioids, barbiturates, and benzodiazepines depress brainstem respiratory and reticular activating system function. Virtually

TABLE 1. Pupillary Changes Caused by Central Nervous System Lesions and Drugs

Lesion/Drug	Size	Reactive/Nonreactive
Midbrain (tectal)	Dilation	Nonreactive
Ipsilateral third nerve	Dilation	Nonreactive
Atropine	Dilation	Nonreactive
Scopolamine	Dilation	Nonreactive
Pons	Constriction	Reactive
Medulla	Constriction	Reactive
Spinal cord	Constriction	Reactive
Hypothalamus	Constriction	Reactive
Opioids	Constriction	Reactive
Barbiturates	Constriction	Nonreactive
Glutethimide	Midpoint	Fixed pupils, frequently unequal

all CNS depressants cause coma before respiratory depression. Respiratory muscle failure may be caused by neuromuscular blocking agents, organophosphates, or rapid administration of fentanyl. Neuromuscular blocking agents cause competitive neuromuscular blockade at the motor endplate. Organophosphates bind acetylcholinesterases, increasing acetylcholine at nicotinic receptors and resulting in skeletal muscle failure. When administered rapidly, fentanyl causes intercostal muscle rigidity.

Several drugs may cause respiratory stimulation. Salicylates, amphetamines, cocaine, and caffeine are central respiratory stimulants. Central stimulants affect the medullary respiratory center[33] and increase both respiratory rate and depth. Respiratory stimulation can occur as a result of metabolic acidosis as seen with carbon monoxide and cyanide poisoning.

Cardiovascular Findings

Hypotension and dysrhythmias are frequent findings in poisoned patients. Patients poisoned by opoids, barbiturates, and tricyclic antidepressants frequently develop hypotension. Blood pressure and perfusion should be aggressively monitored in these patients. Digoxin, cocaine, methylxanthines, and tricyclic compounds may produce cardiac dysrhythmias, which must always be monitored and then treated as necessary.

Certain dysrhythmias, including supraventricular tachycardia, ventricular tachycardia, conduction delays, and bradycardia have each been described in poisoned patients (Table 2). Tachydysrhythmias result from increased sympathetic tone, inhibition of cholinergic tone, enhanced ventricular irritability, and re-entry phenomena. Conduction delays may result in a prolonged QRS due to slow ventricular depolarization or from prolongation of the QT interval. Bradydysrhythmias are the result of decreased sympathetic tone, increased cholinergic tone, or decreased ventricular automaticity.

TABLE 2. Dysrhythmias in Poisoned Patients

Type of Dysrhythmia	Mechanism	Causative Toxins
Tachydysrhythmias	Increased sympathetic tone	Methylxanthines
		Caffeine
		Theophylline
	Inhibition of cholinergic tone	Anticholinergics
	Enhanced ventricular irritability	Amphetamines
		Cocaine
	Re-entry phenomena	Tricyclic antidepressants
		Digoxin
Conduction delays	Prolongation of the QRS	Tricyclic antidepressants
		Phenothiazines
		Quinidine
		Procalnamide
	Prolongation of the QT interval	Tricyclic antidepressants
		Type I antidysrhythmics
		Phenothiazines
		Digoxin
Bradycardia	Decreased sympathetic tone	Beta blockers
	Increased cholinergic tone	Organophosphates
		Physostigmine
		Digoxin
	Decreased ventricular automaticity	Lidocaine
		Lithium

Movement Disorders

Movement abnormalities can be helpful when identifying toxic agents. Poisoned patients may present with muscular weakness, flaccidity, hyperkinesis, or seizures. One should observe the symmetry, quantity, control, and strength of the muscular activity. Poisoned patients and those with metabolic disease tend to display symmetrical movements. Asymmetry suggests a localized lesion consistent with a structural abnormality.

Poisoned patients commonly present with seizures. Toxic causes of seizures include theophylline, tricyclic antidepressants, isoniazid, amphetamines, phencyclidine, and cocaine. Seizures following tricyclic antidepressant ingestion are frequently preceded by a widened QRS.[5] Theophylline-induced seizures frequently are difficult to control.[32] Reduction of the theophylline level is the most effective means. Charcoal hemoperfusion or repeated doses of activated charcoal are effective methods to reduce the serum theophylline level. Isoniazid-induced seizures require pyridoxine for control. Cyanide, fluoride, and organophosphate poisonings each require specific antidotes to control seizures.

Dopaminergic blockade results in rigidity, bradykinesia, and parkinsonian posturing. Antipsychotic agents, metoclopramide, and 1-methyl-4-phenyl-1,2,5,6-tetrahydropyridine (MPTP) cause dopaminergic blockade. MPTP is found as a contaminant of illegal opioid synthesis and may cause permanent parkinsonism by destroying cells in the substantia nigra.[1]

Hyperkinesis manifests as rigidity, dyskinesia, myoclonus, or chorea. Drugs used to treat dystonia (e.g., anticholinergics and antihistamines) may cause dyskinesia[4] Hyperkinetic dyskinesias (e.g., myoclonic jerks, twitching, facial grimacing, head tossing, and rapid tongue movements) are caused by increased dopaminergic activity. Levodopa, amphetamines, tricyclic antidepressants, anticholinergics, and antihistamines increase dopaminergic activity.[33]

Muscular rigidity can be caused by many mechanisms. Black-widow bites cause neurotransmitter release, persistent muscular contraction, and localized painful rigidity.[33] Strychnine poisoning interferes with inhibitory neurons in the spinal cord.[50] Patients are alert but rigid and unable to move.

Toxidromes

Anticholinergic poisoning is a common toxidrome that presents following ingestion of tricyclic antidepressants, phenothiazines, antihistamines, and anti-parkinsonism agents. Anticholinergic poisoning can present with psychosis, tachycardia, mydriasis, vasodilation, hyperpyrexia, ileus, urinary retention, decreased salivation, decreased sweating, amnesia, agitation, and seizures. Excessive anticholinergic activity may occur when treating organophosphate poisoning with atropine.

The cholinergic toxidrome is caused by agents that poison serum and red blood cell cholinesterases, leading to increased cholinergic activity. It is seen with organophosphate insecticides, carbamates, and nicotine. Patients present with a decreased level of consciousness, pinpoint pupils, fasciculations, incontinence, salivation, bronchorrhea, lacrimation, and bradycardia.

Opioid intoxication frequently presents with a symptom complex consisting of depressed sensorium, hypotension, hypothermia, and pinpoint pupils. Patients who have ingested Lomotil or Darvon present similarly.

Cocaine causes tachypnea, agitation, and occasionally hallucinations (see below). Unlike patients poisoned by opioids, cocaine abusers manifest with dilated pupils. Hemodynamic consequences may result in sudden death. Tachycardia, tachydysrhythmias, and hypertension may be noted. Poisonings from methyl-xanthines (theophylline and caffeine) and amphetamines present with symptoms similar to those of cocaine.

Patients poisoned by sedatives or hypnotics present with depressed sensorium, depressed ventilation, dilated pupils, hypotension, decreased reflexes, and hypothermia.

MONITORING AND LABORATORY TESTS

Cardiorespiratory monitoring is essential as many agents cause disturbances of cardiac rhythm and respiratory function. It is essential to monitor repeatedly each patient's level of consciousness, responsiveness to various stimuli, and the character of their motor movements. Pupillary size and reactivity should be monitored as well. Blood pressure must be monitored continuously. Every poisoned patient will not require arterial catheterization, but blood pressure should be followed very frequently, using noninvasive methods during transport even in those cases having seemingly trivial ingestions. Ideally, oxygen saturation should be monitored during transport to a tertiary care center. Oxygen saturation measured by pulse oximetry is a sensitive indicator of impending respiratory failure.

Metabolic derangements should be carefully assessed by evaluating serum electrolytes and arterial blood gases. Significant derangements should be treated. Measuring serum levels of the ingested agent may be appropriate in certain circumstances, as might serum or urine drug screening. Delays in obtaining serum levels in referring hospitals may be substantial. Delaying departure from the referring hospital while awaiting serum levels or screening test results is unwarranted. As previously mentioned, the history is a more important method of identifying toxic agents than toxicologic screens.[9] Even when initial clinical impressions and toxicologic assays disagree, discovery of an unexpected agent rarely leads to changes in therapy. Numerous accounts suggest that toxicologic screening is not a diagnostic panacea. Before ordering a battery of tests, the physician should determine which toxic agents are the most likely. History, prevalence of drugs in the community, and physical examination will be most helpful in guiding the selection. Toxicologic assays may require large sample volumes and may be time-consuming and expensive. The more the clinician can narrow the scope, the greater the likelihood of success.

TREATMENT

Transport teams should remember that the general precepts for resuscitation and stabilization apply to the poisoned patient as well. *It is more important to treat the patient than the poison.* One must first stop any deterioration in the patient's condition and treat life-threatening problems and organ failure. An efficient resuscitation-oriented physical examination must be performed with attention to airway patency, ventilation, and perfusion. Upper airway obstruction may occur as a result of pharyngeal muscle relaxation in patients poisoned by opioids, barbiturates, and sedatives. Emesis may result in upper airway obstruction by gastric contents.

The goals of treatment for any poisoning are to limit toxin absorption, enhance toxin elimination, and provide supportive care until the toxic effects of the substance resolve.[46] Emetics, gastric lavage, activated charcoal, and cathartics are currently used to remove toxic agents from the gastrointestinal tract and limit absorption. Antidotes are available for some toxic agents and are discussed below.

Gastric Decontamination

Several recent reports[6,20,21,40,41] suggest that traditional methods of removing gastric contents are ineffective. Induced emesis using syrup of ipecac and gastric lavage fail to remove gastric contents completely when used for gastric decontamination.[40,41] For greatest utility, syrup of ipecac should be administered soon after ingestion,[6,21] as it appears to have less effect if administered after 90 minutes. Some authors believe that early administration of ipecac may delay administration of activated charcoal,[20] which may be superior in its ability to remove toxins by limiting absorption. The case for using ipecac in children, however, remains strong. Children who are accidentally poisoned usually present for treatment within 2 hours of ingestion,[12] and many poisons delay gastric motility. Because children frequently vomit as a result of the initial ingestion and ingest nontoxic substances and nontoxic amounts of toxic substances, the need for aggressive gastric emptying is limited.[36] Emesis is contraindicated with most hydrocarbons, when rapid onset of CNS depression is likely, and for infants less than 6 months old.[36]

Gastric lavage accomplishes gastric emptying by instillation of a liquid through an orogastric or nasogastric tube with subsequent drainage. Lavage is indicated if the patient has a depressed sensorium, cannot protect the airway, or is actively convulsing. If the patient has ingested an agent that might rapidly lead to convulsions or CNS depression,[22] gastric lavage should be considered. In addition, gastric lavage offers the ability to alter a toxin's bioavailability.[22] In adults, lavage is most effective when performed within an hour of the ingestion. Lavage is contraindicated when there is a reliable history of an insignificant ingestion,[22] alkali or acid ingestions, hydrocarbons, or when ingested particles exceed the luminal size of the largest orogastric tube that can be placed.[36] It should be noted that gastric lavage is more difficult in very young children and that indications for lavage in this group of patients are less clear. Treatment delays significantly diminish the usefulness of gastric lavage. A postingestion time of more than 3 hours has been said to limit its effectiveness severely.[22] More time is allowed if the ingested substance delays gastric emptying and/or is neurotoxic.

Once the airway is secured and the largest possible orogastric or nasogastric tube is placed, patients being lavaged should be positioned with the left side down. Lavage should be started with warm normal saline in small aliquots. Hyponatremia and hypothermia have been noted with improper lavage fluids. Therefore, lavage should be performed with a warm isotonic solution. Warm fluid may delay gastric emptying and improve yield.[22] Lavage is safest when performed by gravity drainage, but manual lavage is more commonly employed. Forceful instillation and large volumes of fluid can push material through the pylorus and aid absorption. The procedure should be continued until the contents are clear and particulate matter is no longer noted. Caution must be exercised during placement of the lavage tube because esophageal or gastric perforation can occur.

Activated Charcoal

Activated charcoal is a product of the pyrolysis of various organic compounds. "Activation" is achieved by exposing the residue to oxidizing agents and high temperatures.[36] Activation increases the adsorptive capacity of the residue by removing impurities and increasing surface area. Essentially, it places a number of depressions on the particle's surface, similar to the "dimples" on a golf ball.

Charcoal alone is as effective as ipecac or gastric lavage,[21] while some studies suggest that it might be more effective.[9,31,47] Activated charcoal can be given either in a single dose or multiple doses. Multiple doses of activated charcoal have been noted to reduce the half-life of carbamazepine,[30] phenylbutazone,[30] phenobarbital,[3] theophylline,[2] digoxin,[34] digitoxin,[34] desmethyldoxepin,[42] nodalol,[11] and sotalol.[19] Drug elimination is enhanced for compounds that undergo enterohepatic recirculation. Activated charcoal in the gastrointestinal tract adsorbs the portion of the compound that is secreted or passively diffused back into the gastric or intestinal lumen.[2,3,23]

Ionization, characteristics of certain toxic agents, and gastric motility alter the ability of activated charcoal to adsorb toxins. Nonionized particles bind more readily to charcoal than do ionized particles.[36] Activated charcoal is less effective on agents highly ionized at gastric pH (mineral acid, alkali, boric acid, cyanide, iron, and lithium ingestions). Gastric motility determines whether any toxin is available for adsorption.[30] If gastric motility is depressed, more toxin is available. Delays in charcoal administration beyond 60 minutes have been shown to diminish its usefulness.[10] Many toxins slow gastric emptying and preserve charcoal's beneficial effects.[48]

Doses of 15–30 grams for small children and 50–100 grams for larger children and adolescents are recommended. Alternatively, 1–2 gm/kg body weight may be used. The charcoal may be given as a slurry with water, but is often combined with the cathartic sorbitol. Cherry syrup, chocolate syrup, saccharin, fructose, and sucrose all have been used as flavoring agents without compromising charcoal's adsorptive capacity. Except for the flavoring agents mentioned, mixing charcoal with foods before administration decreases its adsorptive capacity and thus its effectiveness.[48]

Specific Antidotes

Table 3 lists certain toxins and their antidotes.

SPECIFIC DRUG INGESTION AND TOXICITY

Aspirin

Salicylate poisoning in children has decreased markedly over the past several decades because of alterations in packaging and product safety information. The statistical relationship between aspirin use and Reye syndrome has received substantial public attention. Acetaminophen and more recently ibuprofen are recommended for common causes of minor pain and fever. Despite a reduction in poisoning occurrences, aspirin and other salicylates are still widely available and continue to be important causes of pediatric poisonings.

Following oral ingestion, aspirin is rapidly absorbed in the upper small intestine and also in the stomach. Absorption rates are influenced by type of preparation, gastric pH, and rates of gastric empting. High luminal pH slows absorption as does the presence of food in the stomach.[45] Aspirin becomes distributed throughout most body tissues, including the brain and CSF. Peak plasma levels usually occur within 8–12 hours following ingestion, but with very large doses peak levels may not be reached until 24 hours.[13] Extensive protein binding occurs, which may slow blood-brain barrier transport.

Hepatic metabolism occurs through glycine conjugation, glucuronidation, and oxidation. At normal pH, about 10% is excreted renally in unchanged form. In alkaline urine, excretion of unchanged drug may increase to 30%, while an

TABLE 3.   Selected Toxins and Their Antidotes

Toxin	Antidote
Opioids	Naloxone: <20 kg use 0.1 mg/kg IV
Morphine	or 0.2–0.5 mg/kg ET
Heroin	>20 kg use 2.0 mg IV
Methadone	or 5 mg ET
Meperidine	
Lomotil	Repeat as often as necessary; if repeated doses are needed, may give as
Fentanyl	continuous IV infusion at 0.1–0.2 mg/kg/hr
Codeine	
Digitalis	Digibind: per package insert; 1 vial = 40 mg Fab fragments, which will bind 0.6 mg
Digoxin	digoxin; to determine number of vials for known amount ingested, use:
Digitoxin	No. vials = digoxin load in mg/0.6
	or
	No vials = digoxin level (ng/ml) × wt (kg)/100
Benzodiazepines	Flumazenil: avoid using if benzodiazepine used in conjunction with tricyclic
Diazepam	antidepressants as seizures may develop
Lorazepam	Dose: 0.2 mg (2 ml) IV over 30 sec, may increase at 1-minute intervals to 0.3 mg
Midazolam	and then 0.5 mg to total dose of 3 mg; no per kg dose has been established
Methemoglobinemia	Dose: 1.0–2.0 mg/kg slow IV; prepare as 1% solution (1 mg/dl) in 0.9% normal
Methylene blue	saline
Organophosphate	Pralidoxime
Acetaminophen	N-acetylcysteine
Iron	Deferoxamine

acidic urine may decrease the amount excreted to as low as 2%.[14] At usual therapeutic doses, elimination follows first-order kinetics, and the half-life is 2–3 hours, but with massive overdoses elimination is by zero-order kinetics and the half-life may increase to as long as 30 hours.[17]

Physiologic derangements from aspirin poisoning are complex and variable. Not all mechanisms of intoxication are well understood. Aspirin may uncouple oxidative phosphorylation, leading to altered heat production and lactic acidosis. As a cyclooxygenase inhibitor, aspirin reduces thromboxane and prostacyclin formation. Amino acid metabolism is inhibited and glucose metabolism is stimulated, with increases in both gluconeogenesis and glycolysis. This in turn may stimulate lipid metabolism and ketone formation. Initial hyperglycemia may be followed by hypoglycemia. As CSF glucose levels fall, respiratory depression may ensue. Vomiting due to both gastric irritation and CNS stimulation is the cardinal sign of aspirin intoxication. Dehydration may follow from vomiting, increased respiratory losses from hyperventilation, and increased heat production. Tinnitus is commonly noted in older children and adolescents, presumably due to increased labyrinthine pressure.

Because aspirin stimulates central respiratory centers, respiratory alkalosis is commonly present. Metabolic acidosis may occur from anaerobic metabolism, dehydration, and/or ketone formation. Interference with platelet aggregation, hypoprothrombinemia, and alterations in thromboxane and prostacyclin regulation may lead to bleeding problems.

Central nervous system alterations may include delirium, agitation, disorientation, convulsions, stupor, and/or coma. A diffuse encephalopathy with increased intracranial pressure clinically indistinguishable from Reye syndrome may develop. This may be exacerbated by hyperammonemia. With doses less than 240 mg/kg, toxicity rarely occurs. Doses greater than 480 mg/kg may cause death. Plasma levels correlate poorly with clinical symptoms, but are helpful in following the course of an ingestion. The severity of CNS symptoms is the best indicator of overall severity.

Initial treatment must include methods to enhance elimination, including forced emesis or gastric lavage followed by activated charcoal administration. Forced alkaline diuresis via bicarbonate infusion will greatly assist renal elimination. Volume expansion must be approached cautiously to avoid cerebral edema. Potassium replacement may be necessary to correct alterations caused by vomiting, dehydration, alkalinization, and diuretic use. Hemodialysis and charcoal hemoperfusion are effective in enhancing aspirin elimination, but these methods should be used only in selected severe cases. Continuous hemofiltration with dialysis is more readily accomplished in many centers and may be as effective.

Further care is supportive and depends on clinical conditions. Vitamin K may help correct bleeding problems, as may fresh frozen plasma. Treatment of cerebral edema and increased intracranial pressure should follow standard techniques, including hyperventilation, sedation, osmolar therapy, and temperature control.

Tricyclic Antidepressants

Tricyclic antidepressants (TCAs) cause a myriad of clinically important symptoms when ingested by small children or consumed in large amounts by adolescents. Clinical conditions may develop rapidly without warning, making these agents dangerous and important causes of pediatric intoxication. Prescribed commonly for adults and adolescents with depressive symptoms, TCAs are also used to treat hyperactivity, school phobia, sleep disorders, and enuresis. This broad range of therapeutic indications makes these drugs widely available in many households.

TCAs get their name from the three rings making up the base compound—two benzene rings and a seven-member central ring. They block presynaptic uptake of neurotransmitters in both the central and peripheral nervous systems, thereby increasing the time norepinephrine and serotonin remain in the synaptic junction.[18] They also block sympathetically-mediated alpha-adrenergic receptors and parasympathetic muscarinic receptors. Early-onset dysrhythmias usually are due to anticholinergic effects, but conduction system prolongation may develop later owing to quinidine-like effects at all levels of the conducting system. This may lead to ectopy, atrioventricular blocks, and wide-complex tachydysrhythmias. Additionally, TCAs are negative inotropic agents.

The high lipid solubility of TCAs allows rapid uptake by the CNS. It also contributes to the long half-life of TCAs, which may range from 10–80 hours. These agents are well absorbed following oral intake, which may be further enhanced by their anticholinergic activity. Their extensive binding to plasma proteins is enhanced at higher pH, whereas increased free drug concentrations occur at lower pH.[15] The drug is metabolized by the liver, with many metabolites retaining the pharmacologic actions of the parent compound.

Early symptoms are often anticholinergic in nature (flushing, dry mouth, fever, mydriasis, urinary retention), although many patients initially will be asymptomatic. Central nervous system changes may include confusion, excitation, delirium, and hallucinations. Obtundation, stupor, or coma may develop. Involuntary twitching, ataxia, myoclonus, and choreoathetosis have been described. Generalized seizures may occur, and respiratory depression may develop. Cardiovascular symptoms may occur with or without CNS manifestations and may be more problematic. Sudden cardiovascular collapse from dysrhythmias, decreased cardiac output, and/or peripheral vasodilatation may ensue. Early tachydys- rhythmias including ventricular tachycardia may be supplanted by ectopy, conduction delays, wide QRS complexes, and even ventricular fibrillation.

Treatment may be quite difficult. The ABCs of basic life support are paramount in patients with life-threatening symptoms. Patients with unstable vital signs should be monitored continuously and may benefit from early endotracheal intubation. Gastric lavage is preferred over forced emesis because of the unpredictable nature of TCAs. Activated charcoal and a cathartic should be used; repeated charcoal administration may help because TCAs undergo some enterohepatic circulation.

Systemic alkalinization should be accomplished with bolus sodium bicar- bonate followed by a continuous infusion of a bicarbonate-containing fluid. The serum pH should be increased to between 7.45 and 7.50 by titration of the bicarbonate infusion. Hypotension should be treated with isotonic volume expansion. If an adequate blood pressure response is not achieved, norepinephrine by continuous infusion in doses ranging from 0.1–2.0 μg/kg/min should be added. Dysrhythmias should be treated initially with bicarbonate. Ventricular ectopy can be managed with lidocaine. Type 1 antidysrhythmics (quinidine, procainamide, disopyramide) should be avoided. Phenytoin may exacerbate hypotension and cause further conduction delays.

TCA-induced seizures should be treated with benzodiazepines (diazepam or lorazepam). Phenobarbital also may be helpful, but may worsen respiratory depression. Phenytoin should be avoided. Physostigmine has been useful but should be given with extreme caution because of its cardiovascular side effects, including asystole and heart block. It should be considered only when other agents fail.

Hemodialysis, charcoal hemoperfusion, and hemofiltration play no role in TCA removal because of high lipid solubility and protein binding. Plasma levels may help determine the severity of the amount ingested, but do not correlate with clinical symptoms. Plasma levels may be of assistance in determining how long to monitor asymptomatic patients. Documented TCA intoxications should have cardiorespiratory monitoring for a minimum of 36–48 hours.

Acetaminophen

Acetaminophen, an over-the-counter analgesic/antipyretic, is used frequently because of its therapeutic efficacy, low cost, and lack of major side effects. It is often prepared in combination with other agents, including codeine, hydrocodone, antihistaminics, and decongestants. Concerns about the safety of aspirin and gastrointestinal upset from ibuprofen have made acetaminophen one of the most widely used of all medications. Despite its wide therapeutic margin, acetamino- phen can cause life-threatening and/or fatal situations when large amounts are ingested.

Peak serum levels are reached within 30–60 minutes of oral ingestion. Rectal absorption is similar. Gastrointestinal absorption is delayed with massive ingestions and may delay peak serum levels up to 4 hours. The drug has a large volume of distribution, suggesting that high tissue levels are achieved.[38]

Acetaminophen is metabolized almost completely by hepatic mechanisms, with just 2% excreted in the urine. Glucuronidation and sulfonation account for most of the hepatic metabolism, but with therapeutic doses a small amount undergoes cytochrome P450 conversion to mercapturic acid. With massive

TABLE 4.   Stages of Acetaminophen Intoxication

Stage 1	Nausea, vomiting, malaise, and diaphoresis develop within 12–24 hr after ingestion. Children younger than 6 years usually vomit earlier and rarely demonstrate diaphoresis. All patients with toxic levels develop symptoms by 14 hr. Transaminases, bilirubin, and prothrombin times are normal at this stage.
Stage 2	24–48 hr after ingestion, the patient usually feels better. If therapy is delayed, transaminases, bilirubin, and prothrombin times increase.
Stage 3	Peak hepatotoxicity is noted 72–96 hr after ingestion. SGOT is elevated (usually greater than 100 IU/L, occasionally with dramatic elevations of 20,000–30,000 IU/L). Even with this degree of toxicity, less then 1% of patients in stage 3 develop fulminant hepatotoxicity.
Stage 4	Resolution begins 7–8 days after ingestion. At this time, the SGOT begins to normalize.

overdose, the glucuronidation and sulfonation pathways are insufficient, and more drug undergoes cytochrome P450 conversion.[38] This conversion creates the toxic intermediate, N-acetyl-p-benzoquinonimine, which binds to hepatocelluar proteins and results in centrilobular hepatatocellular necrosis. Renal and cardiac toxicity may develop also from N-acetyl-p-benzoquinonimine binding to renal tubules and myocardial cells, respectively. Acute renal failure has been reported in the absence of hepatic injury,[7] but myocardial dysfunction and dysrhythmias appear to occur only with concomitant hepatic dysfunction.

The clinical stages of acetaminophen intoxication are described in Table 4. Patients presenting with altered sensorium should be examined for other causes. Plasma levels should be drawn upon initial presentation and also at 4 hours after ingestion. Levels should be plotted using the Rumack-Matthew nomogram (Fig. 1) to determine whether N-acetylcysteine should be used.

Gastric emptying via forced emesis or gastric lavage should be initiated independently of plasma level determinations. Activated charcoal should be used if N-acetylcysteine will not be used or pending plasma level determinations. If N-acetylcysteine is to be used based on the nomogram, activated charcoal should be withheld because it binds N-acetylcysteine. If charcoal has been administered previously and N-acetylcysteine is to be given, attempts should be made to remove the charcoal.

Use N-acetylcysteine when plotted levels indicate "possible" hepatic toxicity, when the ingestion occurred within 24 hours, or when the history strongly suggests more than 140 mg/kg (7.5 gm in adolescents) was ingested. The agent is given orally or via nasogastric tube as a 5% solution mixed in citrus juice, carbonated beverages, or water. The initial dose should be 150 mg/kg followed by 17 additional doses of 70 mg/kg given every 4 hours. Intravenous preparations are not available in the United States, but where they are available, only 12 maintenance doses are recommended. Should hepatic failure develop, therapy is supportive. Vitamin K and fresh frozen plasma may be needed to avert bleeding. Lactulose or neomycin may help control hyperammonemia, and intravenous dextrose via continuous infusion is indicated to prevent hypoglycemia.

Hydrocarbons

Hydrocarbons are a heterogeneous group of chemical compounds derived from crude oil or pine oil. For clinical purposes, they should be divided into two groups. Aromatic hydrocarbons, including benzene, toluene, and xylene, cause visceral organ injury following gastric absorption and have little propensity for aspiration. Following an early excitatory phase, the aromatic hydrocarbons may cause CNS depression, respiratory depression, or frank respiratory arrest. Renal

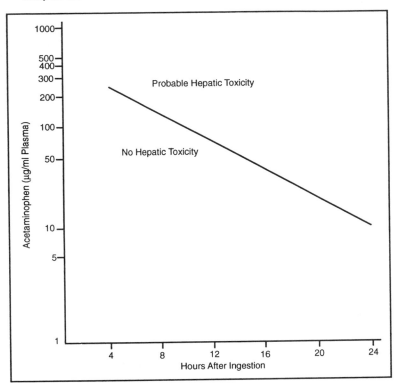

FIGURE 1. Rumack-Matthew nomogram of plasma acetaminophen level versus time. Time refers to time after ingestion. Similar figures have included a range of "possible hepatic toxicity," which is not included here. (From Pediatrics 55:1975, with permission.)

and hepatic insults may follow. Hematopoietic abnormalities, pulmonary edema, and myocardial sensitization to catecholamines may also be noted.

The more commonly ingested group of hydrocarbons includes aliphatic compounds and the pine oil distillates, including turpentine. Gasoline, mineral spirits, kerosene, lubricating oils, lighter fluids, pine oil, and turpentine produce primarily pulmonary injuries. These substances are highly irritating to mucosal surfaces, and their foul taste leads to a burning sensation, coughing, and choking before sustained volumes can be consumed. The ability of these compounds to cause pulmonary disease is based on their viscosity, surface tension, and volatility. Viscosity is the resistance to flow or change in form, and surface tension is the molecular cohesiveness along air-liquid interfaces. Low viscosity and low surface tension favor spread of hydrocarbons along mucosal surfaces. Volatility, the tendency for liquids to become gases, is equally important. Highly volatile substances such as gasoline and kerosene are readily "vaporized" when they contact warm mucosal surfaces. Although turpentine and pine oil may cause gastrointestinal and CNS disturbances, the other compounds in this group undergo minimal gastrointestinal absorption.

When aspirated hydrocarbons reach the lower respiratory tract, they create early inflammation, edema, hemorrhage, and necrosis. This acute alveolitis may be apparent upon initial presentation or may take up to 6 hours to manifest. Patients asymptomatic for 6 hours are unlikely to develop any clinically significant disease and may be discharged home. Patients symptomatic before

6 hours after ingestion should be admitted, if only for observation. The acute alveolitis generally peaks in 3 days and may be followed by a more chronic, proliferative alveolitis, which develops around 10 days and may include alveolar thickening or hyaline membrane formation. Pneumothorax, bronchiectasis, secondary bacterial pneumonia, and/or pneumatocele formation may develop.

Initial coughing, choking, and vomiting may be followed by dyspnea, tachycardia, and cyanosis. Patients with these symptoms should be provided supplemental oxygen early in their course. Gastric emptying via induced emesis is contraindicated except for the aromatic hydrocarbons or if mixed with other highly toxic substances such as heavy metals, organophosphates, or camphor. Gastric lavage may precipitate vomiting and/or aspiration and should not be performed. Activated charcoal is not helpful. Cathartics may be used with the aromatic hydrocarbons. Adding mineral oil or olive oil to alter the viscosity of an ingested hydrocarbon is discouraged and may actually increase the likelihood for aspiration. Corticosteroids play no role in the early treatment of these patients. Those likely to develop pulmonary fibrosis may benefit from short-term corticosteroids later in the course of therapy.

Supplemental oxygen and intravenous fluids may be all that is necessary in mild or moderate cases. Those with severe symptoms wherein adequate oxygenation cannot be maintained in 60% inspired oxygen will require endotracheal intubation, mechanical ventilation, and positive end-expiratory pressure (PEEP). Neuromuscular blockade along with intravenous sedation should be used in the early period of mechanical ventilation to control minute ventilation and peak inspiratory pressure. PEEP will help improve oxygenation, but must be used judiciously to minimize the chances for pneumothorax and/or cardiovascular compromise. Excess hydration should be avoided because increased capillary hydrostatic pressure worsens gas exchange in experimental animals.[51] Monitoring central venous pressure or pulmonary capillary wedge pressure may help guide therapy. Newer methods of respiratory support including high-frequency ventilation and extracorporeal lung support (ECMO, ECCO$_2$R) have been successfully employed and are reserved for the most severe cases.

Organophosphates

Chlorinated hydrocarbons were banned from regular use as insecticides in the 1970s. Since then, organophosphate compounds have become common for agricultural and domestic uses. Although household preparations usually are very dilute, toxic ingestions still occur. Agricultural products containing substantially higher concentrations of organophosphates make those residing in rural areas more susceptible to the toxic effects of these compounds. Products have been classified as highly toxic and moderately toxic (Table 5).

Organophosphates can be absorbed by ingestion, inhalation, through the skin, through mucous membranes, and through the conjunctivae. They bind

TABLE 5.   Relative Toxicity of Organophosphate Compounds

Highly Toxic	Moderately Toxic
Tetraethyl pyrophosphate	Malathion
Methyl parathion	Diazinon
Ethyl parathion	Dichlorvos
Bomyl	Fenthion*

* Long-acting agent.

TABLE 6.   Organ System Effects of Organophosphates

Central effects	Apathy, obtundation, convulsions, coma
Nicotinic effects	Muscle fasciculations, cramps, incoordination, weakness, paralysis
Muscarinic effects	Miosis, salivation, lacrimation, diaphoresis, bronchospasm, bronchorrhea, diarrhea, vomiting, bradycardia, hypertension

irreversibly to cholinesterases, thus allowing acetylcholine to persist following release from the nerve terminus. Acetylcholinesterase (true cholinesterase) is found in neurons and red blood cells, whereas pseudocholinesterase (plasma or serum cholinesterase) is found in liver, serum, and other organs. Cholinesterases terminate the effects of acetylcholine centrally at the respiratory and cardiovascular control centers and peripherally at nicotinic and muscarinic receptors. Symptoms occurring from organophosphate absorption therefore are classified as central, nicotinic, or muscarinic (Table 6).

Ingestions often occur concomitantly with cutaneous exposure. Health care workers must take care to avoid contact with organophosphate residues on a patient's skin or clothing. Inducing emesis usually is indicated in the absence of CNS symptoms, provided there is no associated hydrocarbon ingestion. Controversy remains as to the role of induced emesis when volatile hydrocarbons are used as a vehicle for organophosphates. Activated charcoal and cathartics should be employed.

Basic life support measures should always be undertaken. Those with early respiratory symptoms, especially bronchorrhea, should be intubated expectantly rather than emergently to avoid hypoxemia. Cardiac monitoring is warranted as dysrhythmias, particularly bradydysrhythmias, are somewhat common. Atropine in high doses should be given for those with more than mild symptoms. An initial dose of 0.5 mg/kg intravenously should be followed by "maintanance doses" of 0.2 mg/kg intravenously every 15–30 minutes while symptoms persist. Atropine will reverse central and muscarinic effects, but not nicotinic effects (muscle weakness, muscle cramps, fasciculations, paralysis). Full atropinization should be achieved as manifest by dry mouth, dilated pupils, increased heart rate, and warm, flushed skin. Atropine toxicity consisting of fever, fasciculations, and delirium is to be avoided.

Pralidoxime iodide (PAM, 2-PAM) and pralidoxime chloride (Protopam) may be used interchangeably. These oximes reactivate cholinesterase enzymes at nicotinic and muscarinic receptors. A dose of 25–50 mg/kg made up in 5% dextrose in 0.45 normal saline should be administered intravenously over 20 minutes. Adolescents may receive up to 1.0 gm over the same time period. A second dose should be given 1 hour after completion of the initial dose. Should cholinergic signs persist, a third dose is given 12 hours after the initial dose. Further therapy is seldom necessary. Side effects of pralidoxime include nausea, dizziness, diplopia, hypertension, and respiratory depression. Pralidoxime therapy should not be delayed while waiting for cholinesterase levels, but rather should be given when symptoms warrant. Most hospitals do not routinely measure acetylcholinesterase levels, while pseudocholinesterase levels are more frequently available. Because pseudocholinesterase levels are not closely associated with the degree of toxicity, their value is in differential diagnosis and in following the course of the illness.

Iron Poisoning

Iron-containing preparations are commonly available in most households. Use by pregnant women who have toddlers around provides an "ideal" setting

TABLE 7.   Stages of Iron Poisoning

Stage	Time	Symptoms
1. Initial	Early, immediate	Vomiting, diarrhea, hematochezia, abdominal pain
2. Quiescent	4–48 hours	Few symptoms, tachycardia
3. Circulatory	24 hours	Shock, acidosis, bleeding, coagulopathy
4. Hepatic	48–96 hours	Hepatic failure, encephalopathy, coma, hyperammonemia, hypoglycemia, bleeding
5. Scarring	2–6 weeks	Gastric obstruction, small bowel stenosis

for a toxic ingestion. Many preparations are formulated as "cartoon characters," making them highly attractive to venturesome youngsters.

Following ingestion, iron is rapidly absorbed from the gastrointestinal tract. It is oxidized to the ferric state and complexed to ferritin for storage. When released into plasma, it is bound to transferrin and can attach to the reticuloendothelial cells in the bone marrow for use in erythropoiesis. Additional iron is stored as ferritin or hemosiderin in liver and spleen. When the total iron binding capacity (TIBC; total available transferrin binding potential) is exceeded, a small amount of iron is bound to albumin. The remainder of any excess iron circulates as free iron, causing postarteriolar vasodilation, increased capillary permeability, metabolic acidosis, and mitochondrial dysfunction.

Iron poisoning is divided into five clinical phases (Table 7). Hypotension, metabolic acidosis, fever, lethargy, and/or coma may develop early in severe cases. The quiescent second phase may be mistaken as resolution, but subtle hemodynamic changes (tachycardia, decreased perfusion) must be looked for. Overt shock may dominate the third phase, as may bleeding from consumption of clotting factors, acidosis, and/or disseminated intravascular coagulation (DIC) syndrome. Fulminant hepatic failure is rare, but may result in death. The fifth phase occurs 2–6 weeks after ingestion, in some cases without previous third- or fourth-stage symptoms.

Treatment includes early gastric emptying. Large pill fragments are seldom cleared by gastric lavage. Therefore, induced emesis plays a major role in early management. The need for induced emesis may be obviated by first-phase vomiting. Gastric lavage is used primarily to remove small pill fragments, for liquid preparations, and for sodium bicarbonate instillation. A 5% sodium bicarbonate solution converts some iron to ferrous carbonate, which is poorly soluble. Activated charcoal does not complex iron and should be avoided. Oral deferoxamine therapy remains controversial and generally is not recommended.

Serum iron levels should be drawn at initial presentation and again at 4 hours after the ingestion. Levels greater than 300 mg/dl should be considered toxic. Hemodynamically stable patients should receive 40 mg/kg of deferoxamine intramuscularly. Patients with circulatory derangements must have intravenous fluids for circulating volume expansion (minimum: 20 ml/kg as an initial bolus). Intravenous deferoxamine via continuous infusion at a rate of 15 mg/kg/hr may then be given while blood pressure and capillary refill are frequently monitored. Hypotensive patients require continuous cardiorespiratory and blood pressure monitoring via an indwelling arterial catheter. Central venous line placement will assist in guiding further therapy. Those with serum iron levels greater than 500 mg/dl should receive deferoxamine intravenously even if they are normotensive. Deferoxamine should be continued until the "vin rose" color of the urine clears. Subsequent tests for serum iron levels also may be helpful. Hepatic failure, should it develop, is treated, as with other causes of acute hepatic injury, with volume replacement, correction of coagulation disorders, glucose provision, and ammonia control.

Cocaine

For more than a decade, cocaine abuse has been commonplace. Deaths from cocaine intoxication among pediatric patients have been reported, as have serious intoxications. The overall pediatric mortality from cocaine use is not known. Its potent cardiovascular and neurologic consequences make it vital that proper care be administered in serious intoxications.

Cocaine is a crystalline alkaloid derived from the leaves of *Erythroxylon coca*. Nonmedicinal use in the United States was banned in 1914, but the drug continues to have some medical utility when applied topically by anesthesiologists, otolaryngologists, and emergency medicine physicians. The crystalline salt may be mixed with adulterants and "snorted" or injected intravenously. Simple chemical conversion of the crystalline salt to the "freebase" alkaloid known as "crack" makes it possible to smoke cocaine, resulting in an immediate "rush" quite similar to intravenous injection.

Cocaine is rapidly metabolized by plasma and hepatic cholinesterases, but nonenzymatic hydrolysis also occurs.[27] The drug has a half-life of 60–90 minutes following inhalation or intravenous injection; intranasal or gastrointestinal uptake results in variable absorption and a longer half-life.

Symptoms arise from stimulation of the autonomic nervous system. Cardiovascular effects include hypertension, tachycardia, palpitations, and chest pain. Dysrhythmias including supraventricular tachycardia, ventricular tachycardia, atrial fibrillation, ventricular fibrillation, complete heart block, or asystole may develop.[29] Intense sympathetic nerve stimulation may result in peripheral vasoconstriction with resulting increased systemic vascular resistance. High myocardial oxygen demand coupled with decreased myocardial oxygen supply due to decreased filling time, coronary vasoconstriction, and/or coronary vasospasm make myocardial infarction very possible even in previously healthy young hearts.

Central nervous system effects may include headache, dizziness, anxiety, confusion, hyperexcitability, and hallucinations. Depression, suicidal ideation, seizures, stroke, and/or encephalopathy may ensue. Coma may develop. Seizures appear to be due to a reduced seizure threshold. Generalized tonic-clonic type seizures are the most common.[35] Differential diagnosis of pediatric patients without another explained cause for seizures should include cocaine. Pulmonary manifestations including pulmonary edema, pneumothorax, and bronchospasm may develop from "crack" smoking or may be secondary to acute congestive cardiac failure. Hyperthermia and rhabdomyolysis may lead to acute renal failure.[37]

History and physical examination along with laboratory screening of blood or plasma are needed for proper diagnosis. Screening for other drugs is usually necessary, particularly with adolescent patients. Social service referral of all pediatric cocaine intoxications is warranted.

Treatment begins with the ABCs of basic life support. Intravenous naloxone may ameliorate effects caused by other intoxicants. Therapy is guided by the severity of symptoms (Table 8).

Marijuana

Marijuana is the most commonly used illicit drug in the United States. Although use has declined slightly over the past several years, it remains a major

TABLE 8. Symptomatic Treatment of Cocaine Intoxication

Symptom	Treatment	Comments
Agitation	Midazolam, 0.05–0.10 mg/kg IV, or Diazepam, 0.1–0.4 mg/kg IV, or Haloperidol 0.1–0.3 mg/kg IM	Only if severe; may lower seizure threshold

Hyperthermia	Tepid sponging, surface cooling
	Neuromuscular blockade
	  Vecuronium, 0.05–0.2 mg/kg IV
	  Pancuronium, 0.1 mg/kg IV
		If mild or moderate; if severe, may require
		continuous EEG monitoring

Seizures	Diazepam, 0.2–0.4 mg/kg IV, plus Phenytoin, 10–20 mg/kg IV over 20 min or Lorazepam, 0.05–0.10 mg/kg IV, plus Phenytoin, 10–20 mg/kg IV over 20 min (or phenobarbital, 10–20 mg/kg IV)	Airway management must be maintained at all times

Hypertension	Propranolol, 0.01–0.05 mg/kg IV, or
	Labetolol, 0.25 mg/kg IV over 3 min
	Phentolamine, 0.05–0.1 mg/kg IV
	  or
	Continuous infusions
	  Labetolol, 25 μg/kg/min
	  Esmolol, 50–200 μg/kg/min (after
	    50 μg/kg loading dose)
	  Sodium nitroprusside, 0.5–5.0 μg/kg/min
		Check blood pressure frequently; use
		arterial line to monitor all continuous
		infusions

Dysrhythmias	Propranolol, 0.01–0.05 mg/kg IV	For tachydysrhythmias, avoid Ca⁺⁺ channel antagonists

Myocardial
  ischemia
	Nitrates
	  Sodium nitroprusside, 0.5–5.0 μg/kg/min
	  Nitroglycerin, 0.5–4.0 μg/kg/min
	Heparinization	

Rhabdomyolysis	Urinary alkalinization via bicarbonate infusion; keep urine pH > 7.5	

health problem. Recent report of toddlers developing coma after accidentally ingesting marijuana have heightened concerns,[26] but critical illness from marijuana intoxication is infrequent.

The active compound, delta-9-tetrahydrocannabinol (delta-9-THC), is found in the flowering tops, leaves, stems, and seeds of *Cannibis sativa*. This rather hearty "weed" grows in most U.S. climates. Hashish, the dried resin from flowering tops, hash oil (a liquid obtained from the nonpolar extraction of plant material), and sensimilla (the seedless flowering tops) have particularly high concentrations of delta-9-THC. Active delta-9-THC readily passes into the blood stream with smoking any of the aforementioned forms. Oral absorption is erratic, but does occur if ingested. Serum levels do not correlate with clinical findings. Uptake into fatty tissues results in very slow release and elimination. CNS receptors appear to bind delta-9-THC and subsequently alter dopaminergic, serotonergic, cholinergic, and GABAergic neurotransmitter functions.[28]

Clinical findings usually are nonspecific and benign. Confusion, short-term memory loss, mild pupillary constriction, conjunctival inflammation, and tachycardia are common. Increased appetite may be a helpful historical feature. Coordination and complex motor ability are often limited. Hypothermia, ataxia, nystagmus, tremor, and coma have been reported in pediatric patients.[49] Care must be taken to diagnose concomitant use of other intoxicants such as phencyclidine, cocaine, ethanol, or sedatives. Usually supportive care is all that is required. Severe anxiety may be treated with midazolam, 0.05–0.10 mg/kg intravenously; diazepam, 0.10–0.30 mg/kg intravenously; or haloperidol, 0.10–0.30 mg/kg intramuscularly.

Other Stimulants

Stimulants may be medically prescribed for narcolepsy, attention deficit disorders, and obesity, but otherwise have very limited clinical utility. Compounds in this group include amphetamines, sympathomimetics, and phenylpropanolamine. These agents have high abuse potential. Chemically, the substances resemble the parent compound phenylethylamine and have similarities to the endogenous catecholamines dopamine, epinephrine, and norepinephrine.

This group of drugs may be taken orally, intranasally, intravenously, subcutaneously, or smoked and inhaled. The duration of action is extremely variable and is affected by the route of intake, dose taken, and the pharmacokinetics of each compound. Centrally, they increase neurotransmitter release, thereby increasing CNS activity of the dopaminergic and adrenergic pathways. Reticular activating system stimulation increases alertness, whereas stimulation of the forebrain reward center accounts for the feelings of euphoria and increased libido. Acute psychosis associated with amphetamine use probably is due to dopaminergic stimulation.[24] Peripherally, stimulants lead to release of neurotransmitters modulating alpha- and beta-adrenergic receptors. Neurotransmitter concentrations in the synapse are further increased by amphetamines, which block catecholamine reuptake.[44]

Clinical manifestations are neurologic and cardiovascular. Agitation, irritability, anxiety, paranoia, hallucinations, delusions, and/or seizures are not uncommon. Rarely, stroke, intracranial hemorrhage, encephalopathy, and even coma may develop. Cardiovascular alterations include palpitations, chest pain, tachycardia, hypertension, and dysrhythmias. Myocardial ischemia may ensue, along with congestive cardiac failure. Other signs and symptoms include mydriasis, tremor, hyperthermia, abdominal pain, diarrhea, vomiting, and, in severe cases, rhabdomyolysis, which may lead to myoglobinuric renal failure. Death has been attributed to intracranial hemorrhage, hypertensive crisis, myocardial failure, or myoglobinuric renal failure.

Treatment is supportive and nonspecific. Gastrointestinal decontamination follows the rules as with other ingestions. Pharamcotherapy is similar to that of cocaine (see above) and includes lorazepam or diazepam plus phenytoin for seizures and midazolam or diazepam for severe agitation. Hypertension is best treated with sodium nitroprusside or esmolol by continuous intravenous infusion. Supraventricular tachycardia can be treated with adenosine in a dose of 50 μg/kg as a very rapid intravenous bolus, which can be increased by 50 μg/kg increments to a maximum of 250 μg/kg. Digoxin loading following successful conversion with adenosine using a total digitalizing dose of 30–40 μg/kg should be given via half the loading dose and then two quarter doses at 4- to 8-hour intervals. Alternatively, esmolol as a loading dose of 50 μg/kg/min followed by a continuous infusion of 50–200 μg/kg/min may be useful. Ventricular tachycardia may respond to intravenous lidocaine (1 mg/kg) followed by a continuous intravenous infusion at 5–30 μg/kg/min. Hyperthermia without muscle rigidity may be treated with tepid sponging, antipyretics, and/or a cooling blanket. For severe refractory cases or in the presence of muscle rigidity, aggressive external cooling along with neuromuscular blockade should be employed. Intravenous dantrolene used as with the malignant hyperthermia syndrome may be life-saving.

Hallucinogens

Included in this group are phencyclidine (PCP), lysergic acid diethylamide (LSD), the phenylalkylamines (e.g., mescaline), and the indolealkylamines (e.g., DMT). These agents are of no clinical value and are strictly drugs of abuse. PCP is the most commonly used of these agents. It can be smoked after being sprinkled or coated into tobacco or marijuana, or can be taken orally, intranasally, or intravenously. Being highly lipid soluble, it readily enters adipose and brain tissue, which accounts for its duration of action and its predominantly CNS effects. PCP interacts with virtually all neurotransmitters in the CNS, resulting in dopaminergic, sympathomimetic, and anticholinergic symptoms.[43] These include tremor, nystagmus, agitation, and panic.

Major neurologic manifestations include hypertension, tachycardia, diaphoresis, and altered consciousness. Extreme agitation and violent behavior may be suddenly followed by unresponsiveness and coma. Other mental status changes include confusion, delusions, disorientation, and hallucinations. Acute schizophrenia, choreoathetosis, dystonia, and opisthotonus also have been described. Self-mutilation, seizures, and/or rhabdomyolysis occur less commonly. Unpredictability and rapidly changing signs and symptoms are hallmarks of PCP intoxication. Interestingly, these findings are seen typically with adolescents and adults; toddlers and young children usually present with lethargy with as the cardinal finding. Staring, agitation, ataxia, opisthotonus, and nystagmus occur with some frequency. Seizures, hypertension, aggressive behavior, and coma are rather infrequent.

Therapy is supportive and may include benzodiazepines such as midazolam (0.05–0.10 mg/kg IV), diazepam (0.1–0.4 mg/kg IV), or haloperidol (0.1–0.3 mg/kg IM) for severe agitation. Phenothiazines should be avoided as they lower seizure threshold. Physostigmine is effective in reversing certain symptoms such as tremors, nystagmus, and agitation, but may worsen cholinergic symptoms. Seizures are treated with lorazepam (0.05–0.10 mg/kg IV) or diazepam (0.2–0.4 mg/kg IV), but most are short-lived and will resolve without therapy. Urinary acidification using ascorbic acid or ammonium chloride has been used to augment excretion, but remains controversial because only 15% of the drug is excreted renally. Forced diuresis using intravenous hydration seems more prudent.

LSD may be taken orally or by insufflation, smoking, or injection. It appears to inhibit CNS serotonin, leading to disinhibition of sensory and other cortical functions, resulting in distorted perception and thought.[16] Signs and symptoms include nausea, flushing, tachycardia, hypertension, and tremors. Altered affect, time distortion, illusions, and synesthesia (feeling colors and seeing sounds) are more common than true hallucinations. Recurrence of symptoms without repeat drug use ("flashbacks") are somewhat common.

Treatment is entirely supportive and seldom requires pharmacotherapy. In severe cases, agitation or severe psychosis may be treated with benzodiazepines or haloperidol in doses similar to those mentioned for PCP or cocaine. No deaths from LSD have been reported. Treatment for other agents in this group also should be supportive and nonspecific.

REFERENCES

1. Ballard PA, Tetrud JW, Langston JW: Permanent human parkinsonism due to 1-methyl 4-phenyl-1,2,3,6-tetrahydropyridine (MPTP). Neurology 35:949, 1985.
2. Berlinger WG, Spector R, Goldberg MJ, et al: Enhancement of theophylline clearance by oral activated charcoal. Clin Pharmacol Ther 33:351, 1983.
3. Bert KJ, Berlinger WG, Goldberg MJ, et al: Acceleration of the body clearance of phenobarbital by oral activated charcoal. N Engl J Med 307:642, 1982.

4. Bianchine JR: Drugs for Parkinson's disease, spasticity and acute muscle spasms. In Gilman AG, et al (eds): The Pharmacological Basis of Therapeutics, 7th ed. New York, Macmillan, 1985, pp 473–490.
5. Boehnert MT, Lovejoy FH: Value of the QRS duration versus the serum drug level in predicting seizures and ventricular arrhythmias after an acute overdose of tricyclic antidepressants. N Engl J Med 313:474, 1985.
6. Bond GR, Requa RK, Krenzelok EP, et al: Influence of time until emesis on the efficacy of decontamination using acetaminophen as a marker in a pediatric population. Ann Emerg Med 22:1403, 1993.
7. Boyd DA, Eling TE: Prostaglandin endoperoxide synthetase dependent cooxidation of acetaminophen to intermediates which covalently bind in vitro to rabbit renal medullary microsomes. J Pharmacol Exp Ther 219:659, 1981.
8. Brett AS: Implications of discordance between clinical impression and toxicology analysis in drug overdose. Arch Intern Med 148:427, 1988.
9. Curtis RA, Barone J, Geacona N: Efficacy of ipecac and activated charcoal cathartic: Prevention of salicylate absorption in a simulated overdose. Arch Intern Med 144:48, 1984.
10. Decker WJ, Corby DG, Ibanez JD: Aspirin absorption with activated charcoal. Lancet i:754, 1968.
11. DuSovich P, Caille G, Larchelle P: Enhancement of nadolol elimination by activated charcoal and antibiotics. Clin Pharmacol Ther 33:585, 1983.
12. Fazen LE, Lovejoy FH, Crone RK: Acute poisoning in a children's hospital: A 2-year experience. Pediatrics 77:144, 1986.
13. Ferguson RK, Boutros AR: Death following self-poisoning with aspirin. JAMA 213:1186, 1970.
14. Flower RJ, Moncada S, Vane JR: Analgesics-antipyretics and antiinflammatory agents: Drugs employed in the treatment of gout. In Gilman AG, Goodman LS, Murad F (eds): The Pharmacological Basis of Therapeutics, 7th ed. New York, Macmillan, 1985, pp 680–689.
15. Frommer DA, Kulig KW, Marx JA, et al: Tricyclic antidepressant overdose: A review. JAMA 257:521, 1987.
16. Glennon R, Titeler M, McKenney J: Evidence for 5HT2 involvement in the mechanism of action of hallucinogenic agents. Life Sci 35:2505, 1984.
17. Hartwig-Otto H: Pharmacokinetic considerations of common analgesics and anti-pyretics. Am J Med 75(Suppl):9, 1980.
18. Horn AS: The mode of action of tricyclic antidepressants. A brief review of recent progress. Postgrad Med 56(Suppl):30, 1983.
19. Karkkainen S, Neuvonen PJ: Effect of oral charcoal and urine pH on sotalol pharmacokinetics. Int J Clin Pharmacol Ther Toxicol 22:441, 1984.
20. Kornberg AE, Dolgin J: Pediatric ingestions: Charcoal alone versus ipecac and charcoal. Ann Emerg Med 20:648, 1991.
21. Kulig K, Bar-Or D, Cantrill SV, et al: Management of acutely poisoned patients without gastric emptying. Ann Emerg Med 14:562, 1985.
22. Lanphear WF: Gastric lavage. J Emerg Med 4:43, 1986.
23. Levy G: Gastrointestinal clearance of drugs with activated charcoal. N Engl J Med 307:676, 1982.
24. Linden CH, Kulig KW, Rumack BH: Amphetamines. Trends Emerg Med 7:18, 1985.
25. Litovitz TL, Schmitz BF, Bailey KM: 1989 Annual Report of the American Association of Poison Control Centers National Data Collection System. Am J Emerg Med 8:394, 1989.
26. MacNab A, Anderson E, Susak L: Ingestion of cannabis: A cause of coma in children. Pediatr Emerg Care 5:238, 1989.
27. Mueller PD, Benowitz NL, Olson KR: Cocaine. Emerg Med Clin North Am 8:481, 1990.
28. Nahas GG: Cannabis: Toxicological properties and epidemiological aspects. Med J Aust 145:82, 1986.
29. Nanji AA, Filipenko JD: Asystole and ventricular fibrillation associated with cocaine intoxication. Chest 85:132, 1984.
30. Neuvonen PH, Elonen E: Effect of activated charcoal on absorption and elimination of phenobarbitone, carbamazepine and phenylbutazone in man. Eur J Clin Pharmacol 17:51, 1980.
31. Neuvonen PJ, Tokala O, Vartiauien M: Comparison of activated charcoal and ipecac syrup in prevention of drug absorption. Eur J Clin Pharmacol 24:557, 1983.
32. Olson KR, Becker CE: Poisoning. In Mills et al (eds): Current Emergency Diagnosis and Treatment, 2nd ed. Los Altos, CA, Lange, 1985, pp 451–482.
33. Olson KR, Pentel PR, Kelley MT: Physical assessment and differential diagnosis of the poisoned patient. Med Toxicol 2:52, 1987.
34. Park GD, Goldberg KJ, Spector R, et al: The effects of activated charcoal on digoxin and digitoxin clearance. Drug Intell Clin Pharmacol 19:937, 1985.

35. Peng SK, Franks WJ, Pelikan PCD: Direct cocaine cardiotoxicity demonstrated by endomyocardial biopsy. Arch Pathol Lab Med 113:842, 1989.

36. Rodgers GC, Matyunas NJ: Gastrointestinal decontamination for acute poisoning. Pediatr Clin North Am 33:261, 1986.

37. Roth D, Alarcon FJ, Fernandez JA, et al: Acute rhabdomyolysis associated with cocaine intoxication. N Engl J Med 319:673, 1987.

38. Rumack BH: Acetaminophen overdose in children and adolescents. Pediatr Clin North Am 33:691, 1986.

39. Rygnestad T, Berg KJ: Evaluation of benefits of drug analysis in the routine clinical management of acute self-poisoning. Clin Toxicol 22:51, 1984.

40. Saetta JP, March S, Gaunt ME, et al: Gastric emptying procedures in the self-poisoned patient: Are we forcing gastric content beyond the pylorus? J R Soc Med 84:274, 1991.

41. Saetta JP, Quinton DN: Residual gastric content after gastric lavage and ipecacuanaha-induced emesis in self-poisoned patients: An endoscopic study. J R Soc Med 84:35, 1991.

42. Scheinen M, Virtanen R, Ilsalo RP: Effect of single and repeated doses of activated charcoal on pharmacokinetics of doxepin. Int J Clin Pharmacol Ther 37:367, 1985.

43. Shepherd SM, Jagoda AS: Phencyclidine and the hallucinogens. In Haddad LM, Winchester JF (eds): Clinical Management of Poisoning and Drug Overdose, 2nd ed. Philadelphia, W.B. Saunders, 1990, pp 749–769.

44. Shields RO: Designer drugs and amphetamines. Part B. Amphetamines. In Haddad LM, Winchester JF (eds): Clinical Management of Poisoning and Drug Overdose, 2nd ed. Philadelphia, W.B. Saunders, 1990, pp 771–780.

45. Sondgrass WR: Salicylate toxicity. Pediatr Clin North Am 33:381, 1986.

46. Steinhart CM, Pearson-Shaver AL: Poisoning. Crit Care Clin 4:845, 1988.

47. Tenenbein M, Cohen S, Sitar DS: Efficacy of ipecac induced emesis, orogastric lavage and activated charcoal for acute drug overdose [abstract]. Vet Hum Toxicol 28:321, 1985.

48. Watson WA: Factors influencing the clinical efficacy of activated charcoal. Drug Intell Clin Pharmacol 21:160, 1987.

49. Weinberg D, Lande A, Holton N: Intoxication from accidental marijuana ingestion. Pediatrics 72:948, 1983.

50. Weiner N, Taylor P: Neurohumoral transmission: The autonomic and somatic motor nervous systems. In Gilman AG, et al (eds): The Pharmacological Basis of Therapeutics. New York, Macmillan, 1985, pp 66–99.

51. Zucker AR, Sznajder JI, Becker CJ, et al: The pathophysiology and treatment of canine kerosene pulmonary injury: Effect of plasmapheresis and positive end-expiratory pressure. J Crit Care 4:184, 1989.

Initial Stabilization and Transport of the Pediatric Trauma Patient

MICHAEL S. SABEL, M.D.
ANGEL B. BASSUK, M.D.

Over the past 20 years, prehospital training and care have focused most strongly on the management of the adult cardiac patient and then the adult trauma patient. Attention is now being turned toward the prehospital approach to the pediatric trauma victim. Several studies have revealed that the most common reason for a child or adolescent to need prehospital care is trauma.[19] Almost 50% of deaths in children aged 1–14 in the United States are caused by trauma.[10] Each year, more than 1.5 million injuries and 500,000 hospitalizations are sustained by children, resulting in more than 50,000 children with permanent disabilities and 15,000–20,000 pediatric deaths.

To care best for the pediatric trauma victim, available community resources must be appropriately organized. Rapid transport by well-trained EMT personnel is mandatory. Although the general principles of trauma care are the same for the child as for the adult, several significant differences must be taken into account in the care of the pediatric trauma patient. Motor vehicle accidents are the most common cause of trauma in both adults and children, but the next most common causes are events that are less common in adults, such as falls, bicycle accidents, sports-related injuries, and abuse. Another important point is that children are still growing and developing, and several anatomic and physiologic differences must be appreciated to assess and treat the pediatric patient. This chapter discusses those factors specific to the initial assessment and transport of the pediatric trauma victim.

INITIAL ASSESSMENT (THE ABCs)

The goal in all patients is definitive care for the specific problem that exists. The trauma patient presents a unique challenge to this goal because of the magnitude and severity of multiple potential injuries. Neither a "load-and-go" nor a "stay-and-play" approach is appropriate to the management of the pediatric trauma patient. The wide variety of mechanisms of injury and potential complications mandate that each patient be assessed thoroughly with appropriate steps being taken in the proper order. Some of these steps must be performed at the scene, others in transport, and others on initial presentation to the emergency department. Each step is a balance between importance and time delay in transporting the patient. Unwanted outcomes can result from both missing crucial steps as well as unnecessarily delaying transport of the patient.

At the scene of the accident, the on-site personnel are dependent on information available from bystanders, police, witnesses, or involved persons. This information often may be limited, and most of the information must be gleaned from the injury pattern and physiologic state. Significant differences exist between children and adults, making the recognition of signs of impending physiologic compromise difficult for personnel without practical experience or training specifically in pediatric trauma. Children have more difficulty expressing pain and describing their complaints. They are often more frightened after an accident, and this fear may give misleading signals. For instance, attention may be turned away from quiet infants or children toward others in more apparent need of medical attention, yet they are often the ones most severely injured. Remarkably quiet or gently whimpering infants and small children must be suspected of having a compromised circulatory or neurologic state.

Definitive evaluation and treatment of severe or complex injuries may be better accomplished at a referral center, but the child with major injuries must be stabilized before transport. A narrow time restraint exists in which to recognize and stabilize those injuries that place the pediatric victim at greatest risk. The primary survey, as described in the Advanced Trauma Life Support course, is designed to identify and simultaneously manage life-threatening conditions. To put it simply, the goal is to recognize remediable life-threatening problems immediately—i.e., those problems that can produce profound systemic hypoxia.

The primary survey consists of *A*irway, *B*reathing, *C*irculation, *D*isability, and *E*xposure. These will be discussed in detail, but this ABC system is a guideline. Management in the field may be narrowed by a dangerous situation or a difficult extrication. Steps may be, and often must be, performed simultaneously and individualized to each patient. The on-site approach to the pediatric trauma patient should consist of (1) a rapid assessment, (2) airway management with cervical spine stabilization, (3) ventilation as appropriate, (4) rapid immobilization of major fractures and extrication, (5) intravenous access and administration of crystalloid fluids, and (6) delivery to the appropriate hospital.

Airway and Cervical Spine Control

Establishing a patent airway and avoiding hypoxia are the highest priority in all trauma patients. This is especially true of pediatric patients, as repiratory failure is the primary etiology for cardiopulmonary arrest in children.[8] Once arrest occurs, the outcome is extremely dismal.[20]

Cervical Spine Stabilization

Problems specific to obtaining a secure airway in a pediatric patient include potential head injuries, maxillofacial injuries, and most importantly, a possible cervical spine injury. When evaluating the airway of the child in the trauma setting, specific attention must be payed to the cervical spine. Protection must be afforded the cervical spine so that an unknown fracture is not manipulated unintentionally, which could result in a spinal cord injury. Spinal injuries occur less often in children than in adults, but the mortality is extremely high when it does occur. The safest approach is to treat all children with traumatic injuries that may have created forces upon the head and spine as if they have a cervical spine injury. Any child who fulfills any of the following criteria should be presumed to have a cervical cord injury until proven otherwise:

- Any evidence or suggestion of injuries to the head and neck
- Any complaints of neck pain, paresthesia, numbness, or weakness

- Depressed level of consciousness
- A mechanism of injury suggesting possible impact to the head or neck
- Any child with other significant injuries, as this may mask cervical spine pain
- Any child who is awake but has flaccid extremities has a spinal cord injury until proven otherwise[1]

If any question exists, erring on the side of overcautiousness is safer. These children need to have their cervical spine protected with in-line immobilization. This should not be achieved with traction.[10] In-line traction has been shown to exacerbate cervical spine instability in patients with unstable cervical spine injuries.

Airway Management

With the cervical spine stabilized, attention must immediately be turned toward the airway. The airway structures of the child are different from those of the adult, and understanding these differences is crucial to the establishment of a patent airway. The child has a small oral cavity in proportion to the tongue. Hence, the tongue alone can cause airway obstruction. Several differences exist that make intubation, if necessary, more challenging in the pediatric population. The larynx is located relatively high in the neck, at a level of C1–C4 in the newborn and young infant, descending to C2–C5 by age 2. The epiglottis in the infant is relatively floppy, narrow, and angled more posterior as compared with adults. The narrowest portion of the airway in adults is the glottic opening, but in children up to age 8–10, it is the cricoid cartilage. These differences mandate that the approach to airway management in the pediatric patient be modified.

Airway obstruction is the most frequent source of ventilatory insufficiency in the pediatric trauma victim and, if not overlooked, usually the simplest to treat. It is observed commonly in unconscious children following severe head trauma, as the oral cavity is relatively small and the upper airway is easily compromised by a lax oropharyngeal musculature in the obtuned, supine patient. The airway is opened by bringing the head slightly forward into the "sniffing position," (head slightly extended and the neck slightly flexed). While the cervical spine is immobilized, the airway should be opened with a jaw-thrust method, as described in the chapter on Pediatric Cardiopulmonary Resuscitation. Extreme care must be taken not to over-extend or over-flex the neck. These simple maneuvers alone may open the airway by lifting the mandible, moving the tongue forward, and drawing the larynx away from surrounding structures, but are often overlooked in the emergency situation.

If this approach is unsuccessful, the next step in airway management is to clear the airway of blood, emesis, and other material. The child's pharynx is cleared by gentle aspiration. Routine suctioning is inappropriate, particularly in a patient with an intact gag reflex, since this may precipitate vomiting and aspiration. Keep in mind that infants are obligate nose-breathers and must have the nasal passages cleared of obstruction. Once the airway has been cleared, oxygen is provided despite the severity of injury.

Upper airway obstruction that persists despite these efforts may be secondary to the presence of foreign material impacted in the larynx. A modified Heimlich maneuver can be performed by placing the heel of the hand midway between the xiphoid and umbilicus and thrusting sharply upward and inward. Although this maneuver may be contraindicated in some pediatric patients depending on the type of trauma, obtaining a patent airway takes precedent over everything else. Failure of all these efforts to clear the airway demands placement of an endotracheal tube or cricothyrotomy.

If the airway is open, an oral airway can be used in the unconscious child to maintain airway patency. These should not be used in the child who is awake, as he or she may vomit and aspirate gastric contents. Nasopharyngeal airways are a better choice in the awake patient. The proper-sized nasopharyngeal tube must be used to ensure that the airway is passed down to the pharynx.

If the airway is opened and easily maintainable, it is safe to proceed and assess the child's breathing. Even if the airway is patent and the patient is breathing, supplemental oxygen should always be provided. Children, while they may be resistant to the effects of severe hypercarbia and respiratory acidosis, do not tolerate even minimal periods of oxygen deprivation. If opening the airway has not been possible, if it cannot be maintained, or if the level of injuries requires ventilatory support, then the patient must be intubated.

Initially, the child should be hyperventilated with a bag-valve-mask device. After the child has been preoxygenated, a rapid sequence induction should be performed, dependent on intravenous access being available. However, in the severely obstructed child or a child in whom consciousness is so depressed that airway management takes precedent, an awake intubation should be performed. The appropriate endotracheal (ET) tube must be chosen. An approximation can be made by the formula (16 + age in years) ÷ 4, giving the internal diameter of the ET tube in millimeters. Other rapid approximations can be made by choosing a tube the size of the patient's fifth finger or nares. Because these are only estimations, one should have ET tubes one-half size smaller and larger immediately nearby. Only uncuffed ET tubes should be used in children less than 8 years of age. This minimizes the subglottic edema and ulceration seen with cuffed tubes.

Nasotracheal intubation was often touted as a preferable route for airway management in trauma patients in order to avoid excessive manipulation of the neck. Blind nasal intubation is spontaneously breathing patients is recommended by some, but it is more difficult to perform in children. It is also more likely to make the awake patient gag, resulting in more neck movement, increased intracranial pressure, and increased risk of vomiting and aspiration. If one is going to perform a blind nasal intubation in an older child or adolescent, it is important to determine if one nostril is more patent than the other. A topical vasoconstrictor and local anesthetic should be applied to both nostrils.

Maxillofacial Fractures

An extremely important factor in the trauma patient is the presence of facial fractures. The airway should be protected early if severe facial trauma is present; before swelling makes visualization more difficult. The nature of the injuries generally dictates the choice of orotracheal versus nasotracheal approach. Nasal intubation must not be attempted when there may be a basilar skull fracture. Orotracheal intubation may be limited by soft tissue obscuring the airway or profuse bleeding limiting visualization. A free-floating maxilla in a LeFort III fracture allows the upper teeth to descend into the mouth, obscuring one's line of vision. Bilateral mandibular fractures allow the tongue to fall into the posterior pharynx and occlude the airway. Soft tissue injuries may compromise the airway due to swelling or hematoma formation. Therefore, the child with severe facial fractures may not be able to tolerate intubation.

If these patients require an airway or, for any reason, cannot be intubated, they must be considered for cricothyrotomy with needle jet insufflation. The head should be stabilized in a neutral position, *not* hyperextended. The cricothyroid membrane should be identified by palpation and the overlying skin prepped. While the cricoid and thyroid cartilages are stabilized with the nondominant hand, puncture the skin and cricothyroid membrane with a 12- or 14-gauge cannula-over-needle attached to a syringe. Apply suction to the syringe while advancing the catheter at a 45° angle. Once air is aspirated, advance the plastic cannula into the trachea and provide oxygen by jet insufflation through a Y-connector. Suture the catheter securely in place and make plans to provide definitive airway control as soon as possible. This is a temporary measure only and can be replaced with more definitive airway control later, such as tracheostomy.

Breathing

The recognition of the child in respiratory distress is vital if early respiratory problems are to be corrected. Initial assessment of the child's breathing may begin with the recognition of abnormal vital signs as well as early patterns of respiratory difficulty, including tachypnea. However, to assess this properly, the health care providers need to be familiar with the normal age variation of respiratory rates in children (Table 1). A normal respiratory rate, however, may still be indicative of respiratory compromise if associated with grunting, nasal flaring, and the use of accessory muscles of respiration.

Assessment of breathing in the child may be easier than in the adult because of the thin chest wall, so simple visualization can tell much about lung expansion. Several life-threatening injuries to the airway and thorax, if identified, must be dealt with immediately and appropriately: e.g., open or tension pneumothorax, hemothorax, flail chest, and pericardial tamponade. Therefore, when looking at the patient, several questions should run through your mind that would suggest these injuries: Is the patient breathing, and are the respiratory efforts adequate? Is the patient cyanotic? Is the breathing labored? Is the trachea in the midline, and is the thorax expanding symmetrically? Auscultation in the child should be performed in the axillae since these are the farthest away from the major airways. Are the breath sounds equal bilaterally? Are the heart sounds of normal intensity and position? If any of these abnormalities are noted, immediate intervention may be required.

Although the pathophysiology and interventions for these injuries will be discussed in later sections, being familiar with the signs and symptoms of these injuries is important so that they can be identified early in the resuscitation. *Pneumothorax* is the most common consequence of thoracic injury in the child. The child may be in severe respiratory distress or may be asymptomatic.

TABLE 1. Normal Respiratory Rates and Hemodynamic Parameters by Age

Age	Respiratory Rate (bpm)	Systolic Blood Pressure (mmHg)	Heart Rate (bpm)
Newborn	60	60	120–180
6 months	30–40	70	110–170
1 year	30	80	100–150
4 years	20–30	80	80–120
6 years	20–30	80	70–100
10 years	15–20	100	70– 90

Abrasions of the chest wall, an absence of breath sounds, subcutaneous emphysema, or hyper-resonance to percussion suggests the diagnosis. Symptomatic pneumothorax requires treatment by needle aspiration of the pleural space and insertion of a thoracostomy tube. *Hemothorax* is an infrequent finding in children but is being seen increasingly with increasing penetrating injuries. Massive hemothorax is a space-occupying lesion that produces both circulatory collapse and respiratory insufficiency. Physical findings include pallor, tachycardia, and hypotension in addition to decreased breath sounds. As opposed to a pneumothorax where hyper-resonance is found on percussion, hemothorax usually gives a dull percussion. Treatment involves tube thoracostomy once blood volume has been restored, so if hemothorax is suggested, tube placement should be delayed until adequate intravenous access has been obtained and fluids begun. If there is exsanguinating hemorrhage from the chest tube, the patient will require emergency thoracotomy upon arrival. If a chest tube is placed on the scene and massive blood is released, this may require clamping of the chest tube in an attempt to tamponade the bleeding.

Tension pneumothorax develops as a result of air entry into the pleural space with elevation of the intrapleural pressure. This pressure shifts the mediastinum to cause compression of the opposite lung. Excessive shift results in angulation of the vena cava, with a decrease in blood return to the right side of the heart, decrease in cardiac output, and potentially lethal cardiovascular collapse. Again, treatment by rapid needle aspiration and insertion of a thoracostomy tube is essential.

Flail chest is less commonly seen in children because of the flexibility of the chest wall, but if multiple rib fractures occur, flail chest is a possibility. Once a flail segment develops, normal respiratory gas exchange is severely compromised. With each inspiration, the unsupported segment of chest wall is displaced inward by the negative pressure. Physical examination usually discloses asymmetry of the hemithoraces. There is a paradoxical movement of the chest wall, most noticeable during inspiration. Stabilization of the mobile portion of the chest may help, but endotracheal intubation and mechanical ventilation are usually required to achieve reliable gas exchange. Also important to keep in mind is that any injury strong enough to produce flail chest in a child is strong enough to result in associated pulmonary or myocardial contusions.

Circulation

Shock is defined as a state in which the heart is unable to provide a sufficient amount of oxygen and nutrients to meet the metabolic tissue demand. Shock is the second leading cause of pediatric mortality, following respiratory compromise, so after stabilization of the airway and breathing, attention is turned toward the circulatory system. While there are several etiologies of shock, hypovolemic shock is the most common type of shock in the pediatric patient, especially the trauma patient.

Several anatomic and physiologic differences between children and adults result in different reactions to blood loss. Most significant is the fact that children can increase their peripheral vascular resistance in response to an acute depletion of their blood volume.[17] Blood pressure can be maintained until there is a 30–40% decrease in intravascular volume, so keep in mind that dangerous volume depletion is important and shock can exist in the presence of a normal blood pressure. Hypotension in the pediatric population is a late manifestation of shock, blood pressure being the last parameter to fall.[15]

TABLE 2.   Systemic Responses to Blood Loss in the Pediatric Trauma Patient

	Early Blood Loss (< 25% blood volume loss)	Prehypotensive (25–40% blood volume loss)	Hypotensive (▷ 40% blood loss)
Cardiac	Weak, thready pulse Increased heart rate	Tachycardia Positive tilt test	Hypotension Tachycardia to bradycardia
CNS	Irritable, combative Confused, lethargic	Decreased consciousness Dulled response to pain	Comatose
Skin	Cool, clammy	Cyanotic, cold extremities Decreased capillary refill	Pale, cold
Renal	Decreased urine output	—	No urine output

The key to the management of shock is to recognize the signs and symptoms at an early point and to intervene appropriately. The earliest stage of shock in children is the "compensated" stage. Failure to intervene during this stage results in the patient progressing to "decompensated" shock, which can rapidly lead to cardiopulmonary arrest unless immediate intervention is undertaken.

The earliest sign of shock in children is *tachycardia.* To identify this, the health care personnel on the scene must be familiar with the normal heart rate and blood pressures that vary with age (Table 1). Other important signs to look for include *delayed capillary refill time* (> 2 sec), *cool extremities, duskiness* or *mottling of the skin,* and *thready* or *diminished peripheral pulses* (Table 2). Any child with a depressed level of consciousness, decreased central pulses, pallor, or hypotension is already in the later stages of shock.

Intravascular volume repletion is of extreme importance in the pediatric patient in shock. Fluid resuscitation should begin with infusions of either lactated Ringer's solution or isotonic saline. These solutions should not include dextrose, as the physiologic response to injury already produces an increase in serum glucose. Hyperglycemia can result in an osmotic diuresis that may worsen the child's hypovolemia and fool you into thinking that an adequate urine output is a sign of good renal perfusion.

The initial fluid resuscitation is based on the weight of the child. This information is usually accessible from the parents, but in the hectic situation in the field, it may not be available. A rough assessment of the age and body weight of the child can be made based on some obvious characteristics that describe developmental landmarks in children (Table 3).

The initial resuscitation should consist of boluses of 20 ml/kg, the first one being given over 5–10 minutes. Two to three such boluses can be delivered in succession with re-evaluation after each intervention. The pulse rate, blood pressure, peripheral perfusion, mentation, and volume of urine output should be monitored, and normalization of these parameters should be expected if blood loss is in the 20–25% range. If a response to these efforts is achieved, maintenance fluid administration can be initiated and vital signs monitored. Failure to respond to these boluses may be an indication of ongoing blood loss, possibly internal.

Pericardial tamponade occurs from accumulation of blood within the pericardial cavity after injury to the myocardium. Decrease in venous return and restriction of cardiac output occur with relatively small volumes of fluid within the pericardium because of the inelasticity of the pericardial membrane. Hypotension despite fluid resuscitation along with neck vein distension and peripheral vasoconstriction suggest the diagnosis. With the rapid respiratory and pulse rates

TABLE 3.   Estimates of Children's Body Weight by Age

Age	Probable Weight (kg)
< 6 months	6–9
12–17 months	10–15
< 3 years	15–20
3–5 years	20–30
6–8 years	25–30
9–11 years	30–35
11–13 years	35–45
13–15	45–55

in a child, pulsus paradoxus may be extremely difficult to appreciate. Distended neck veins may not be present in a hypovolemic child. If suspected, diagnostic pericardiocentesis is performed. The same left subxyphoid approach is used as in the adult patient. Aspiration of blood or air results in immediate cardiovascular improvement. Any child who has blood aspirated from a pericardiocentesis will require a thoracotomy to identify the source of the pericardial bleeding.

Persistent hypotension despite adequate volume administration may be an indication for application of a pneumatic antishock garment (MAST trousers). This garment increases systemic vascular resistance peripherally and translocates venous blood from the extremities to the central circulation. Application of the abdominal portion of the garment may be helpful in tamponading retroperitoneal bleeding in patients with pelvic fractures. However, inflation of the abdominal portion can negatively affect the patient's respirations, and thus it should be left deflated if possible. If it is used, the child must be closely monitored for respiratory compromise. Another advantage of using the pediatric MAST with inflation of the leg compartments to 60–70 mmHg is to provide tamponade of blood flow to the lower extremities, allowing identification of a venous access site in the upper extremities.

Hemorrhage control is also part of the circulatory survey. Most areas of external bleeding can be controlled with elevation and direct pressure. The use of hemostats to control hemorrhage is to be discouraged, as is the use of tourniquets.

Critical to fluid resuscitation is obtaining venous access. Placing two large-bore cannulas is of the highest priority. However, this is often difficult in the healthy child, let alone the child in hemorrhagic shock. Two stable intravenous lines are recommended because loss of intravenous access during transport could be a life-threatening situation.

A significant problem arises in the on-site management of the pediatric trauma patient, and that is how much time to spend at the scene trying to obtain intravenous access. On one hand, cannulation of veins will probably be easiest within the first few minutes following trauma, as opposed to arrival at a hospital after a variable delay where ongoing hemorrhage may result in severely collapsed vessels. On the other hand, unnecessary delay of the patient to initiate intravenous fluid resuscitation can be extremely detrimental. The on-site team therefore must have an established protocol on how to address intravenous access in the trauma patient, which takes into account the mechanism of injury, rate of ongoing hemorrhage, experience of the personnel on the scene, hemodynamic stability of the patient, and transport time to an appropriate hospital. Neglect of the airway, ventilation, and adequate oxygenation is dangerous to the patient, and so to move the patient before achieving airway management is incorrect. On the other hand, intravenous access can be obtained in the ambulance as easily as in the field. If, after 90 seconds or two attempts, peripheral cannulation fails, more definitive vascular access must be obtained in critical situations. The patient should be moved and loaded into the ambulance, and other means for intravenous access attempted, such as intraosseous lines, saphenous cut-downs, and central venous access.

Peripheral Venous Access

Potential sites for access are the veins on the dorsum of the hand or foot, the major saphenous vein anterior to the medial malleolus, and the cephalic vein posterolateral to the wrist. Scalp veins may be used effectively in infants younger than 1 year. A tourniquet may be placed around the head just above the ears to facilitate identification of these veins. Antecubital veins are often easier to cannulate, if necessary, but have the risks of accidental cannulation of the artery and become kinked by flexion of the elbow joint. The use of the external jugular is normally a popular choice in pediatric patients, However, in the pediatric trauma patient, this route is often limited by the cervical collar as well as the need to place the patient in the head-down position to find it, which is deleterious to head trauma.

Central Venous Access

The use of central lines in the initial resuscitation stage is usually not necessary, nor is it recommended. Catheters of this sort have low flow rates and so are not appropriate for rapid volume replacement, and placement is difficult and time-consuming. If, however, venous access cannot be obtained, a central line may need to be placed. Many trauma patients will be in cervical spine immobilization, so the internal jugular approach is not available. The subclavian vein is a more difficult approach and should be performed only by practitioners confident in its use. It carries a significant risk of pneumothorax and hemothorax. If this route is to be used, the recommendation is that it be placed on the side of any potential chest injury.

The best choice for central venous access in this situation is the femoral vein. It is readily accessible in the immobilized patient, has fewer risks, and remains relatively large despite increased systemic vascular resistance.

Intraosseous Access

The intraosseous route may be used by trained prehospital personnel for the initial management of the patient before arrival at the emergency department. This route has become an increasingly popular choice among emergency physicians and paramedics as the vascular access of choice in the critically ill child. The bone marrow represents a noncollapsible network of medullary sinusoids that drain into the venous circulation. Intraosseous infusion is extremely successful with minimal complications. Complications include local cellulitis, osteomyelitis, fat emboli, fractures, growth plate damage, and leakage from multiple sticks. While the rate of complications in the hands of experienced personnel is acceptably low, these complications can be significant, and so this procedure should not be performed by inexperienced hands. The use of an intraosseous line is contraindicated if there is a possibility of a femoral or tibial fracture or a vascular disruption in that particular leg.

Intraosseous puncture should be reserved for children under 5 years of age. After this age, the cortex of the long bones becomes harder and the medullary space smaller. The two recommended sites of intraosseous insertions in children are the proximal tibia and distal femur. The needle may be inserted either 2 cm distal to the tibial tuberosity, on the flat medial aspect of the proximal tibia, or in the midline of the distal femur, 3 cm proximal to the femoral condyle. A screwing motion is used to advance the needle until resistance gives way, indicating that the marrow has been entered. Volume resuscitation as well as emergency drugs may be administered this way. Bear in mind, however, that infusions will not usually flow freely; a three-way stopcock and large syringe should be used to push fluid boluses.

Disability

After the patient's cardiopulmonary status has been stabilized, an extremely quick assessment of the neurologic status should be obtained. A further evaluation will be performed later, but at this point two factors should be assessed. The first is the pupils, including the pupillary size and reactivity to light. The pupils should be looked at with a bright light, and their size, equality, and responsiveness determined. The second is the level of consciousness. This can be rapidly assessed using the AVPU method:

A —Alert and responsive
V —Responsive to Verbal stimuli
P —Responsive to Painful stimuli
U —Unresponsive

This initial evaluation is directed at not only determining the neurologic state of the patient but also establishing a baseline. Any change in neurologic status is of significance and may indicate either a worsening cardiopulmonary status or need for neurosurgical intervention. The injured child must always be assumed to have suffered multisystem rather than single system injury. A more detailed neurologic assessment is not needed at this point, as it will be addressed during the secondary survey. Although the central nervous system (CNS) is the most frequently injured organ system that results in death of the child, the best treatment for a head injury at this point is to ensure that the brain is well perfused with adequately oxygenated blood. For this reason, careful attention must be payed to the breathing and circulation during the resuscitation and transport.

A basic concept of CNS trauma that is important to anyone responsible for initial care of the injured child is understanding primary and secondary brain injuries. Primary injuries involve those at the time of trauma and include cerebral contusions, bleeds, and lacerations. Definitive management of these are the responsibility of the neurosurgeon. Secondary CNS damage may occur as a result of hypoxia, hypotension, or hypercarbia. Protection of the patient from these sources of CNS disability is the responsibility of those providing initial trauma care.

If the ABCs are adhered to, then control of intracerebral pressure, maintenance of adequate CNS perfusion, and prevention of hypoxia will be achieved. Prevention of cerebral edema is most reliably achieved by hyperventilation. The intracranial pressure (ICP) is directly proportionate to the volume of the intracranial space, which includes the brain parenchyma (80%), blood (10%), and cerebrospinal fluid (10%). An increase in the volume of one of these components must be matched by a decrease in another to maintain a normal ICP. Hypocarbia induces cerebral vasoconstriction and thereby reduces the cerebral blood flow and edema. Hypocarbia in the range of 25 mm Hg is desirable and should reduce cerebral blood flow up to 500%; this can acutely lower an increased ICP.[12] Other practical measures may be elevation of the head of the bed to decrease venous pressure, restriction of intravenous fluids to two-thirds maintenance, and the use of paralysis in intubated patients to prevent coughing. These measures are only appropriate for hemodynamically stable patients and should be avoided if there is any question of the hemodynamic status.

Also important to consider in the use of paralysis in pediatric trauma is the effect on the ability to assess the patient. There exists the potential for a progressive neurologic injury without the knowledge of the medical treatment team, because the physical examination would be ablated by the neuromuscular blockade.

Exposure

The final stage of the primary survey is to disrobe the patient completely in order for the trauma team to assess the extent of injuries fully. All possible sites of injury need to be evaluated so that definitive care can be rendered quickly and appropriately. However, exposure in the pediatric patient carries greater risk than in the adult patient. Because children have an increased ratio of body surface area to mass, they are more prone to the development of hypothermia. This becomes increasingly true in the younger age groups, especially infants. Hypothermia has negative effects on coagulation and the inotropic effect of the heart, and it may worsen metabolic acidosis.[8] Because of the detrimental effects, measures should be taken to avoid hypothermia in the pediatric trauma patient. Lactated Ringer's and normal saline solutions should be kept warm. Overhead warming lamps and blankets should be used to keep the child warm during and after the resuscitation.

INITIAL TRANSPORT

Once the patient has been stabilized as best they can under the circumstances, they should be transported to the nearest facility capable of managing the specific injuries. This transport may be several hundred yards or several hundred miles depending on the location of the nearest appropriate special care unit. In any circumstance, the patient should be transported with (1) qualified personnel in attendance who are specifically experienced in the care of pediatric patients and (2) advanced life support technology in place.

Determining where to transport the patient is of utmost importance. Many factors come into play in this decision. Distance and geography, safety, expense, available transport vehicles, and personnel are important considerations. The most important factor, however, is the severity of the injuries, and assessing this quickly and efficiently is crucial. The National Pediatric Trauma Registry was established in 1985 to collect data on injured children and report that data to both the medical communicty and public.[18] These data were used to develop a trauma score for rapidly assessing the severity of the pediatric trauma patients. Previous scores had been based on adult trauma victims and were not completely appropriate to the pediatric population.

The Pediatric Trauma Score (PTS) has six components (Table 4). These have been identified by regression analysis as those most predictive of death and disability. Each of these is scored by either +2 for a minor or no injury, +1 for a major injury, or –1 for a critical, life-threatening injury. The totals are added and range from either 12 for no or only minor injuries to –6 for universally fatal injuries.

This score can be used as a simple yet effective triage tool. Essentially no deaths are reported in patients with a PTS of 9 or more. The possibility of morbidity begins at scores of 8 and increases as the PTS drops. Thus, any patient

TABLE 4. Pediatric Trauma Scoring System

Component	Add 2 Points	Add 1 Point	Subtract 1 Point
Size of child	> 20 kg	10–20 kg	< 10 kg
Airway	Normal	Maintainable	Unmaintainable
CNS status	Awake	Obtunded	Comatose
Systolic blood pressure	> 90 mmHg	50–90 mmHg	< 50 mmHg
Open wounds	None	Minor	Major
Fractures	None	Single, closed	Open or multiple

Adapted from Tepas JJ, et al: National Pediatric Trauma Registry. J Pediatr Surg 24:156–158, 1989; with permission.

with a PTS score of 8 or less must be transported to an institution capable of providing the the highest level of care.[14]

Besides the pediatric trauma score, other criteria exist for identifying the seriously injured child for whom transfer to a pediatric trauma center should be considered. Some of these criteria are based on the mechanism of injury. Examples are motor vehicle accidents that were rollovers or had evidence of high-impact velocity (shattered windshield, bent steering wheel, passenger cabin invasion), pedestrian versus automobiles, and accidents in which the victim was thrown from the vehicle, another passenger died, or the extrication took longer than 20 minutes. Falls from > 15 ft (> 10 ft for children under 14) or accidents involving hostile environments (e.g., excessive heat, cold water) should also warrant transfer to a tertiary facility. Many physical findings should direct your transport, including multiple injuries, two or more long bone fractures, amputation, persistent hypotension, severe head or spinal cord injury, burns, blunt or penetrating injury to the chest or abdomen, and penetrating injury to the groin or neck.

Prior to transport, all fractures should be stabilized with splints, and a circulatory examination proximal and distal to the fracture should be documented. Stabilizing the fracture will decrease the amount of pain and discomfort for the child, as well as decrease the amount of blood loss. If there is an absence of distal pulses or massive swelling, compartment syndrome is a risk, and the time of transport becomes a more crucial factor.

The child should be secured to a backboard. The cervical spine has already been stabilized in a semirigid collar and should be further immobilized by securing to the backboard. Because placement on the backboard results in some degree of spine flexion (resulting from the child's large occiput), a folded blanket or pad under the back at the level of the chest will help. This should align the external auditory meatus with the shoulders and prevent unintentional flexion.

SECONDARY SURVEY

The purpose of the secondary survey is to identify all coexisting injuries that may not be an immediate threat to the life of the patient but, if not identified, could result in increased mortality and morbidity. Although a patient may seem stable during the initial ABCs, the secondary survey may reveal injuries that require transport to a more specialized center. The secondary survey involves a head-to-toe physical examination and the planning of definitive treatment on arrival. It is essential that the patient's vital signs be reevaluated frequently during the secondary survey, with a priority on ensuring a stable condition and looking for new problems as they arise, adjusting management as necessary. Additional history should be obtained at this point, once the child has been stabilized. A full, detailed history is not necessary. Instead the following information should be obtained, easily remembered with the mnemonic AMPLE:

A —Allergies

M —Medications

P —Past medical and surgical history

L —Last meal eaten

E —Events preceding the accident

Once the patient has been stabilized, a more comprehensive neurologic assessment can be performed. This includes repeating the evaluation of the level of consciousness and pupillary responses to see if there has been a change. Motor and sensory evaluations should be performed. At this time a Glasgow Coma Scale (GCS) Score can be determined (Table 5). The GCS provides an accurate method of following the changes in the patient's level of consciousness and neurologic function. Accurately assessing the GCS during transport is important so that miscommunication does not occur between the personnel in the field and those in the hospital. One significant arm of the GCS is the verbal response; this has been modified for children under the age of 4.

It is recommended that severely head-injured patients, especially those with GCS scores less than 8, undergo early endotracheal intubation to avoid hypoxemia and a worsening of secondary ischemic brain injury. Intubation ensures optimal gas exchange and controlled hyperventilation.

Although a thorough examination of the head and neck may be difficult in transport, it can reveal many signs of possible CNS injury that will determine the most appropriate care center. Careful attention should be paid to any lacerations or abrasions on the head and face. The head should be palpated for any skull

TABLE 5. Glasgow Coma Scale for Children

Eye opening	
Spontaneous	4
As a reaction to speech	3
As a reaction to pain	2
No response	1
Best motor response	
Spontaneous	6
Localizes pain	5
Withdraws to pain	4
Flexion to pain (decorticate)	3
Extension to pain (decerebrate)	2
No response	1
Best verbal response (for > 2 years of age)	
Appropriate words and phrases	5
Inappropriate	4
Persistent cries/screams	3
Grunts	2
No response	1
or	
Best verbal response (for < 2 years of age)	
Smiles, coos appropriately	5
Cries, but consolable	4
Persistent crying	3
Grunts, agitated, restless	2
No response	1
TOTAL	3–15

fractures or subgaleal hematomas. Blood or cerebrospinal fluid behind the ear-drum, around the orbit, or in the nose (Battle's sign) is presumptive evidence of basilar skull fractures. An otoscopic examination should be performed to note the presence of blood or cerebrospinal fluid draining from the ear or nose. Palpation along the maxilla and mandible will detect fracture-dislocations. Maxillofacial trauma is not uncommon in the pediatric population, and these must be noted early in conjunction with establishing a patent airway. If these injuries are stable and not interfering with the airway, then they should be treated after the patient has been completely stabilized and life-threatening injuries have been treated.

From the very beginning of the resuscitation, the cervical spine must be treated as if it were injured until proven otherwise. This approach should be maintained throughout the entire transport. Removal of the cervical spine immobilization to examine the neck should not be done en route because of the possibility of trauma from unexpected motion.

The chest has already been carefully examined to assess the patient's breathing, but this examination is usually hurried and directed at those injuries specifically life-threatening. The chest should be reexamined to reevaluate injuries not identified in the primary survey. The position of the trachea with respect to the midline should be noted. Repeat ausculation should be performed constantly to assess the patient's breathing. Integrity of the ribs is tested by placing an examining hand on the lateral aspects of the left and right chest and exerting pressure toward the sternum to elicit tenderness. Heart sounds should be clear and distinct. Also important at this point is to "logroll" the patient to evaluate the back. This maneuver takes at least two people to roll the patient and stabilize the neck, and if this cannot be done safely, it should be postponed until the patient has arrived at the hospital. If it can be done, the back should be palpated while looking for spinal fractures or tenderness, hematomas, and other injuries.

The abdomen can be the site of significant occult blood loss and may result in hemodynamic compromise. Careful inspection and palpation of the abdomen and flanks should be performed. After an injury, the child may be upset and swallow large amounts of air. This air can result in significant gastric distention, which can decrease effective respiration and mimic an intra-abdominal injury. Thus, the abdomen should be decompressed with a nasogastric tube. It is important to note any maxillofacial trauma, and if present, an orogastric tube should be used to avoid the possibility of inserting the tube through a cribriform plate fracture.

The perineum should also be evaluated and a rectal examination performed. Blood at the urethral meatus or a "high-riding" prostate on rectal exam may indicate urethral disruption. In this case, the catheterization of the bladder should be delayed until a urethrogram can be performed. Blood may be present in the scrotum or labia majora, indicative of a hemoperitoneum or pelvic fracture.

A thorough extremity examination should assess deformity contusions, abrasions, penetration, and perfusion, including pulse palpation. Soft tissue injuries should be inspected for both wound foreign bodies and the presence of devitalized tissue. These wounds should not be probed with any instruments. Long bones should be palpated with rotational or three-point pressure for tenderness, crepitation, or abnormal movement. Pressure must be applied to the pubis and anterior iliac spines to assess for the presence of a pelvic structure. Torus and greenstick fractures, which are unusual in adults, may be typical fractures found in children. Compound fracture sites should be covered with sterile dressings. Any severe extremity angulations should be straightened, the joints immobilized, and traction splints applied. Various traction devices are available in the prehospital settings. Stabilization of the injured limb can be achieved with splinting devices ranging from simple boards and pillows to Hare traction devices and Thomas splints. The goal of management of extremity trauma during transport is to avoid subsequent neurovascular compromise.

SPECIFIC INJURIES

Head Injury

Head trauma is extremely common in the pediatric population and is the leading cause of morbidity and mortality in pediatric trauma victims. Motor vehicle accidents are the leading cause of pediatric head injury, followed by falls. Children have an increased head-to-body ratio and thus a higher center of gravity, contributing to the increased incidence of head trauma in motor vehicle collisions. In an automotive deceleration event, the child, unless restrained, tends to fly through the air, hitting the dashboard or windshield. Adults tend to "submarine" beneath the dashboard. The neck muscles in children are weaker, absorbing less force, and rendering the brain more vulnerable to shearing stress. While the open sutures and fontanelles in younger children afford some protection by permitting expansion with expanding subdural and epidural hematomas, the thinner cranial bones in children place the brain parenchyma at an increased risk. Another major difference is that children are more prone to development of reactive cerebral hyperemia in response to significant head trauma. As discussed, management of cerebral edema is even more important in children to avoid secondary injury.

Spinal Cord Injuries

With the relatively short and more flexible necks in young children, cervical spine injuries are relatively rare. Motor vehicle accidents are the most frequent cause of cervical spine injuries in children of all ages. Most spinal cord injuries in children younger than 8-12 years tend to occur in the upper three cervical segments. This results because of a relatively larger inertial mass of the head of the infant and young child. While the fulcrum of cervical motion occurs at C5-C6 in the adult, it occurs at C2-C3 in the young child. Other differences, including the facet joints being in a more horizontal plane, wedge-shaped vertebral bodies, and incompletely developed uncinate processes, allow subluxation to occur more easily. Many of the injuries are ligamentous in nature. As children get older, their patterns of injury increasingly resemble those of adults. The incidence of injury increases in children over age 12, as does the frequency of lower cord injuries. Older children are more likely to have bony fractures as opposed to ligamentous injuries.

Despite the decreased frequency, it is important to have a high index of suspicion of spinal cord injuries in children because of the devastating results of missing one. Children with injuries to the cervical spine are extremely susceptible to spinal cord injury and neurologic deficit; this is especially true of subluxations. Reflexive neck muscle spasms may spontaneously reduce traumatic subluxations on the radiographic examination. Therefore, any child with head and neck injuries and a history of even transient paresthesias or extremity weakness should be presumed to have a spinal cord injury until proven otherwise. Urinary retention is a common finding with spinal cord injuries, and hence it should raise a red flag.[19]

Another reason to be highly suspicious of cervical spine trauma is the phenomenon of "spinal cord injury without radiologic abnormality" (SCIWORA). This occurs with a much higher incidence in children, the reasons for which are not completely understood. It is more frequently seen in younger children and is associated with a high incidence of complete neurologic injury. The neurologic deficit sometimes occurs in a delayed fashion (2 days) and often after what is considered to be a trivial injury. Once initiated, there is often rapid evolution to severe and irreversible neurologic injury. Hence, when considering a child for interhospital transport, cervical spine immobilization should be used in any patient with suspicion of head or neck trauma, even if the initial radiologic examination demonstrated no injuries.

Thoracic Injuries

Most thoracic injuries are blunt, with motor vehicle accidents being responsible for most of these. Thoracic trauma often accompanies other injuries. Waddell's triad describes an injury pattern frequently seen in pedestrian children—i.e., the combination of head, thoracic, and extremity injuries. The prognosis worsens with the presence of associated injuries. Penetrating trauma is becoming more common, especially in urban areas where violent crimes are becoming the number one killers of young men. Penetrating injuries are associated with an increased mortality secondary to disruptions of the mediastinal vessels and myocardium.

Blunt thoracic injuries are less common in children, owing to the fact that the pediatric chest wall is more compliant than the adult's. With this increased elasticity and compliance, the incidence of rib fractures, sternal fractures, and flail chest is much lower in children. The chest wall may be exposed to high amounts of force without obvious external signs of serious injury. This permits traumatic forces to be transmitted to deeper thoracic structures. Thus, significant pulmonary and myocardial contusions may be present in the absence of rib fractures.

Many thoracic injuries are life-threatening and hence need to be identified during the initial assessment. However, they may develop or become apparent in transport, and so constant reassessment of the child's breathing is essential. As mentioned, pneumothorax is the most common consequence of thoracic trauma. A pneumothorax in a child may be more prone to progress to a tension pneumothorax due to the increased mobility of the mediastinal structures.[4] The tension pneumothorax is a life-threatening complication and must be treated immediately upon recognition. Spontaneous pneumothorax is a complication of mechanical ventilation. Both spontaneous pneumothorax and tension pneumothorax can occur during transport. It is therefore extremely important during transport of the mechanically ventilated patient to assess the hemodynamic and respiratory status continuously and to be prepared to correct these complications. While tube thoracostomy is the definitive therapy, this procedure may not be readily available in transit. If not, needle aspiration must be initiated promptly, before waiting for radiographic evidence of a pneumothorax. Placing a small needle into the second intercostal space at the midclavicular line of the anterior chest wall allows for the escape of trapped air. The rush of air may be heard as the pressure inside the chest is relieved.

Hemothorax is a rare consequence of blunt trauma, but is rising in incidence with the increased frequency of penetrating traumas. Blunt chest trauma, however, can result in hemothoraces from injury to the intercostal arteries. Large volumes of blood (up to 40% of the total blood volume) can accumulate in the pleural space.[6] It is important to keep in mind, in the child who is hemodynamically unstable and not responding to fluids, that while an abdominal source of onoging blood loss is most likely, a thoracic source must not be overlooked. Pulmonary contusions cause respiratory distress and failure secondary to parenchymal damage with intra-alveolar hemorrhage and edema. The increase in pulmonary capillary membrane permeability impairs gas exchange. Children with significant hypoxia require intubation and ventilation to support their respiratory status.

Abdominal Injuries

Several anatomic differences between adults and children increase the possibility of abdominal trauma in the pediatric patient. The size of the abdominal cavity is smaller, thus bringing all the organs into closer proximity. There is decreased protective muscle and adipose tissue mass, and the protective rigidity of the rib cage is less, providing less protection to abdominal organs and increasing the risk of abdominal injuries. The child's diaphragm is in a more horizontal orientation, thus forcing the liver and spleen into a more anterior and caudal position. Blunt forces on the abdomen are thus more likely to injure these organs. The liver and spleen are the two most commonly injured organs.

Abdominal injury occurs in more than 25% of children suffering multisystem trauma.[11] The mortality rate for children sustaining abdominal trauma is 14%,[13] with the great majority of abdominal trauma being blunt. Children suffer trauma primarily as a result of motor-vehicle accidents, falls, or abuse. Blunt trauma in children also often occurs with sports-related injuries. The mechanisms of injury in blunt trauma are varied and may be secondary to crushing of solid organs (such as the spleen, liver, or kidney), rupture of hollow viscera (stomach, bladder), or the shearing of tubular structures (ureters, blood vessels). Blunt abdominal trauma associated with child abuse deserves special mention, because while it occurs less frequently, it is associated with a high mortality rate. Frequently, the history of abuse is withheld, and there is a delay from the time of injury until treatment is sought.[3] It thus becomes important, if child abuse is suspected, to consider the possibility of abdominal trauma and carefully assess the abdomen. Penetrating wounds to the abdominal cavity are infrequent but are becoming more common as violence involving children increases. These may be the result of gunshot or stab wounds or impalement on an object. Penetrating trauma may also occur when a fractured bone pierces an abdominal structure—for instance, the laceration of the spleen by a fractured rib.

During the initial resuscitation of the trauma patient, it is more important to identify a possible abdominal injury as opposed to defining exactly which organ is injured. While most children have mild, blunt trauma without serious sequelae, those with penetrating trauma, multiple trauma, or isolated severe abdominal trauma require transport to a more specialized care center. It is important in the field to have a high index of suspicion for abdominal injuries, as many serious intra-abdominal injuries can present with subtle clinical findings. Many children who have an unstable cardiovascular status or who fail to stabilize during the initial fluid resuscitation phase often have intra-abdominal injuries. These patients very likely require surgical exploration and intervention upon arrival at the hospital. Other significant factors to look for include abdominal tenderness, distension, significant bruising, contusions and abrasions on the abdomen, and flank, gross hematuria or a mechanism or pattern of injuries that suggest a high risk of intra-abdominal injury.

Physical examination and the physiologic status of the patient are keys to identifying abdominal injuries. However, the initial evaluation of the abdomen in children is more difficult than in adults. The frightened child tends to tighten his or her rectus muscles, possibly giving a false impression of intra-abdominal injury. Gastric dilatation and reflex ileus are far more common in children than in adults after a major injury, thus distending the abdomen. This distension can affect the respiratory patterns of the child; therefore, a nasogastric tube should be inserted early. This tube will not only reduce the risk of aspiration pneumonia and improve respiration but also allow more accurate physical examination of the abdomen. Also, the return of blood in the aspirate can help diagnose intra-abdominal injury. In a similar fashion, decompression of the bladder with a Foley catheter makes examination of the abdomen easier.

The spleen is the most commonly injured organ in children with blunt trauma. Classically, the findings associated with splenic injury are those of a hemoperitoneum (shock, tachycardia, and abdominal distension); however, children with an injury to the spleen present like this only 10% of the time.[16] Often, patients complain of left upper quadrant pain and left shoulder pain, and they may have bruising to the left chest wall or left upper quadrant of the abdomen. Splenic lacerations can be associated with left rib and femur fractures and pelvic fractures with bladder or rectal injuries.[9] Most children with splenic and hepatic injuries who are hemodynamically stable are managed nonoperatively. This management includes close observation in a pediatric intensive care unit. In transporting the pediatric trauma patient, despite hemodynamic stability, any patient with left upper quadrant pain, ecchymosis over the left quadrant, or possible left lower rib fractures should be suspected of a possible splenic injury and transported to a trauma center for close observation. There, immediate surgical intervention is possible should the child become a surgical candidate or the hemodynamic status decompensates.

The liver is the second most commonly injured organ. The liver is relatively larger in the child, and the fibrous stroma of the liver is decreased. The child's flexible rib cage provides the liver with less protection, hence the susceptibility to injury from blunt abdominal trauma or from right lower chest trauma. Like splenic trauma, many hepatic injuries can be managed nonoperatively but require close observation in an intensive care setting, so any suspected liver injury should be transported accordingly.

Although the use of seatbelts greatly reduces the number of deaths from motor vehicle collisions, a number of injuries may result from their use. Hollow viscus injury is rare in children but has become more frequently noted in lap-belted children.[7] This injury is often referred to as the "lap belt complex." Symptoms of these injuries often become apparent later in the clinical course, but it is important to identify those children in motor vehicle accidents who were restrained and the type of restraint device used. A high level of suspicion should be maintained in those children using lap belts who have abdominal wall ecchymosis.

Pelvic Injuries

Pelvic fracture is uncommon in children, most often occurring as a result of blunt trauma from motor vehicle/pedestrian injuries. Also fortunate is that unlike with pelvic fractures in the adult, death from uncontrolled hemorrhage or sepsis is unusual in children. The presence of a pelvic fracture should alert the clinician to a possible concomitant visceral or genitourinary injury. The incidence of intra-abdominal injury in children with an isolated pubic ramus fracture is approximately 6%.[2] However, the risk increases with the complexity of the pelvic fracture. This incidence rises to 33% for isolated iliac or sacral fractures. The presence of multiple fracture sites within the pelvic circle results in visceral injury in 80% of children.[5]

INTERHOSPITAL TRANSPORT

Sometimes, the location and severity of the injured child dictate that he or she be brought to the nearest facility capable of stabilization. Also, because the evaluation of the severity of injury in the pediatric population is more difficult, injuries requiring more advanced care may be missed during the initial evaluation and the patient transported to a center incapable of providing appropriate management. Thus, a pediatric trauma patient often must be transported from one facility to another. This transport carries some inherent risks. Although the patient has theoretically been stabilized, these transports are often long and may put the child at increased risk of deterioration. No matter how sophisticated the method of transport, it represents at the very least a disruption of the in-hospital critical care environment.

Regarding interhospital transport, risks versus benefits must be strongly considered, and the level of care must reflect the severity of the injury. The indications for transport are an inability to provide the necessary definitive care or a need for specialized testing or treatment not available in the current hospital. As with the initial transport of the patient, strict adherence to the transport guidelines is imperative.

Identifying common transport problems, and dealing with them prior to transport, can avoid potentially preventable causes of patient deterioration. The dislodgement of intravenous catheters can be a devastating problem during transport. Securing these prior to transport is essential, and restraint of the patient's extremities is needed. As discussed, the avoidance of hypothermia is crucial in children, so a neutral thermal environment is necessary. The need for sedation to avoid the loss of endotracheal tubes or intravenous lines must be weighed against the need to evaluate the neurologic status of the patient. If it is necessary, short-acting agents such as fentanyl, midazolam, or morphine can be used.

In the intubated patient, securing the endotracheal tube is of paramount importance. After taping, the final position at the lips or nares should be recorded in case it is dislodged. Manual stabilization may be necessary even in a well-taped endotracheal tube. Plugged endotracheal tubes are a common occurrence in tubes smaller than 4.5 mm and can occur in any size tube. Instillation of 1 to 2 ml of saline and suctioning prior to departure and at intervals during transport (roughly every 30 minutes) may prevent this. During long transports, humidification of gas may further alleviate this problem.

Patients with chest tubes can be extremely frustrating during transport. The tubes must be sutured and taped securely, and care provided not to overturn the attached apparatus. Children with pneumothorax are at risk of recurrent or ongoing air leaks. The patient's tolerance for having the tubes disconnected from suction should be assessed prior to moving. If necessary, a portable suction machine may be necessary during transport.

An extremely important factor in transfer is impeccable communication. Interhospital transfer requires that responsibility for the child is being transferred twice; first to the transport team and then to the receiving hospital staff. Before the transfer, there should be a complete history and summary of the physical findings, laboratory, or radiographic findings, procedures done, and medications given communicated to the receiving physicians. This should be updated with any change in the patient's status. The medical record and copies of all radiographs should accompany the child. A lack of suitable communication can counteract all the excellent work done at the first institution and possibly result in ignoring an already identified injury. Also, to improve quality of care, follow-up information should be given back to the referring facility after the patient is transferred.

REFERENCES

1. American Academy of Pediatrics, American College of Emergency Physicians: Advanced Pediatric Life Support Manual.
2. Bond SL, Gotshall CS, Eichelberger MR: Predictors of abdominal injury in children with pelvic fracture. J Trauma 31:1169-1173, 1991.
3. Cooper A, et al: Major blunt abdominal trauma due to child abuse. J Trauma 28:1483-1487, 1988.
4. Eichelberger MR: Trauma of the airway and thorax. Pediatr Ann 16:307-316, 1987.
5. Gausche M, Seidel JS, Henderson DP, et al: Pediatric deaths in emergency medical services in urban and rural areas. Pediatr Emerg Care 5:158-162, 1989.
6. Golladay ES: Thoracic injuries. In Ehrlich FE, Heldrich FJ, Tepas JJ (eds): Pediatric Emergency Medicine. Rockville, MD, Aspen, 1987, pp 69-83.
7. Hoffman MA, Spence LJ, Wesson DE, et al: The pediatric passenger: Trends in seatbelt use and injury patterns. J Trauma 27:974-976, 1987.
8. Inaba AS, Seward PN: An approach to pediatric trauma: Unique anatomic and pathophysiologic aspects of the pediatric patient. Emerg Med Clin North Am 9:523-548, 1991.
9. King DR: Trauma in infancy and childhood: Initial evaluation and management. Pediatr Clin North Am 32:1299-1311, 1985.
10. McCarty DL, Surbure JS: Pediatric trauma: Initial evaluation and stabilization. Pediatr Ann 19:584-596, 1990.
11. Miller R, Leno T: Advances in pediatric emergency department procedures. Emerg Med Clin North Am 9:639-652, 1991.
12. Moront ML, Williams JA, Eichelberger MR, Wilkinson JD: The injured child: An approach to care. Pediatr Clin North Am 41:1201-1226, 1994.
13. Peclet MH, Newman KD, Eichelberger MR, et al: Patterns of injury in children. J Pediatr Surg 25:85-91, 1990.
14. Ramenofsky ML: The predictive validity of the PTS. J Trauma 28:1039-1042, 1988.
15. Rieger A, Berman JM, Striebel HW: Initial resuscitation and vascular access. Int Anesthesiol Clin.
16. Ross AJ: The delicate matter of the spleen. Contemp Pediatr 8:111-122, 1989.
17. Schwaitzberg SD, Bergman KS, Harris BH: A pediatric trauma model of continuous hemorrhage. J Pediatr Surg 23:605-609, 1988.
18. Tepas JJ, Ramenofsky ML, Barlo B, et al: National Pediatric Trauma Registry. J Pediatr Surg 24:156-158, 1989.
19. Thompson AE, Mettler FA, Royal HD: Environmental emergencies. In Fleisher GR, Ludwig S (eds): Textbook of Pediatric Emergency Medicine, 3rd ed. Baltimore, Williams & Wilkins, 1993, pp 612-616.
20. Zanitsky A: Selected topics of controversies in pediatric cardiopulmonary resuscitation. Crit Care Clin 4:735-750, 1988.

CHAPTER 24

Central Nervous System Injuries

YOON S. HAHN, M.D.

Successful experience with prehospital stabilization and treatment of adults with life-threatening cardiac illness in the early 1970s led to the development of the Emergency Medical Service (EMS) system. Analysis of that early prehospital experience with advanced life support (ALS) suggested that field treatment could also improve the survival of patients with traumatic cardiac arrest, blunt trauma, major intraabdominal vascular trauma, and falls from heights.[2,3,11,20,31] The time spent on vascular access was minimal and had no adverse effect on mortality.[24] Now it is standard practice to perform medical stabilization in the field on patients with multiple system injuries.

Prehospital care is predicated on the notion that there is a clear survival advantage in receiving care in a tertiary referral center where sophisticated experienced resources are readily available. There has been ample evidence that rapid transport to a place of definitive care results in a better outcome for a patient with immediately life-threatening injuries.[10,14] Epidemiologic evidence has shown that survival after a motor vehicle accident is greater in areas where ALS is available.[1,36]

Prehospital advanced life support appears to be effective in children[27] as well as adults.[8,21,38] However, children are not simply small adults; their anatomy, physiology, and epidemiology are different. The different mechanisms of injury to which a child is typically exposed and the unique features and physiologic responses of a child are distinct from those observed in adults.

Prehospital care and field management are intended to supply adequate supportive measures, including resuscitation. The same concerns—establishing the airway, breathing, circulation, and administering medications as needed, possibly including hydration—are critically essential for a small child who has lost body fluid or blood from trauma during transport to a definitive care center.

Regionalization is an integral part of care and at least as important as prehospital interventions. The field triage should include a hospital bypass procedure so that a child can be transported directly from the field or accident scene to an appropriate tertiary center without risk of critical deterioration en route.

The chain of survival starts with the caregiver's ability to recognize critical illness and the medical urgency of the situation, followed by the ability to access the EMS system. Next, the system must be able to reach the child in a timely manner, provide appropriate interventions for stabilization, and transport the child to an emergency department for definitive care or further stabilization before transport to a tertiary referral center for definitive management. All parts of this process are critical; if any part of the sequence fails, the child's potential for positive outcome will be compromised.

Longer transport times may require a greater degree of stabilization prior to transportation. This should include airway stabilization, vascular access, intravenous access, placement and inflation of a pneumatic antishock garment where applicable, or administration of beta-agonist therapy. The length of time needed to reach the nearest emergency department will determine the type and sequence of interventions. Inserting an IV may be unnecessary when a hospital is only minutes away. However, if a child with respiratory difficulty is hours away from definitive care, establishing an airway for proper oxygenation, an intravenous line, and delivering intravenous fluid can prevent hypoxic injury to an already critically contused and swollen brain. Children with moderate to severe head injuries and respiratory difficulty can easily deteriorate without proper airway, making field stabilization critical to maintaining an opportunity for survival and a positive outcome.

An initial assessment for a child with a head injury must include rapid but efficient stabilization of cardiopulmonary status. It is often best to intubate in anticipation of interhospital transport if a child has severe head injuries (Children's Coma Scale 8 and under),[19] airway obstruction, abnormalities in the respiratory rate or rhythm, associated chest injury, central nervous system (CNS) signs of lethargy, vomiting, or seizures, with respiratory compromise. Special airway management may be needed for children with facial, oromaxillary, or airway injuries, or cervical spine injuries. Threading an endotracheal tube through the nose can be done with fiberoptic flexible bronchoscopy. The alternatives are emergency tracheostomy or cannulation of the cricothyroid membrane. After intubation, an aerogastric tube should be placed, especially in children with CNS injuries. The nasal route should be avoided in children with basal skull fracture with cerebrospinal fluid (CSF) rhinorrhea and in clinically suspected cases lest the cannula go into the brain.

Because manipulation of the airway may produce a severe cholinergic response, care should be taken to achieve complete cholinergic blockade with atropine. Laryngoscopy after atropine (0.01–0.02 mg/kg IV), even in an unconscious child, may lead to a rise in intracranial pressure.[7] Therefore, intravenous pentothal (3–5 mg/kg IV) or lidocaine (1 mg/kg IV) and muscle relaxants may be needed to prevent or attenuate this response.[4,34]

Establishment of intravenous access is almost mandatory, not only for administration of fluids but also to administer anticonvulsants as indicated. However, this may be difficult, especially in younger children. Intraosseous cannulation can be performed in these cases, using special cannulas or spinal needles. Cannulation of the intraosseous space can be performed about 2 or 3 cm below the tibial tuberosity. The appropriate space can be recognized easily because of the sudden decrease in resistance when the needle goes through the cortical bone into the marrow space. Placement can be confirmed by aspiration of blood from the bone marrow and free flow of fluid by gravity. This access can be used during the field care and transportation for fluids, blood, crystalloids and colloids, and anticonvulsants, as well as antibiotics.

Initial fluid management may include a crystalloid such as Ringer's solution or normal saline, or colloid such as 5% albumin, or blood if there has been traumatic loss. Euvolemia is the main goal of fluid management, particularly in children with CNS injuries. Fluid management in the head-injured patient has been the subject of heated controversy.[39,40] The side arguing for fluid restriction to achieve intracranial dehydration has been pitted against the need to achieve euvolemia rapidly. The appropriate management objective must be to minimize the risks of overhydration, thus precipitating cerebral edema in an already injured brain that may have lost some ability for autoregulation. However, it has been very clear that euvolemia must be maintained to avoid fluctuations in blood pressure, particularly hypotension that could lead to a decrease in the perfusion pressure or cerebral hyperemia, which, in turn, would make the cerebral edema worse and put the brain in jeopardy of herniation. Because both fluid overload and excess free water are detrimental to the patient, as are fluctuations in serum osmolarity, a reasonable starting point is an isotonic solution given at a maintenance rate. However, therapy is best guided by central venous pressure (CVP). Acceptable values are 5–10 mmHg. Other findings such as electrolytes, serum osmolarity, urine output, and specific gravity, can be performed at a later time at the trauma center where the patient receives definitive care.

In the field, a quick physical examination always provides very important information. The appearance, color, and temperature of the skin, quality and rapidity of capillary refill, and peripheral pulses supply the observer with necessary information. Children with head injuries commonly have alterations in peripheral perfusion, heart rate and rhythm, and blood pressure. These changes may emanate from the brain injury itself, or may be an associated complication from traumatic injuries of other organs. The cornerstone of hemodynamic management in all children with head injuries must be the maintenance of an adequate mean arterial pressure.

Central venous pressure is monitored at the level of the right atrium and provides an estimate of cardiac preload. The catheter is threaded to the junction of vena cava and right atrium and then attached to a transducer for continuous monitoring. The preferred site of catheter introduction in infants or younger children is either the femoral or subclavian vein. The Trendelenburg position is not recommended for the procedures lest it increase venous congestion and increase the intracranial pressure. Establishing a central catheter line is also useful for children with severe head injury who may require hyperalimentation, frequent blood sampling, and monitoring of blood gases. In trained hands there should be few complications, although superficial or deep infections, pulmonary embolism, and intrathoracic perforations have been reported.

A pressure of 5–10 mmHg is acceptable under most circumstances; however, children with impaired myocardial contractility may require pressures as high as 16 mmHg. Low right atrial pressures imply hypovolemia, and this should be vigorously corrected.

In all cases, the intravascular volume must be adequate, even if this requires repeated fluid challenges with isotonic solutions. When the patient remains hemodynamically unstable even after intravascular volume is adequately administered, the use of inotropic/vasoactive agents is indicated. Therefore, hemodynamic monitoring is essential for all children with severe head injury. The degree of monitoring should be proportionate to the severity of injury, the amount of hemodynamic compromise, and the complexity of treatment.

Fluid and electrolyte imbalance is frequently associated with severe head injury. The syndrome of inappropriate secretion of antidiuretic hormone (SIADH) can be a serious problem in patient management because the patient's mental state may be worsened in association with convulsion, simulating a mass lesion of the brain. Children with SIADH may have decreased urine output, increased urine sodium and specific gravity, subnormally decreased serum sodium level, and decreased osmolarity. Central venous pressure (CVP) may remain elevated. It is best managed by fluid restriction; the degree of restriction can be determined by CVP and osmolarity of urine and serum, as well as serum urine sodium levels. When a serum sodium level is lower than 125 mEq/L, supplemental sodium may be used to prevent worsening of the neurologic status.

Diabetes insipidus is another form of fluid imbalance that can occur after a severe head injury. It may appear transiently in injuries involving the base of the brain, as a consequence of edema, or as a vascular effect such as vasospasm. Urinary output usually is copious and crystal clear, and the urinary specific gravity is less than 1.005. The serum sodium level is rising and the urinary sodium is less than 10 mEq/L. The CVP is usually low or decreasing. To avoid dehydration or fluid overload, fluid management consists of replacing daily insensible losses (400 ml/m^2 or for infants under 10 kg, 30 ml/kg) and urinary output once euvolemia is reestablished. The pharmacologic replacement of antidiuretic hormone is not usually indicated, especially within the first few days, so long as there is adequate fluid management. When fluid management fails, either short-acting vasopressin (Pitressin) or long-acting (DDAVP) can be used, depending on whether the condition is viewed as temporary or permanent. A short-acting agent is recommended when there is doubt.

Respiratory care in children with head injuries differs in subtle but important ways from the usual respiratory protocol in adults. Oxygen supplementation is recommended for all children with brain injuries in an attempt to avoid sudden unpredictable episodes of hypoxemia.[46] A slight degree of airway obstruction or hypercarbia should be treated vigorously by endotracheal intubation and mechanical ventilation. Evidence of cerebral dysfunction or signs of impending cerebral herniation, such as unstable vital signs with bradycardia, respiratory irregularities, or clouding of consciousness, are an indication for intubation and mechanical ventilation, regardless of carbon dioxide partial pressure (PCO_2).

Once a patient is intubated, mechanical ventilation is adjusted to a PCO_2 of about 30–35 mmHg. Unless otherwise indicated, initial ventilator parameters usually approximate a tidal volume of 10–14 ml/kg and a respiratory rate slightly higher than physiologic parameters for age. Positive end-expiratory pressure (PEEP) and FiO_2 are adjusted to achieve a partial pressure of oxygen (PO_2) of 100 mmHg. If PEEP is inadequately aligned, it can contribute to an increase in intracranial pressure. If this occurs, it usually can be counteracted by judicious positioning of the patient in bed. The head of the bed should be elevated about 30°, and the patient's head should be kept in neutral position.

It is often necessary to sedate or chemically paralyze children with severe head injuries to avoid unwanted movement caused by bucking, gagging, coughing, and/or agitation, all of which may serve to increase intracranial pressure (ICP). In addition to minimizing movement or turning of the children, pulmonary toilet is kept at a minimum. It may be necessary to premedicate a child with a short-acting barbiturate (e.g., pentothal, 1 mg/kg IV, or lidocaine, 1 mg/kg IV) to minimize movement that might increase ICP about 1 minute before suctioning or other manipulation. The use of a kinetic bed may eliminate the effect of stasis and prevent some of the complications caused by its effect on cerebral hemodynamics. Respiratory monitoring of a child with severe head injury can be done by invasive or noninvasive methods. Continuous monitoring of arterial oxygen saturations by pulse oximetry is recommended for all severely head-injured children. The use of end-tidal exhaled carbon dioxide measurements ($ETCO_2$) as an index of arterial PCO_2 has become increasingly popular because it is noninvasive and because continuous, real-time information is gained.[42] The limitations of this device in some clinical settings (lung disease, large air leak around the endotracheal tube) must be recognized in order for it to be an effective monitoring strategy. Transcutaneous CO_2 monitoring may be substituted for $ETCO_2$ in some circumstances. Ultimately, periodic sampling of arterial blood for measurement of blood gas tensions (usually from an indwelling arterial catheter) is the most precise tool, and it also allows monitoring the child's acid-base status.

The clinical manifestations of increased ICP are different in children, depending on age and whether or not the sutures are open or closed. Normally there is a rather delicate balance between the volume of the intracranial space and the volume of its contents. After the sutures and anterior fontanelle close, the cranium becomes a rigid container with limited capability for effective volume management should an intracranial mass lesion develop. The intracranial contents include the meninges, brain parenchyma, cerebrospinal fluid, blood vessels, and the blood within them. In order to maintain the pressure relationships between these intracranial contents, enlargement of any one of these structures must be accompanied by a reduction in volume of one or more of the others; this principle is known as the Monro-Kellie doctrine. The buffering system that compensates for increased intracranial pressure due to a mass lesion is relatively limited. The CSF usually is the first to be displaced from the skull into either the spinal thecal sac or from the ventricles into the subarachnoid space. In addition, there may be a temporary increase of CSF absorption across the arachnoid villi. However, when the maximal amount of CSF displacement is exceeded, clinical manifestations of increased ICP emerge. These are affected by several factors: (1) age of the child (cranial sutures, anterior fontanelle open or closed) and (2) onset of the mass lesion. With acute lesions such as cerebral edema and intracranial hematomas, the adaptability is marginal, resulting in a quick increase in pressure. With slower growing lesions such as meningioma, the mass can achieve a remarkably large size with only minor symptoms or signs.

Experimental studies in animals have shown that the injection of a small volume of normal saline (1 ml) into the closed intracranial space initially results in little or no elevation of pressure and a rapid return to baseline. With additional instillations of small quantities over a short period, a point is reached where one further injection of a very small volume gives rise to a marked rise in the intracranial pressure that does not subsequently return to baseline.[26] The clinical application of these studies is pertinent to the problem of mass lesions in humans, such as a neoplasm, which slowly increases in size, gradually displacing intracranial CSF and shifting of (regional) brain. At the point of maximal compensatory displacement, even a slight increase in the intracranial volume or brain water content will result in exponential pressure changes. In the early decades of this century Cushing-Kocher observed the following vital sign changes when the ICP increased: slowing of the pulse, alteration of the respiration rate, and elevation of the blood pressure. This sequence of changes of vital signs is called Cushing phenomenon.

The classic symptom triad of increased ICP is headaches, nausea-vomiting, and papilledema. Headaches alone are rather nonspecific, but headaches and papilledema together are virtually diagnostic of increased intracranial pressure. The headache may be persistent, but is more often intermittent and frequently associated with vomiting. The vomiting usually occurs in the early morning, shortly before rising from sleep, and can be projectile, especially in children with posterior fossa lesions. This phenomenon is due to an intermittent pressure increase during the rapid eye movement phase (REM stage) of sleep, a decrease of venous return with subsequent increase of intracranial pressure, and a decrease in gravity drainage of CSF from the ventricular system while in the supine position throughout the night.

In the chronic stages of increased ICP, infants and toddlers become irritable and agitated, showing personality and behavior changes. As a result of loss of appetite, compounded by recurrent attacks of vomiting, there can be a significant loss of body weight. An increase in head circumference usually progresses to macrocephaly; the sutures become separated, and the anterior fontanelle becomes full and tense; the scalp stretches and takes on a shiny appearance, and the scalp veins engorge; the eyeballs look like a "setting sun" because of the paralysis of upward gaze. Seizure disorders can occur in up to 30% of children. Older children frequently are noted to become indifferent, drowsy, or show a lack of interest. School performance may decline, and physical activity may diminish.

Increased ICP in the newborn is usually the result of either congenital hydrocephalus, perinatal asphyxia, or periventricular-intraventricular hemorrhage associated with low birth weight. Tentorial or falx laceration secondary to distortion of the skull during passage through the birth canal can result in traumatic subarachnoid or subdural hemorrhage. These complications of labor and delivery can evolve into progressive hydrocephalus. Increased intracranial pressure in infants and toddlers can be associated with brain tumors, meningitis, infection of brain, head trauma, severe craniosynostosis, or bleeding associated with an arteriovenous malformation of the brain.

The management of children with increased intracranial pressure will be explained in reference to the child with severe head injury.

When a child has proven increased ICP, the focus of therapy changes dramatically, and all aspects of care are realigned. Elevated ICP should be suspected in a patient with a Children's Coma Scale score below 8 or in any head-injured child with progressive deterioration of neurologic status. The indications for ICP monitoring in children include: (1) deep coma; (2) a Children's Coma Scale score of 8 or less (severe head injury); (3) head injury with respiratory difficulties or pulmonary injury requiring mechanical ventilation, sedation, and paralyzation; and (4) systemic injuries requiring mechanical ventilation and paralyzation.

Although the most frequently used method of CSF sampling and pressure measurement is the lumbar puncture, this method is seldom, if ever, indicated in the management of acute head injury. Its complications include infection, CSF leakage, hematoma, and brain herniation. Direct ventricular pressure measurement remains the gold standard of ICP monitoring. A ventricular catheter is advanced through a small trephination (usually in the frontal region) through the brain parenchyma to the frontal horn of the lateral ventricle. It can be connected through a pressure transducer to a monitor, a manometer, and drainage system or both. The advantages of this method are its accuracy and the ability to drain CSF and thereby decrease ICP. Disadvantages include the risk of infection, especially ventricultis, intraventricular bleeding, and obstruction of the catheter, which requires surgical revision.

The intracranial bolt to measure ICP through the subarachnoid space once enjoyed great popularity, but its use is less common now. It is a simple device; however, malfunction of the system is relatively common because of disruption of the fluid column (e.g, air bubble) or occlusion of the lumen by blood clot or brain debris.

A more frequently used device is intraparenchymal pressure monitoring (Camino Laboratories, San Diego). This fiberoptic monitor is introduced into the brain parenchyma through a small trephination, usually in the frontal area close to the coronal suture. Pressure readings are displayed as a digital readout and a waveform so that 8-hour or 24-hour trend information can be obtained. This device is reliable even though there is a minimal drift of 0.5–1 mmHg a day, and it can be used easily even in infants and toddlers. It can be kept in place from a few days to weeks, and infection is rare. Management of a patient with acute brain injury must focus on prevention of cerebral herniation, minimizing secondary neuronal damage or restoring already damaged neurons by control of ICP, proper ventilation, and preservation of cerebral perfusion pressure. At present, there is no reliable clinical or physiologic indicator that accurately predicts patient outcome. It is clear that patients whose ICP exceeds 30 mmHg fare poorly, yet maintaining ICP below 20 mmHg does not necessarily guarantee a better outcome. Physiologic parameters that herald a good outcome should include intracranial pressure less than 20 mmHg and cerebral perfusion pressure (equals systemic blood pressure minus ICP) of 50–70 mmHg. All management decisions should be influenced by maintaining these parameters.

In the clinical setting, ICP may be influenced by removing an extracerebral mass lesion, decreasing intracranial blood volume or intraparenchymal extracellular water, draining CSF, decreasing cerebral water, and, rarely, by reducing parenchymal mass by surgical decompression.

The most expedient method to control ICP is hyperventilation (PCO_2 25–27 mmHg), which, through its effects on PCO_2 and pH of the cerebral blood vessels, causes vasoconstriction, a 4% decrease in cerebral blood flow (CBF) for each mmHg drop in the PCO_2, and a decline in blood volume and ICP almost immediately. However, extreme hyperventilation (less than 20 mmHg) can reduce CBF below the ischemic threshold, thus promoting secondary damage in an already traumatized brain. Although hyperventilation is a very effective acute intervention, it loses its effectiveness after a time (usually days to weeks) because of acid-base reequilibration or vasomotor paralysis.[9] When the degree of hyperventilation is relaxed, even after days, there are intracranial volume changes and ICP increases. For these reasons, extreme hyperventilation should not be used as a routine maintenance therapy. Elevating the head of the bed about 30° promotes venous return, thus decreasing the ICP, and is very widely used and effective tool.

Diuretic therapy often is used to decrease ICP, and osmotic diuretic agents have been used extensively. The most frequently used today is mannitol.[28,29,41] Recently, its use has been questioned because (1) mannitol does not cross the intact blood-brain barrier but exerts its dehydrating influence mainly on unhealthy brain, making it possible to hyperfuse the traumatized portion of the brain and aggravate edema in the injured parts, and (2) mannitol has a direct effect on the cerebral blood vessels and, under most circumstances, causes vasoconstriction.[23,37] However, mannitol may at times cause an increase in intravascular volume and precipitate an acute rise in ICP, particularly in vasoparalyzed brain.[33] Mannitol may be given as bolus of 0.25–1 gm/kg/dose or via a continuous drip. Therapy is titrated to ICP response and is limited by rising serum osmolality and serum sodium. The desired serum osmolality during mannitol therapy is 300 mOsm/L, and efforts must be made to limit osmolality to below 320 mOsm/L. Renal failure can occur at osmolality of 340 mOsm/L. Furosemide is a loop diuretic used occasionally in the management of ICP. It is believed to augment the effect of mannitol and to cause extracellular water loss. It is a mild inhibitor of CSF production and thus may transiently decrease control of ICP.

Cerebrospinal fluid drainage or external ventricular drainage (EVD) for ICP control appears to be a simple and logical procedure, but many times the volume needed to decrease ICP is too small for a brain that is generally edematous or contused. Often, tapping the ventricle is not feasible because the brain is edematous and the ventricles are collapsed so that there can be catheter obstruction even after a line is established. Moreover, the production of CSF is often suppressed, especially when the ICP is elevated.

Barbiturates have been used extensively in neurosurgery to reduce ICP.[43,47] Pentobarbital and phenobarbital have been used for this purpose in the pediatric intensive care unit. Both require large doses to maintain their effect, dosages that can cause hemodynamic instability and may lead to an increase in systemic infections. Large doses of barbiturates increase short-term morbidity; at this time, there are no systematic data supporting their use in pediatric head injury.

Glucocorticoids influence brain function and activity in many ways. Their mechanism of action is incompletely understood, even though their effects on cerebral edema have been studied extensively.[15,32] Briefly, they exert the greatest influence on vasoactive edema. They are most effective in peritumoral vasoactive edema and least effective in head injury and cerebral edema. Although the use of high-dose steroids was shown to be effective in acute traumatic spinal cord injuries[5] and perhaps in some subgroups of traumatic head injury, their benefits remain unproven and their use in acute head injury remains controversial.

Several small clinical series have suggested that survival from very severe head injury can be improved by performing large decompressive craniectomies.[6,12,16] This form of therapy remains controversial. The author believes that a swollen traumatized brain is best managed medically in an intensive care setting. Very rarely, a decompressive craniectomy coupled with a resection of contused cerebral tissue is required to regain control of ICP, but there is almost no role for this procedure.[13]

A number of exciting developments are taking place in research laboratories where the roles of neurotransmitters, calcium, oxyradicals, prostaglandins, and a host of mediators of cellular injury are being investigated.[35,44] In all probability, it will be possible in the future to block some of these mechanisms and to prevent cellular injury in a specific and elegant fashion. For now, these preliminary investigations must be limited to the laboratory. Therapeutic efforts, therefore, remain targeted at the organ system level.

It is well known that even minor head injuries can cause serious neurologic sequelae and long-term neuropsychological deficits.[18,25,26,45] Fortunately, the injury to the nervous system is insignificant in the vast majority of cases. Occasionally, the brain is the primary site of injury, or processes are set in motion that cause secondary injury to the CNS. Little can be done about primary brain injury, aside from prevention, but a great deal can now be done to treat secondary damage that results from cerebral ischemia, hypoxia, raised intracranial pressure, intracranial mass lesions such as epidural or subdural hematomas, and associated systemic hypotension. These problems compound the primary damage to the brain and can initiate a process leading to irreversible brain damage or death if medical-surgical intervention is not prompt.

Trauma accounts for about one-third of all pediatric surgical admissions, and half of these children have sustained a head injury. Mortality figures for head injury in children vary widely. There about 100,000 accidental deaths per year in North America, and approximately 25,000 of these are children. Previous studies have shown that one-half to three-fourths of children who are admitted to the hospital in coma die. Recent studies paint a somewhat more optimistic picture, with a mortality rate of 20–40%.[19,22,30]

Under the general plan of management for children with head injuries, the first step is deciding whether to admit an injured child for further care in a hospital setting or to leave the patient in the hands of the caretaker. A hospital that can adequately treat children with head injuries will have an area for constant observation, personnel knowledgeable in trauma care, emergency equipment appropriate for pediatric patients, a CT scanner, and a readily available neurosurgeon. Lack of any of these capabilities precludes admission and demands transfer of the child to another hospital.

Children not admitted to a hospital should be watched closely at home by caretakers (usually parents) who have been instructed to return to the hospital if the child's level of consciousness deteriorates or if the child develops such signs or symptoms as seizures, persistent vomiting, irritability, or headaches. Not all caretakers can or will follow instructions as given, a fact that must be kept in mind. The reliability of the caretakers has been the subject of several studies; in the author's own study, only one in three caretakers followed instructions as directed. Therefore, admission is recommended for children who have sustained seemingly minor head injuries and have any one of the following: (1) loss of consciousness or lethargy; (2) skull fracture; (3) vomiting or irritability; (4) seizures; (5) caretakers who appear unable to observe a child properly at home; or (6) lack of an adequate history or mechanism of injury.

The author believes that all children admitted with a diagnosis of head injury, whether minor or severe, should have CT examination of the skull and the brain.

REFERENCES

1. Alexander RH, Pons PT, Krischer J: The effect of advanced life support and sophisticated hospital systems on motor vehicle mortality. J Trauma 24:486–490, 1984.
2. Aprahamian C, Darin JC, Thompson BM: Traumatic cardiac arrest: Scope of paramedic services. Ann Emerg Med 14:583–586, 1985.
3. Aprahamian C, Thompson BM, Towne JB: The effect of a paramedic system on mortality of major open intra-abdominal vascular trauma. J Trauma 23:687–690, 1983.
4. Bedford RF, Persing JA, Pobereskin L: Clinical practice; secondary insults during intrahospital transport of head-injured patients. Lancet 335:327–330, 1990.
5. Bracken MB, Shepard MJ, Collins WF: A randomised, controlled trial of methylprednisolone or naloxone in the treatment of acute spinal cord injury. Results of the Second National Acute Spinal Cord Injury Study. N Engl J Med 322:1405–1411, 1990.
6. Britt RH, Hamilton RD: Large decompressive craniotomy in the treatment of acute subdural hematoma. Neurosurgery 22:195–200, 1978.
7. Burney RG, Winn R: Increased cerebrospinal fluid pressure during laryngoscopy and intubation for induction of anesthesia. Anesth Analg 54:687–690, 1975.
8. Cwinn AA, Pons PT, Moore EE: Prehospital advanced trauma life support for critical blunt trauma victims. Ann Emerg Med 16:399–403, 1987.
9. Darby JM, Yonus H, Marion DW: Local "inverse steal" induced by hyperventilation in head injury. Neurosurgery 23:84–88, 1988.
10. Fischer RP, Jelense S, Perry JF: Direct transfer to operating room improves care of trauma patients: A simple, economically feasible plan for large hospitals. JAMA 240:1731–1732, 1978.
11. Fortner GS, Oreskovich MR, Copass MK: The effect of prehospital trauma care on survival from a 50-metre fall. J Trauma 23:976–981, 1983.
12. Gaab M, Knoblich OE, Fuhrmeister U: Comparison of the effects of surgical decompression and resection of local edema in the therapy of experimental brain trauma. Child's Brain 5:484–498, 1979.
13. Gaab M, Rittierodt M, Lorenz M: Traumatic brain swelling and operative decompression: A prospective investigation. Acta Neurochir 51(Suppl):326–328, 1990.
14. Gervin AS, Fischer RP: The importance of prompt transport in salvage of patients with penetrating heart wounds. J Trauma 22:443–448, 1982.
15. Giannotta SL, Weiss MH, Apuzzo MLJ: High dose glucocorticoids in the management of severe head injury. Neurosurgery 15:497–501, 1984.
16. Goetting MG, Preston G: Jugular bulb catheterization: Experience with 123 patients. Crit Care Med 18:1220–1223, 1990.

17. Hahn YS, Fuchs S, Flannery AM, et al: Factors influencing posttraumatic seizures in children. Neurosurgery 22:864–867, 1988.
18. Hahn YS, McLone DG: Risk factors in the outcome of children with minor head injury. Pediatr Neurosurg 19:135–142, 1993.
19. Hahn YS, McLone DG, Chyung CH, Barthel M: Head injuries in children under 36 months of age. Childs Nerv Syst 4:34–40, 1988.
20. Hedges JR, Sacco WJ, Champion HR: An analysis of prehospital care of blunt trauma. J Trauma 22:989–993, 1982.
21. Honigman B, Rohweder K, Moore EE: Prehospital advanced trauma life support for penetrating cardiac wounds. Ann Emerg Med 19:145–150, 1990.
22. Humphreys RP, Jamimovich R, Hendrick B, Hoffman H: Severe head injuries in children. Concepts Pediatr Neurosurg 4:230, 1983.
23. Jafar JJ, Johns LM, Mulligan SF: The effect of mannitol on cerebral blood flow. J Neurosurg 64:754–759, 1986.
24. Kaweski SM, Sise MJ, Virgilio RW: The effect of prehospital fluids on survival in trauma patients. J Trauma 30:1215–1219, 1990.
25. Klauber MR, Marshall LF, Luerssen TG, et al: Determinants of head injury mortality: Importance of the low risk patient. Neurosurgery 24:31–36, 1989.
26. Langfitt TW, Bruce DA: Microcirculation and brain edema in head injury. In Vinken PJ, Bruyn GW (eds): Handbook of Clinical Neurology, vol. 23. Amsterdam, North-Holland, 1978, pp 133–161.
27. Lavery RF, Tortella BJ, Griffin CG: The prehospital treatment of pediatric trauma. Pediatr Emerg Care 8:9–12, 1992.
28. Levin AB, Duff TA, Javid MJ: Treatment of increased intracranial pressure: A comparison of different hyperosmotic agents and the use of thiopental. Neurosurgery 5:570–575, 1979.
29. Levin HS, Williams D, Crofford MJ: Relationship of depth of brain lesions to consciousness and outcome after closed head injury. J Neurosurg 69:861–866, 1988.
30. Mahoney WJ, D'Souza BJ, Haller JA: Long-term outcome of children with severe head trauma and prolonged coma. Pediatrics 71:75, 1983.
31. McSwain GR, Garrison WB, Artz CP: Evaluation of resuscitation from cardiopulmonary arrest by paramedics. Ann Emerg Med 9:341–345, 1980.
32. Molofsky WJ: Steroid and head trauma. Neurosurgery 15:424–426, 1984.
33. Muizelaar JP, Marmarou A, DeSalles AAF: Cerebral blood flow and metabolism in severely head-injured children. Part I: Relationship with GCS score, outcome, ICP, and PVI. J Neurosurg 71:63–71, 1989.
34. Nagao S, Murota T, Momma F: The effect of intravenous lidocaine on experimental brain edema and neural activities. J Trauma 28:1650–1655, 1988.
35. Nemoto EM, Shiu GK, Nemmer J, et al: Attenuation of brain fatty acid liberation during global ischemia: A model for screening potential therapies for efficacy? J Cereb Blood Flow Metab 6:332, 1986.
36. Ornato JP, Craren EJ, Nelson NM: Impact of improved emergency medical services and emergency trauma care on the reduction in mortality from trauma. J Trauma 25:575–579, 1985.
37. Ostrup RC, Luerssen TG, Marshall LF: Continuous monitoring of intracranial pressure with a miniaturized fiberoptic device. J Neurosurg 67:206–209, 1987.
38. Potter D, Goldstein G, Fung SC: A controlled trial of prehospital advanced life support in trauma. Ann Emerg Med 17:582–588, 1988.
39. Prough DS: Fluid resuscitation in head-injured patients: Unresolved issues. J Intens Care Med 5:53–56, 1990.
40. Rabow L, DeSalles AAF, Becker DP: CSF brain creatine kinase levels and lactic acidosis in severe head injury. J Neurosurg 65:625–629, 1986.
41. Ravussin P, Abou-Madi M, Archer D: Changes in CSF pressure after mannitol in patients with and without elevated CSF pressure. J Neurosurg 69:869–876, 1988.
42. Rubenstein JS, Hageman JR: Monitoring of critically ill infants and children. Crit Care Clin 4:621–639, 1988.
43. Shapiro K: Head injury in children. U.S. Government Central Nervous System Trauma Status Report, NINCDS. Bethesda, MD, National Institutes of Health, 1985, pp 243–253.
44. Siesjo BK, Wieloch T: Brain ischemia and cellular calcium homeostasis. In Godfraind T (ed): Calcium Entry Blockers and Tissue Protection. New York, Raven Press, 1985, p 139.
45. Singer HS, Freeman JM: Head trauma for the pediatrician. Pediatrics 62:819–825, 1978.
46. Taylor MB, Whitman JG: The current status of pulse-oximetry; clinical value of continuous noninvasive oxygen saturation monitoring. Anaesthesia 41:943–949, 1982.
47. Traeger SM, Henning RJ, Dobkin W: Hemodynamic effects of pentobarbital therapy for intracranial pressure. Crit Care Med 11:697–701, 1983.

CHAPTER 25

Cardiothoracic Injuries in Children

MICHAEL N. ILBAWI, M.D.
LOU M. SMITH, M.D.
PHILIP C. SMITH, M.D.

Trauma continues to exact an inordinate toll on children, accounting for more deaths in individuals between ages 1 and 15 than all other causes combined. In addition to the 20,000 annual pediatric deaths in the United States, over 50,000 children are left with a disability.[33] The billions of dollars spent annually in hospital, medical, and rehabilitative costs pale in comparison to the incalculable losses in productivity and the disrupted lives and emotional upheaval of victims and their families.

Thoracic trauma in children is infrequent but potentially lethal. Most reports suggest that thoracic injuries account for 10% of pediatric trauma admissions and for 15–25% of pediatric trauma deaths, second only to head injury.[17] Frequently, children with thoracic injuries have coexisting head, abdominal, and skeletal involvement. The potential lethality of this spectrum of injury mandates meticulous evaluation of any child presenting with thoracic injury. As such, chest trauma has proved a valid marker for injury severity.[14]

Prompt management of chest trauma in children in the field and hospital is sometimes hindered by lack of experience with this population and difficulties with diagnosis due to the subtle findings on routine history, physical examination, and supine chest radiographs. Focused efforts to detect the nature and extent of disease are of utmost importance, as many life-threatening thoracic injuries can be treated effectively during the initial phase of evaluation and resuscitation.

PATHOPHYSIOLOGIC AND ANATOMIC CONSIDERATIONS

Despite all the devastating effects of trauma in children, fewer resources and less attention have been directed toward the injured child. Although the principles of resuscitation are similar to those for adults, appreciation of differences in cardiorespiratory variables, airway anatomy, response to blood loss, and thermoregulation is necessary for optimum care. Some of these factors are not well emphasized, leading to insufficient training of emergency medical personnel and, hence, lack of expertise in management. It is important that differences in the child be recognized to minimize death and disability.[19]

The physiologic response of the child to injury differs from that in the adult in several aspects, some of which are advantageous. Children have larger cardiac and pulmonary reserves and better tolerance to hypoxia. Acute blood loss is compensated for by increased heart rate and peripheral vascular resistance, making it possible to maintain blood pressure within a normal range with blood loss up to 25% of the total blood volume.[18] Unfortunately, these compensatory mechanisms can lull one into a false sense of security and lead to delay in proper volume replacement. If hypovolemia continues, blood pressure tends to drop in a more precipitous fashion than in the adult and may be more difficult to recover, even when appropriate fluids are then administered. For this reason, continuous surveillance for tachycardia and cool extremities is essential, and the threshold for insertion of adequate venous access should be low.

The high ratio of body surface area to weight in the child also leads to a more rapid development of hypothermia.[22] This effect is even more pronounced in the infant, in whom the thermoregulatory system is immature. Hypothermia complicates shock by worsening the acidosis, shifting the oxygen-hemoglobin dissociation curve, and exerting a negative inotropic effect on the myocardium. Cool ambient temperatures in trauma rooms and administration of cold and room-temperature fluids further exacerbate the problem. Overhead and fluid warmers, as well as in-room temperature controls, are needed in the care of these patients.

Another concern in pediatric trauma is the airway. The infant has a small oral cavity with a larger tongue and a more cephalad and anterior laryngeal position. This situation makes visualization of the cords more challenging. The vocal cords and trachea are also shorter. The length of the trachea in the newborn is 4–5 cm and in the 18-month-old is 7–8 cm. Thus, right main stem intubation is not uncommon and should be suspected when poor ventilation and oxygenation occur. Also, the prominent occiput in the smaller child leads to flexion of the head and neck when the child is supine. This, in and of itself, can cause airway obstruction and/or exacerbate obstruction due to trauma. Placement of a small towel or pad under the shoulders and upper back opens the airway and maintains more proper cervical alignment as well.

Very important to any discussions of chest trauma in the pediatric patient are the differences in the chest wall that affect the patterns of injury and subsequent management. The child has more elasticity and resilience in the chest wall; this makes fractures of the ribs and sternum and flail chest less common than in adults but results in the transmission of greater kinetic energy to the internal thoracic structures.[9] Therefore, the child can have severe internal injuries with little or no external signs and with a normal initial chest radiograph. The compliant sternum allows retrosternal structures such as the heart, which has little other protective mechanisms, to be traumatized. Pain and discomfort are also less common. The greater mobility of the heart and mediastinum may decrease the likelihood of injuries to the tracheobronchial tree and great vessels, but is more likely to produce translocation of the heart, transection or angulation of the great vessels, and tracheal compression. Moreover, it results in cardiovascular and ventilatory compromise more readily due to mediastinal shift. Pulmonary and cardiac contusions and rupture of the diaphragm are also more likely. In addition, the child has weaker chest musculature and is more reliant on the diaphragm for effective breathing. Not only diaphragmatic injury but also gastric distension and tight spine board straps may impair ventilation.[1]

Traumatic asphyxia occurs almost exclusively in children due to their flexible thorax and absence of valves in the superior and inferior vena cava. The direct sudden compression of the compliant thoracic cage against a closed glottis causes a dramatic rise in intratracheal and intrapulmonary pressures and concomitant temporary caval obstruction, with capillary extravasation, cerebral hemorrhage, and with possible bleeding in other organs. This can easily be confused with central nervous system injury, as the child typically presents with disorientation, loss of consciousness, seizures, facial cyanosis, subconjunctival hemorrhage, vascular engorgement, petechiae of the chest, head, and neck, hepatomegaly, and respiratory failure. Misdiagnosis leads to misdirection of therapy and subsequent complications.

Hypoxemia and hypotension produced in children is extremely serious in light of their increased metabolic demands, which lead to an oxygen demand three times greater than that of the adult. The normal compensatory mechanism of increasing minute ventilation may be severely compromised by chest injury. Tachypnea caused by chest trauma may exaggerate fluid and heat loss and accelerate hypothermia and hypovolemia.

Add to all of these anatomic and physiologic differences the obvious developmental, emotional, intellectual, and social differences, and one easily understands that the pediatric patient is more difficult to assess, monitor, and treat. Recognition of the differences and incorporation of these concepts into the plan of trauma management is essential to good outcome.

PREHOSPITAL CARE

The most common reason for emergency medical services in the pediatric population is trauma. Some issues in the prehospital care of the child remain unresolved and lack adequate scientific investigation. Much literature has been generated in the last 5 years regarding whether patients should go to a designated pediatric trauma center or an adult trauma center for care. The answer remains unresolved, but in all but large urban centers, the eventual point may be moot.[32]

The extent of prehospital care is also a divided issue. Ivatury et al. believe that because of limitation to resuscitative efforts in the field, a "scoop and run" approach is best for the child with thoracic injury, especially in an urban setting.[15] Gervin and Fischer contend that delay in the field, particularly for intubation and intravenous access, contributes to an increase in mortality.[11] Evidence indicates that for transport times of < 20 minutes, the volume of fluid infused for resuscitation does not significantly influence final outcome. Nakayama et al. indicate that airway complications in the field are common and usually associated with multiple attempts.[25] Misadventures included right main stem intubation, massive barotrauma, inadequate preoxygenation, esophageal intubation, attempted nasotracheal intubation through a facial fracture, and extubation during transport—all potentially life-threatening. Confusion at the scene, inadequate lighting, limitation in personnel, and distracting influences all exacerbate the already difficult management in children.

Even in light of these points, many feel that prehospital care administered by well-trained paramedical and medical staff, in communication with an experienced hospital-based team, has increased survival in the pediatric population by as much as 30%.[7,16,20] However, it is generally agreed that efficient, knowledgeable staff can and should provide care before and during transport.

Another issue in prehospital management of pediatric trauma concerns which procedure should be attempted in the field or during transport.[28] Losek and colleagues noted that intubation is 78% successful in the arrested pediatric patient in the field, a rate that compares favorably with statistics in adults. However, the success rate dropped 48% in the nonarrested patient.[21] Ornato et al. have shown that mortality can be further reduced when additional airway skills and guidelines are aggressively implemented.[26] Vascular access can be a challenge in the child, even under the best of circumstances; prehospital personnel should be familiar with intraosseous as well as intravenous techniques for fluid administration. Studies have demonstrated that emergency personnel can successfully place an intraosseous access on the first attempt in 80% of cases.[23] Using all forms of access, success rates as high as 93% in the prehospital setting have been cited. Moreover, procedures that can be performed with reasonable success in the field can also be done equally effectively en route to the definitive care facility, thereby alleviating the delay and still reaping the benefits of well-executed resuscitative efforts.[4]

Obviously, these areas need further scientific investigation. In some instances, these controversies are more apparent than real, particularly in large urban areas with multiple trauma centers and short transport times. Field resuscitation must be tailored to the special circumstances of each community, taking into account the nature of the injury and geographic location of the nearest trauma center. Physicians must assume an active role in recognizing which hospitals are equipped to handle major pediatric trauma, maintaining quality assurance of scene attempt and procedural success, proper dispatch of air and ground transport, and development and continuing education of specialized pediatric prehospital teams. In the child with chest injuries, skilled, well-educated prehospital care indeed can make a real difference in outcome, as the basic ABC's of resuscitation can be life-preserving.

INITIAL ASSESSMENT AND RESUSCITATION

A systematic approach to the injured child minimizes morbidity and mortality. The care provider must develop the knowledge and skill to correctly and expediently assess and intervene in the critical early stages, while bearing in mind that the patient is a dynamic entity who requires frequent reevaluation. Attention to the anatomic and pathophysiologic differences in the pediatric population are particularly important in the chest-injured child, as many of the therapeutic interventions performed during a primary survey can be life-saving. Inspection of the child's chest for brusing, wounds, signs of respiratory obstruction, asymmetry of movement, or certain patterns suggestive of a particular type of injury is essential. Bruises from seat belts may indicate a tear in the thoracic aorta or pulmonary contusion. In older children, the marks of a steering wheel suggest sternal fracture and cardiac contusion.[8] The importance of supplying and maintaining appropriate equipment to perform the ABC's in this patient group cannot be overemphasized.

Airway

Establisment and maintenance of a patent airway are of the utmost priority. One-hundred-percent mask oxygen should be administered initially to all unintubated trauma victims. The basic "look, listen, and feel" approach is helpful in establishing if an airway exists. Clearing the airway of oral secretions, debris, and foreign material can be performed with suctioning devices. In the infant, an obligate nasal breather, obstructed nares and oropharynx make breathing more difficult due to the large head and tongue. Simple changes in positioning and support can often alleviate the difficulties. Chin-lift and jaw-thrust maneuvers also can be helpful but must be used with caution in any child with suspected cervical spine injury.[31] Cervical spine immobilization, if necessary, can make airway intervention more challenging.

Nasopharyngeal airways can be employed in children without facial fractures. Oropharyngeal airways are recommended only in the unconscious child, as their use in children with an intact gag reflex may lead to choking, laryngospasm, or vomiting and further complicate matters. In general, the recommended airway for the unconscious child is an uncuffed endotracheal intubation, particularly in victims with Glasgow Coma Scores of 8 or less.[5] Proper equipment for intubation, ventilation, and monitoring is required. If these methods fail, needle cricothyroidotomy with jet insufflation can temporize airway management until more definitive airway control can be secured.

Breathing

Assessment of breathing encompasses not only rate, pattern, depth, symmetry, and observation for nasal flaring and retraction, but also includes evaluation of the effectiveness of the process. The chest should be completely disrobed and inspected for external signs of injury. Contusions on the chest indicate strong kinetic forces which may affect major internal structures and lead to significant injuries, such as pulmonary or cardiac contusion. The trachea should also be observed for shift from the midline. The chest should be palpated for crepitus associated with sternal and rib fractures and for subcutaneous emphysema, which may herald injury to the lung parenchyma, tracheobronchial tree, and/or esophagus. Auscultation assesses effectiveness of bilateral air movement. Unilateral absence of breath sounds aids in the diagnosis of pneumothorax, hemothorax, and hemopneumothorax.

During this portion of the initial assessment, open, closed, and tension pneumothoraces, large hemothorax, flail chest, and sucking chest wounds should be recognized and treatment instituted.[38] Treatment of these specific entities is discussed in the following sections.

Circulation

Due to the tremendous compensatory mechanisms, volume loss, the most common cause of shock in the injured child, is frequently underestimated. Adequate large-bore (16 gauge or larger) intravenous access should be placed early in any child whose mechanism of injury is sufficient to be life-threatening, regardless of the vital signs on presentation. The onset of hypotension portends a volume loss of at least 25%. Careful observation for mild tachycardia and tachypnea, cool extremities, pale coloration, narrowing of the pulse pressure, and delays in capillary refill in the patient with an otherwise normal examination will lead to earlier resuscitative efforts and avert disastrous outcomes. Knowledge of the normal values for heart rate and blood pressure in a given pediatric age range is needed, and these values should be available for the resuscitating team at the field or in the emergency room. Peripheral, central, and intraosseous vascular access capabilities must be readily available. A rapid, 20-ml/kg isotonic crystalloid bolus should be administered in the face of even subtle signs of volume loss and can be repeated up to four times. If the child's condition does not stabilize, colloids may need to be administered in the same volume. Whole blood or packed red cells should be prepared at the destination hospital for immediate use at the time of the child's arrival at the emergency room.[18]

Disability

The field team should make a rapid assessment for neurologic trauma, particularly brain injury, by checking pupillary reflex and mental alertness. The mnemonic AVPU reminds one to note if the child is Alert or responsive to Voice or Pain or Unresponsive. Further detailed neurologic assessment is not a part of the primary survey but will be performed during the secondary assessment.[39]

Exposure

The child should be completely disrobed to allow observation for external signs of trauma and to aid in a thorough evaluation. However, precautions against hypothermia should be enacted immediately, as children are prone to rapid heat loss and significant hypothermia.

Ideally, the process of primary survey and resuscitation placed simultaneously should be by a team of skilled individuals with preassigned tasks. In the chest-injured child, a well-executed initial assessment and management can literally elude mortality.

SPECIFIC INJURIES AND THEIR MANAGEMENT

Thoracic trauma may produce injuries to the heart, great vessels, tracheobronchial tree, lungs, esophagus, diaphragm, or chest wall. These injuries may present alone, in combination, or in conjunction with extrathoracic injuries.

Cardiac Injury

The heart lies behind the sternum and is suspended within the fluid cushion of the pericardial sac. Although it appears to be well-protected, the heart is highly vulnerable to both penetrating and blunt injury in the child.

Penetrating Trauma

Most penetrating cardiac trauma is now due to gunshot wounds. Over half of these victims die soon after due to exsanguination or cardiac tamponade. The survivors, if recognized and promptly treated, are likely to experience a complete recovery.

The acute manifestations of cardiac injuries depend on the state of the pericardial wound.[10] If the injury drains freely through the pericardium into the pleural space or outside the body, the patient will present with hemothorax and/or signs and symptoms of hypovolemic shock. When the pericardial wound is obliterated by blood clot or adjacent structures, the patient presents with cardiac tamponade, distended neck veins, muffled heart tones, hypotension, narrowed pulse pressure, pulsus paradoxus, increased central venous pressure, and decreased amplitude of the waveform on EKG.

Cardiac injury should be suspected in patients with lower neck, precordial, and upper abdominal wounds who present with signs of tamponade, hypotension, and distended veins or with hemothorax, hypotension, and decreased breath sounds. Current trends in management emphasize early suspicion, with diagnosis in the operating room by pericardial window, followed by urgent thoracotomy.[36] However, in view of diagnostic difficulty, there should be a low threshold for performing a percutaneous pericardial aspiration in the field for both diagnosis and temporary management prior to thoracotomy. If one does find nonclotting intrapericardial blood, the catheter thould be left in place for further aspirations, if needed.

The diagnosis of penetrating cardiac injury can be made easily at the site of accident. No attempt to maintain normal systemic pressures should be made in penetrating cardiac trauma, as this may exacerbate hemorrhage and tamponade. If penetrating objects, such as a knife, are still inside the patient upon presentation in the field, they should not be manipulated except by the surgeon in the operating room. In the preparation of the patient for operative intervention, positioning and sterile prep and drape should occur prior to induction of a general anesthetic, when circumstances allow the luxury of time.

Blunt Injuries

The vast majority of cardiac injuries are due to motor vehicle trauma. The mechanism of injury is direct compression of the sternum and overlying chest wall on the heart and/or shearing injuries caused by deceleration. Blunt forces may injure the heart, causing contusion, rupture of the cardiac wall, septum, or valves, or injuries to the coronary arteries.

Cardiac contusion as a cause of death from blunt trauma in children has been quoted to range from 9.4–76%. The degree of cardiac involvement varies from subepicardial petechial hemorrhage to full-thickness myocardial hemorrhage and fiber disruption. Some contend that the very diagnosis of cardiac contusion is suspect and rarely represents a significant clinical entity. Others, however, emphasize that it should be ruled out in any patient with a significant deceleration chest injury, as with the classic history of the bent steering wheel in adults. Nonetheless, contusion is a real entity, and though it may only be a serious process in a minority of patients, the unfortunate complications of death, dysrhythmia and septal rupture do not permit its complete dismissal.

Although the most children are asymptomatic and may have mild tachycardia as the only sign, others present with hypotension, cardiac failure, shortness of breath, and chest pain. The EKG, if performed in the field, may show nonspecific ST-T changes and a variety of atrial and ventricular dysrhythmia.[14] Initial management at the accident site is directed at cardiac support and may include the administration of inotropes and, if there is evidence of right heart failure, volume expansion. Standard antidysrhythmic therapies should be employed when needed. Two-dimensional echocardiography may be used to evaluate the degree of myocardial dysfunction on the patient's arrival to the emergency room.

In patients who sustain cardiac rupture, few survive to undergo operative intervention, although there are various case reports of survivors. If this injury is suspected in the patient with evidence of tamponade, blood loss, or congestive failure, management in the field should be similar to that for penetrating injury.

Injuries to the Great Vessels

Penetrating injuries to the great vessels in children are frequently fatal unless the hole is quite small or surrounding structures result in tamponade. Any of the great vessels may be involved. Frequently, these patients present in shock and go directly to the operating room after chest tube insertion, without any further diagnostic testing. In these cases, thoracotomy may be diagnostic as well as therapeutic. In patients who do not present in extremis, one may see developing hemothorax and signs of hypovolemia or signs and symptoms of pericardial tamponade if the intrapericardial portions of the vessels are affected. Another presentation is a widened mediastinum on chest film (Fig. 1). Angiography remains the gold standard for diagnosis of great vessel injury, but computed tomographic (CT) scans have been touted by some.

Blunt injuries to the great vessels most commonly involve the aorta. Eighty-five percent of victims of this injury have free rupture and succumb at the scene. The remaining 15% survive due to containment of the hematoma within the adventitia of the aorta and parietal pleura. These patients are at risk for rupture within hours of arriving at the hospital, if not appropriately diagnosed and treated. The most common site of rupture is at the takeoff of the left subclavian artery; therefore, the patient generally presents with a widened mediastinum with or without concomitant hemothorax. Aortic injuries associated with blunt trauma rarely occur alone and coexisting trauma may mask or distract attention

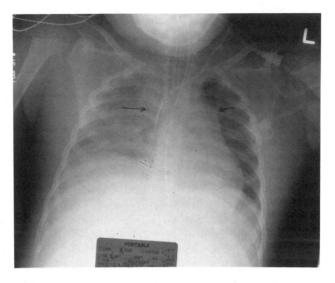

FIGURE 1.   Mediastinal widening secondary to injury to the great vessels.

from an aortic injury. A high index of suspicion should be maintained in patients with rapid deceleration from vehicular trauma or falls from a height. Clinical signs include those of hypovolemia and pericardial tamponade, as well as decreased pulses and blood pressure in the lower extremities and intrascapular systolic murmur.[34]

Initial therapeutic intervention is directed at maintaining adequate vital signs without excessive fluid replacement. Hypertension may result from inappropriate baroreceptor responses and catecholamine release, but should be avoided as it may lead to exsanguination. The use of antihypertensives, such as nitroprusside, is recommended to maintain the blood pressure at a systolic pressure < 100 mmHg. Diagnosis is made by aortography or CT scan. The role of transesophageal echocardiography is being explored extensively in adults but has not been adequately studied in the pediatric population. Upon diagnosis, operative intervention should occur expediently. Because paraplegia is a potential complication of the repair, ideally the patient should undergo cardiopulmonary bypass with cooling. If it is necessary to transfer a patient to another institution to provide the services of a pediatric chest surgeon, the patient should be intubated and well-sedated for transport.[37]

Injuries to the Lung

Simple Pneumothorax

Simple pneumothorax can be due to either blunt or penetrating trauma. With penetrating trauma, air may be sucked into the chest cavity by negative pressure during inspiration or, more likely, may escape from injured lung parenchyma, esophagus, or tracheobronchial tree. In blunt injury, it is frequently associated with parenchymal injury due to rib or chest fractures, or it may be due to rupture of congenital or acquired blebs. The symptoms are usually chest pain with inspiration and/or shortness of breath. Unilateral decreased breath sounds are the diagnostic hallmark, although if < 20% of the hemithorax is filled with air, the finding may be subtle and the diagnosis made only after a chest x-ray is obtained. Hyper-resonance to percussion and increased fremitus are also clinical indicators of pneumothorax.

Chest radiography is neither necessary nor recommended prior to definitive treatment. Unnecessary delay in therapy for this condition, which can be accurately defined clinically, may allow time for a simple pneumothorax to convert to a tension penumothorax, a much more deadly entity. A tube thoracostomy is the treatment of choice.[12]

Tension Pneumothorax

The same mechanisms that result in simple pneumothorax can also produce tension pneumothorax. This condition results when air leaking into the pleural space creates a flap-valve effect. Continued accumulation of air in the pleural space with no route of escape eventually leads to an increase in intrapleural pressures with complete collapse of the lung and shifting of the mediastinal structures (Fig. 2); this condition not only impedes adequate ventilation but also interferes with venous return to the heart and, if left untreated, causes death.[3] In addition to the signs and symptoms of simple pneumothorax, shifting of the mediastinal structures will lead to tracheal shift to the side, away from the pneumothorax, and distention of the neck veins.

Tube thoracostomy remains the mainstay of therapy. Insertion of a needle into the second intercostal space of the affected side can provide temporary relief of tension. Chest tube insertion cannot be performed at the accident site.

Open Pneumothorax

Disruption of the continuity of the chest wall, resulting in free communication of the pleural space with the ambient atmosphere, is called open pneumothorax. It may be due to either blunt or penetrating chest trauma and is often associated with injury of the underlying lung parenchyma. Depending on the

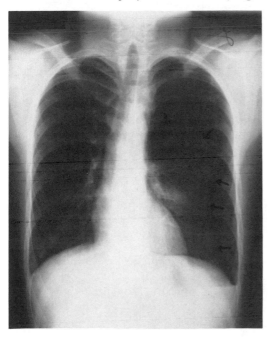

FIGURE 2. Left pneumothorax with collapse of lung, displaced diaphragm, and mild shift of mediastinal structures to the right.

size of the communication and the presence or absence of lung injury, the patient may be asymptomatic or severely dyspneic.

Diagnosis is easy, as the patient presents with a defect filled with frothy bleeding and audible air entering and leaving the pleural space.[27] This is referred to as a "sucking chest wound." Due to the inability to generate a negative intrathoracic pressure, the lung will collapse and the patient will have decreased breath sounds.

Treatment in the immediate stages consists of covering the wound with a Vaseline gauze. It should be taped on three sides rather than four, so that if intrapleural pressure increases, the dressing can act as a flutter-valve rather than allowing the creation of a tension pneumothorax. Tube thoracostomy should be performed at the earliest feasible time, but the most important component of treatment is closure of the chest wall. In general, this should be done in the operating room with adequate debridement. If there is gross contamination, the wound may be left partially open and covered with a dressing.

Hemothorax

Hemothorax is defined as blood in the pleural space. Although small accumulations of blood may result with nearly any intrathoracic injury, large collections are usually associated with injuries to the great vessels, pulmonary hilum, and/or systemic vessels, such as the internal mammary or intercostal artery. Massive hemothorax presents with a decrease in breath sounds on the affected side, dullness to percussion, and signs and symptoms of volume loss. Chest x-ray shows a variable degree of opacification of the hemithorax, depending on the organ injured and the volume of blood loss. Concomitant pneumothorax is not unusual.

Tube thoracostomy should be placed early for assessment of the amount and rate of bleeding. It can be useful in guiding replacement fluids also. Whenever possible, an autotransfusion device should be attached to the drainage system to minimize the need for blood products.

Although the overwhelming majority of hemothorax patients do not need operation, particularly in cases of low-velocity penetrating injuries, blood losses of > 20% of the estimated blood volume of the child would, under most circumstances, prompt exploratory thoracotomy.[34] Continued blood loss over several hours may also require surgical procedures. Since the pulmonary parenchyma is a low-pressure system with a pressure rarely exceeding 15 mmHg, massive losses and continuing hemorrhage should suggest arterial bleeding.[30] In any patient presenting with a hemothorax, regardless of the size, appropriate measures to rule out injury to the heart, aorta, and other great vessels should be considered.

Flail Chest and Pulmonary Contusion

Fractures of three or more ribs in at least two sites each can lead to flail chest. In this entity, the chest wall moves paradoxically—inward during inspiration and outward during expiration. The pathophysiologic features of the injury are dependent on three factors: the premorbid condition of the respiratory system, the severity of the underlying pulmonary contusion, and concomitant injuries. Pendulum movement of mediastinal structures was once thought to be the major etiology of respiratory distress; although now thought to play almost no role in adults, it may still be a contributing factor in children with a compliant chest wall and mobile mediastinum.

Pulmonary contusion, caused by compression of the chest wall against the lung parenchyma and a common chest injury in the pediatric trauma population, leads to decreased lung compliance, increased airway resistance, and increased intrapulmonary shunting.[29,30] The chest wall injury causes splinting and decreases in tidal volumes and inability to clear secretions. This may result in hypoxemia, carbon dioxide retention, respiratory insufficiency, and even adult respiratory distress syndrome. Excessive administration of blood products and crystalloid will further compound the problem. The addition of a hemothorax, pneumothorax, or both can further compound hypoxemia and acidosis. Low cardiac output can result from bleeding, tamponade, and profound metabolic derangements. With large flail segments in the child, the mediastinum may swing with breathing and produce hypoventilation, atelectasis, decreased tidal volume, arteriovenous shunting, and hypoxemia. Within the initial 72 hours after presentation, the clinical condition of the patient may worsen rather than improve, due to retained secretions, pulmonary edema, increased shunting, and more work of breathing.

Flail chest is relatively easy to diagnose, as the segment can be seen making paradoxical motion. It is important that all trauma victims have their back thoroughly examined, as flailing can occur posteriorly. Pulmonary contusion may present with a chest radiograph showing consolidated-appearing areas of lung parenchyma; however, the diagnosis is a clinical one, as chest x-ray findings may not be abnormal initially.

Management spans several levels. The foremost concern is treatment of hypoxia. Although many patients can be managed with humidified mask O_2, some require intubation; and one should not hesitate to intubate if indicated, as it provides the benefits of airway control, adequate ventilation, and internal splinting of the flail segment due to positive pressure. Another aspect of care is adequate pain relief. In addition to intravenous narcotics and rib block, epidural catheters have also been employed effectively to help the patient with increasing tidal volume and pulmonary toilet. Fixation of the chest wall is also needed in some cases. Temporary use of sandbag and weights in the field can be helpful in cases with large flailed segments until intubation takes place. Operative fixation is still needed in some extreme cases, although in general, internal splinting with intubation and positive pressure ventilation has supplanted surgical therapy.

Supportive care in this group is also extremely important. Although "drying" the patients with diuretics is not really beneficial, avoidance of excessive hypotonic solutions and use of diuretics to maintain normal central venous pressures and osmolality can be useful. Controversies still exist regarding diuretics, steroids, and administration of colloids. In brief, the patient should be in a euvolemic state, and hypervolemia can be detrimental. Use of central venous catheters and Swan-Ganz catheters may be indicated, especially in considering that this injury is common in the multiply injured child with concomitant head, abdominal, and/or skeletal injury in whom tight intravascular control is essential. Furthermore, prompt attention to concomitant injuries is needed. Surveillance for pneumonitis and other intensive care unit–associated infections is also key in ensuring a complete recovery in this very challenging patient group.

Pulmonary Injury

Injury to the lung may be due to penetrating, blunt, compressive, or decelerating trauma. It may result from penetration, laceration, contusion of the parenchyma, or a combination. Penetrating trauma generally presents as pneumothorax, hemothorax, or hemopneumothorax. Depending on the amount of air or blood in the pleural space, the patient may be asymptomatic or have significant cardiorespiratory embarrassment. Hemoptysis is another common presenting complaint.

Treatment of penetrating pulmonary trauma depends on the presenting clinical picture, and these entities have been discussed previously in the chapter. In general, parenchymal injuries may produce significant pneumothorax but rarely cause large hemothorax due to the low pressures in the pulmonary vasculature. Massive hemorrhage should suggest that the pulmonary injury is not isolated.

Blunt pulmonary injury and its therapy were discussed with pulmonary contusion. Generally therapy is supportive in nature.

Tracheobronchial Injuries

Injury to the trachea and major bronchi is fortunately relatively uncommon and can be due to either blunt or penetrating mechanisms. The unprotected cervical segment of the trachea is most susceptible to penetrating injuries, while the distal segment within 2 cm of the carina is most frequently involved in blunt trauma.[13] A single transverse injury is the most typical (78%), longitudinal along the membranous segment of the airways is second most common (18%), while combination injuries occur in only 4%. Blunt injuries result from traction at the level of the carina, caused by a sudden decrease in the anterior/posterior diameter of the trachea, sudden increase in the intrabronchial pressure against a closed glottis, and/or shearing forces of rapid deceleration.

The presentation varies with the location and extent of injury, but tracheobronchial injury should be suspected in any patient who presents with respiratory distress, subcutaneous emphysema, and hemoptysis. Nearly all patients will have a pneumothorax of variable severity. Tension pneumothorax in this population should make one suspicious of injury to a larger airway. Large air leaks at the time of chest tube insertion can also be an alerting finding.

Airway management can be particularly challenging in this population. If the patient is alert and breathing, bronchoscopic examination with concomitant intubation is recommended. Rigid equipment may be required and is generally applied in the operating suite. If the patient does not have an airway and bronchoscopic capabilities are not readily available, initial treatment consists of intubation with attempts to pass the tube beyond the area of injury. Expedient chest tube placement is essential in this circumstance, as tension pneumothorax develops rapidly with positive pressure ventilation. The option of visualized bronchoscopic intubation, however, is always the preferred method. Operative intervention is nearly always needed for primary repair of the injury. In small tears, a conservative approach with appropriate supervision may be attempted.

Diaphragmatic Injuries

Again, either a blunt or penetrating mechanism is possible. Blunt injuries occur more commonly on the left side, allowing the abdominal contents to herniate into the chest cavity.[35] Penetrating injuries are small and may take longer to manifest. Commonly, the abdominal component of the penetrating diaphragmatic wound may produce the majority of symptoms.

Diagnosis is not always easy. A high index of suspicion should be maintained in any patient with a deceleration injury or with a penetrating wound of the upper abdomen or in the thorax below the nipple anteriorly or the scapula posteriorly. In most cases, the injury can be seen on routine chest film due to the absence or upward displacement of the diaphragmatic border with the stomach and/or other hollow viscus in the chest.

Initial management includes insertion of a nasogastric tube to decompress the stomach and to treat or avoid respiratory distress. Definitive management is operative. Most surgeons would initially approach this injury through the abdominal cavity, as the likelihood of concomitant abdominal injuries is high. In cases that are discovered "late," days to years after the event, many prefer a thoracic approach.

Esophageal Injury

Most esophageal wounds are penetrating, although blunt rupture is possible. Due to the lack of protective elements, the cervical esophagus is the area most commonly involved.[34] Although symptomatic in the early stages, esophageal injuries are rarely isolated and can be overlooked while other equally life-threatening complaints are attended. The usual presentation is that of neck or chest pain with crepitance. Most children will also resist movement of the neck and may drool and avoid swallowing. With esophageal injuries in the chest, the patient may present with a fever and pneumomediastinum, pleural effusion, and/or pneumothorax. Soft tissue neck films in the cervical esophageal injury also can reveal subcutaneous emphysema. Many childhood injuries are due to swallowing foreign bodies and ingestion of caustic material.[2]

Diagnosis can be made with a Gastrografin (meglumine diatrizoate) or thin barium swallow. Endoscopy is also very reliable but less available in most locations.[6]

Treatment consists of early operative intervention for debridement, repair, and drainage. In caustic ingestions, therapy is guided by the extent and depth of the burns and must be individualized. Early consultation with a pediatric or trauma surgeon avoids potential morbidity and mortality in this injury.

SUMMARY

Trauma is the leading cause of death of children aged 1–15 in this country. Chest trauma alone accounts for one-fourth of these deaths. The primary focus of the medical community with regard to pediatric trauma should be prevention. Legislation concerning seat belt, car seat, and bicycle helmet use should be supported and enforced. Other methods of preventing accidents and injuries and providing safety education in school and homes deserve investigation and implementation. When injuries are not prevented, skilled prehospital and hospital care provided by well-trained professionals who have a familiarity with pediatric injury patterns and their treatment saves lives. Many issues in the care of this patient group are the subject of ongoing scientific research, but much future study is required to better manage this very challenging group of patients.

REFERENCES

1. American College of Surgeons: Advanced Trauma Life Support Manual. Chicago, American College of Surgeons, 1988.
2. Beaver BL, Laschinger JC: Pediatric thoracic trauma. Semin Cardiothor Surg 4:255–2623, 1992.
3. Blaisdell FW: Pneumothorax and hemothorax. In Blaisdell FW, Trunkey DD (eds): Trauma Management: Vol. 3. Cervico Thoracic Trauma. New York, Thieme, 1986, pp 150–166.
4. Bonler J, Lewis F, Aprahainian C, et al: Pre-hospital trauma care-stabilization or scoop and run. J Trauma 28:708–711, 1983.
5. Bruce DA, Schuik L, Bruno LA, et al: Outcome following severe head injury in children. J Neurosurg 48:679–688, 1978.
6. Cheadle W, Richardson JA: Options in management of trauma to the esophagus. Surg Gynecol Obstet 155:380, 1982.

7. Don SP, Honigman B, Moore E, et al: Pre-hospital advanced trauma life support for critical penetrating wounds to the thorax and abdomen. J Trauma 25:828–832, 1985.
8. Driscoll P, Sinner D: ABC of major trauma, initial assessment and management: Secondary survey. BMJ 300:1329–1333, 1990.
9. Eichelberger MR, Randolph JG: Thoracic trauma in children. Surg Clin North Am 61:1181–1197, 1981.
10. Evans J, Gray LA, Rayner A, et al: Principles for management of penetrating cardiac wounds. Am Surg 189:777, 1979.
11. Gervin AS, Fischer RP: The importance of prompt transport in salvage of patients with penetrating heart wounds. J Trauma 22:443–448, 1982.
12. Hammond S: Chest injuries in the trauma patient. Nurs Clin North Am 25:35–43, 1990.
13. Hankcock BJ, Wiseman NE: Tracheobronchial injuries in children. J Pediatr Surg 26:1316–1319, 1991.
14. Ildstad S, Tollerud D, Weiss R, et al: Cardiac contusion in pediatric patients with blunt thoracic trauma. J Pediatr Surg 25:287–289, 1990.
15. Ivatury RR, Nallathamhi MN, Roberge RJ, et al: Penetrating thoracic injuries in field stabilization vs. prompt transport. J Trauma 27:1066–1073, 1987.
16. Jacobs LM, Sinclair A, Beiser A, et al: Pre-hospital advanced life support: Benefits in trauma. J Trauma 24:8–12, 1984.
17. Keen T: Nursing care of the pediatric multitrauma patient. Nurs Clin North Am 25:13, 1990.
18. King DR: Trauma in childhood: Initial evaluation and management. Pediatr Clin North Am 32:1299, 1985.
19. Kissoon N, Dreyer J, Walis M: Pediatric trauma: Differences in pathophysiology, injury patterns, and treatment compared with adult trauma. Can Med Assoc J 142:27–34, 1990.
20. Lavery R, Torlella B, Griffin C: The pre-hospital treatment of pediatric trauma. Pediatr Emerg Med 8:9–12, 1992.
21. Losek JD, Bondio WA, Walsh KC, et al: Pre-hospital pediatric endotracheal intubation performance review. Pediatr Emerg Care 5:1–4, 1989.
22. Mayer TA: Management of hypovolemic shock. In Mayer TA (ed): Emergency Management of Pediatric Trauma. Philadelphia, W.B. Saunders, 1985, pp 39–51.
23. Miner WF, Corneli HM, Bolte RG, et al: Pre-hospital use of interosseous infusion by paramedics. Pediatr Emerg Care 5:5–7, 1989.
24. Nakayama DK, Copes WS, Sacco WJ: The effect of patient age upon survival in pediatric trauma. J Trauma 31:1521–1526, 1991.
25. Nakayama DK, Gardner MJ, Rowe MI: Emergency endotracheal intubation in pediatric patients by paramedics. Ann Emerg Med 18:489–494, 1989.
26. Ornato JP, Craven TJ, Nelson NM: The impact of improved emergency medical services in emergency trauma care on the reduction in mortality from trauma. J Trauma 24:674, 1984.
27. Pate J: Chest wall injuries. Surg Clin North Am 69:59–70, 1989.
28. Ramenofsky ML: Emergency medical services for children and pediatric trauma system components: J Pediatr Surg 24:153–155, 1989.
29. Richardson JD, Adams L, Flint CM: Selective management of flail chest and pulmonary contusion. Am Surg 196:481, 1982.
30. Roux P, Fisher RM: Chest injuries in children: An analysis of 100 cases of blunt chest trauma from motor vehicle accidents. J Pediatr Surg 27:551–555, 1992.
31. Schafermeyer R: Pediatric trauma. Emerg Med Clin North Am 11:187–205, 1993.
32. Seidel JS, Hornbein M, Yoshiyama K, et al: Emergency medical services and the pediatric patient: Are the needs being met? Pediatrics 73:769–772, 1984.
33. Smyth BT: Chest trauma in children. J Pediatr Surg 14:41–47, 1979.
34. Symbas P: Cardiothoracic trauma. Curr Probl Surg (Nov):747–797, 1991.
35. Symbas P, Vlasis S, Hatcher C: Blunt and penetrating diaphragmatic injuries with or without herniation of organs into the chest. Ann Thor Surg 42:158–162, 1986.
36. Trinkle JJK, Toon RS, Franz JC, et al: Affairs of the wounded heart: Penetrating cardiac wounds. J Trauma 19:467, 1979.
37. Vasko JS, Roess DH, Williams TE, et al: Non-penetrating trauma of thoracic aorta. Ann Surg 24:38, 1986.
38. Westaby S: Thoracic trauma—1. BMJ 300:1639–1643, 1990.
39. Yaster M, Haller JA: Multiple trauma in the pediatric patient. In Rogers C (ed): Textbook of Pediatric Intensive Care, vol 2. Baltimore, Williams & Wilkins, 1987, pp 1265–11322.

CHAPTER 26

Abdominal Anomalies

ASCENSION M. TORRES, M.D.

Many congenital anomalies of the abdominal wall and gastrointestinal (GI) tract require surgical management. This chapter focuses on abdominal wall defects and some of the causes of GI obstruction in the neonate. Awareness of these conditions leads to prompt investigation, rapid diagnosis, and appropriate treatment to achieve a decrease in infant mortality.

ABDOMINAL WALL DEFECTS

The embryologic origin of abdominal wall defects remains controversial. Although there are divergent views as to the embryology and pathogenesis of these defects, most would agree that the integrity of the abdominal wall and the development of the peritoneal cavity depend on the return of the midgut along with proper development of fusion of the cephalic, caudal, and lateral embryonic folds as they come together at the umbilicus.

Omphalocele is a rare condition estimated to occur in approximately 1 in 6000 births. This condition was first described in the 16th century by Ambroise Paré, who recognized the severity and poor prognosis of this condition. Over the next several centuries, little progress was made in the management of this disease, with most series in the 1960s reporting a mortality of 80%.[14] In the last 30 years, with the development of neonatal transport, anesthesia, neonatal critical care, and total parenteral nutrition, the overall mortality for omphalocele has fallen to approximately 30%.[6,21,40]

Omphalocele is a defect of the central abdominal wall covered by a sac composed of amnion and peritoneum (Figs. 1 and 2). It is thought to result from partial or complete arrest in the development of one or more of the embryonic folds. Cephalic fold arrest leads to "epigastric omphalocele," which frequently is associated with lower thoracic wall malformations such as sternal clefts, diaphragmatic, pericardial, and cardiac anomalies. This constellation of defects is referred to as the pentalogy of Cantrell.[5] Infants affected with this upper midline syndrome usually exhibit a bifid sternum, anterior diaphragmatic hernia, pericardial defects, and cardiac malformations ranging from atrial septal defects to ectopia cordis. Caudal fold arrest leads to "hypogastric omphalocele" and abnormalities of the hindgut, such as imperforate anus, or lower abdominal wall defects, such as bladder exstrophy or cloacal exstrophy. The most common condition is lateral fold arrest leading to "midabdominal omphalocele" with evisceration of the intraabdominal organs including liver, spleen, stomach, and intestines. As a consequence of these different forms of developmental arrest and

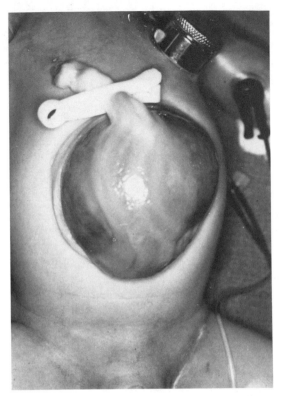

FIGURE 1. Omphalocele. Note the central abdominal wall defect covered by an intact sac.

failure of midgut return, omphalocele is characterized by nonrotation of the intestines and failure of normal formation of the umbilical ring.

In contrast to omphalocele, hernia of the umbilical cord is an umbilical defect with a diameter less than 4.0 cm and a sac that contains only loops of intestine (Fig. 3). The developmental abnormality resulting in hernia of the umbilical cord presumably occurs later in gestation during the 8th and 10th week and is secondary to failure of contracture of a normally formed umbilical ring.

Clinically, gastroschisis may mimic a ruptured omphalocele; however, the two conditions are different. Gastroschisis is a congenital defect of the periumbilical body wall through which abdominal contents protrude. The protruding viscera are not covered by skin or peritoneum (Figs. 4 and 5). Gastroschisis is a failure of vascularization of the abdominal wall, probably secondary to complete dissolution of the right umbilical artery at a time before collateral circulation can maintain integrity of the mesenchyme.[8] Omphalocele is a failure of fusion and therefore is associated with a far higher incidence of associated malformations. Gastrointestinal, cardiac, neurogenic, genitourinary, skeletal, and chromosomal anomalies are common and explain the marked increase in morbidity and mortality found with omphalocele as compared with gastroschisis. Chromosomal abnormalities associated with omphalocele are reported in one-third of cases, with trisomy 13, 18, and 21 being the most common. Cardiovascular malformations are reported in 10–25% of the cases, with the most common lesions being tetralogy of Fallot and septal defects.[6,21,25,33,40]

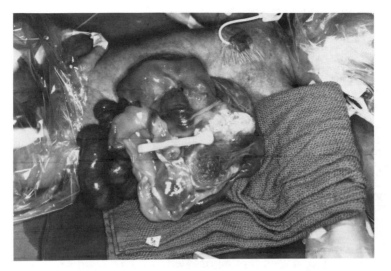

FIGURE 2. A large omphalocele with a ruptured sac.

In contrast, gastroschisis and hernia of the umbilical cord are rarely associated with other serious malformations. The most common associated malformation in these patients is intestinal atresia.[22,35] These are usually jejunoileal and presumably related to ischemia of the protruding intestines. The

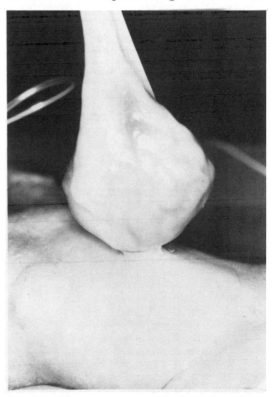

FIGURE 3. Hernia of the umbilical cord. Note the small fascial defect and a sac containing only loops of intestine.

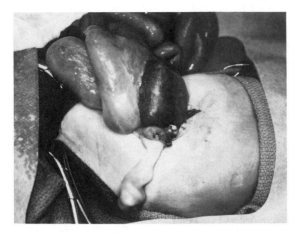

FIGURE 4.   Gastroschisis.

overall mortality rate for gastroschisis is about 10% and is related to the complications of sepsis and prolonged intestinal dysfunction.

The prenatal diagnosis of omphalocele is now possible, so it is important to know the incidence and prognostic significance of the associated malformations. Prenatal sonography can make the diagnosis of omphalocele as early as in the 12th week of gestation and reliably differentiate it from gastroschisis. The prenatal diagnosis of omphalocele should not automatically dictate a cesarean section because of the risk of rupture. Sac rupture does not significantly influence the final outcome.[10,25,27]

The initial care of the omphalocele by the pediatrician or obstetrician in the delivery room is of major importance. Clamping of the cord should be done distally to prevent crushing of intraabdominal viscera. Every effort should be made to avoid contamination of the exposed viscera. Sterile gloves should be used for inspection and dressing the defect. The omphalocele should be covered

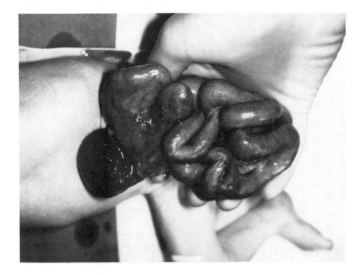

FIGURE 5.   The eviscerated organs are not covered by a sac in gastroschisis. Note the edematous and thickened intestine.

with a layer of sterile gauze moistened with warm normal saline. The baby should be placed in a sterile plastic bag to cover the lower half of the body. This impermeable membrane will decrease loss of moisture and heat.

The initial evaluation of the infant determines the priorities of subsequent management. If the tongue is enlarged, the blood sugar should be monitored immediately because of possible association with Beckwith-Wiedemann syndrome (macroglossia, hypoglycemia, and gigantism).[3] Unrecognized hypoglycemia can lead to permanent neurologic injury; therefore, intravenous administration of dextrose should be started immediately for any infant with an omphalocele. Concomitant immediate management involves nasogastric decompression, ventilatory support (if necessary), aggressive fluid resuscitation, and systemic intravenous antibiotics. A nasogastric, 10-French sump tube should be inserted to prevent further GI distention by swallowed air and to avoid aspiration of vomitus. Mask ventilation should be avoided because it is likely to contribute to the distention of the intestines. Peripheral cyanosis associated with omphalocele should alert the physician to look for intracardiac malformations or perhaps associated diaphragmatic hernia.[5] Therefore, careful auscultation of the lungs and heart is indicated. These infants have marked heat, fluid, and protein losses from their exposed viscera, especially if the sac is ruptured. Intravenous fluid infusion and temperature control must be closely monitored because this large surface area is subject to evaporative losses. The combination of exposed viscera and decreased immune resistance due to low serum proteins places these infants at high risk for contamination and sepsis. Therefore, broad-spectrum antibiotics should be initiated. Initial exam should include a careful inspection of the intestines. Cyanosis, venous congestion, or ischemia of the intestines may be secondary to a mechanical problem. The weight of the intestines hanging over the abdominal wall can lead to midgut volvulus, caval compression, or hepatic vein kinking. These problems can be avoided by positioning the infant on his or her side and supporting the intestinal mass. One can also look for caliber difference in the intestines, which may be secondary to associated atresia.

The ideal repair is primary fascial and skin closure (Fig. 6). If the reduction of the viscera causes bowel discoloration or marked decrease in pulmonary compliance, a staged repair is indicated. Primary fascial closure carries the risk of placing the abdominal contents under pressure, which may produce a reduction in cardiac output, bowel ischemia, and postoperative respiratory and renal failure. A staged repair using only skin closure or construction of a silo is a viable alternative (Figs. 7 and 8).[2,16,31] Clinical judgment should be the best guide to the type of repair.

Nonoperative treatment consists of protecting the omphalocele sac for weeks to allow skin to grow over the defect. It is sometimes advisable for huge omphaloceles with an intact sac or in the event of severe associated anomalies. Escharotic agents used for this purpose include alcohol, Mercurochrome, and benzalkonium chloride (Zephiran).[1,13]

The most severe of the abdominal wall defects is cloacal exstrophy, also termed vesicointestinal fissure, ileovesical fistula, or exstrophia splanchnica. The lesion was first described by Littre in 1709. Rickham reported "successful" surgical management in 1960; before then most children with cloacal exstrophy were allowed to die.[30] Through the 1970s and 1980s, staged correction and aggressive supportive care resulted in salvage of most of these patients.[9,29,41]

Classic cloacal exstrophy consists of an omphalocele superiorly, below which is an open plate of mucosa consisting of two posterior walls of hemibladders on

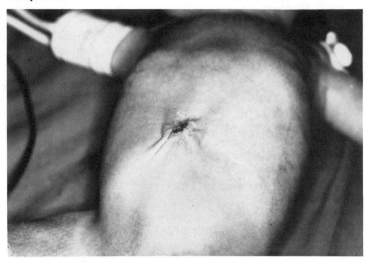

FIGURE 6. The postoperative appearance of a small omphalocele after primary fascial and skin closure.

either side of the central intestinal wall. The exstrophic lesion represents abnormal embryogenesis of the cloacal membrane. The Marshall-Muecke theory attempts to describe embryologically the anatomy found in cloacal exstrophy. An abnormal overdevelopment of cloacal membrane produces a wedge effect, serving as a mechanical barrier to mesodermal migration and resulting in impaired development of the abdominal wall, failure of fusion of the genital tubercles, and diastasis pubis.[28]

Associated anomalies are present in 75–95% of the patients.[9,41] Omphalocele and imperforate anus are nearly always present. Upper urinary tract anomalies are found in two-thirds of patients. Spinal dysraphism may be found in up to 50% of the patients, and musculoskeletal anomalies in another one-fourth.

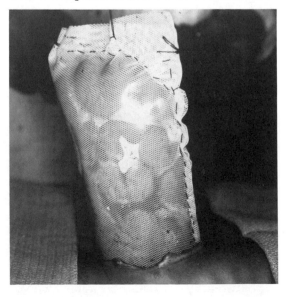

FIGURE 7. Construction of a silo.

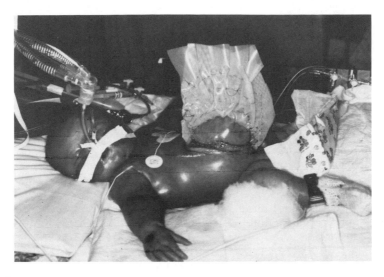

FIGURE 8. Sequential reduction of the viscera is done at bedside using aseptic technique.

Immediate management of cloacal exstrophy should include careful monitoring of fluid and electrolytes. Losses from exposed bowel may be quite significant. Evaluation of the upper genitourinary system in conjunction with baseline BUN and creatinine should be done prior to surgical intervention. An urgent neurosurgical consult should be obtained in patients with associated spinal dysraphism to rule out leakage of cerebrospinal fluid. Gender assignment, even though it is not part of the immediate management, should be discussed with the parents early in the course. Although there is a male genotype predominance in cloacal exstrophy, it is generally recommended that these children be reared as females. The severe anomalies of the phallus preclude reconstruction of satisfactory male genitalia. The gender assignment conversion is best performed in the neonatal period. In patients who do not have anomalies incompatible with life, a staged repair is indicated. The first stage involves management of the GI tract and closure of the omphalocele. Subsequent stages include closure of the bladder exstrophy, a colonic pull-through via a posterior sagittal approach, and correction genitoplasty. Quality of life rather than survival is now the major factor affecting decision making and management of patients with cloacal exstrophy.[9,29,41]

GASTROINTESTINAL OBSTRUCTION IN THE NEWBORN PERIOD

Bile-stained emesis should be considered a sign of mechanical bowel obstruction in the newborn until proven otherwise. Abdominal distention and failure to evacuate meconium in the first 24 hours of life should also raise the possibility of a mechanical obstruction requiring surgical intervention. The degree of distention depends on the level of obstruction. The more distal the obstruction, the worse the abdominal distention. In pyloric and duodenal obstruction, distention may be minimal. The diagnosis of obstruction is confirmed by radiologic studies. Plain abdominal films in the supine and upright or decubitus position indicate the level of obstruction. Contrast studies delineate the caliber of the bowel and whether the colon is used or unused.

The newborn child with a GI obstruction should have fluid resuscitation first. Intravenous fluids are given until adequate urine output (greater than 1 ml/

kg/hr) is achieved. Nasogastric decompression is essential prior to induction of anesthesia to prevent aspiration of vomitus. Systemic intravenous antibiotics (ampicillin, 100 mg/kg, and gentamicin, 2.5 mg/kg) are given preoperatively.

Gastric volvulus and pyloric atresia are rare causes of gastric outlet obstruction. Gastric volvulus in the newborn is a rare life-threatening emergency.[4,19] Epigastric distention and failure to pass a nasogatric tube beyond the esophagus should raise suspicion. An upper GI series is diagnostic, and these patients should undergo emergency surgical detorsion accompanied by anterior gastropexy—preferably before progressive ischemia leads to necrosis and perforation of the stomach, in which case a resection may be required.

Duodenal obstruction may be the result of an intrinsic anomaly or extrinsic compression. Intrinsic anomalies include duodenal atresia, stenosis, or web. Extrinsic compression may be secondary to an annular pancreas, a preduodenal portal vein, or malrotation from Ladds bands or midgut volvulus. Infants with intrinsic duodenal obstruction present early with bilious emesis and little or no abdominal distention.

Duodenal atresia occurs in 1 in 10,000–40,000 births.[23] Pathogenesis is thought to be due to a failure of recanalization of the solid core stage of intestinal growth. Plain radiographs demonstrate the characteristic "double bubble" sign. Down syndrome may be seen in 30–40% of patients with duodenal atresia.[12,23] A duodenoduodenostomy is the preferred repair. Infants with this condition should remain NPO with nasogastric decompression and be supported with total parenteral nutrition until surgical correction is undertaken. Survival rates in these patients are usually greater than 80%.

Duodenal obstruction caused by malrotation and midgut volvulus constitutes a true surgical emergency. Malrotation of the intestine occurs when the normal rotational process and fixation of the intestine fail to take place. The incidence is approximately 1 in 500 live births.[34] Two-thirds present in the newborn period, and males predominate in this age group. Associated anomalies include abdominal wall defects, diaphragmatic hernia, and intestinal atresias. Bilious emesis is the hallmark of malrotation and midgut volvulus. Physical exam may be normal in half of the patients. An expeditious work-up in conjunction with resuscitation measures should be instituted. Upper GI series is diagnostic, and surgical exploration should follow immediately. Outcome in these patients is excellent if intervention is done prior to frank midgut gangrene.[37]

Jejunoileal obstruction usually is due to atresias or stenosis. Meconium ileus should also be considered in the differential diagnosis. Atresias ocur in 1 in 330 live births in the United States[17] and are due to a mesenteric vascular insult in utero. Bilious emesis and abdominal distention usually are the presenting signs; abdominal radiographs reveal multiple dilated loops of bowel with air fluid levels and very little distal air. A contrast enema will show a small unused "microcolon" in most cases. The preoperative treatment is the same as described earlier for any newborn with intestinal obstruction. Operative treatment depends on the type, location, and total bowel length. Tapering enteroplasty with end-to-end anastomosis is done in those with borderline or insufficient bowel length. Improved survival in these patients is now expected with the use of long-term total parenteral nutrition. Death is from infection, pneumonia, and sepsis.

Distal large bowel obstruction in the newborn may be due to colonic atresia or congenital colonic aganglionosis in the presence of a normally located and patent anus. Colonic atresia is a rare form of congenital obstruction. Diagnosis is made by a contrast enema that fails to fill the entire colon, and only a blind-ending segment of microcolon is visualized. Treatment consists of primary end-to-end anastomosis if technically feasible—otherwise, a colostomy with subsequent anastomosis months later.

The earliest description of megacolon was by Frederick Ruysch in 1691. In 1887, Harold Hirschsprung reported the abnormality that is referred to clinically as Hirschsprung disease.[18] The pathology of Hirschsprung disease is a lack of ganglion cells in both the mysenteric (Auerbach's) and the submucous (Meissner's) plexuses in the distal bowel. In addition to the lack of ganglion cells there is an increased number of coarse, tortuous nerve fibers within the wall of the narrowed distal bowel. The extent of aganglionic, diseased bowel is variable, ranging from "ultra-short" segments of the distal rectum to total colonic aganglionosis. The extent of the disease is always from the anus to the segment where ganglion cells reappear. This caudal-to-cranial orientation of the disease process follows the embryology of gut innervation.

The incidence of Hirschsprung disease is 1 in 5000 live births. Most of the babies are healthy, full-term white males, and the diagnosis should be considered in infants who fail to pass meconium in the first 48 hours. Vomiting and abdominal distention also may be present. A barium enema may demonstrate a transition zone (between the normal dilated and abnormal narrowed bowel). Other radiographic findings include a sawtooth appearance of the colon due to spasm, retained barium for 2 or 3 days, or a rectal-to-sigmoid diameter ratio of less than 1. The definitive diagnostic procedure is a rectal biopsy that demonstrates absence of ganglion cells and an associated increase in nerve fibers. Increased acetylcholinesterase activity usually is demonstrated in histochemical studies.[11]

The initial goal of treating Hirschsprung disease is the correction of fluid and electrolyte abnormalities. Preoperative antibiotics, ampicillin, gentamicin, and clindamycin, are also given to cover the colonic flora. A diverting colostomy is performed as the first stage in the treatment. The definitive procedure is deferred until the child is about 12 months of age or weighs 10 kg. The Swenson, Duhamel retrorectal transanal pull-through and the Soave endorectal pull-through are the options available to the surgeon at the time of the definitive correction.[24] The greatest risk of Hirschsprung disease in the neonate is the development of enterocolitis. Delayed diagnosis beyond one week of age and the presence of trisomy 21 appear to increase the risk of developing enterocolitis in these patients.[36]

Necrotizing enterocolitis (NEC) is the most common diagnosis in the newborn infant requiring emergency surgical intervention. It generally affects infants who are premature, of low birth weight, and have been formula fed; but it also can occur in full-term infants, especially in association with cyanotic heart disease, severe diarrhea, and in those who have never been fed. The pathogenesis of NEC is unknown, but three main factors appear to be necessary for its development: (1) ischemic damage to the gut; (2) bacterial colonization; and (3) the presence of intraluminal substrate.[7]

Necrotizing enterocolitis is characterized by diffuse or patchy intestinal necrosis (Fig. 9). The terminal ileum and the ascending colon are the most common sites involved. The lesions can be encountered throughout the intestines, and mucosal ulcerations progressing to necrosis and perforation are seen with disease progression. No one specific microorganism can be implicated in NEC. Peritoneal cultures done at the time of laparotomy show a predominance of gram-negative enteric rods, especially Klebsiella and Enterobacter and coagulase-negative staphylococcus.[26] Some evidence indicates that a defective gut immunity allows the usually noninvasive enteric flora to invade the intestinal wall.[39] Early

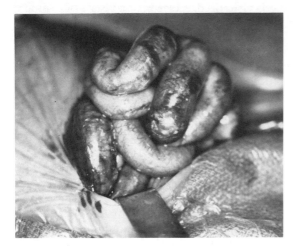

FIGURE 9. Laparotomy findings in a baby with necrotizing enterocolitis. Note the diffuse, patchy involvement of the intestine, with intramural and subserosal blebs.

symptoms include increase in gastric aspirate, ileus, bilious emesis, abdominal distention, and heme-positive stools. As the disease progresses, patients become more lethargic, hypothermic, and apneic, at which time intubation, ventilatory support, and external heat sources as well as warming of intravenous fluids are indicated. Erythema and edema of the abdominal wall usually are associated with major intraabdominal bowel involvement. Plain films of the abdomen may reveal pneumatosis intestinalis, dilated "fixed" loops of bowel, portal venous air, ascites, or pneumoperitoneum (Fig. 10).

Initial management consists of keeping the patient NPO with nasogastric decompression, correcting the hypotension by intravenous fluid resuscitation, reversal of acidosis, and coagulopathy in those with overwhelming sepsis. Intravenous fluid resuscitation with lactated Ringer's (10–20 ml/kg) bolus is preferred over normal saline due to a lower sodium concentration (130 mEq/L vs. 154 mEq/L) and the presence of bicarbonate (28 mEq/L). Fresh-frozen plasma, platelets, and fibrinogen often are employed to correct the coagulopathy. Intravenous antibiotics, ampicillin, gentamycin, and clindamycin, are given. Serial blood counts are done every 6 hours to monitor the white blood count, the hematocrit, and the platelet count. Serial abdominal films looking for fixed loops of bowel or free air also are obtained every 6–8 hours. Hyperalimentation should be instituted early in the course to prevent nutritional depletion in these highly stressed infants. Surgical intervention usually is indicated for pneumoperitoneum or failure of medical management. At exploration, after peritoneal cultures are sent, the necrotic bowel is resected, and exteriorization of the ends of the bowel is done as an ostomy and mucous fistula. Postoperative management employs the guidelines for treatment of neonatal critical patients. The patients are given systemic intravenous antibiotics for a 10-day course. Nutrition is maintained by total parenteral nutrition, while enteral feeds are slowly introduced using hypoosmolar formulas after 2 weeks' NPO status. Prior to ostomy closure, a contrast enema is recommended to rule out strictures of the distal bowel. Strictures are noted in 25% of the patients treated medically.[20]

In summary, the preoperative care of the neonatal surgical patient follows the same guidelines of resuscitation as in other medically ill infants. The airway and breathing are secured in the standard fashion, except that patients with a surgical abdomen benefit from early intubation rather than mask ventilation to prevent

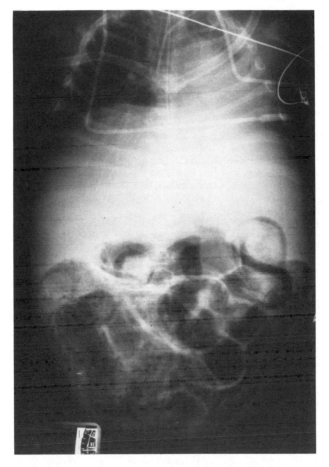

FIGURE 10.   Pneumatosis intestinalis as seen on plain abdominal radiograph in a patient with necrotizing enterocolitis.

further abdominal distention. Owing to "third space" fluid losses, aggressive fluid resuscitation rather than pharmacologic support is indicated to maintain circulation. Nasogastric decompression is essential to prevent further worsening of the abdominal distention and the aspiration of vomitus during transport and anesthetic induction. Certain surgical conditions do call for some added measures, especially those dealing with abdominal wall defects, as previously described. Early recognition and expeditious work-up of these patients are essential. They should be transported early in their care to a facility where pediatric surgical services are immediately available, so that treatment can be instituted without delays.

REFERENCES

1. Adam AS, Corbally MT, Fitzgerald RJ: Evaluation of conservative therapy for exomphalos. Surg Gynecol Obstet 172:394, 1991.
2. Allen RG, Wrenn EL: Silon as a sac in the treatment of omphalocele and gastroschisis. J Pediatr Surg 4:3, 1969.
3. Beckwith JB, Wang CL, Donnell GN: Hyperplastic fetal visceromegaly with macroglossia, omphalocele, cytomegaly of adrenal fetal cortex, post natal gigantism, and other abnormalities: Newly recognized syndrome. Proc Am Pediatr Soc Seattle, June 1964.
4. Cameron AEP, Howard ER: Gastric volvulus in childhood. J Pediatr Surg 22:944, 1987.

5. Cantrell JR, Haller JA, Ravitch MM: A syndrome of congenital defects involving the abdominal wall, sternum, diaphragm, pericardium, and heart. Surg Gynceol Obstet 107:606, 1958.
6. Chang PY, Yeh ML, Sheu JC, Chen CC: Experience with treatment of gastroschisis and omphalocele. J Formosan Med Assoc 91:447, 1992.
7. Cheromcha DP, Hyman PE: Neonatal necrotizing enterocolitis. Inflammatory bowel disease of the newborn. Dig Dis Sci 33:78S, 1988.
8. DeVries PA: The pathogenesis of gastroschisis and omphalocele. J Pediatr Surg 15:245, 1980.
9. Diamond PA, Jeffs RD: Cloacal exstrophy: A 22-year experience. J Urol 133:779, 1985.
10. Evans MI, Drugan A, Greenholz SK, et al: Development of a program for planned cesarean delivery and immediate pediatric surgical repair of ventral wall defects. Fetal Ther 3:84, 1988.
11. Garrett JR, Howard ER, Nixon HH: Autonomic nerves in rectum and colon in Hirschsprung's disease. A cholinesterase and catecholamine histochemical study. Arch Dis Child 44:406, 1969.
12. Ghory MJ, Sheldon CA: Newborn surgical emergencies of the gastrointestinal tract. Surg Clin North Am 65:1083, 1985.
13. Grob M: Conservative treatment of exomphalos. Arch Dis Child 38:148, 1963.
14. Grosfeld JL, Weber TR: Congenital abdominal wall defects: Gastroschisis and omphalocele. Curr Probl Surg 19:159, 1982.
15. Grosfeld JL, Rescorla FJ: Duodenal atresia and stenosis: Reassessment of treatment and outcome based on antenatal diagnosis, pathologic variance, and long term follow up. World J Surg 17:301, 1993.
16. Gross RE: A new method for surgical treatment of large omphaloceles. Surgery 24:277, 1948.
17. Hays DM: Intestinal atresia and stenosis. Curr Probl Surg Oct 1969.
18. Hirschsprung H: Stuhltragheit neugeborener in folge von dilatation und hypertropie des colons. Jahrb Kenderh 27:1, 1887.
19. Idowu J, Aitken DR, Georgeson KE: Gastric volvulus in the newborn. Arch Surg 115:1046, 1980.
20. Janik JS, Ein SH, Mancer K: Intestinal stricture after necrotizing enterocolitis. J Pediatr Surg 16:438, 1981.
21. Knight PJ, Sommer A, Clatworthy HW Jr: Omphalocele: A prognostic classification. J Pediatr Surg 16:599, 1981.
22. Luck SR, Sherman JO, Raffensperger JG, Goldstein IR: Gastroschisis in 106 consecutive newborn infants. Surgery 98:677, 1985.
23. Lynn HB: Duodenal obstruction: Atresia, stenosis and annular pancreas. In Ravitch MM, et al (eds): Pediatric Surgery, Chicago, Year Book, 1979.
24. Martin LW, Torres AM: Hirschsprung's disease. Surg Clin North Am 65:1171, 1985.
25. Molenaar JC, Tibboel D: Gastroschisis and omphalocele. World J Surg 17:337, 1993.
26. Mollitt DL, Tepas JJ, Talbert JL: The role of coagulase staphylococcus in neonatal necrotizing enterocolitis. J Pediatr Surg 23:60, 1988.
27. Moretti M, Khoury A, Rodriguez J, et al: The effect of mode delivery on the perinatal outcome in fetuses with abdominal wall defects. Am J Obstet Gynecol 163:833, 1990.
28. Muecke EC: The role of cloacal membrane in exstrophy: The first successful experimental study. J Urol 92:659, 1964.
29. Ricketts RR, Woodard JR, Zwiren GT, et al: Modern treatment of cloacal exstrophy. J Pediatr Surg 26:444, 1991.
30. Rickham PO: Vesicointestinal fissure. Arch Dis Child 35:97, 1960.
31. Schuster SR: A new method for the staged repair of large omphaloceles. Surg Gynecol Obstet 125:837, 1967.
32. Seiber WK: Hirschsprung's disease. In Welch KJ, et al (eds): Pediatric Surgery, 4th ed. Chicago, Year Book, 1986.
33. Smith WR, Leix I: Omphalocele. Am J Surg 111:450, 1966.
34. Stewart DR, Colodny AL, Daggett WC: Malrotation of the bowel in infants and children: A 15 year review. Surgery 79:716, 1976.
35. Swartz KR, Harrison MW, Campbell TJ, Campbell JR: Selective management of gastroschisis. Ann Surg 203:214, 1986.
36. Tietelbaum DH, Qualman SJ, Caniano DA: Hirschsprung's disease, identification of risk factors for enterocolitis. Ann Surg 207:240, 1988.
37. Torres AM, Ziegler MM: Malrotation of the intestine. World J Surg 17:326, 1993.
38. Touloukian RJ: Diagnosis and treatment of jejunoileal atresia. World J Surg 17:310, 1993.
39. Wijesinha SS: Neonatal necrotizing enterocolitis: New thoughts for the eighties. Ann R Coll Surg 64:406, 1982.
40. Yasbeck S, Ndoye M, Khan AH: Omphalocele: A 25 year experience. J Pediatr Surg 21:761, 1986.
41. Ziegler MM, Duckett JW, Howell CG: Cloacal exstrophy. In Welch JK, et al (eds): Pediatric Surgery, 4th ed. Chicago, Year Book, 1986.

CHAPTER 27

Skeletal Injuries

JOHN W. GRANETO, D.O.
DAVID F. SOGLIN, M.D.

Up to one-third of all pediatric prehospital transports involve motor vehicle accidents and other trauma.[12,15,21] Both blunt and penetrating trauma are occurring with increasing frequency to pediatric victims. Specialized transport and stabilization of a patient who has sustained a skeletal injury occurs in conjunction with the general care given any transported patient. Extremity injuries alone usually are not life-threatening, and care given the skeletal injury is directed toward preventing further injury during transport.[4,9] The attention given to extremity injuries in the acute care of trauma and in stabilization prior to and during transport should come only after significant stepwise care has been addressed in the "primary survey" of airway, breathing, and circulation (ABCs). Caution should be exercised to remain attentive to the ABCs when there is a potentially distracting injury, e.g., a dramatic deformity or open fracture of a long bone.[5,11]

Of all pediatric prehospital trauma transports, one-fourth have a skeletal injury.[8] Injuries of the extremity should not be overlooked when performing a complete secondary survey of the traumatized patient. In such cases, the child's life-threatening injuries may distract care away from the affected extremity because of the overwhelming magnitude of the injuries being addressed during the primary survey of trauma.

Direct application of prehospital protocols originally designed for adults and then later adapted to children is impractical.[19] Specific protocols for pediatric patients should be addressed and will be discussed. The general steps in assessment and stabilization of injured extremities will be outlined. The areas of blunt trauma (including fractures and crush injuries), amputations, and penetrating trauma will be discussed.

To assess the extent and nature of the patient's injuries appropriately, it is essential that the extremities be exposed. Generally, it is better to cut clothes off rather than try to pull them off because even minimal movement can cause excruciating pain to the injured child. Because children, particularly infants, are highly susceptible to hypothermia, the exposure must be brief and the patient's body temperature protected.

BLUNT TRAUMA

Blunt trauma is defined as a blow of force significant enough to produce injury to the skin without necessarily breaking the skin. It may occur as a large object strikes the body with a strong force, or if the patient is subjected to a rapid deceleration into a fixed object, e.g., a motor vehicle accident or a fall from a height.[1] Bony contusions resulting from direct blows to the bone, even without a fracture, are significant injuries and can be very painful. In a child, pain accounts in great part for general discomfort and, therefore, lack of cooperation. Prior acknowledgement of this can allow the transporting health care provider to understand the nature of the child's difficulty in remaining calm.

Regardless of the injured extremity involved or the type of injury, the general initial approach will begin with the assessment of the distal portion of the injured extremity (Table 1). Emergency medical services (EMS) scene time is frequently under scrutiny. Only a few minutes of observation will be needed for any extremity injury.[16,18]

Any obvious hemorrhage or severely open wounds such as an open fracture should be covered with a pressure dressing or sterile occlusive bandages before performing an elaborate assessment. Prevention of further blood loss and minimizing infectious complications are achieved by this simple yet effective initial step.

Locating the specific area of the bone that is fractured or dislocated may be difficult. Some clues are swelling, ecchymosis, tenderness, and deformity. After locating the specific area of injury or suspected injury, assessment of function should follow. The neurologic/sensory function can be assessed through the patient's ability to feel light touch or pain. Simple assessment can be accomplished with the end of a pen or even a plastic catheter/needle. Both medial and lateral surfaces should be tested for comparison and completeness. Assessment of motor function and strength testing can be good markers for the severity of the injury to nerves or tendons. Assessment can range from observing spontaneous motor activity to more elaborate active range of motion strength testing against resistance at each joint distal to the injured area. Careful evaluation of the vascular supply is initiated with comparison of pulses from the noninjured side. Capillary refill times are an excellent way of comparing the vascular integrity of the injured side with the noninjured side. The injured area should be splinted or immobilized. The area should be reassessed after the placement of the splints to ensure that no injury was caused by the placement of the immobilization equipment.

Treating any affected extremity should involve splinting the affected areas. This stabilization step should occur prior to transport to help maintain the integrity of the area while preventing further movement and possible further damage. Children can tolerate immobilized areas longer than adults, as postimmobilization stiffness generally occurs less often in children. Splints are available from the very simple to the more elaborate commercial products (Fig. 1). Types range from very rigid splints made from cardboard or preformed plastics to formable materials and the recently developed air splints with inflatable

TABLE 1. Extremity Injury Checklist

Treatments addressing the ABCs with hemorrhage control
History of injury and mechanism
Physical exam for tenderness, swelling, ecchymosis, and deformity
Initial assessment of motor function, vascular supply, and sensation
Splint, immobilizaton, and compression
Application of ice
Elevation of the injured area
Reassessment of motor function, vascular supply, and sensation

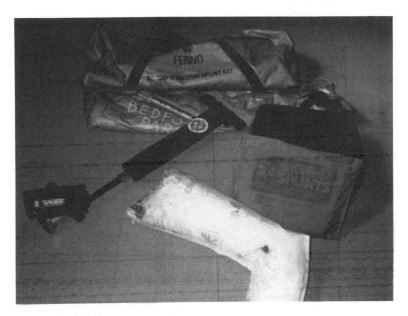

FIGURE 1.   Various types of splints currently available.

compartments.[3,5] All ambulance transport vehicles should be equipped with the most basic splinting devices to fit pediatric patients.[2]

Compression wraps also should be applied early to prevent or minimize edema formation.[7] Swelling is the most common response to injury.[1] Whenever possible, ice or cold packs should be applied early to aid in the reduction or prevention of swelling.

CRUSH INJURIES

Crush injuries can occur from a great force applied to a specific body area over a prolonged period. Examples include an arm being caught in a "wringer" or a leg trapped under a heavy object for several hours. The problems with crush injuries are that delayed injury to the underlying area may not be apparent for several hours after the initial insult. During transport attention is centered on recognizing the mechanism that could lead to this type of injury. The pathophysiologic problem with crush injuries is that soft tissue damage can result in edema and blood entrapment without a portal for drainage. Significant injury with a large hematoma or soft tissue swelling can result in compartment syndrome, e.g., neurovascular or muscular symptoms of pain and/or paresthesias. These injuries have no specific treatment during transport other than the assessments and immobilization, as outlined in Table 1.

CHILD ABUSE

Motor vehicle accidents account for the majority of isolated long bone fractures in children. However, patients with injuries to the humerus or femur, isolated from other serious trauma, or with multiple rib fractures, should raise the suspicion of child abuse.[11] Diaphyseal fractures are the most common in child abuse. They can result from a direct blow or bending force applied to the center of the long bone, resulting in a transverse fracture. Torsional forces applied during a twisting or rotational movement result in a spiral fracture. A careful history should be obtained in any cases of suspected abuse. Transport personnel should attempt to obtain a thorough history without being judgmental toward the historian. It is not necessary to prove that child abuse has occurred—only to suspect it and be careful to obtain detailed historical findings prior to transport in order to begin to piece together the possible reason for the fractures.[11]

FRACTURES AND DISLOCATIONS

General Approach

The child who has sustained either dislocations or fractures may present with the same initial appearance—that is, deformity and/or angulation of the injured area. Fractures of long bones may accompany general trauma or may occur as isolated injuries. In general, the approach to the the injured segment will be the same in either case. Even if subtle findings are the only clues to a possible fracture, and if doubt exists as to whether a fracture has occurred, the patient should be treated as if there were indeed a definite fracture to that area.[13]

Lower Extremity

Femur fractures occurring alone are less likely to produce hemodynamic instability in children than in adults, but splinting is still indicated to avoid possible arterial rupture during transport.[9] Various traction splint devices are available, the most common being the Hare traction device (Fig. 2). Femur and tibial splinting may be accomplished simply with two long boards as well. Regardless of the splinting method used, careful palpation of the dorsalis pedis and posterior tibial pulses should be performed when assessing the distal vascular supply both before and after splint application. Gentle continuous traction may be applied during the splinting procedure initially to reduce pain. Pneumatic antishock garments (PASGs) are generally discouraged, especially for shorter transport times.[16]

Knee dislocations and suspected fractures should be splinted in the position in which they are initially found. No traction or attempts at reduction are necessary in the prehospital or interhospital settings. Stabilization for transport should consist only of the initial assessment, splinting and hemorrhage control, and the final reassessment.

Ankle fractures are common in older children and adolescents. These are most commonly and effectively splinted with commercially available air splints. A simpler rigid supporting immobilization certainly is acceptable. The same general principles of assessment and postsplinting reassessment apply here as well.

Upper Extremity

The arm found in a straightened or extended position should be splinted in that position. If the arm is angulated or deformed, care should be taken to leave the extremity in the position found. No attempts at straightening or reducing the angulation are necessary prior to transport. Palpation to locate pinpoint tenderness may be a clue to the location of the specific fracture. Other signs may include ecchymosis and swelling. When in doubt about the specific site of the fracture, immobilization of the entire extremity should be the goal.

Greater fracture angulation during transport is tolerated than in adults. This is important to remember if the transport system usually deals with adult

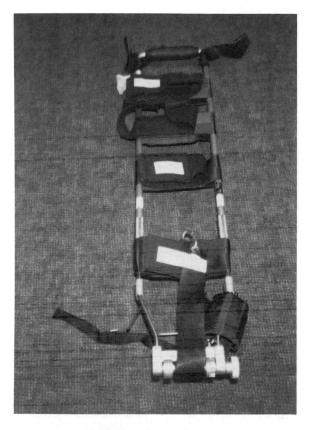

FIGURE 2.   Hare traction splint.

patients and protocols are simply adapted to fit children.[19] Humerus fractures should be splinted with a rigid splint. Rigid splints are also applicable to the distal portion of the arm; however, air splints also are acceptable for wrist and hand injuries. Once again, careful assessment of distal function should occur before and after splinting devices are placed. A description of this "pre- and post-" procedure should be documented clearly in the transport records.

PENETRATING INJURIES

Penetrating injuries of the extremities are rarely life-threatening and generally should be identified and addressed during the secondary survey. Because of the potential for massive bleeding with arterial disruption or extensive injuries, as might occur from a shotgun blast, volume resuscitation and control of hemorrhage become major priorities. In the absence of life-threatening injuries that demand immediate transport, management in the field should include bandaging with dry, sterile dressings to reduce further contamination and immobilization of the affected limb. Splinting can provide pain relief, reduce the risk of additional soft tissue, nerve, and/or blood vessel injury, and will make moving the patient significantly easier. Although splinting is important, transport of the critical patient should not be delayed just to secure immobilization. It is vital that neurovascular integrity distal to the wound be assessed carefully before and after any manipulation of the extremity. Distal pulses, capillary refill, and sensation can be evaluated quickly and easily. With penetrating trauma near major vessels, there is concern for vascular integrity.

GUNSHOT WOUNDS

More and more frequently, children are victims of firearm injuries.[6] Gunshot wounds are frequently "multiple," and patients with gunshot wounds to the extremity are at risk for other injuries that may be a more immediate threat to life. Therefore, with the exception of hemorrhage control, management of the gunshot wound to the extremity should be undertaken during the secondary survey. The extent of the injury from a gunshot is related to the velocity of the bullet. It is important for the person treating the patient in the field to note the type of gun used, if that information is available. A small entrance wound may belie significant internal injury. Exit wounds are frequently more extensive than entrance wounds and may bleed vigorously; therefore, careful inspection of the patient, both front and back, is vital. There may be bony injury from the force of the bullet, creating an open fracture with subsequent risk of infection. All extremity wounds should be managed conservatively. Bandaging to reduce contamination and to aid in the control of bleeding is important, as is splinting of the extremity. A careful assessment of neurovascular function distal to the wound can be performed quickly by assessing sensation, motor function, pulses, and capillary refill. This should be done before and after any manipulation of the extremity.

STAB WOUNDS

When the skin is punctured with a knife, glass, or other sharp object, the injury to the deep tissue is frequently more severe than is apparent from the surface laceration. Rarely, however, are such wounds life-threatening; thus, they should be managed as part of the secondary trauma survey. Initial management is focused on control of hemorrhage and reduction of contamination. Unlike closed soft tissue injuries, once the skin has been disrupted there is significant potential for bacteria to "seed" the deeper tissues, resulting in such infections as cellulitis or osteomyelitis. Splinting extremities that have penetrating wounds often will reduce bleeding and provide pain relief, even in the absence of an underlying fracture. Sensation, motor function, capillary refill, and pulses should be carefully assessed and documented distal to the stab wound. Evidence of vascular injury such as bleeding with arterial pulsations, diminished pulse, or an overlying bruit or thrill indicates that the patient has a limb-threatening injury and mandates prompt transport to an appropriate center. If a partial avulsion or skin flap has been produced, the tissue is dependent on blood flow through this remaining attached portion, or pedicle. It is vital that the wound be bandaged with the pedicle in good position to avoid kinking, twisting, and the attendant lack of blood supply to the flap.

An object—for example, a knife or sharp piece of glass—that has remained in the wound should not be removed. Removal can cause additional soft tissue injury and serious bleeding that could be difficult to control in the field. Instead, bleeding should be controlled with direct pressure while avoiding application of force to the impaled object or the immediately involved tissues. A bulky dressing should be applied that protects the wound and encompasses the impaled object to keep it stationary. This reduces the risk of further injury to the surrounding tissues, nerves, or vessels.

AMPUTATIONS

Potentially life-threatening injuries that accompany an amputation should not be overlooked because of the dramatic presence of an amputated part. However, like pelvic and femur fractures, amputation of extremities may cause profound blood loss, and hemorrhaging wounds must be controlled. Generally, direct pressure and elevation are sufficient to control bleeding. Tourniquets are rarely indicated.

The stump should be bandaged to prevent further contamination of the wound and to aid in control of bleeding. If there is a partial amputation, the distal portion should be maintained with the stump if at all possible. A bulky pressure dressing and careful splinting can prevent inadvertent completion of the amputation.

If the amputation is complete, the amputated part should be transported along with the patient to a center skilled in microsurgical technique and reimplantation. The likelihoood of successful reimplantation depends on the nature and extent of the initial injury and the length of time prior to surgery. Sharp amputations with little surrounding tissue destruction are more likely to be successfully reattached than are crush or tearing injuries. In children, amputations of the hand are often successfully reimplanted;[14] rarely can lower extremity amputations be reimplanted with good functional results. The rate of successful reimplantation diminishes with time, although proper handling of the amputated part can lengthen viability from 6–8 hours to 12–18 hours.[5] To maximize the potential for reimplantation, the amputated part should be gently wrapped in a sterile dressing. No attempt to scrub the part clean should be made prior to transport; this can cause additional tissue damage. The protected part should be placed in a plastic bag and then on ice. The part should never be in direct contact with the ice nor should "dry ice" be used. Freezing can lead to extensive tissue damage.

CONCLUSION

Regardless of the type of injury, the approach to the injured extremity is basically very similar and stepwise. All extremity injuries first require attention to the mechanism of injury and the history. Timely treatments addressing the ABCs are the next steps. Assessment of distal function as outlined above is important in the overall documentation and care of the patient. Ultimately, splinting, immobilization, and reassessment of the injured area complete the assessment.

Careful attention to the extremity injuries, including adequate immobilization, is necessary to prevent further, secondary injury during transport.

REFERENCES

1. American Academy of Orthopedic Surgeons: Emergency Care and Transportation of the Sick and Injured, 4th ed. Park Ridge, IL, American Academy of Orthopedic Surgeons, 1987.
2. American College of Emergency Physicians: Minimum pediatric prehospital equipment guidelines. ACEP News January insert, 1992.
3. Butnam AM, Paturas JL: Prehospital Trauma Life Support Emergency Training. Akron, OH, 1986.
4. Bledshoe BE, Porter RS, Shade BR: Paramedic Emergency Care. Englewood Cliffs, NJ, Prentice-Hall, 1991.
5. Campbell JE: Extremity trauma. In BTLS: Basic Prehospital Trauma Care. Englewood Cliffs, NJ, Prentice-Hall, 1988.
6. Christoffel KK: Violent death and injury in US children and adolescents. Am J Dis Child 144:697, 1990.
7. Dyment PG: Initial management of minor acute soft-tissue injuries. Pediatr Ann 17:99, 1988.

8. Eichelberger MR, Mangubat EA, Sacco WS, et al: Comparative outcomes of children and adults suffering blunt trauma. J Trauma 28:430, 1988.
9. Graneto JW, Soglin DF: Transport and management of the pediatric trauma patient. Pediatr Clin North Am 40:365, 1993.
10. Gillespie DL, Woodson J, Kaufman J, et al: Role of arteriography for blunt and penetrating injuries in proximity to major vascular structures: An evolution in management. Ann Vasc Surg 7:145, 1993.
11. Hayden PW, Gallagher TA: Child abuse and intervention in the emergency room. Pediatr Clin North Am 39:1053, 1992.
12. Jaffe D, Wesson D: Emergency management of blunt trauma in children. N Engl J Med 324:1477, 1991.
13. Henry MC, Stapleton ER: EMT Prehospital Care. Philadelphia, W.B. Saunders, 1992.
14. Jaeger SH, Tsai T, Kleinert HE: Upper extremity replantation in children. Orthop Clin North Am 12:897, 1981.
15. Keen TP: Nursing care of the pediatric multiple trauma patient. Nurs Clin North Am 25:131, 1990.
16. Lavery RF, Tortella BJ, Griffin CC: The prehospital treatment of pediatric trauma. Pediatr Emerg Care 8:9, 1992.
17. Lynch K, Johansen K: Can Doppler pressure measurement replace "exclusion" arteriography in the diagnosis of occult extremity arterial trauma? Ann Surg 214:737, 1991.
18. Rouse A: Study to examine the timeliness of care received by patients with open fractures of the lower limb. J Public Health Med 13:267, 1991.
19. Sachetti A, Carraccio C, Feder M: Pediatric EMS transport: Are we treating children in a system designed for adults only? Pediatr Emerg Care 8:4, 1992.
20. Trooskin SZ, Sclafini S, Winfield J, et al: The management of vascular injuries of the extremity associated with civilian firearms. Surg Gynecol Obstet 176:350, 1993.
21. Tsai A, Kallsen G: Epidemiology of pediatric prehospital care. Ann Emerg Med 16:284, 1987.

CHAPTER 28

Burns and Inhalation Injuries

RICHARD J. KAGAN, M.D.
MARILYN E. JENKINS, R.N., M.B.A.

Burn injuries are responsible for over 500,000 emergency department visits and approximately 70,000 acute hospital admissions in the United States each year.[2] Loss of the functional skin barrier after thermal injury results in increased susceptibility to infection and is the major cause of morbidity and mortality postburn. In addition, factors such as age, associated injuries, and inhalation injury may have an adverse effect on clinical outcome.

Regional burn care facilities, enhanced communication networks, and emergency medical systems have helped provide a highly sophisticated level of care for thermally injured children. Most of these children are treated initially in hospitals not equipped to care for the complicated problems arising secondary to burn injury. The need for rapid and expert transport of these patients to burn treatment centers has contributed to the development of specialized programs in many areas of the country. The transport teams bring expertise to the referring center to assess and stabilize the patient both before and during transport and provide support until the patient arrives at the specialized burn treatment center.

PATHOPHYSIOLOGY

In order to assess and stabilize the burn-injured child properly, it is important to have an understanding of the basic pathophysiologic events that occur following thermal injury. These include, but are not limited to, burn shock, inhalation injury, and the burn wound.

Burn Shock

Burn shock is both a hypovolemic and cellular shock. It is characterized by hemodynamic changes that include decreased plasma volume, extracellular fluid, cardiac output, and oliguria. The primary goal of therapy is to restore and preserve tissue perfusion; however, resuscitation is complicated by obligatory burn edema. The most significant factor in the etiology of burn shock is the increase in total body capillary permeability.[4] Water, electrolytes, and protein freely escape from the intravascular space into the interstitial space. Generalized edema develops, with predominance at the burn site. Maximal edema forms 8–12 hours after small burns and 12–24 hours following major injuries. The magnitude of tissue edema depends on the adequacy of resuscitation.

Multiple mediators have been proposed to explain the changes in vascular permeability postburn. Much of the vascular damage is thought to be due to such vasoactive substances as histamine, serotonin, kinins, and the products of arachidonic acid metabolism.[28] The end-result of these changes is a disruption of normal capillary barriers and rapid equilibrium of the intravascular and interstitial compartments. In addition, after major thermal injury there is a breakdown of the energy-dependent sodium pump, resulting in an increase in intracellular sodium concentration.

Inhalation Injury

Three components of inhalation injury may be present alone or in combination: (1) thermal injury to the airway; (2) carbon monoxide poisoning; and (3) inhalation of toxic gases and smoke. Heated air usually results in burns limited to the face, oropharynx, and upper airway. Superheated air rarely causes parenchymal damage because of efficient heat dissipation in the upper respiratory tract. Steam inhalation may cause lower airway injury owing to its markedly increased heat capacity.[6]

Carbon monoxide poisoning is the most common immediate cause of fire-related deaths. The affinity of hemoglobin for carbon monoxide is approximately 200 times greater than for oxygen. Carboxyhemoglobin is unable to bind oxygen, resulting in a left shift of the oxyhemoglobin dissociation curve and reduced oxygen delivery to peripheral tissues. The predominant mechanism for carbon monoxide toxicity is altered oxygen transport, not a direct cytotoxic action of heme-containing proteins.[13]

Smoke damage to the lower airway is caused by the toxic products of combustion, such as aldehydes, ketones, polyurethanes, and organic acids.[10] Within minutes of exposure, the cilia of the respiratory mucosa cease functioning and inflammatory mediators are released. This response results in bronchospasm, mucosal edema and de-epithelialization, obstruction, and a deficiency in surfactant activity. Bronchial blood flow is markedly increased, leading to interstitial edema, shunting, and a reduction in pulmonary compliance.[25]

Burn Wound

Tissue loss following thermal injury is a consequence of coagulation necrosis. The depth of injury is related to heat intensity, duration of exposure, and tissue conductance. The burn wound has been described as having three concentric zones.[11] The zone of coagulation represents the area of most intense thermal injury and tissue destruction. It is surrounded by a zone of stasis, or ischemia, which may or may not survive. The outer layer, or zone of hyperemia, is the least injured area and may be confused by the inexperienced caregiver with cellulitis. The hyperemia typically resolves within 7–10 days postinjury.

The injury process remains dynamic during the first 24–48 hours after the burning process has been arrested. Studies have shown that capillary occlusion can progress during this time and support the clinical impression that skin necrosis progresses during the first 48 hours postburn.[5] This phenomenon is not considered a continuation of the burning process but a pathophysiologic event that may be the consequence of tissue edema, dermal ischemia, inadequate resuscitation, or desiccation.

FIELD MANAGEMENT

Appropriate administration of first aid is extremely important in minimizing morbidity and mortality from burn injuries. An organized systematic approach should be used to assess and stabilize the burn patient prior to initiating transport. Because the size and depth of the burn are key determinants of the magnitude of injury, the first step should be to stop the burning process and begin the ABCs of resuscitation. All clothing and jewelry should be removed and the patient wrapped in a clean or sterile sheet to minimize contamination. Although the use of cool solutions has been reported to reduce the pain of partial-thickness injuries, their use should be limited to small wounds since this treatment may be associated with a significant reduction in core temperature and possible ventricular fibrillation.[18] Application of topical antimicrobial agents is not necessary at this time. Multiple layers of blankets and a warm transport environment should be used to prevent hypothermia, especially during cold weather.

Chemical burns should be copiously irrigated with water because the concentration of the burning agent and the length of exposure determine the depth and extent of tissue damage. Time should not be wasted searching for a neutralizing agent. Patients with electrical injuries initially should be assessed for functional cardiac activity. If cardiopulmonary arrest has occurred, CPR must be initiated immediately. All patients with electrical injury should undergo cardiac monitoring since dysrhythmias are not uncommon. In addition, patients with electrical injury should be evaluated for fractures secondary to falls or tetany.

Baseline vital signs including respiratory rate, pulse, temperature, and blood pressure should be obtained at the scene prior to initial transport. Maintenance of an adequate airway is mandatory. High-flow oxygen should be administered to all patients with fire-related injuries because of the likelihood of carbon monoxide poisoning. Although upper airway obstruction due to laryngeal edema usually does not develop until 12–24 hours after the injury, it may be necessary to insert an endotracheal tube to maintain airway patency. If it is necessary to travel more than 30 minutes to the nearest hospital, a large-bore intravenous catheter should be inserted percutaneously through unburned skin and a balanced salt solution infused. Fluid needs may be estimated based on the child's weight and the extent of burn.

For patients with small wounds, burn size can be estimated using the principle that the palmar surface of the patient's hand represents approximately 1% of the total body surface area (TBSA). Wounds greater than 10–15% TBSA can be quickly estimated in the field using the Rule of Nines, which divides the body area into multiples of 9% TBSA;[17] however, this method of estimating wound size may be inaccurate in small children and infants because it does not account for the differences in proportional surface area between children and adults. Since most children sustaining thermal injuries are stable in the immediate postburn period, they should be transported to the nearest health care facility, particularly if the time necessary for transport to the regional burn center hospital is lengthy.

PRETRANSPORT HOSPITAL ASSESSMENT

Once the child arrives at the first hospital, it is important to perform a more in-depth assessment of the injuries in order to avoid unnecessary delay in transport to a specialized care facility. The decision whether to transfer the thermally injured child to a specialized burn care facility is based not only on the extent, depth, type, and location of the burn, but also on the presence of other complicating factors and the capabilities of the referring hospital. In general, children should be transferred to burn centers when the referring hospital lacks the personnel and/or facilities to provide optimal and complete pediatric burn care. The indications for referral should be based on medical necessity rather than socioeconomic or time considerations.

Burn injuries are typically classifed according to severity. *Minor* burns in children are defined as partial-thickness injuries less than 10% TBSA and full-thickness injuries less than 2% TBSA that are not caused by electric current, do not involve critical areas of the body (such as the hands, face, feet, or perineum), and that are not ocmplicated by inhalation injury or other risk factors. *Moderate* burns are defined as partial-thickness injuries involving 10–20% TBSA and full-thickness injuries less than 10% TBSA, also excluding electric etiology, inhalation injury, or associated risk factors. *Major* burns are defined as partial-thickness wounds greater than 20% of TBSA and full-thickness wounds greater than 10% TBSA or wounds due to electricity, involving critical body areas, or with associated risk factors.[18] Recently, however, the American Burn Association and the American College of Surgeons Committee on Trauma have advocated that patients meeting the criteria outlined in Table 1 be referred to specialized burn care facilities to ensure optimal outcomes.[2,3]

Inhalation Injury

A history of closed-space injury in patients with decreased level of consciousness is strongly correlated with inhalation injury. Physical examination may reveal facial burns, singed nasal vibrissae, carbonaceous sputum, hoarseness, and wheezing. Carbon monoxide poisoning is best diagnosed by measuring the carboxyhemoglobin content of arterial blood. Values greater than 2–6% are diagnostic. Fiberoptic bronchoscopy is the best modality for assessment of the upper respiratory tract.[19] Although small airway injury is best evaluated by demonstrating trapping of 133-xenon on lung scanning,[14] a $pO_2{:}FiO_2$ ratio less than 300 is considered by many to be diagnostic of pulmonary injury.

TABLE 1. Burn Center Referral Criteria

Second- and third-degree burns greater than 10% TBSA in patients under 10 or over 50 years of age
Second- and third-degree burns greater than 20% TBSA in other age groups
Second- and third-degree burns that involve the face, hands, feet, genitals, perineum, and/or major joints
Third-degree burns greater than 5% TBSA in any age group
Electrical burns including lightning injury
Chemical burns
Inhalation injury
Burn injury in patients with preexisting medical disorders that could complicate management, prolong recovery, or affect mortality
Any patients with burns and concomitant trauma (such as fractures) in which the burn injury poses the greatest risk of morbidity of mortality; in such cases, if the trauma poses the greater immediate risk, the patient may be treated initially in a Trauma Center until stable before being transferred to a Burn Center; physician judgment will be necessary in such situations and should be in concert with the regional medical control plan and triage protocols
Hospitals without qualified personnel or equipment for the care of children should transfer children with burns to a Burn Center with these capabilities
Burn injury in patients who require special social, emotional, and/or long-term rehabilitative support, including suspected child abuse, substance abuse, and the like.

Adapted from American Burn Association: Guidelines for operation of burn centers. J Burn Care Rehabil 16(1):20A–29A, 1995, and American College of Surgeons Committee on Trauma: Resources for optimal care of patients with burn injury. In American College of Surgeons: Resources for Optimal Care of the Injured Patient. Chicago, American College of Surgeons, 1993, with permission.

Burn Wound

Estimation of burn depth remains subjective even among experienced burn surgeons. Depth of burn is categorized as partial-thickness and full-thickness. Superficial partial-thickness wounds are characterized by a blistered, painful, moist erythematous surface that exhibits capillary refill. Deep dermal wounds are typically waxy-white and are less painful. Full-thickness burns are characterized by a pale, dry, leathery insensate surface that fails to demonstrate capillary refill.

Estimation of the extent of injury is nearly as variable as the determination of burn depth. Partial- and full-thickness wounds are identified and an age-specific grid, such as the Lund-Browder diagram,[12] should be completed to calculate accurately the extent of body surface area involved (Fig. 1). As a rule, when triaging patients for referral to the regional burn care facility, it is better to overestimate rather than underestimate the extent and depth of injury.

PRETRANSPORT HOSPITAL MANAGEMENT

As in all forms of injury, airway maintenance is of paramount importance. Vital signs, including core body temperature, should be maintained and intravenous access established. Once the burn wound size has been determined, the fluid requirements for resuscitation can be calculated. A nasogastric tube should be placed because ileus is a common sequela of burn injury and may be associated with vomiting and aspiration of gastric contents. A Foley catheter should be placed to monitor hourly urine output in all patients requiring fluid resuscitation. Tetanus prophylaxis is mandatory. Patients not previously immunized should receive both tetanus toxoid and tetanus immune globulin. Pain medications and sedatives should be given intravenously in small incremental doses because drug absorption from subcutaneous and intramuscular sites is erratic during the immediate postburn period.[23]

Routine laboratory tests should include a complete blood count, serum electrolytes and albumin, blood urea nitrogen (BUN), urinalysis, and arterial blood gas with determination of the carboxyhemoglobin (CO:Hb) level. Chest radiography generally is valuable only to assess the position of central venous catheter tips and/or the endotracheal tube and the presence of other chest trauma such as pneumothorax and rib fractures.

Management of Inhalation Injury

Treatment of inhalation injury must be initiated before its diagnosis can be confirmed. High-flow 100% O_2 should be administered until the CO:Hb levels return to normal. The role of hyperbaric O_2 therapy in inhalation injury remains controversial.[10,13] Although it may be beneficial in patients with isolated carbon monoxide poisoning, it should not be instituted in burn patients with suspected inhalation injury until they are first assessed at the burn center.

Patients with signs and symptoms of impending airway obstruction must have upper airway control established. In general, it is prudent to intubate the patient prophylactically once the clinical diagnosis of inhalation injury is made.[8] In general, nasotracheal intubation is preferred over oral intubation and tracheostomy. Once the tube is in place, suctioning, aerosolized bronchodilators, humidification, and continuous positive airway pressure should be administered.

Systemic antibiotics have been demonstrated to be of no benefit in the prevention of pneumonia and respiratory distress syndrome.[20] In addition, systemic corticosteroids have been shown not only to have little utility, but also to be associated with a threefold increase in the incidence of pneumonia and death.[21,29]

Burn Estimate and Diagram
Age vs Area

Initial Evaluation

Cause of burn_____

Date of Burn_____

Time of Burn_____

Age _____

Sex _____

Weight _____

Date of Admission _____

Signature _____

Date_____

Burn Diagram

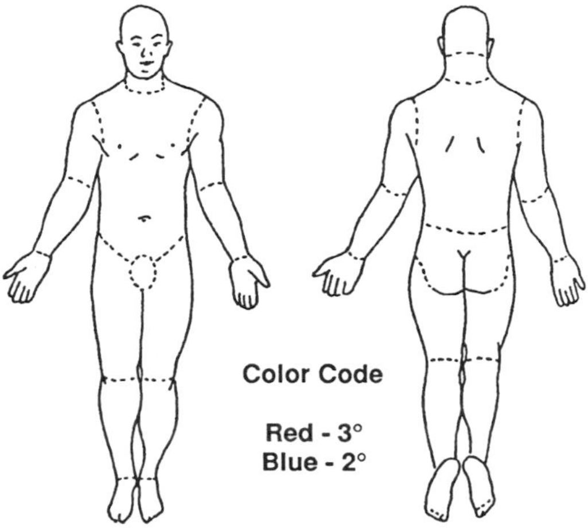

Color Code

Red - 3°
Blue - 2°

Area	Birth 1 yr.	1-4 yrs.	5-9 yrs.	10-14 yrs.	15 yrs.	Adult	2°	3°	Total	Donor Areas
Head	19	17	13	11	9	7				
Neck	2	2	2	2	2	2				
Ant. Trunk	13	13	13	13	13	13				
Post. Trunk	13	13	13	13	13	13				
R. Buttock	2 1/2	2 1/2	2 1/2	2 1/2	2 1/2	2 1/2				
L. Buttock	2 1/2	2 1/2	2 1/2	2 1/2	2 1/2	2 1/2				
Genitalia	1	1	1	1	1	1				
R.U. Arm	4	4	4	4	4	4				
L.U. Arm	4	4	4	4	4	4				
R.L. Arm	3	3	3	3	3	3				
L.L. Arm	3	3	3	3	3	3				
R. Hand	2 1/2	2 1/2	2 1/2	2 1/2	2 1/2	2 1/2				
L. Hand	2 1/2	2 1/2	2 1/2	2 1/2	2 1/2	2 1/2				
R. Thigh	5 1/2	6 1/2	8	8 1/2	9	9 1/2				
L. Thigh	5 1/2	6 1/2	8	8 1/2	9	9 1/2				
R. Leg	5	5	5 1/2	6	6 1/2	7				
L. Leg	5	5	5 1/2	6	6 1/2	7				
R. Foot	3 1/2	3 1/2	3 1/2	3 1/2	3 1/2	3 1/2				
L. Foot	3 1/2	3 1/2	3 1/2	3 1/2	3 1/2	3 1/2				
Total										

Shriners Hospitals
for crippled children

. Form

Burns Institute

Burn Diagram

FIGURE 1. The modified Lund-Browder chart for estimating body surface area burned. Differences in surface areas are age-dependent.(From Shriners Burns Institute, Cincinnati Unit, with permission.)

Management of Burn Shock

The primary goal of resuscitation is to replace the fluid lost from the circulatory volume as a result of increased capillary permeability. Because of their limited physiologic reserve, burned children require more precise resuscitation than do adults with the same extent of burn. Studies have demonstrated that children require 40% more fluid during burn shock than adults.[16] In addition, the presence of inhalation injury increases the fluid requirements for resuscitation.[24]

Many burn centers administer lactated Ringer's (LR) solution in accordance with the Parkland formula (4 ml/kg/% TBSA burn) with the addition of basal fluid needs (1500 ml/m² body surface area) to the calculated resuscitation volume. For patients with thermal injuries equal to or greater than 40% TBSA, a resuscitation fluid containing 180 mEq of sodium (100 ml LR + 50 mEq $NaHCO_3$) is recommended until metabolic acidosis has been reversed. This usually is achieved approximately 8 hours postburn. After correction of the acidosis, LR is infused for the second 8 hours, and LR with 5% albumin added is given to complete resuscitation. The key to optimal resuscitation is the frequent adjustment of the rate of fluid administration to maintain adequate urine output and vital signs. Increasing the rate of infusion is preferred to the sporadic administration of fluid boluses, and diuretics should be avoided. Resuscitation is deemed complete when the rate of administration is equal to the calculated maintenance fluid rate: basal (1500 ml/m²) + evaporative water loss (35 + % TBSA burn × m² × 24).

Because fluid replacement formulas provide only a rough guideline for resuscitation, monitoring the patient's response is critically important. Hourly urine output should be maintained between 0.5 and 1.0 ml/kg/hr and above 1.0 ml/kg/hr in the presence of hemoglobinuria or myoglobinuria. Adequacy of resuscitation also can be monitored with serial hematocrits, electrolytes, BUN, and blood pH. Invasive hemodynamic monitoring is rarely necessary in the pediatric burn patient.[9,16]

Management of the Burn Wound

Traditional management of the burn wound involves careful debridement of loose necrotic tissue and gentle cleansing of the wound with a bland soap. Controversy still exists regarding the debridement of blisters. This decision must be based not only on the location and size of the blister but also on the reliability of the patient. In general, it is safer and more practical to debride all blisters.

Circumferential full-thickness and deep partial-thickness burns are often associated with increased tissue pressures because of inelasticity and the increased capillary permeability that accompanies tissue trauma.[27] Capillary circulation should be monitored because nerve entrapment and venous obstruction occur before obliteration of the arterial pulse. The presence of delayed capillary refill, cyanosis, paresthesias, and/or decreased chest wall excursion are clinical indications for the performance of an escharotomy and/or fasciotomy. Another modality that is extremely helpful is subeschar compartment pressure measurement.[26] This may be easily performed at the patient's bedside by inserting an 18-gauge needle, that is connected to an arterial pressure monitor, beneath the eschar into the subcutaneous tissue or subfascial space. If tissue pressure is greater than 30 mmHg, a surgical release is required. This technique also is helpful in determining the adequacy of escharotomy, the need for fasciotomy, and the need for escharotomies in unburned extremities in which subfascial edema may develop because of diffuse capillary permeability changes.

If escharotomies are required, they should be performed by an experienced physician. The incisions should be made along the medial and lateral aspects of the extremity for the entire length of the burn and should extend deep into the subcutaneous tissue. Chest wall escharotomies may be necessary following circumferential torso burns if chest wall excursion is diminished and there is difficulty maintaining adequate ventilation. These incisions are typically made along the anterior axillary lines, the infraclavicular lines, and the subcostal margin.

TRANSPORT

Once the decision has been made to transport the patient to a specialized burn care facility, the optimal mode of transport must be determined. This choice is based on patient acuity, resources of the referring and receiving hospitals, optimal interhospital transport time, carrier and personnel availabiity, regional geography, weather and traffic conditions, and cost.

Transport Team Composition

Transport of critically ill pediatric burn patients to specialized treatment centers is now a widely accepted practice. The transport team must be composed of experienced individuals who have diagnostic and treatment skills in intensive care, pediatric care, and burn care. There should be a small number of individuals who perform all transports. This will optimize familiarity with equipment and protocols and will ensure competency maintenance of team members in patient transport management.[14]

The medical director of the transport team should be a specialist in burn care and/or pediatric critical care who has an understanding of transport physiology. There is considerable debate whether physicians are needed for the transport of critically ill patients.[7] With standardized protocols and communication at the burn center, it is rarely necessary to include a physician on the pediatric burn transport team. Our team consists of a burn nurse and a respiratory therapist with pediatric burn/critical care experience. Team members function as agents of the receiving burn center such that, upon their arrival at the referring institution, the patient's care becomes the responsibility of the receiving hospital.

Transport Team Responsibilities

Thermally injured pediatric patients meeting referral criteria should be transported to the regional burn center as soon as possible following injury, initial assessment, and stabilization. It is essential that the transport coordinator obtain baseline information (Fig. 2) from the referring center regarding the patient's condition; this may be an important factor in determining the composition of the transport team.

The transport team is responsible for assessing, stabilizing, and preparing the patient for transport. The team should function as an extension of the burn center and should follow its clinical protocols for care of the burned child. In general, the time spent by the transport team at the referring hospital is dictated by the condition of the patient; however, it is the responsibility of the registered nurse, in consultation with the burn center, to determine the appropriateness of delaying transport for stabilization of the patient and/or the performance of needed procedures. If the team is only minutes away from the receiving hospital, the team leader may elect to delay certain procedures, such as escharotomies, until the patient has arrived at the burn center.

PATIENT INFORMATION

Date/Time of Injury: _____ Cause: _____   * Patient Weight: _____

Estimated TBSA: _____ %   Full Thickness: _____ %   Partial Thickness: _____ %

Areas Involved: _____ Head   _____ Face   _____ Trunk (post.)

_____ RUE   _____ LUE   _____ Trunk (ant.)

_____ RLE   _____ LLE   _____ Genitals

_____ Right Hand   _____ Left Hand   _____ Other

Areas of Circumferential Burns/Swelling: _____

Compartment Pressure Measurements: _____   _____   _____   _____

Escharotomies/Fasciotomies Preformed: _____   _____   _____   _____

Topical Agents Used: _____   Associated Injuries: _____

Respiratory Inhalation Injury: _____   Carboxyhemoglobin: _____   Time Obtained: _____

Oxygen Therapy: _____   Artificial Airway: _____   SaO2: _____

Ventilator Settings	Last ABG Results			
Mode _____	Time _____	WBC _____	Na _____
F1O2 _____	pH _____	RBC _____	K _____
Tidal Volume _____	pCO2 _____	HgB _____	Cl– _____
Rate _____	pO2 _____	HCT _____	Ca _____
Peep\CPAP _____	B.E. _____	Platelets _____	CO2 _____
Vent Pressure: _____	HCO3 _____	PT _____	BUN _____
	O2 Sat _____	PTT _____	Glucose _____

Other _____

Vitals: HR_____   R_____   BP_____   Temp_____

Invasive Lines   Site/Fluids/Rate

Arterial Line   _____

Central Line   _____

Peripheral Line _____

* TOTAL FLUIDS

In   Out

NGT: _____

Tube Feedings: _____

PO Intake: _____   Foley: _____

                                 UOP: _____ cc / hr

Pt NPO and gastric
feeding off 2 hours
prior to transport: _____

Medications: Drug _____   Dose _____   Route _____

              Drug _____   Dose _____   Route _____

              Drug _____   Dose _____   Route _____

Allergies: _____   Prior Medical History: _____

Exposure To Contagious Disease: Yes ____ No ____   Tetanus Toxoid Given: Yes ____ No ____

Immunizations Up To Date: Yes ____ No ____   Date: _____

Reason For Transfer: _____

Recommendations For Changes In Treatment: _____

Parent/Guardian To Accompany Patient: _____

Withdrawal of Application/Reason: _____

REF# 123\INQUIRY.WK1   rev 11/93   (page 2 of 2)   RN Signature: _____

FIGURE 2. Medical information obtained by the transport coordinator at the time of referral of the burned child. (Shriners Burns Institute, Cincinnati Unit, with permission.)

Communication between the transport coordinator, transport team, and the referring physician is essential.[1] Furthermore, there should be physician-to-physician communication whenever possible in order to ensure prompt airway management, appropriate resuscitation, and continuity of optimal burn care.

Patient Name		Age	Sex
Ref. Institution	Ref. Inst. Phone #		
Ref. Doctor			
% Burn Wgt.	Hgt. Allergies		

Report from Ref. Inst. Nurse Name:

Parent/ Guardian Name

Records Rec. from Ref. Inst.

Case Summary   H & P
Labs   Other Diag.
RN Notes (opt)   Resuscitation Hx

Resuscitation Calculations

Resuscitation

A.   Calculated Resuscitation & Basal Requirement

(4cc x _____ kg x_____ % burn) + (1500cc x_____ m^2) = cc / 24 hours

(_____) + (_____) = _____ cc / 24 hours

B.   Resuscitation Fluid per 8 hours

1st 8 hours = _____ cc, _____ cc/ hr.

2nd 8 hours = _____ cc, _____ cc/ hr.

3rd 8 hours = _____ cc, _____ cc/ hr.

Maintenance Fluids

A.   Basal fluid requirement - 1500 cc/ m^2

1.   Total body surface area = _____ / m^2

2.   24 hours = _____ cc

3.   Hour - _____ cc/ hr.

B.   Evaporative water loss

1.   Adults - (25 + % Burn) m^2 = cc/ hr.

Children - (35 + % burn) m^2 = cc/ hr.

2.   Calculated evaporative water loss

a. (_____ + _____ % burn)_____ m^2 = _____ cc/hr; _____ cc/ 24 hours

C.   Total maintenance fluids - Basal requirement & evaporative water loss

1.   24 hours = _____ cc

2.   Hour = _____ cc

	Estimate	Actual
Take-off Lunken	_____	_____
Land Ref. City	_____	_____
Arrive Ref/ Inst.	_____	_____
Depart Ref/ Inst.	_____	_____
Take-off Ref City	_____	_____
Land Lunken	_____	_____
Depart In Grd/ Amb	_____	_____
Arrive SBI	_____	_____

Safety Checklist

Litter Secure	_____	_____
Safety Belts on Pt.	_____	_____
Seat belts on crew	_____	_____
Equip. strapped/		
stowed	_____	_____
Cardiac Monitor on	_____	_____
Pulse Oximeter on	_____	_____
Doors/ Latch Locked	_____	_____
No Smoking Materials	_____	_____
Outflow Vent Clear	_____	_____

Shriners Hospitals   Cincinnati Unit
for crippled children   **Transport Record**

Form

FIGURE 3.   Transport team record for documentation of resuscitation calculations, demographic data, and transport times. (Shriners Burns Institute, Cincinnati Unit, with permission.)

Documentation during the transport process should include the initial assessment, evidence of the plan of care, and the treatment instituted (Figs. 3, 4, and 5). Monitoring of vital signs, hemodynamic and respiratory condition, and fluid balance provide ongoing evaluation of the patient's response to treatment. It is important to provide documentation of any alteration in therapy as well as patient response during transport.

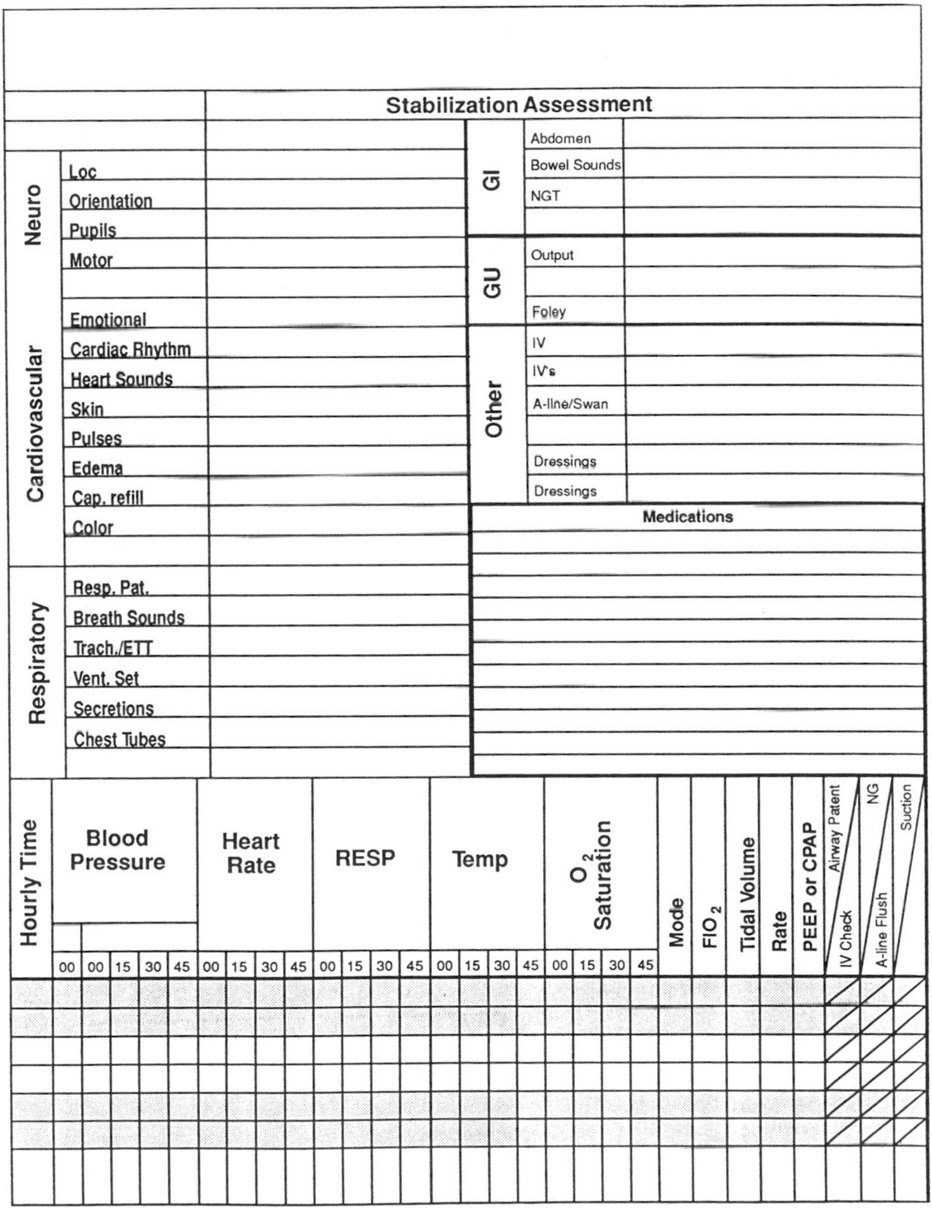

FIGURE 4. Transport team record of assessment, stabilization, and vital signs documentation. (Shriners Burns Institute, Cincinnati Unit, with permission.)

Hourly Time	Intravenous						Total IV	Other	Total I & O		Urine	Emesis	Stool	NG
									Hourly Intake	Hourly Output				
								·						
Total														

SBI Report called prior to leaving Hospital	Safety/ Orientation to parent or significant other

Narrative Notes: (Date/Time)

_____

_____

_____

_____

_____

_____

_____

_____

_____

_____

_____

_____

_____

Report Given to:	
SBI RN Receiving Pt.	
Transport Team Sig.	
Transport Team Sig.	
Transport Team Sig.	

FIGURE 5.   Transport team intake/output records and narrative observational documentation. (Shriners Burns Institute, Cincinnati Unit, with permission.)

Transport Equipment

The selection of equipment for transporting the burned child is determined by the patient's condition and the mode of transport. All medical supplies, monitoring and respiratory equipment, and suction devices should be evaluated for completeness and function prior to transport. There must be capability for providing continuous critical care monitoring including blood pressure, temperature, EKG, pulse oximetry, and capnography. Supplies should include medications necessary for cardiopulmonary resuscitation, pain control, comfort management, and patient safety.

INTRATRANSPORT MANAGEMENT

Regardless of the mode of transport, the referring physician is responsible for ensuring that the patient has been properly prepared for transfer. Prior to departing from the referring hospital, the patient's condition should be thoroughly assessed. Necessary changes in therapy should be made and the patient's condition stabilized.[15] Vital signs should be within normal limits for age or supported appropriately. Any patient demonstrating symptoms or having a high probability of developing airway compromise should be intubated in the controlled hospital environment prior to movement since endotracheal tube placement is extremely difficult once airway edema has developed. The tube should be adequately secured with adhesive tape, umbilical tape, and/or staples in order to avoid accidental extubation during transport (Fig. 6). The patient should also be placed on the transport ventilator and adequate gas exchange documented prior to departure. Intravenous catheters should be checked for adequacy and patency and secured to prevent dislodgment during transport. If the patient has undergone subclavian or internal jugular venous catheterization, a radiograph should be obtained prior to movement to rule out pneumothorax or hemothorax. Urine output should be monitored hourly via an indwelling catheter since the rate of fluid administration may require frequent adjustment during transport.

It is also important that a nasogastric tube be placed prior to transport. Ileus is a common occurrence after burn injury and may be associated with aspiration and acute gastric dilatation. Adequacy of gastric decompression should also be assessed during transport.

Maintenance of core body temperature during transport is mandatory. Gauze dressings should be applied to the wounds and the patient covered with

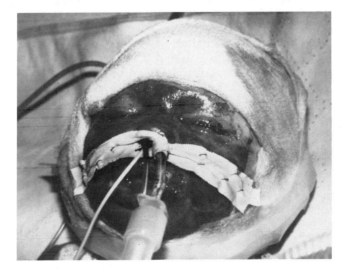

FIGURE 6. A child with facial burns and edema. The endotracheal tube must be secured adequately before movement and transport.

warm blankets, thermal hats, and drapes to minimize heat loss. Squad and cabin temperatures are increased to maintain core body temperature. In-flight warming should continue with the goal of maintaining a temperature of 38.3°C.

MANAGEMENT OF POTENTIAL COMPLICATIONS

The most life-threatening complication that can occur during transport of a burned child is acute airway obstruction. If there is airway compromise during transport, a cricothyroidotomy may be quickly performed with a large-bore intravenous catheter or a percutaneous cricothyroidotomy tube. Attempts to replace a dislodged endotracheal tube often result in a serious delay in reestablishing the airway, even in the hands of experienced professionals.

Patients developing sudden hypoxia during transport should be treated initially by increasing the FiO_2 to 100%. One should first check the status of the O_2 supply and all ventilator tubing. Auscultation of the chest should be performed quickly. If breath sounds are diminished, the diagnosis and treatment of pneumothorax can be ruled out by needle aspiration of the pleural cavity. If a pneumothorax is present, a large-bore plastic angiocath should be placed in the pleural space to prevent a tension pneumothorax. If breath sounds are not diminished, one may consider adding or increasing the positive end-expiratory pressure.

The development of hypercapnia should also be assessed by careful lung auscultation. If pneumothorax is suspected, treatment should be instituted as outlined above. If breath sounds are not diminished, a diagnosis of hypoventilation should be entertained and treated by increasing either the tidal volume or ventilatory rate.

Hypotension developing during the course of transport of the burn patient is most often due to hypovolemia. Initial assessment should include an evaluation of intravenous access and luminal patency. If the catheter has become displaced, intravenous access should be reestablished promptly percutaneously. The femoral and jugular veins are the preferred routes of access if no peripheral sites are available. If intravenous access is intact, the rate of fluid administration should be increased. If sudden severe hypotension develops, it may be necessary to give a bolus of balanced salt solution or colloid. It is rarely necessary to administer vasopressors during resuscitation from burn shock.

Oliguria is most often secondary to hypovolemia. Initial evaluation should include an assessment of proper positioning of the Foley catheter within the bladder. If the catheter can be demonstrated to be functioning properly, it should be left in place and the rate of fluid administration increased. Diuretics should not be administered because they will cause a further reduction in intravascular volume.

REFERENCES

1. American Academy of Pediatrics Committee on Hospital Care: Guidelines for air and ground transportation of pediatric patients. Pediatrics 78:943, 1986.
2. American Burn Association: Guidelines for operation of burn centers. J Burn Care Rehabil 16(1):20A–29A, 1995.
3. American College of Surgeons Committee on Trauma: Resources for optimal care of patients with burn injury. In American College of Surgeons: Resources for Optimal Care of the Injured Patient. Chicago, American College of Surgeons, 1990.
4. Arturson G: Microvascular permeability to macromolecules in thermal injury. Acta Physiol Scand (Suppl) 463:111, 1979.
5. Boykin JV, Eriksson E, Pittman RN: In-vivo microcirculation of a scald burn and the progression of postburn dermal ischemia. Plast Reconstr Surg 66:191, 1980.

6. Cahalane M, Demling RH: Early respiratory abnormalities from smoke inhalation. JAMA 251:771, 1984.

7. Day S, McCloskey KA, Orr R, et al: Pediatric interhospital critical care transport: Consensus of a national leadership conference. Pediatrics 88:696, 1991.

8. Demling RH, LaLonde C: Airway and pulmonary abnormalities. In Demling RH, LaLonde C (eds): Burn Trauma. New York, Thieme, 1989.

9. Hanumadass M, Kagan RJ, Matsuda T: Management of pediatric burns. In Vidyasagar D, Sarnaik AP (eds): Neonatal and Pediatric Intensive Care. Littleton, MA, PSG Publishing, 1985.

10. Herndon DN, Langner F, Thompson P, et al: Pulmonary injury in burned patients. Surg Clin North Am 67:31, 1987.

11. Jackson DM: The diagnosis of the depth of burning. Br J Surg 40:588, 1953.

12. Lund CC, Browder NC: The estimate of area of burns. Surg Gynecol Obstet 79:352, 1944.

13. Madden MR, Finkelstein JL, Goodwin CW: Respiratory care of the burn patient. Clin Plast Surg 13:29, 1986.

14. McCloskey KA, Johnston C: Pediatric critical care transport survey: Team composition and training, mobilization time, and mode of transportation. Pediatr Emerg Care 6(11):1, 1990.

15. Merk T, Jenkins M, Scheidt L, et al: Air transport of pediatric burn patients. Proc Am Burn Assoc 23:207, 1991.

16. Merrell SW, Saffle JR, Sullivan JJ, et al: Fluid resuscitation in thermally injured children. Am J Surg 152:664, 1986.

17. Moncrief JA: Burns. I: Assessment. JAMA 242:72, 1979.

18. Moylan JA: First aid and transportation of burned patients. In Artz CP, Moncrief JA, Pruitt BA Jr (eds): Burns: A Team Approach. Philadelphia, W.B. Saunders, 1979.

19. Moylan JA, Adib K, Birnbaum M: Fiberoptic bronchoscopy following thermal injury. Surg Gynecol Obstet 140:541, 1975.

20. Moylan JA, Alexander G Jr: Diagnosis and treatment of inhalation injury. World J Surg 2:185, 1978.

21. Moylan JA, Chan CK: Inhalation injury—an increasing problem. Surgery 188:34, 1978.

22. Moylan JA, Wilmore DW, Mouton DE, et al: Early diagnosis of inhalation injury using 133-xenon lung scan. Ann Surg 176:477, 1972.

23. Munster AM: The early management of thermal burns. Surgery 87:29, 1980.

24. Navar PD, Saffle JR Warden GD: Effect of inhalation injury on fluid resuscitation requirements after thermal injury. Am J Surg 150:716, 1985.

25. Robinson NB, Hudson LD, Robertson HT, et al: Ventilation and perfusion alterations after smoke inhalation injury. Surgery 90:352, 1981.

26. Saffle JR, Zeluff GR, Warden GD: Intramuscular pressure in the burned arm: Measurement and response to escharotomy. Am J Surg 140:825, 1980.

27. Salisbury RE, McKeel DW, Mason AD Jr: Ischemic necrosis of the intrinsic muscles of the hand after thermal injuries. J Bone Joint Surg 56:1701, 1974.

28. Warden GD: Burn shock resuscitation. World J Surg 16:16, 1992.

29. Welch GW, Lull RJ, Petroff PA, et al: The use of steroids in inhalation injury. Surg Gynecol Obstet 145:539, 1977.

CHAPTER 29

Infectious Disease

ROBERT M. LEVIN, M.D.

Children may require transport for many reasons. Some are moved from one hospital to the next simply because they need a CT scan. Such referral patterns are bound to change as outlying hospitals acquire newer technology. At the other end of the spectrum are children who will always need referral from such places as rural hospitals or institutions with limited pediatric services because of illness so severe they cannot be handled on site.

Thompson and co-workers[1] looked at Emergency Department records of all pediatric cardiopulmonary arrests at seven rural hospitals from 1980 to 1986. Of 95 cardiopulmonary arrests, 11 (12%) were due to infectious diseases (8 pneumonias, 1 tracheitis, 1 meningitis, 1 sepsis).

Remarkably consistent proportions of newborns sent from outlying hospitals to centers for intensive care are transported for reasons of an infectious disease.[2-4] While most of these transports (7.5–11.0%) were diagnosed as neonatal sepsis, some were for meningitis and pneumonia and rare admissions were for *Toxoplasma, Rubella, Cytomegalovirus, Herpes* (TORCH) syndrome. Very low birth weight infants ($\leq$ 750 gm) admitted to the neonatal unit of Kyushu University Hospital in Fukuoka, Japan, were evaluated for characteristics on admission. Of the 20 infants $\leq$ 750 grams admitted from January to December 1987, two (10%) were septic.[5]

A report on air transport of pediatric emergency cases[6] analyzed the data on 752 transported over a 32-month period to Primary Children's Medical Center in Salt Lake City, Utah. Patients' ages ranged from three weeks to 16 years. One-third of patients were $\leq$ one year, one-half between one and six years, and the remainder over six years of age. Interpretation of the results is clouded by an illogical lumping of infectious disease information with other categories. One classification of diagnosis is called respiratory infection (141 patients); another is called metabolic/infection (53 patients). It can be concluded then that no more than 194 of 752 (25.8%) of these pediatric patients were transported for an infectious disease-related problem.

THE INITIAL CALL FOR HELP/WHAT TO DO BEFORE LEAVING

Evaluation/Diagnosis

One of the most commonly misrepresented features of the history is fever. Much of what is called fever—often by the parents, and sometimes by doctors and nurses—isn't fever. Fever can arbitrarily be said to begin at 100.5° F rectally. Also, the length of time that a patient has had a fever is commonly exaggerated or blurred. Most patients said to be febrile for a prolonged period usually have had a couple of febrile episodes separated by a distinguishable afebrile period. This can only be brought out by careful questioning. The distinction is important in separating a fever of unknown origin from other distinct illnesses.

One element of the physical exam that can be misleading is descriptions of rashes reported over the phone. Determining whether a lesion is petechial or not by asking "Do the lesions blanch when you press them?" may not be fool-proof.

Before accepting a diagnosis over the phone that is based on a laboratory test, you must explore the specifics of that test. A patient does not have acute mononucleosis just because the Epstein-Barr virus (EBV) IgG is positive. A diagnosis of mononucleosis depends on the EBV IgM being positive. A positive latex agglutination test (what used to be CIE in many hospitals) for group B Streptococcus does not mean that a newborn has group B streptococcal sepsis. A baby that is colonized, a frequent and usually benign event, will have a positive latex agglutination test in blood and urine for group B Streptococcus. All too frequently, clinicians rule out the possibility of strep throat because the rapid strep test is negative. Many such patients still have positive throat cultures (the more sensitive test) for group A beta-hemolytic Streptococcus.

Advice/Recommendations

If it is apparent to you that a certain therapeutic intervention is important, make your expectations very clear. If you think that the patient may be septic and antibiotics have not been started yet, make certain that they are started. Talk to the doctor and tell him or her what antibiotics you think are necessary, at what dose, and then ask how long it will be before they will be infused into the patient.

Be judicious in your requests for further evaluations. Only ask for tests that are absolutely necessary or that may lose validity after the passage of time. Make sure that good-quality cultures of the blood and urine are obtained (and of the CSF and stool when indicated) before antibiotics are started. Always be certain that the urine culture is a catheterized or suprapubic specimen.

In anticipation of the transport team's arrival, ask that the parents be available to discuss their child's state after the initial assessment. Aside from reassuring them, it is a good opportunity to clarify or expand on some of the historical issues that have come to mind now that you are better acquainted with their child.

Diagnosis-Specific Precautions

Experience would indicate that the risk of acquiring an infection from transported patients by ambulance personnel is extremely low.[7] However, the actual risk in any given transport is directly related to the infection from which the patient is suffering and the immunity to that specific agent in each member of the transport team. In 1980, The London Ambulance Service requested that the British Society for the Study of Infection develop guidelines to protect ambulance personnel from contracting transmissible diseases.[7] The Society noted that while transported patients do not necessarily carry a precise diagnosis, those with fever, rash, or diarrhea are more likely to have an infectious disease. Patients with these symptoms are of special concern if they have recently arrived from a foreign country.

Taking into consideration the Society's recommendations, criticisms of those recommendations,[8] and the more recent universal precautions,[9] two

TABLE 1.   Examples of Problems that Require Routine Precautions Only

Fever of unknown origin	Encephalitis	Influenza	Rubella
Anthrax	Food poisoning	Measles	Scabies
Chickenpox	Gastroenteritis	Meningitis	Scarlet fever
Cholera	Impetigo	Mumps	Tuberculosis
Diphtheria	Hepatitis A, B, C, delta, and E	Pertussis	Typhoid fever
Dysentery	Herpes zoster	Poliomyelitis	Typhus

categories of infectious diseases can be delineated, each with its own guidelines for transport personnel safety.

Routine Precautions

At a minimum, these should be in effect for transport personnel involved in the conveyance of patients with all infection-related problems (Table 1). These rules should apply to all members of the health care team who accompany the patient on the ambulance. Any member of the transport team who comes in contact with the following body fluids or procedures should wear disposable gloves, a nonporous disposable gown, a disposable surgical mask, and, if spattering is likely, barrier eye protection:

Blood	Vascular catheter placement
Blood-contaminated fluids	Tracheostomy or endotracheal suctioning
Intubation	Handling of used instruments
Wound discharge	Lumbar puncture
Phlebotomy	Puncture of other cavities
Arterial Puncture	(e.g., pleural or peritoneal)

Transport personnel should wear gloves only when they are involved in direct patient contact with blood-contaminated fluids and the above procedures. As soon as the task is completed, the gloves should be removed and hands should be washed. Failure to remove gloves immediately following their appropriate use facilitates the transmission of infection. The wearing of gloves should not be seen as a substitute for hand-washing.[10]

Body fluids and procedures for which only hand washing is recommended (when no blood is present):

Urine	Nasal secretions
Stool	Oral secretions
Vomitus	Diaper change
Tears	

Hand-washing is the single best method of protecting the patient from a nosocomial infection and of protecting transport personnel from acquiring the patient's infectious disease.

Maximum Precautions

These should be in effect for transport personnel when patients are known or suspected to have certain virulent and particularly transmissible infections. Full protective clothing should be worn that will be incinerated or autoclaved after use. The outfit should include ventilated head gear such as a hepa-filtered, battery-powered, air-purified hood, latex gloves, and fluid-impervious boots. A list of the names, addresses and phone numbers of any person who has contact with the patient from the moment the transport team arrives should be maintained by the transport nurse or designee. Following the transport, the ambulance should be subjected to the most rigorous cleaning regimen available to the transport company.[11] These precautions should be taken for patients suspected of having the following infections:

Lassa fever Plague
Marburg virus disease Smallpox (research laboratory employees)
Ebola hemorrhagic fever Crimean-Congo hemorrhagic fever
Rabies

Luckily, these infections are quite rare in the United States. However, air travel places any of them within the realm of the possible. When in doubt, the transport team should use the most aggressive sanitary precautions available to them.

Pre-exposure Prophylaxis

All members of transport teams should be fully immunized against measles, rubella, polio, diphtheria, tetanus and hepatitis A and B. After the hepatitis B series has been completed, bloodwork should be performed to confirm development of an antibody response. Yearly immunization against influenza is also a necessity. Neither meningococcal nor pneumococcal vaccines are routinely indicated for transport personnel. Should meningococcal disease become epidemic in a given area, then strong consideration should be given to that vaccine. Given the low rate of tuberculosis transmission by pediatric patients, vaccination with BCG is not necessary for protection from children, even in areas of high prevalence.

Prior to employment, members of the transport team should have their antibody status determined for varicella, rubella, measles (rubeola), and hepatitis B. Each member should have a PPD placed, which, if < 10 mm of induration, should be repeated two weeks later. The repeat "boosted" response is the more reliable of the two and is the one that should be recorded as the true test result. The PPD should be retested yearly.

THE TRIP TO THE REFERRING HOSPITAL

Most transport vehicles have an adequate light source available for reading. If the diagnosis of the patient is clear, read about that disease entity. Take time to consider what kinds of scenarios may occur with the patient you'll be transporting. If all the information the team has received is some symptoms and signs, work through a differential diagnosis. Are there some ways to distinguish between meningococcemia and Rocky Mountain spotted fever when evaluating the patient? What antibiotics would be administered for each condition? If, after the patient is examined, a diagnostic decision cannot be made, is there one antibiotic that will treat both conditions? Is there a specimen to collect before starting therapy? Is there something about the contagiousness of the diseases in question that would lead the team to approach the patient with certain caution? It should be mentioned to the health care providers at the referring hospital that they might need prophylaxis if the patient proves to have (or does have) a certain infection.

ARRIVAL AT THE REFERRING HOSPITAL

History

The neonatal history would not be complete without a thorough understanding of the mother's pregnancy, delivery, and postpartum period. Particular attention should be paid to issues that might be related to maternal infection. Look for a history of fever, duration of ruptured membranes, and the amount and character of the amniotic fluid (clear, cloudy, foul-smelling, or purulent). Is there a past or current history of vaginal herpetic lesions? Was the mother ill during her pregnancy? Was screening for carriage of the group B Streptococcus performed? Did she have a positive VDRL, and, if so, was it treated adequately? Determine whether the mother received any antibiotics either during her labor or in the days immediately before delivery.[12]

Aside from the maternal aspects, there is little difference between gathering the history about a sick newborn and that of an older child. There is a tendency in collecting historical data about a hospitalized newborn or child to rely on data already present in the chart. Did the referring physician think to ask the mother what she meant by "fever"? Were the parents asked whether the child had been handling a hamster recently (lymphocytic choriomeningitis virus), been around a new litter of kittens (Q fever), or recently traveled to the American southwest where the child might have been exposed to a dead squirrel (plague)?

Physical Examination of Laboratory Results

A complete physical examination should be performed by the transport team. Aspects of the physical exam that prove particularly influential in shaping a diagnosis or determining a patient's status include an evaluation of the patient's irritability and mental status, a search for subtle seizures, an honest view of the tympanic membranes, a careful look at the throat (even in the youngest child), a search of the neck, axillae, and inguinal region for enlarged lymph nodes, auscultation of the lungs, palpation of the abdomen for enlargement of the liver and spleen, and a careful investigation of the skin.

Methodically review all laboratory data for pertinent clues to an infectious process present or developing.

Impression

In formulating a clinical impression, give particular thought to infectious diseases that are circulating in the community at the time. What illnesses have been seen back at your own hospital? Is it Respiratory Syncytial Virus (RSV) season? Has influenza appeared? Don't overlook the uncommon presentation of a common disease.

Plan

After the initial evaluation the clinician may feel that additional cultures are necessary. Most laboratories distinguish between herpes cultures (which grow only herpes simplex) and viral cultures (which grow out many viruses, including herpes, in the same way that a routine bacterial culture will grow many different bacteria). Most viral cultures can wait until the patient is transported back to the tertiary institution. As a general rule, the less time that specimens for viral culture spend in transport the more likely they are to grow. A possible exception to this would be herpes cultures when antiviral therapy is started before leaving the referring hospital. In that case, it would be prudent to collect a set of herpes cultures before leaving the referring hospital, begin acyclovir therapy, and get another set of herpes cultures immediately after having stabilized the patient in the PICU. If herpes is not suspected, then obtain general viral cultures of the throat, stool, and CSF (if the CNS is clinically suspect).

The decision to get bacterial cultures before the patient is transported will depend on several factors. If a different antibiotic will be started before leaving the referring hospital, it will be important to repeat key cultures. If the patient was started on antibiotics just prior to the team's arrival and critical cultures were left out, by all means collect them before leaving.

Viral cultures collected at the referring hospital should be sent through that hospital's microbiology system. In general, viral cultures are so fragile that to transport them could easily destroy the virus inside the transport tube. On the other hand, most bacterial cultures withstand the trip back to the referral center without any significant loss in viability.

Therapy—and whether to begin before leaving or to wait until the patient is transported to the PICU—will be based on the clinician's best judgment. If the organism has not yet been identified, the appropriate empiric therapy for the patient's clinical syndrome should be administered. One of the most common pitfalls into which a clinician stumbles is to narrow the antibiotic therapy from the usual broad-spectrum agents based on a Gram stain. Gram stains should never cause the clinician to focus empiric therapy—only to broaden the coverage.

DISEASE ENTITIES

The disease entities discussed here were selected from all infectious diseases as being most likely to result in transport to a tertiary care center. Not all of them are likely to be encountered during a career in pediatric transport medicine (Table 2). A minority will account for most of the infectious disease-related transports performed. The limited information given below is selected because of its potential utility to members of a transport team. More detailed information about each of these disease entities is readily available in standard pediatric infectious disease textbooks.[13-16] The first section deals with the major neonatal infections. This is followed by infectious diseases affecting all children.

NEONATAL (< 1 month)

Pneumonia

Clinical Manifestations

The infant with pneumonia usually will present with nonspecific signs, such as decreased appetite, irritability or lethargy, and cyanosis or a pale color. More obvious indications of respiratory disease are tachypnea, grunting, flaring of the nasal alae, retractions, dyspnea, cough, and temperature instability. On physical examination the patient often will have decreased air movement over part or all of the lung fields. Rales and/or wheezing may or may not be present.

Etiology

Pneumonia usually arises in the early neonatal period from aspiration of contaminated amniotic fluid or from exposure to organisms in the birth canal. Resultant pneumonias are due to group B Streptococci, *E. coli,* and *Listeria monocytogenes.* Pneumonia acquired transplacentally may be due to one of the TORCH organisms. Infants who have been on a ventilator for other reasons, such as the respiratory distress syndrome, can get pneumonia from contaminated equipment. *Staphylococcus aureus* and gram-negative enteric rods such as *Pseudomonas aeruginosa* are usually implicated in these often very resistant infections. Since neonates are handled by nurses, doctors, respiratory therapists, and parents who live in the outside world, they can get whatever viral infections are affecting the general population. Thus, neonates get infections with common viral organisms such as respiratory syncytial virus, influenza A and B, parainfluenza, and adenovirus.

TABLE 2.   Infectious Disease Entities in Pediatric and Neonatal
Transport Medicine

Neonatal	Pneumonia (including group B streptococcal and others) Meningitis Encephalitis and aseptic meningitis Sepsis Necrotizing enterocolitis Omphalitis (see under Skin)
Central Nervous System	Meningitis, septic versus aseptic Encephalitis Guillain-Barré syndrome Infant botulism Tetanus Febrile seizures

Respiratory	Upper respiratory tract infections
	   Epiglottitis
	   Croup (laryngotracheobronchitis)
	   Acute bacterial tracheitis
	   Retropharyngeal abscess
	   Peritonsillar abscess
	Lower respiratory tract infections
	   Pneumonia (including bacterial, viral, mycobacterial, fungal, and others)
	   Pleural effusions
	   Aspiration pneumonia
	   Adult respiratory distress syndrome (ARDS)
	   Chest syndrome in sickle cell disease
	   AIDS—associated pneumonias, including pneumocystis, pneumonia,
	     and lymphoid interstitial pneumonitis (LIP)
	   Bronchiolitis
	   Pertussis syndrome

Gastrointestinal	Necrotizing enterocolitis (see under Neonatal) Peritonitis
Cardiac	Pericarditis (myocarditis), pericardial effusion, and cardiac tamponade

Systemic	Sepsis (versus bacteremia) with and without shock
	Meningococcemia
	Toxic shock syndrome
	   Staphylococcal
	   Streptococcal
	Rocky Mountain spotted fever
	Leptospirosis
	Acquired immunodeficiency syndrome (AIDS) presenting with sepsis and septic shock
	Hemolytic-uremic syndrome
	Malaria
	Plague
	Ebola hemorrhagic fever
	Marburg disease
	Lassa fever

Skin	Meningococcemia (see under Systemic) Rocky Mountain spotted fever (see under Systemic) Omphalitis and Fournier's gangrene Smallpox (research laboratory employees)
Ocular	Periorbital cellulitis Orbital cellulitis

Epidemiology

Pneumonias acquired prepartum and intrapartum usually manifest within the first seven days of life. Infections acquired postnatally usually present after the first week of life. These infections can occur in seriously ill prematures or in healthy babies who have already gone home. The nosocomial bacterial infections that occur in heavily instrumented, hospitalized neonates also tend to occur after the first week of life.

Diagnostic Tests

The chest radiograph can serve both to document pneumonia and to indicate the etiologic agent. In group B streptococcal disease, the chest radiograph is distinguished with difficulty from that of respiratory distress syndrome. Listeria monocytogenes infection will tend to appear as a pneumonitis with a miliary pattern. Lobar consolidation with pneumatoceles is indicative of infection with *Staphylococcus aureus*.

White blood cell counts are not particularly reliable in distinguishing bacterial from viral pneumonias. The exception to this may be the premature infant with group B streptococcal pneumonia who will usually be leukopenic with an increased proportion of bands. A positive blood culture should reflect the true etiology of the pneumonia, though blood cultures usually are negative in bacterial pneumonias.[13] Some reliance may be placed on the endotracheal aspirate if the specimens for culture and Gram stain are collected within four hours of intubation. The Gram stain is useful in interpreting the results of the culture. A positive endotracheal aspirate culture for Klebsiella pneumonia has less significance when the Gram stain shows polymorphonuclear leukocytes and gram-positive cocci in pairs and chains.

Urine antigen detection tests cannot be relied upon for definitive diagnosis. Owing to lack of both sensitivity and specificity, these tests are at best only indicators of disease. The most useful of the urine antigen detection tests in the neonatal period is that for group B Streptococcus.

Viral respiratory cultures can wait until the patient has been transported back to the referral center.

Management

Pneumonia occurring in the first month of life should be treated with ampicillin and gentamicin. Modification of this regimen should be based on the patient's clinical course, the instrumentation the patient has been exposed to, previous antibiotic therapy, and laboratory studies such as Gram stain and culture of recent endotracheal aspirates. If the patient is intubated, on ampicillin and gentamicin when clinical deterioration occurs, vancomycin paired with a third generation cephalosporin would be a good choice. Base the choice of cephalosporin on what is growing out of the endotracheal tube culture.

Before transporting the patient, supplemental O_2 or intubation and assisted ventilation may be required. Rarely, a thoracentesis will be needed to stabilize the patient before moving into the transport vehicle.

Isolation

No specific precautions are necessary.

Meningitis, Bacterial Versus Aseptic

Clinical Manifestations

The neonate with meningitis, whether bacterial or aseptic, shares many symptoms with the newborn who has sepsis (see section on Sepsis). Signs common in older children with bacterial meningitis may be unusual in neonates. Mustafa and co-workers[17] point out that a bulging fontanelle is seen in only 17% of newborns with meningitis, opisthotonos in 33 percent, stiff neck in 23%, and convulsions in only 12%.

Etiology

The most common agent of bacterial meningitis among neonates is the group B Streptococcus (*Streptococcus agalactiae*). The next most common organism seen in purulent neonatal meningitis is *Escherichia coli*, followed by *Listeria monocytogenes*. Additional cases are attributable to the group D Streptococcus, the Klebsiella-Enterobacter group of organisms, *Citrobacter diversus*, and, rarely, *Haemophilus influenzae*, *Staphylococcus aureus*, and *Streptococcus pneumoniae*.

Aseptic meningitis is the generic name given to meningeal inflammations that are not the result of infection by pyogenic bacteria.[13] Strictly speaking, then, such nonviral agents as *Myobacterium tuberculosis*, leptospirosis, the borrelia of Lyme disease, the spirochete of syphilis, fungi, and mycoplasma, as well as viruses, are causes of aseptic meningitis. The enteroviruses are the most common cause of aseptic meningitis in neonates.[18] Viruses are more common causes of meningitis in the newborn period than are bacteria.[16] Another increasingly common agent of aseptic meningitis in the first two months of life is congenital neurosyphilis.

Epidemiology

The incidence of bacterial meningitis varies between two and ten cases per 10,000 live births in North America. In one recent study of neonatal meningitis, Shattuck and co-workers showed that over a 15-year period, from 1974 to 1988, the incidence of bacterial meningitis decreased, aseptic meningitis remained the same, and enteroviral meningitis, specifically, increased.

Diagnostic Tests

Viral cultures from various sites of the patient's body usually can wait until return to the referrral center. Any cerebrospinal fluid (CSF) still in the laboratory should be collected, put into a leak-proof sterile container, and brought back with the patient on the transport vehicle.

The spinal fluid in neonatal viral meningitis demonstrates significant variability in both cell count and chemistries. The CSF protein is commonly above 100 mg/dl. It should be kept in mind, though, that the upper limit of normal CSF protein in neonates on the first day of life is 175 mg/dl. In one study of seven newborns with coxsackie B5 meningitis, the mean CSF protein value was 244 mg/dl and the mean CSF white blood cell count was 1069 cells/mm³, with 67% of the cells being polymorphonuclear leukocytes.[19] Normally, no more than 29 white blood cells/mm³ are seen in the CSF of healthy newborns. Cell counts and chemistry patterns of viral meningitis may present with values similar to bacterial invasion of the spinal fluid, especially in neonates with enteroviral meningitis.

The high normal values in the CSF of newborns can lead to confusion in the diagnosis of bacterial meningitis. Sarff and co-workers[20] reported 30% of newborns with group B streptococcal meningitis presented with "normal" CSF white blood cell counts. Taking all CSF parameters into account, the chances of a culture-documented bacterial meningitis with all CSF values being normal is less than 1%.

The concentration of organisms in the CSF is dependent, in part, on how long the host has been infected. In order for a Gram stain to be positive under high-power oil immersion field, there must be ≥ 100,000 organisms/ml. It should not be surprising, then, that the Gram stain is positive only 80% of the time in culture-documented bacterial meningitis in neonates. For example, owing to the low concentration of bacteria in the CSF of a patient with Listeria meningitis, the Gram stain usually is negative.

Antigen detection tests performed on spinal fluid are of two main types: countercurrent immunoelectrophoresis (CIE) and latex agglutination. While the term CIE is still common, most hospitals where the term is used have long since changed over to the labor-saving latex agglutination test. Both tests detect group B Streptococcus, *E. coli, S. pneumoniæ, N. meningitidis,* and *H. influenzæ.*

Blood cultures are positive 50% of the time in neonates with bacterial meningitis.[18] If there is a pathogen growing from either the spinal fluid or blood, a sample of the specimen should be brought back to the referral center. Cord blood, if available, should be collected and transported with the neonate.

Management

Newborns suspected of having meningitis should be started on intravenous ampicillin and gentamicin. Specific dosing depends on the age and weight of the neonate (Table 3). (For the management of such problems as fluid administration, increased intracranial pressure, and disseminated intravascular coagulation see below under Infants and Children (> 1 month), meningitis, bacterial versus aseptic.) And, of course, transport personnel who have patient contact should practice universal precautions.

Encephalitis

Clinical Manifestations

Initial clinical findings in neonates with encephalitis include fever, anorexia and lethargy, which are indistinguishable from those seen in any nonspecific febrile illness. Jaundice and vomiting may be present. Affected newborns may become jittery, develop apnea, have increased tone, develop seizures (focal and/or generalized), and may present with a bulging fontanelle. Among patients with herpes encephalitis, only about half have skin vesicles.[14] Involvement of the brain in herpes infection can occur alone or can be a part of disseminated disease with hepatic and adrenal systems primarily involved. Other organs that may be affected include the lungs, larynx, trachea, stomach, esophagus, bowel, spleen, kidneys, pancreas and heart.

Suspect herpes infection of the CNS in any infant who has evidence of acute neurologic deterioration with the onset of seizures. Since seizures can be very subtle in the newborn, the clinician must maintain a very high index of suspicion. Most infants with neonatal herpes present between six days and three weeks of age, with some infants beginning their illness at birth and others as late as six weeks. The reason for the focus on herpes is that it is the only encephalitis virus with specific and effective antiviral therapy available.

Etiology

The etiologic agents of the TORCH syndrome can cause an encephalitis in newborn infants. Unusually, encephalitis may be seen with Chagas' disease, measles, and, in a quite malignant form, listeriosis. While the enteroviruses (echovirus and coxsackievirus) frequently are mentioned as causes of viral meningitis in the neonatal period, little reference is made to them as significant causes of encephalitis in newborns. The premier agent of encephalitis in the neonatal period, then, is herpesvirus. The more significant of the herpesviruses in this role is herpesvirus type 2.

Epidemiology

Most neonatal herpes infections are derived from contact with the maternal genital tract during delivery. Additional cases arise as a result of spread from

TABLE 3. Table of Antibiotic Dosages for Neonates

Antibiotics	Routes	Dosages (mg/kg) and Intervals of Administration				
		Weight < 1200 gm	Weight 1200–2000 gm		Weight > 2000 gm	
		Age 0–4 wk	Age 0–7 days	Age > 7 days	Age 0–7 days	Age > 7 days
Amikacin	IV,IM	7.5 q18–24 h	7.5 q12–18h	7.5 q8–12h	10 q12h	10 q8h
Ampicillin	IV,IM					
Meningitis		50 q12h	50 q12h	50 q8h	50 q8h	50 q6h
Other diseases		25 q12h	25 q12h	25 q8h	25 q8h	25 q6h
Aztreonam	IV,IM	30 q12h	30 q12h	30 q8h	30 q8h	30 q6h
Cefazolin	IV,IM	20 q12h	20 q12h	20 q12h	20 q12h	20 q8h
Cefotaxime	IV,IM	50 q12h	50 q12h	50 q8h	50 q12h	50 q8h
Ceftazidime	IV,IM	50 q12h	50 q12h	50 q8h	50 q12h	50 q8h
Ceftriaxone	IV,IM	50 q24h	50 q24h	50 q24h	50 q24h	75 q24h
Cephalothin	IV	20 q12h	20 q12h	20 q8h	20 q8h	20 q6h
Chloramphenicol	IV,PO	25 q24h	25 q24h	25 q24h	25 q24h	25 q12h
Clindamycin	IV,IM,PO	5 q12h	5 q12h	5 q8h	5 q8h	5 q6h
Erythromycin	PO	10 q12h	10 q12h	10 q8h	10 q12h	10 q8h
Gentamicin	IV,IM	2.5 q18–24h	2.5 q12–18h	2.5 q8–12h	2.5 q12h	2.5 q8h
Imipenem	IV,IM	20 q18–24h	20 q12h	20 q12h	20 q12h	20 q8h
Kanamycin	IV,IM	7.5 q18–24h	7.5 q12–18h	7.5 q8–12h	10 q12h	10 q8h
Methacillin	IV,IM					
Meningitis		50 q12h	50 q12h	50 q8h	50 q8h	50 q6h
Other diseases		25 q12h	25 q12h	25 q8h	25 q8h	25 q6h
Metronidazole	IV,PO	7.5 q48h	7.5 q24h	7.5 q12h	7.5 q12h	15 q12h
Mezlocillin	IV,IM	75 q12h	75 q12h	75 q8h	75 q12h	75 q8h
Oxacillin	IV,IM	25 q12h	25 q12h	25 q8h	25 q8h	25 q6h
Nafcillin	IV	25 q12h	25 q12h	25 q8h	25 q8h	25q6h
Netilmicin	IV,IM	2.5 q18–24h	2.5 q12–18h	2.5 q8–12h	2.5 q12h	2.5 q8h
Penicillin G	IV					
Meningitis		50,000 U q12h	50,000 U q12h	75,000 U q8h	50,000 U q8h	50,000 U q6h
Other diseases		25,000 U q12h	25,000 U q12h	25,000 U q8h	25,000 U q8h	25,000 U q6h
Penicillin G	IM					
Benzathine			50,000 U (one dose)	50,000 U (one dose)	50,000 U (one dose)	50,000 U (one dose)
Procaine			50,000 U q24h	50,000 U q24h	50,000 U q24h	50,000 U q24h
Ticarcillin	IV,IM	75 q12h	75 q12h	75 q8h	75 q8h	75 q6h
Tobramycin	IV,IM	2.5 q18–24h	2.5 q12–18h	2.5 q8–12h	2.5 q12h	2.5 q8h
Vancomycin	IV	15 q24h	15 q12–18h	15 q8–12h	15 q12h	15 q8h

Recommendations for infants weighing < 1200 gm based on Prober et al., Pediatr Infect Dis J 9:111, 1990. From Nelson JD: Pocketbook of Pediatric Antimicrobial Therapy 1993–1994, 10th ed. Baltimore, Williams & Wilkins, with permission.

health care workers and family members. Asymptomatic infection with herpes virus is rare; it is almost always symptomatic and frequently lethal.[16] Precautions have been taken to avoid exposing newborns to active maternal genital lesions. The majority of neonatal herpes infections are from exposure to mothers with recurrent, often asymptomatic infection, rather than to women with primary and symptomatic disease. Based on antibody documentation, only one out of every eight women with herpesvirus infection recalls having a prior episode of genital herpes.[21]

Diagnostic Tests

The CSF examination in newborns with encephalitis is identical to that described above under aseptic meningitis. Cultures of the CSF grow herpesvirus 25–40% of the time. Rarely, the CSF will have absolutely normal parameters. If skin lesions are present, these may be cultured for herpesvirus. The vesicular fluid is the most productive sample to send for a culture of the lesion, while a scraping of the base of the vesicle should be sent for a direct fluorescent antibody stain; Tzanck smears are not reliable studies on which to build a diagnosis. Other sites that may be cultured include the conjuctivae, the nasopharynx, the throat, stool, and urine. If herpes is being considered, treatment will most likely be started. These cultures, therefore, should be collected before the infant is transported. Serologic studies are not helpful in making a diagnosis of neonatal herpes.

Management

When herpesvirus is a possible cause of neonatal encephalitis, acyclovir should be started at a dose of 30 mg/kg/day divided into three daily doses IV, each to run in over one hour. (For the management of such problems as fluid administration, increased intracranial pressure, and disseminated intravascular coagulation see below under Infants and Children (>1 month), meningitis, bacterial versus aseptic.) As in all cases of handling potentially infected patients, universal precautions apply.

Sepsis

Clinical Manifestations

Affected newborns manifest symptoms ranging from subtle to dramatic. Perhaps the most sensitive sign of newborn sepsis is a clinician's impression that an infant "just doesn't look right." Other findings may include irritability, poor feeding, abdominal distention, vomiting, temperature instability (hyperthermia or hypothermia), tachycardia,[22] jaundice, and lethargy. While not limited to sepsis, poor peripheral perfusion, respiratory distress, apnea, and bruising also may be seen. Onset may be from the moment of birth to weeks later. Group B Streptococcus and Listeria are well known for having both an early and a late onset presentation. The early onset infection manifests itself within the first few days of life and usually is characterized by septic shock and sometimes persistent fetal circulation.[13] The late-onset disease occurs between four and 21 days and usually presents as meningitis.[13]

Etiology

The agents of neonatal sepsis, groups B and D streptococcus, *E. coli*, *Listeria monocytogenes,* and *Staphylococcus aureus,* usually are acquired by passage through a birth canal colonized with one of these organisms.[16] The group B Streptococcus accounts for 50% of all bacterial meningitis and 40% of all blood culture isolates in neonates.[23] An increasing proportion of newborn sepsis cases due to coagulase negative staphylococci are derived from neonates who acquire their infection from a contaminated in-dwelling vascular catheter.

Epidemiology

Sepsis occurs in neonates (bacterial meningitis or bacteremia within the first 30 days of life) in 0.1-1% of all live births in the United States.[23] Risk factors include prematurity, rupture of membranes for longer than 24 hours, maternal fever, urinary tract infection, chorioamnionitis, and intrapartum asphyxia. Severe viral disease (most often due to a herpesvirus, an enterovirus, coxsackievirus, or echovirus) may be indistinguishable from bacterial infection.

Diagnostic Tests

Cultures of blood, CSF, and urine are of greatest significance in identifying a pathogen. The lumbar puncture (LP) may be postponed if the baby is in severe respiratory distress or hemodynamically unstable. Positioning the infant for this procedure could further compromise a precarious respiratory status and lead to cardiopulmonary embarrassment. A bagged urine culture is inappropriate. Collection of urine in this manner often leads to a delay in starting antibiotics and gross contamination of the specimen. If antibiotics are going to be started, an invasive (suprapubic tap or catheterized) urine specimen must be collected. Of lesser significance is a culture of sputum collected through an endotracheal tube immediately after the tube has been placed. While having some validity, this specimen is prone to contamination by colonizing organisms in the throat. Cultures from such sites as the axillae, groin, umbilicus, ear canal, nasopharynx, rectum, and stomach should not be performed.[24] A chest radiograph may show a pattern of lobar infiltrates or, in the case of group B streptococcal pneumonia, an appearance indistinguishable from that of respiratory distress syndrome. An antigen detection test (usually latex agglutination) of the CSF, positive for a known pathogen, is significant. Latex agglutination tests are positive in the presence of an organism's antigen. Since antigen from an organism may be present in the blood and urine of a patient who is only colonized with an organism, a positive latex agglutination test from one of these sites is not evidence of invasiveness. Septic newborns often have absolute neutrophil counts of ≤ 1800 or ≥ 6000 cells/mm^3 and absolute band counts of ≥ 1100 cells/mm^3 at birth. Septic newborns may have thrombocytopenia and evidence of disseminated intravascular coagulation (DIC).

Management

A newborn should have a septic work-up done (blood and urine cultures, LP, complete blood count, and chest radiograph) and should receive treatment for sepsis if the neonate fits the above-mentioned criteria, or if a health care team member, after careful examination, feels that the patient "looks septic." While this may seem like a "soft" indication to many health care workers new to neonatology, its merit has been borne out rather consistently.[26] Other indications for starting antibiotics after the septic work-up has been performed include:

1. Any of the previously mentioned clinical manifestations, especially in the presence of any abnormal diagnostic tests. Antibiotics may be withheld if there is another indisputable explanation for the symptom.

2. If the infant is pre-term and any of the previously mentioned clinical manifestations, diagnostic test abnormalities or epidemiologic risk factors are present.

When treatment is begun for one of these reasons, it may be stopped after three days if the septic work-up proves to be negative (no pathogens isolated) and the patient did not appear septic at the outset. This knowledge should reassure the medical team on transport that the decision to start antibiotics does not necessarily commit the newborn to a prolonged course of therapy. Newborns with sepsis should receive ampicillin and gentamicin at doses appropriate for their weight and age (Table 3).[27]

Intravenous immune globulin (IVIG) has been studied in the management of sepsis of the newborn. Several studies support the administration of IVIG to the septic-appearing newborn weighing less than 2000 grams. A single dose of 750 mg/kg probably is useful, especially if the neonate has shock and neutropenia.[28]

At least as important as the antibiotics in managing a case of neonatal sepsis is the admininstration of fluids, vasoactive agents, and oxygen.[29]

At this time, the use of dexamethasone may be recommended only in the presence of bacterial meningitis due to either *Haemophilus influenzae*[30,31] and probably *Streptococcus pneumoniae*.[32] The dose of dexamethasone is 0.6 mg/kg/day IV divided into four daily doses for four days. The first dose should be given with or just before the first dose of antibiotics. The use of steroids for sepsis without associated meningitis, is currently not recommended and probably is harmful.[33] An investigation is currently underway to determine whether steroid administration to children with sepsis syndrome before giving antibiotics will prove to be beneficial.

The transport team would be well-advised to know the nonantibiotic aspects of sepsis management thoroughly. The first dose of antibiotics, especially beta-lactam antibiotics such as the penicillins and cephalosporins, can send a flush of cell wall fragments into the bloodstream with the large initial destruction of microorganisms. This can cause an exaggerated host response, and has been associated, in some cases, with a sudden deterioration of the patient's clinical condition.[34] The parenteral dose of antibiotics given before leaving the referring institution may occasionally need to be met with aggressive fluid and cardiorespiratory management on the return trip. Adequate monitoring and therapeutic agents must be in place.

Necrotizing Enterocolitis

Clinical Manifestations

Abdominal distention, bloody stools, emesis, or other manifestations of feeding intolerance are some of the classic symptoms of necrotizing enterocolitis (NEC). Infants with this condition requiring transport most often will be more severely compromised. They may have abdominal wall tenderness and erythema, ascites, respiratory compromise, apnea, bradycardia, and poor perfusion.[35]

Etiology

Precisely what events lead to NEC are unclear. The vast majority of patients have been premature infants who have received formula feedings. Ultimately, what seems to be responsible is the simultaneous presence of altered intestinal mucosal integrity and bacteria.[35] Epidemics of NEC have been found in nurseries in the United States; most cases, though, seem to be sporadic.

Diagnostic Tests

Laboratory evaluation may show acidosis, thrombocytopenia, disseminated intravascular coagulation, anemia, hypoproteinemia, electrolyte abnormalities, and abnormal white blood cell count. Abdominal radiographs may confirm the diagnosis by demonstrating intramural air in the intestinal tract (usually seen in the distal ileum and proximal colon), air in the portal vein, and free air in the peritoneum when perforation occurs. The absence of these radiographic findings does not exclude the diagnosis of NEC.

Management

The management of NEC is primarily medical. Feedings should be discontinued as soon as the condition is suspected. A nasogastric tube should be placed for gastric decompression and appropriate parenteral antibiotic coverage started. The combination of ampicillin and gentamicin is most commonly used, but if the patient has recently had these antibiotics administered, then vancomycin and cefotaxime are acceptable. If the patient has evidence of systemic toxicity, intravenous clindamycin should be added. (For doses of these antibiotics, see Table 3.) The infant should be carefully monitored for evidence of poor perfusion, hypotension, and respiratory compromise. Treatment of these conditions would include fluids, blood products, inotropic agents, and either supplemental O_2 or endotracheal intubation and mechanical ventilation, if clinically indicated. Appropriate central vascular access must be established.

Surgical intervention should be considered for such findings as free air in the abdomen, unremitting metabolic acidosis, erythema of the abdominal wall, and persistently nonchanging dilated loops of bowel on radiography. Other possible indications for surgery are air in the portal vein, falling platelet counts, and a palpable right lower quandrant mass.

The transport team should consider this clinical entity a medical/surgical emergency; and the patient should be stabilized and transported to the referral center as soon as possible.

Isolation

Gowns are indicated if soiling is likely. Gloves should be worn when changing diapers. Hands must be washed after touching the patient or potentially contaminated articles in the area of the patient.

Control Measures

The infection control officer at the referral center should be notified that a patient with a potentially contagious enteric disease is being admitted and enteric precautions should be taken.

INFANTS AND CHILDREN (> 1 Month)

Meningitis, Bacterial Versus Aseptic

Clinical Manifestations

The most common symptoms in a patient with meningitis are fever, lethargy, irritability, photophobia, and vomiting. At about three years of age children can usually verbalize that they have a headache. Seizures are relatively common, especially with bacterial meningitis, occurring in 20% of patients prior to admission. Nuchal rigidity and Kernig's and Brudzinski's signs usually are not present before 15 months of age. Kernig's sign is elicited if there is flexion of any of the joints of the lower extremities when the examiner firmly flexes the head at the neck in a patient in the supine position. Brudzinski's sign is present when the examiner is unable to extend the patient's leg at the knee while the upper leg is flexed at the hip.

Hemiparesis may occur in severe cases of meningitis. Focal neurologic signs involving cranial nerves III or VI also may be found. An abducens nerve palsy or dilated pupil often means uncal herniation and is an ominous sign. When papilledema is present (being unusual in bacterial meningitis) consider the possibility of brain abscess, venous sinus occlusion, subdural empyema, or acute hydrocephalus. In more advanced or severe cases of meningitis, patients may be obtunded or, occasionally, have decerebrate or decorticate posturing. Advanced disease results in hyperventilation, Cheyne-Stokes respirations, apnea, posturing, and/or fixed and dilated pupils.

Etiology

The vast majority of bacterial meningitis is caused by three organisms: *H. influenzae* type b (HIB), *S. pneumoniae*, and *N. meningitidis*. Since the advent of the HIB vaccine, the number of patients with invasive HIB disease has plummeted. One study indicates that it is no more common, and perhaps less common now, than pneumococcal and meningococcal meningitis.[36]

Most aseptic meningitis is caused by one of the enteroviruses; echovirus or coxsackievirus, which is responsible for 70–80% of all viral meningitis in infants. Arbovirus and herpes simplex virus also are relatively common causes of aseptic meningitis.

Epidemiology

The preponderance of bacterial meningitis occurs in children ≤ 5 years of age. An increased risk accrues to those who have been exposed to someone with meningococcal disease and, to a lesser extent, invasive HIB infection. Patients with splenic dysfunction are at increased risk from severe pneumococcal disease, and those with deficiencies of complement components 5–9 are at increased risk from meningococcal infections.

Viral meningitis occurs more frequently than bacterial meningitis, especially in the summer and fall, when outbreaks of both enteroviral and arboviral (mosquito-borne) meningitis occur.

Diagnostic Tests

A lumbar puncture is the definitive test for distinguishing between aseptic and bacterial meningitis. Nonviral agents such as *Mycobacterium tuberculosis*, leptospirosis, the borrelia of Lyme disease, the spirochete of syphilis, fungi, and mycoplasma, as well as viruses, are causes of aseptic meningitis. If one equates aseptic meningitis only with viral meningitis, these treatable causes of CNS infection likely will go undiagnosed.

The Gram stain, the bacterial culture, and the antigen detection tests are the methods employed in the diagnosis of bacterial meningitis. If the patient has not received either oral or parenteral antibiotics in the days before the lumbar puncture is performed, a negative CSF culture result should be relied upon as ruling out pyogenic bacterial meningitis. One of the only exceptions to this is if the blood culture is positive for a known pathogen and there is CSF pleocytosis. When the CSF culture is positive for an unlikely cause of meningitis, such as coagulase-negative staphylococcus or a viridans streptococcus, the result can usually be discounted if there is no CSF pleocytosis. Such saprophytic organisms are extremely unlikely agents of disease unless the patient is a premature infant, is severely immunocompromised, or has foreign material in his body from a previous surgery or indwelling catheter. The blood culture is positive 85% of the time with bacterial meningitis (beyond the neonatal period).

Aseptic Meningitis

Aseptic meningitis is characterized by spinal fluid that fails to grow bacteria in a patient with characteristic symptoms, abnormal CSF, and no pretreatment with antibiotics. The blood culture also should be negative. The classic CSF findings in aseptic meningitis are fewer than 300 WBCs, with a predominance of mononuclear cells, normal CSF glucose, protein, Gram stain, and antigen detection tests negative for bacteria. These CSF parameters occasionally are transgressed in documented viral meningitis, where any one or more of the following may be seen: high WBCs (sometimes with greater than 60% polymorphonuclear leukocytes); high CSF protein; or low glucose. Currently there are no rapid diagnostic tests on spinal fluid available for the diagnosis of viral meningitis; therefore, viral cultures should be sent from the CSF.

If the lumbar puncture already has been performed at the referring institution, ask someone to retrieve any remaining fluid so that it might be sent for viral culture, or bring it back on wet ice to be sent from your laboratory. Other viral cultures usually can wait until the patient is admitted at the referral center. A positive viral culture of the throat or stool makes for a presumptive identification of etiology in an aseptic meningitis case. Other sites that may be cultured for viruses include the conjuctivae, the nasopharynx, skin lesions, urine, and endotracheal tube aspirate. Rapid diagnostic studies for viruses (ELISA) are available on nasopharyngeal (NP) secretions for respiratory syncytial virus (RSV) and influenza A, and for standard panels with direct fluorescent antibody (DFA) stains, usually composed of influenza A and B, parainfluenza 1, 2 and 3, adenovirus, RSV, and sometimes cytomegalovirus (CMV).

Management

Dexamethasone should be given along with appropriate antibiotic therapy for meningitis due to *Haemophilus influenzae*,[30,31] and has also been recommended for Streptococcus pneumonia meningitis.[32] The dose of dexamethasone is 0.6 mg/kg/day IV, divided into four daily doses for four days, with the first dose given with or just before the first dose of antibiotics. Since the definitive diagnosis of *H. influenzae* or *S.pneumoniae* meningitis is based on a positive culture of spinal fluid, and this cannot be known with certitude at the time of the initial lumbar puncture, steroid therapy may be inappropriately started for other pyogenic and viral meningitides. Whenever possible, the Gram stain and the antigen detection test should be relied upon to detect infection with one of these two organisms. Dexamethasone, if stopped as soon as possible, has not been shown to cause harm in these other forms of meningitis.

Starting at one month of age throughout childhood and the teen years, patients should receive cefotaxime, 200 mg/kg/day, divided into four daily doses IV; or ceftriaxone, 100 mg/kg/day, divided into two daily doses IV. Between one and three months of age, children should also receive ampicillin, 200–400 mg/kg/day, divided into four daily doses IV. Penicillin-resistant and cephalosporin-resistant pneumococci have been reported more frequently in the United States. Vancomycin (60 mg/kg/day, divided into four daily doses IV) should be added if Gram-positive cocci are seen on CSF Gram stain or if the patient has received antibiotics in the prior month.

Controversy exists in the frequency and occurrence of the syndrome of inappropriate antidiuretic hormone (SIADH) in bacterial meningitis. Depending on the organism and the criteria used in the diagnosis of SIADH, anywhere from 4 to 88%[37,38] of children with bacterial meningitis are affected. Powell and co-workers[39] demonstrated that an elevated level of ADH usually is a natural consequence of volume depletion, often unrecognized. Recommendations for fluid management appear in *The Report on Pediatric Infectious Diseases.*[40]

When in doubt about the safety of performing a LP, owing to the possibility of increased intracranial pressure, administer the dexamethasone and antibiotics and postpone the LP until the patient shows signs of clinical stability.

If the patient has evidence of disseminated intravascular coagulation (DIC) (petechiae, pupura, bleeding from mucous membranes, bleeding from venipuncture sites), clotting studies should be drawn and appropriate blood products should be administered. Indicated blood tests include a partial thromboplastin time, prothrombin time, thrombin time, a platelet count, fibrinogen level, and fibrin split products. Blood products useful in the management of DIC are platelet concentrates, fresh frozen plasma, and cryoprecipitate.

There is no specific therapy for viral meningitis. If the etiologic agent proves to be herpes simplex virus, but the disease presentation at the time of the transport is that of a herpes meningitis and not an encephalitis, the decision to treat or not could be deferred until after the patient is at the tertiary institution. Virtually all other causes of aseptic meningitis (tuberculosis, fungal, mycoplasma, etc.) may have decisions made about treatment postponed until the patient is admitted to the PICU.

Isolation
Health care workers on the transport team having direct contact with the patient should wear masks and gloves. These precautions will protect them from the patient with unidentified contagious diseases.

Control Measures
Rifampin prophylaxis is recommended for health care workers who have intimate contact, such as mouth-to-mouth resuscitation, intubation, or suctioning, with the patient who has documented meningococcal disease.

Encephalitis
Encephalitis differs from meningitis in that there is parenchymal brain infection marked by impairment of mental function. There is a change in the patient's affect and level of consciousness, resulting in confusion, hallucination, stupor, or coma, often with focal neurologic deficits. Seizures usually are generalized, although uncommon, in meningitis; in encephalitis seizures are common and often focal.

Etiology
In the United States, each year, the etiologic agent of 75% of all cases of encephalitis remains undiagnosed. Most cases are thought to be due to enteroviruses (coxsackievirus and echovirus) and arboviruses. The most dreaded common cause of encephalitis is herpesvirus. Another dreaded, but much less common, cause of encephalitis in the United States is rabiesvirus. Chickenpox may be associated with encephalitis, but more commonly presents with cerebellitis. The following organisms account for a modest proportion of cases in the United States each year: *Mycoplasma pneumoniae*, lymphocytic choriomeningitis

virus, spirochetes (syphilis, leptospirosis, Lyme disease, Borrelia spp. infections), and Rickettsia (Rocky Mountain spotted fever, Q fever, ehrlichiosis). While many other agents are capable of causing encephalitis, most do so only rarely.

Epidemiology

The enteroviruses are spread by fecal-oral contamination and occasionally by the respiratory route. In the United States, arboviruses are transmitted by mosquitoes and ticks. Encephalitis caused by both of these groups of viruses occurs mostly in the late summer and fall. Skunks, raccoons, and bats are most likely to be infected with and transmit rabiesvirus in the United States. Foxes, coyotes, cattle, dogs, and cats are less likely culprits. Herpesvirus type I is the usual cause of herpes encephalitis and can cause this disease following either the primary infection (which may or may not be symptomatic) or reactivation.

Diagnostic Tests

The clinician should be aware that there are differences between laboratory features of herpes encephalitis in neonates and in older children. One difference is that it is unusual to identify the virus directly in herpes encephalitis after the neonatal period. However, a commercially available, more sensitive polymerase chain reaction test to detect herpesvirus in the CSF may now be used. Herpes cultures of all the body orifices are not very helpful. If a culture of the throat or vagina is positive, it could be correctly argued that any severe disease will cause a nonspecific reactivation of a person's herpesvirus infection. And while herpesvirus grows from the CSF up to 40% of the time in neonatal herpes encephalitis,[16] it does so only 1% of the time in the form that affects children beyond the neonatal period.[13] The other feature that differs between the two age groups is that the usual focus of inflammation of the brain in the older child, whether detected by EEG, MRI, or CT, is in one or both temporal lobes and the orbital region of the frontal lobes.[13] In the neonate, the pattern of inflammation is patchy and scattered throughtout the brain. The CT scan is positive in only 60% of cases, but the MRI is significantly more sensitive.[41]

The spinal fluid in herpes encephalitis may have up to 2000 WBCs/mm³. A LP perfomed early in the course of the disease may have a predominance of polymorphonuclear leukocytes, though lymphocytes usually predominate. Up to 85% of patients have red blood cells in their spinal fluid.[41] Some have decreased CSF glucose, and many have an elevated protein. Three percent of affected children will have normal CSF parameters.[41]

There are no serologies for any of the agents that cause encepahlitis that cannot wait to be drawn back at the referral center.

The two most practical specimens that can be provided by the laboratory at the referring hospital are spinal fluid and a Wright—stained peripheral blood smear (most labs keep these for one week) obtained before antibiotic therapy. The CSF can be sent for viral cultures, and the Wright stain can be reviewed for unusual organisms (such as borrelia).

Management

If herpesvirus is a possible cause of a patient's encephalitis, acyclovir should be started at a dose of 30 mg/kg/day, divided into three daily doses intravenously, each to run in over one hour and making sure that the patient is well-hydrated. An excessively rapid infusion—or dehydration—may cause crystallization of the acyclovir in the kidneys leading to renal damage.

Isolation
Universal precautions apply.

Sepsis Syndrome and Septic Shock

Etiology and Clinical Manifestations
Classically, the word "sepsis" incorporates the concept of a bacterium as fundamental to the process. The deleterious effect that the septic host suffers is collateral damage from an inflammatory response aimed at an invading microorganism. This response can proceed, once established, independent of that microorganism.[41] It is no longer clear that the organism has to be a bacterium.[29]

Following infection, some patients develop sepsis. Such patients show clinical evidence of infection, such as temperature instability, tachycardia, tachypnea, WBC count abnormalities, hypoxemia, acidosis, and oliguria. These signs and symptoms make up the sepsis syndrome. Progression to septic shock includes the development of poor capillary refill, impaired organ perfusion, disseminated intravascular coagulation, adult respiratory distress syndrome, acute renal or hepatic failure, and acute CNS dysfunction.

Epidemiology
Cases of sepsis syndrome and septic shock rarely arise from within the community. Most such patients come from the ranks of hospitalized patients.[29] Premature neonates and highly instrumented sick children are two of the more familiar categories of pediatric patients with sepsis.

Diagnostic Tests
Blood, CSF, and urine cultures should be obtained. If the patient has deep lines, such as multiple-lumen central line, a percutaneous venous catheter (PCVC), or a more permanent central line (Broviac, Hickman, etc.), it is important to collect blood cultures from these as well. A lumbar puncture may be postponed until after return to the referral center and until the patient shows hemodynamic and pulmonary stability. If new antibiotics are started before the return trip, consideration should be given to doing the lumbar puncture before boarding the transport vehicle. This procedure should be attempted only if the patient's condition permits. If antibiotics are to be administered, a suprapubic tap or catheterized urine specimen should be collected first.

Chest radiographs and any other pertinent films should be copied. If any cultures from normally sterile sites are positive, ask the microbiology laboratory to prepare specimens to bring back to the tertiary center.

Management
The patient with sepsis should receive antibiotics based on such factors as age, status of having a community-acquired infection versus nosocomial, any known focus of infection (urinary tract, pulmonary, abdominal), and results of cultures that are already known.

Infants between one and three months of age should receive ampicillin (200 mg/kg/day divided into four daily doses) and cefotaxime (200 mg/kg/day divided into four daily doses) IV. These antibiotics are active against the likely (*Haemophilus influenzae*, *Streptococcus pneumoniae*, *Neisseria meningitidis*, and *Listeria monocytogenes*) agents of infection at that age.

From three months of age through adolescence, these organisms continue to prevail, but Listeria is no longer a significant threat. Ceftriaxone (100 mg/kg/

day divided into two daily doses; maximum dose 4 gm/day) or cefotaxime (200 mg/kg/day divided into two daily doses; maximum dose 123 gm/day) should be administered IV. After six years of age Haemophilus is not likely to pose a problem, but these two cephalosporins have excellent CNS penetration and should be administered until meningitis has been ruled out.

When children have been hospitalized for a period of time prior to becoming septic, consideration must be given to such issues as prior antibiotic usage, indwelling intravascular catheters, nosocomial infections with unusual organisms from other patients, and infections with organisms with unusual sensitivity patterns. If the child has had an indwelling vascular catheter (peripheral or central), consideration should be given to the possibility of an infection with Staphylococcus aureus, coagulase negative Staphylococci, Pseudomonas, or Candida. Review the laboratory results to see if there is a positive blood culture that has been disregarded because it was assumed to be a contaminant. The chances that the catheter is the source of the infection are increased if the patient has been receiving parenteral hyperalimentation through that line. This is presumed to be due to the fact that hyperalimentation fluid is a good growth medium for microorganisms. The catheter may be infected, or the process may have progressed to the next step—the establishment of an endovascular infection. In such a setting it would be appropriate to draw two more blood cultures from two different sites and treat the patient with vancomycin (40 mg/kg/day divided into four daily doses; the usual adult maximum is 2 gm/day, but the dose is ultimately based on peak and trough levels. If meningitis is suspected, treat the patient with 60 mg/kg/day divided into four daily doses), ceftazidime (150 mg/kg/day) divided into three daily doses, and amikacin (15-20 mg/kg/day) divided into three daily doses, to be modified later based on peak and trough levels. The broad spectrum coverage will be narrowed over the next several days by the PICU team as more is learned about the patient and the infecting agent.

If the patient has a urinary tract infection associated with the sepsis syndrome, administer intravenous ampicillin (200 mg/kg/day) divided into four daily doses and gentamicin (6 mg/kg/day) divided into three daily doses. An alternate antibiotic would be trimethoprim-sulfamethoxazole (6 mg TMP–30 mg SMX/kg/day) IV divided into two daily doses.

In patients with concomitant pneumonia older than three months, cefuroxime (240 mg/kg/day) IV divided into three daily doses should be administered.

Patients presenting with peritonitis and other potentially life-threatening abdominal infections should be treated with ampicillin, gentamicin (see doses above), and clindamycin (40 mg/kg/day) divided into four daily doses, or metronidazole (30 mg/kg/day) divided into four daily doses.

Finally, never let a result of a Gram stain or culture from a site that is not normally sterile limit the empiric choice of antibiotics; only let it expand the coverage. For instance, if a Pseudomonas is growing out of the endotracheal tube of a patient with pneumonia and the clinician feels that it might be playing a role in the patient's deterioration, by all means choose antibiotics that are active against Pseudomonas—but don't sacrifice the coverage of the usual organisms that cause pneumonia. Instead of cefuroxime, which covers S. aureus, H. influenzae, Pneumococcus and Klebsiella, consider ticarcillin/clavulanic acid and tobramycin, which cover all of these plus Pseudomonas aeruginosa. If a definitive diagnosis has already been established (by blood or other cultures), then focused therapy may be undertaken.

Isolation and Control Measures

Respiratory isolation should be provided for 24 hours if the patient is under seven years of age (for the possibility of *H. influenzae*). Universal precautions apply.

Meningococcemia

Clinical Manifestations

Meningococcemia is a form of sepsis syndrome. There is an acute onset with fever, chills, malaise, and a classic rash that is petechial in nature (nonpalpable and nonblanching); These lesions may grow larger and become sizable purpura. In patients who continue to deteriorate, there is disseminated intravascular coagulation, shock, and coma. All of this can occur over just a few hours. Only a proportion of these patients develop meningitis. Other pyogenic complications include arthritis, pneumonia, pericarditis, myocarditis, and endophthalmitis.

Etiology

Virtually all disease caused by *Neisseria meningitidis* in the United States is endemic; occasional outbreaks are seen. Meningococci of serogroups B, C, Y, and W135 are those most commonly found in the United States. These organisms are among those included in most antigen detection test panels.

Epidemiology

The highest incidence occurs in infants between 6 and 12 months of age; most meningococcal disease occurs in children under five. Asymptomatic upper respiratory tract colonization exists and leads to spread, by infected droplets, from person to person. Individuals with a deficiency of one of the terminal components of complement (C5 through C9) or properdin deficiency are at increased risk of recurrent meningococcal disease. Most patients who present with meningococcemia are unaware that they have one of these conditions.

Diagnostic Tests

Patients with suspected meningococcemia should have a blood culture drawn and, if the patient is clinically stable, a lumbar puncture performed as well. Clinical stability should be affirmed by documenting acceptable hemodynamic and pulmonary parameters, and normal clotting factors. If possible, ask the laboratory for two chocolate or Thayer-Martin agar plates. When blood cultures are drawn, make sure a drop of blood is placed onto one of these plates. *Neisseria meningitidis* is a fastidious (hard to grow) organism. This, coupled with the fact that the preservative added to most blood culture bottles is toxic to meningococci, makes it difficult to grow the organism. Whenever possible, cultures should be collected before starting antibiotics. But if an obstacle arises (no blood culture bottles or LP kits available), don't wait! Administer the antibiotics. Another useful procedure for making the definitive diagnosis is to open, with sterile technique, one of the petechial lesions. The contents should be gram-stained and inoculated directly onto the second agar plate. This procedure can wait, if it will delay therapy, until immediately after the antibiotics are being infused.

Antigen detection tests may be performed on the CSF, blood, and urine. Owing to less than ideal sensitivity and specificity, these tests should be considered circumstantial and not relied on to provide a definitive diagnosis.

Management

All patients with suspected meningococcemia should have blood and CSF cultured, when clinically feasible, and antibiotics administered within 30-45 minutes of the presumptive diagnosis. The initial choice should be ceftriaxone (100 mg/kg/day) divided into two daily doses.

Isolation

The patient should have respiratory isolation for 24 hours after starting antibiotic therapy.

Control Measures

Routine prophylaxis for transport personnel is not recommended unless there has been intimate contact such as mouth-to-mouth resuscitation, intubation, or suctioning. Rifampin prophylaxis administered at 10 mg/kg/dose (with a maximum dose of 600 mg) every 12 hours for four doses (two days). Review these guidelines with the referring hospital's personnel. Also, have that hospital's infection control committee work with the parents of the patient in identifying and prophylaxing with rifampin all household, day-care center, and nursery school contacts.

BEFORE LEAVING THE REFERRING HOSPITAL

Laboratory

Have copies of all the data sheets summarizing the information collected. If a pathogen has already been isolated, whether it has been identified specifically or not, the lab should inoculate it onto an agar plate, a screw-capped slant tube, or into broth for transport with the child, if possible. Most relevant are isolates from deep or clinically significant sites (e.g., blood, spinal fluid, pleural fluid). As a rule, surface cultures collected from infants, such as those from the ear canal, umbilicus, or axilla do not provide useful information.

A particularly valuable specimen may be serum from early in the hospital course. This is useful for antibody studies in general (Mycoplasma IgG and IgM, etc.), before the blood has been contaminated with packed cells, platelets, fresh frozen plasma, or intravenous immunoglobulin, and for early "acute" specimens for acute and convalescent antibody titers. Most hospitals don't routinely save an acute specimen of blood from early in the patient's hospital course. But almost all hospitals have serum samples in their refrigerators, conveniently labeled, from blood draws over the previous week for electrolytes and other serum studies. In the case of a newborn, cord blood serves this purpose well. When the possibility of a TORCH syndrome exists, ask for the placenta. If it's available, place it in a plastic bag and set it on top of wet ice in a styrofoam box. Also, collect Gram and acid-fast bacilli (AFB) stains and slides of tissue, positive or negative. These materials are convenient to have when returning to the referral hospital, since they may save a few days of needless antibiotics or call into question a previous diagnosis.

Copies of all pertinent radiologic studies should be brought back to the referral center, including MRIs, CT scans, and bone and Gallium scans.

Accumulating these materials is a worthy goal, but not worth holding up the transport of a critically ill child. They can always be retrieved later by cab, mail, or messenger.

THE TRIP BACK TO THE TERTIARY CARE CENTER

Whether the patient makes the trip back to the referral center in a transport incubator or under blankets in the internal environment of the ambulance, it is essential that adequate thermal protection be maintained. Unless extremely low temperatures are reached (cold water immersion), a cold environment does not decrease the metabolic rate. Rather, moderate degrees of cold increase oxygen consumption, adding an additional burden to the infected child who is already metabolically stressed from infection.[12]

RETURN TO THE TERTIARY CARE CENTER

Post-Exposure Prophylaxis

Transport personnel who are exposed to patients with meningococcal disease require no special prophylaxis unless they have had intimate exposure. Prophylaxis should begin within 24 hours, if possible, and cultures of the resiratory tract should not be used in making this decision. Rifampin should be given in a dose of 600 mg by mouth, twice a day for two days.

Children with primary tuberculosis are considered noncontagious. The exception to this rule is children and adolescents who can be documented to have reactivation (cavitary) pulmonary tuberculosis or whose sputum is AFB positive. These exceptions are quite rare. While there is no recommended drug prophylaxis for transport personnel following exposure to patients with active tuberculosis, PPD skin testing should be a part of regular medical evaluations of transport personnel.

There is no generally accepted prophylactic regimen for health professionals exposed to the Human Immunodeficiency Virus (HIV). While the risk of HIV infection is quite low following needlestick and mucosal exposure to infected blood, many hospitals have research protocols using the drug azidothymidine (AZT). These programs usually are accessible 24 hours a day through the hospital's emergency department.

With any needle stick, laceration, bite, ocular, or mucous membrane exposure to a patient's blood, that patient's hepatitis B surface antigen (HBsAg) status should be determined immediately by review of the medical record or by blood test. If the exposed member of the transport team has not previously been vaccinated or has not completed the vaccination series, he/she should receive HBIG, 0.06 ml/kg, as soon as possible within 24 hours of the exposure. Hepatitis B vaccination should then be started or completed. If the exposed member is a known responder with an adequate titer [(the anti-HBs is $\geq$ 10 SRU by radioimmunoassay (RIA)] or positive by enzyme immunosorbent assay (EIA), no treatment is necessary. There are three other possible scenarios for immunized, exposed personnel (Table 4). When a repeat dose is indicated in one of these situations, HB vaccine 1.0 ml intramuscularly should be administered, regardless of the vaccine manufacturer.

Prophylaxis is not required following exposure to patients with invasive *Haemophilus influenzae* disease.

Decontamination of Materials

Following the transport of patients, where routine precautions were taken, the ambulance should be aired for 20 minutes, bedding should be laundered or steam disinfected, and the mattress and pillow wiped with a dilute bleach solution. Any spilled blood or blood-contaminated fluid should be wiped up, and the surface cleaned with a solution of dilute bleach.

Following the transport of patients who require maximum precautions, the ambulance should be subjected to the most rigorous cleaning regimen available to the transport company. This should include fumigation with formalin vapor

TABLE 4. Recommendations for Hepatitis B Prophylaxis after Percutaneous or Permucosal Exposure

Exposed Person	HBsAG-Positive Source	Source Not Tested or Unknown	HBsAG-Negative Source
Unvaccinated	HBIG × 1* and initiate HB vaccine†	Initiate HB vaccine†	Initiate HB vaccine†
Previously vaccinated known responder	Test exposed for anti-HBs‡ If adequate, no treatment If inadequate, HB vaccine† booster dose	No treatment	No treatment
Known nonresponder	HBIG × 2 or HBIG × 1 plus 1 dose HB vaccine†	If known high-risk source, may treat as if source were HBsAg-positive	No treatment
Response unknown	Test exposed for anti-HBs‡ If inadequate, HBIG × 1 plus HB vaccine† booster dose If adequate, no treatment	Test exposed for anti-HBs‡ If inadequate, HB vaccine booster dose If adequate, no treatment	No treatment

* HBIG dose 0.06 ml/kg IM.
† HB vaccine dose: 1.0 ml of either Recombivax or Energix-B.
‡ Adequate anti-ABs is ≥ 10 SRU by RIA or positive by EIA.
From Centers for Disease Control and Prevention: Hepatitis B Virus: A comprehensive strategy for eliminating transmission in the United States through universal childhood vaccination: Recommendations of the Immunization Practices Advisory Committee (ACIP). Morbidity and Mortality Weekly Report 1991:40 (RR-13): 22.

or some comparable procedure and then thorough cleaning and washing with a phenolic solution of sodium hypochlorite (household bleach). The bedding should be steam disinfected or incinerated.

REFERENCES

1. Thompson JE, Bonner B, Lower GM: Pediatric cardiopulmonary arrests in rural populations. Pediatrics 86:302–306, 1990.
2. Cunningham MD, Smith FR: Stablilization and transport of severely ill infants. Pediatr Clin North Am 20:359–366, 1973.
3. Gellman EF, Flannery MM: Infant Transport: Two years' experience, Missouri Med 79–80, Feb 1974.
4. Blake AM, McIntosh N, Reynolds EOR, et al: Transport of newborn infants for intensive care. Br Med J 13–17, 4 Oct, 1975.
5. Kukita J, Yamashita H, Minami T, Fujita I, Koyanagi T, Ueda K: Improved outcome for infants weighing less than 750 grams at birth; Effects of advances in perinatal care, infection prevention and maternal transport for fetus, Acta Pediatr Japan 32:625:632, 1990.
6. Black RE, Mayer T, Walker ML, Christison EL, Johnson DG, Matlak ME, Storrs B, Clark P: Special report: Air transport of pediatric emergency cases. N Engl J Med 307:1465–1468, 1982.
7. Emond RTD, Payne DJH, Galbraith SG: Recommended code of practice for the transport by ambulance of persons suspected of suffering from transmissible infection, J Infect 2:289–291, 1980.
8. Wood MJ, Geddes AM: Recommended code of practice for the transport by ambulance of persons suspected of suffering from transmissible infection; Letters to the Editor, J Infect 3:192–193, 1981.
9. Centers for Disease Control: Guidelines for prevention of transmission of human immunodeficiency virus and hepatitis B virus to health-care and public safety workers. MMWR 38:No. S-6; 9–10, 1989.
10. Hoyt NJ: Infection control and emergency medical services: Facts and myths. MMJ 37:551–557, 1988.
11. Clausen L, Bothwell TH, Isaacson M, et al: Isolation and handling of patients with dangerous infectious disease. S Afr Med J 53:238–242, 1978.
12. Segal S: Manual for the Transport of High-Risk Newborn Infants: Principles, Policies, Equipment, Techniques. Quebec, Canadian Pediatric Society, 1972.
13. Feigin RD, Cherry JD: Textbook of Pediatric Infectious Diseases, 3rd ed. Philadelphia, W.B. Saunders, 1992.

14. Committee on Infectious Diseases: Report of the Committee on Infectious Diseases (AKA "The Red Book"), 23rd ed. Elk Grove Village, IL, American Academy of Pediatrics, 1994.
15. Krugman S, Katz SL, Gershon AA, Wilfert CM: Infectious Diseases of Children, 9th ed. St. Louis: Mosby, 1992.
16. Remington JS, Klein JO: Infectious Diseases of the Fetus and Newborn Infant, 3th ed. Philadelphia, W.B. Saunders, 1995.
17. Mustafa MM, McCracken GH: Perinatal bacterial diseases. In Feigin RD, Cherry JD (eds): Textbook of Pediatric Infectious Diseases, 3rd ed. Philadelphia, W.B. Saunders, 1992, pp 891–924.
18. Shattuck KE, Chonmaitree T: The changing spectrum of neonatal meningitis over a fifteen-year period. Clin Pediatr 31:130–136, 1992.
19. Swender PT, Shott RJ, Williams ML: A community and intensive care nursery outbreak of coxsackievirus B5 meningitis. Am J Dis Child 127:42–45, 1974.
20. Sarff LD, Platt LH, McCraken GH: Cerbrospinal fluid evaluation in neonates: Comparison of high-risk infants with and without meningitis. J Pediatr 88:473–477, 1976.
21. Prober CG, Sullender WM, YUasakawa LL, et al: Low risk of herpes simplex virus infections in neonates exposed to the virus at the time of vaginal delivery to mothers with recurrent genital herpes simplex virus infections. N Engl J Med 316:240–244, 1987.
22. Graves GR, Rhodes PG: Tachycardia as a sign of early onset neonatal sepsis. Pediatr Infect Dis J 3:404–406, 1984.
23. Siegel JD, McCracken GH: Sepsis neonatorum. N Engl J Med 304:642–647, 1981.
24. Fulginiti VA: Body surface cultures in the newborn infant. Am J Dis Child 142:19–20, 1988.
25. Manroe BL, Weinberg AG, Rosenfeld CR, Browne R: The neonatal blood count in health and disease. I. Reference values for neutrophilic cells. J Pediatr 95:89–98, 1979.
26. Squire E, Favara B, Todd J: Diagnosis of neonatal bacterial infection: Hematologic and pathologic findings in fatal and nonfatal cases. Pediatrics 64:60–64, 1979.
27. Nelson JD: Pocketbook of Pediatric Antimicrobial Therapy, 10th ed. Baltimore, Williams & Wilkins, 1993.
28. Hill HR: Intravenous immunoglobulin use in the neonate: Role in prophylaxis and therapy of infection. Pediatr Infect Dis J 12:549–559, 1993.
29. Saez-Llorens X, McCracken GH Jr: Sepsis syndrome and septic shock in pediatrics: Current concepts of terminology, pathophysiology and management. J Pediatr 123:497–508, 1993.
30. Lebel MH, Freij BJ, Syrogiannopoulos GA, et al: Dexamethasone therapy for bacterial meningitis: Results of two double-blind, placebo-controlled trials. N Engl J Med 319:964–971, 1988.
31. Odio CM, Faingezitch I, Paris M, et al: The beneficial effects of early dexamethasone administration in infants and children with bacterial meningitis. N Engl J Med 324:1525–1531, 1991.
32. Kennedy WA, Hoyt MJ, McCracken GH Jr: The role of corticosteroid therapy in children with pneumococcal meningitis. Am J Dis Child 145:1374–1378, 1991.
33. Bone RC, Fisher CJ, Clemmer TP, et al: A controlled clinical trial of high-dose methylprednisolone in the treatment of severe sepsis and septic shock. N Engl J Med 317:653–658, 1987.
34. Mertsola J, Ramilo O, Mustafa MM, et al: Release of endotoxin after antibiotic treatment of gram-negative bacterial meningitis. Pediatr Infect Dis J 8:904–906, 1989.
35. Faix RG, Adams JT: Neonatal necrotizing enterolitis: Current concepts and controversies. In Aronoff SC, Hughes WT, Kohl S, et al (eds): Advances in Pediatric Infectious Diseases, Vol. 9, 1994, pp 1–36.
36. Michaels RH, Ali O: A decline in Haemophilus influenza type B meningitis. J Pediatr 122:407–409, 1993.
37. Prince AS, Neu HC: Fluid management in Haemophilus influenzae meningitis. Infection 8:5–7, 1980.
38. Feigin RD, Stechenberg BW, Chang MJ, et al: Prospective evaluation of treatment of Haemophilus influenza. J Pediatr 88:542–548, 1976.
39. Powell KR, Sugarman LI, Eskenazi AE, et al: Normalization of plasma arginine vasopressin concentrations when children with meningitis are given maintenance plus replacement fluid therapy. J Pediatr 117:515–522, 1990.
40. Smith A: Fluid management during bacterial meningitis. Report on Pediatric Infectious Diseases 3:10–11, 1993.
41. Schlossberg D: Infections of the Nervous System. New York, Springer-Verlag, 1990.
42. Saez-Llorenz X, Lagrutta F: The acute-phase host reaction during bacterial infections in children. Pediatr Infect Dis J 12:83–87, 1993.

CHAPTER 30

Temperature Regulation and Management

MICHAEL H. LeBLANC, M.D.

Maintaining control of body temperature is important in all living creatures. All multiple enzyme systems that maintain a living cell function best over a narrow range of temperatures. Poikilothermic vertebrate organisms, such as fishes, amphibians, and reptiles, are aware of the temperature of their surroundings and seek comfortable environments. This is why the best fishing is in deep, cold water on hot days. Higher vertebrates, birds, and mammals do the same, but also actively control their body temperature. That is, they have mechanisms for increasing heat production in a cold environment and for increasing heat loss in a hot environment.

Adult humans regulate their temperature preferentially by behavioral means; that is, if it is cold they put on a coat or go indoors, and if it is hot they wear less clothing or go into an air-conditioned building. In addition, adult humans can increase their heat production by shivering and can reduce their heat loss by constricting blood flow to their skin in a cold environment. In a warm environment adult humans dilate the blood vessels in their skin and increase their evaporative heat losses by sweating.

Small animals or humans have more difficulty in balancing heat losses with heat production. Heat losses are proportional to the body's surface area, and heat production is proportional to the body mass or volume. The smaller an organism is, the more surface area it has per unit volume. Thus, a small animal, such as a hummingbird, shrew, or infant, has great difficulty in staying warm, whereas a large animal such as an elephant has trouble with staying cool. Before birth, temperature regulation is provided by the mother. The fetus swims in a heated pool. Metabolic heat production per kilogram of a fetus is only slightly higher than that of its mother, whereas its surface area is many times larger.

At birth, the term baby has a surface area-to-volume ratio four times that of its parents and a heat production only one and one-half times as high. In addition, the infant's ability to increase heat production in the face of cold stress is only about one-third that of the parents. Thus, a newborn baby requires a warmer environment than the parents do for thermal comfort. The newborn infant's ability to maintain temperature in a cold environment is also much less than that of an adult. Preterm infants are smaller and thus are more susceptible to heat loss than a term infant. In addition, preterm infants, because of an incompletely developed stratum corneum (the surface layer of the skin), have increased evaporative heat losses. Because of this, much warmer temperatures are necessary to keep them warm. Babies are comfortable at warmer temperatures than adults are and are sensitive to changes in temperature that adults would have difficulty detecting. Because of their large surface areas, infants cool or heat much more rapidly than adults, and this makes even brief exposure to inclement weather dangerous. We must worry about keeping babies warm even in the controlled environment of a hospital. Keeping them warm in the much less controlled environment of transport is even more difficult.

PHYSICS OF HEAT LOSS

Body temperature is a reflection of the heat produced within a body and the heat lost from a body. If a body is producing more heat than it is losing, its temperature will gradually increase. Because the rate of heat loss is proportional to the difference in temperature between the environment and the temperature of the body, as the body's temperature goes up it will lose more heat. When it reaches the point that heat loss equals heat gain, the rise in temperature will stop. If the body loses more heat than it produces, its temperature will fall. Because the rate of heat loss is proportional to the difference in temperature between that of the body and that of the environment, as the body temperature falls the heat losses will decrease. The body temperature will eventually stabilize at a point where heat loss again equals heat production. It is important to realize that temperature will change gradually in the face of too much or too little heat loss. Thus, the direction and rate of change of temperature is more important than actual temperature in determining appropriate management. In general, babies' temperatures change much more rapidly than adults' because they are much smaller, but even a baby's temperature change is not instantaneous. The mechanisms of heat loss are basic physical processes that we learned about in physics. They are reviewed below.

Conduction

Conduction is the flow of heat through a solid body. It is proportional to the difference in temperature across the solid body, the area involved, and the thermal conductivity of the body. Thermal conductivity here is very important, because thermal conductivity varies by a factor of 10,000 from the best thermal conductors to the best thermal insulators. In general, metals or fluids are good thermal conductors, and substances like foam rubber, styrofoam, and plastic are good thermal insulators. This is why on a cold day a metal hand rail feels so much colder than a wooden hand rail, even if both are the same temperature. Snow or water feels colder than dirt of the same temperature because heat flows faster from your hand to the better conductor.

Convection

In convective heat transfers, an object heats the air around it; hot air expands and thus becomes lighter than the cool air surrounding it. The cool surrounding air pushes the hot air upward, much as a hot-air balloon rises. Eventually the hot air is swept away in the wind currents of the room. Convective heat losses are proportional to the difference in temperature between a body and the air surrounding it. They are higher if the wind velocity is high and lower in still air. In cold weather we feel colder if the wind is blowing, because we lose more heat by convection.

Radiation

All objects of greater than –273°C or –459°F emit electromagnetic radiation. The sun emits electromagnetic radiation in the visible range, allowing us to see. Most familiar objects emit electromagnetic radiation in the infrared region. Exchange of heat goes on between cold objects and warm objects, provided the medium separating them is transparent to infrared radiation. Net heat flow follows the temperature gradient and is from hot to cooler objects. Air is transparent to infrared radiation. Plexiglass, which is used to make the hoods of infant transport incubators, is transparent to visible radiation, allowing one to see the infant; but it is opaque to infrared radiation, thus preventing losses of radiation directly from baby to the environment. Radiant energy is lost indirectly as the walls of the incubator are cooled by the environment within the ambulance; thus, heat radiated from the baby to the walls of the incubator is lost gradually through the walls of the incubator to the walls of the ambulance. We are much warmer standing in the sunshine than in the shade because in the sunshine we absorb radiant heat energy from the sun.

Evaporation

People are moist on the inside and dry on the outside. The stratum corneum, a waxy layer of dead skin cells, helps keep the moisture inside the body from getting outside. Premature babies may have a very thin stratum corneum that is ineffective in preventing evaporation of body moisture through the skin. In addition, term babies are born soaking wet; until thoroughly dried, they will lose heat as this water evaporates. The heat loss from water evaporation is approximately what it would take to boil the water. Evaporative heat loss is decreased by increasing the local humidity; it is increased by a flow of dry air over the baby or by increased wind velocity. By decreasing the flow of air over a baby, a baby will, to a degree, humidify his or her local environment. Think of what makes you hotter or cooler in hot weather when you are sweating and losing a lot of heat by evaporation. High humidity makes a warm day feel warmer because you lose less heat by evaporation. A breeze is always welcome on a hot day, because it increases evaporative heat loss.

Understanding the physics of heat exchange is important in attaining a thorough understanding of how to keep babies warm. Most of us instinctively know, however, that moving to a warmer place or putting on a coat or blanket will help us to warm up.

PHYSIOLOGY

Core temperature is the temperature deep inside a person. We measure temperature in the axilla or rectum to determine core temperature. The basic control mechanisms in an adult or an infant are designed to try to maintain the core temperature within a narrow range. The first mechanism for doing this is changing the skin's blood flow. In a hot environment skin blood flow is high, and the skin is warm to touch; thus, the skin radiates more heat than it would if its blood flow were diminished. In a cold environment, skin blood flow is reduced, causing the hands and feet to become cold and sometimes even to turn blue. This decreases the temperature gradient between the skin and the environment, thus reducing heat losses. In addition, a vigorous term baby in a cold environment will flex its arms and legs and make itself into a ball, thus reducing the surface area exposed to the environment and reducing heat loss. In a hot environment, the baby will extend its arms and legs and increase its surface area of exposure. Sick or premature babies are much less able to do this and typically will lie spread-eagle in any sort of an environment. In a hot environment, adults will sweat; term newborns will produce beads of sweat on their brow, but not over the rest of their bodies; premature babies will have no visible sweat. Most babies will become slightly tachypneic as well. In a cold environment, the baby's metabolic heat production will increase, exhausting fuel stores needed for other purposes.

Depending on the size of the baby, the core temperature will be maintained and defended much better than the skin temperature. Thus, to seek out a thermal comfort zone, it is important to measure both the core and the skin temperature of a baby in transport. An appropriate core temperature for a baby is about 37°C or 98.6°F. This is usually measured by placing a thermometer in the axilla (arm pit) and holding it there for about five minutes. Alternatively, a glass thermometer or flexible thermistor can be inserted gently into the anus to obtain the rectal temperature. If rectal temperature is used, the examiner must be careful to avoid rectal perforation—a rare but catastrophic complication. If the baby is face up, skin temperature is usually taken on the upper abdomen over the liver by taping a thermistor to the skin (it should be approximately 36.5°C or 97.7°F). If the baby is prone, the skin temperature probe should be placed on its back. If the skin temperature probe is placed on the baby's skin against the mattress, it will reflect core temperature rather than skin temperature.

Most transport monitors will support a skin thermistor. Because skin temperature can be measured continuously rather than intermittently, and because it changes more rapidly than core temperature, it provides great advantages for temperature monitoring during transport. In a baby who is too cold and is warming, first the air around the baby warms, then its skin temperature gradually warms, and lastly the core temperature slowly warms. Similarly, in an overheated baby the skin will cool first, followed by the core.

PRETRANSPORT HOSPITAL MANAGEMENT

Usually a sick infant is placed in an incubator or under a radiant warmer. An incubator is a heated box, the infant compartment of which is made of plexiglass that is opaque to infrared radiation and keeps the inside air of the incubator warmer than the outside air and insulates the baby from radiant heat losses. The incubator can either be set to control the baby's skin temperature at 36.5°C or to control the air temperature within the incubator at an appropriate temperature for the age and gestation of the baby. Another common device for keeping babies warm prior to transport is the radiant warmer. In this case, a skin probe is attached to the baby's skin, and the radiant heater automatically adjusts its heat output to maintain the skin temperature at approximately 36.5°C.

INTRATRANSPORT MANAGEMENT

Babies are normally transported in transport incubators, which are heavily insulated boxes that have a plexiglass window to allow visualization of the baby and small plexiglass portholes through which procedures can be done. The box temperature is controlled by a knob so that the internal air temperature can be set by the user. Appropriate settings for babies of various ages and weights are shown in Table 1. This table is appropriate if the inside air temperature of the ambulance is approximately 75–80°F or approximately 25°C. In a colder environment, the air temperature should be increased 1° for each 5° decrease in ambient temperature if a single-walled incubator is used and 1° for every 12°

TABLE 1. Incubator Air Temperature*

Age and Weight of Infant	Single-walled incubator	Double-walled Incubator‡
0–12 hr		
<750	41.5 (39)†	39.5 (37.5)
750–1000	40.5 (38.5)	39.0 (37)
1000–1200	39 (37.0)	37.5
1200–1500	37.5	36.5
1500–2000	36.5	35.5
>2000	35	34
12 hr–3 days		
<1000	40.5 (38.0)	38 (37)
1000–1200	38	37
1200–1500	37	36
1500–2000	36	35
>2000	34	33
3–14 days		
<1000	37.5	36
1000–1200	35	34.5
1200–1500	34.5	34.0
1500–2000	34.0	33.5
>2000	33.5	33
2–4 weeks		
<1000	36	35
1000–1500	34.5	34
1500–2500	34.0	33.5
4–8 weeks		
<1200	35.0	34.0
1200–1500	32.5	32.0
1500–2500	31.5	31.0

* Temperature is in °C by age and weight for single- and double-walled incubators, assuming an ambient temperature of 25°C and a PH_2O of 13. Temperatures given are for AGA infants. Temperatures for SGA infants will be lower. Increase single-walled air temperature by 1° for each 5° drop in ambient temperature below 25°C. Increase double-walled incubator 1° for each 12° drop in ambient temperature below 25°C.
† The numbers in parentheses are the suggested air temperatures for humidified incubators or for babies covered with plastic. The required temperature for dry incubators in these cases exceeds the capability of most incubators.
‡ Plexiglass shield over infants may be used instead of double wall.
Adapted from Scopes J, Ahmed I: Arch Dis Child 41:417, 1966; Sauer PJJ, Dane HJ, Visser HKA: Arch Dis Child 59:18–22, 1994; and LeBlanc MH: Med Instrum 1:11–15, 1987.

if a double-walled incubator is used. Transport incubators typically take 20–30 minutes to heat; thus, they should be preheated before placing the baby within.

Because the transport incubator, like all incubators, will lose its heat very rapidly if the hood is open, the hood should not be opened unless absolutely necessary. Frequently it is possible to place a small infant in the infant compartment through the portholes without opening the hood of the incubator. The hot air within an incubator will escape within seconds after the lid is opened. When possible, procedures should be done through the portholes with the lid in place. Since transport incubators are typically small and cramped, making procedures difficult, it is important to do all procedures likely to be needed in transport before leaving the hospital of origin. Normally a skin probe would be attached to the baby's abdomen and plugged into the infant heart-rate monitor to keep track of the skin temperature. The baby's skin temperature will be noted, as will the rate and direction of change of the temperature.

If the baby's skin temperature is too low and is not rising, the incubator air temperature should be increased slightly, usually about 0.5°C every 5–10 minutes. Similarly, if the baby's skin temperature is too hot and is not falling, the air temperature should be adjusted downward. It is important to note not only the temperature but also the direction of change. If the temperature is moving in the correct direction, leave the incubator temperature where it is. Sometimes when transporting very immature babies, or in a cold environment, it may not be possible to get the incubator warm enough to keep the baby warm. Additional methods must then be used to reduce heat loss or to increase heat production. A plexiglass shield placed between the baby and the walls of the incubator will reduce radiant heat losses, because the shield is warmer than the incubator walls, and helps to keep the baby warm. Small babies, especially those under 28 weeks' gestation, will have very high evaporative water losses. These can be reduced by placing a sheet of plastic over the baby, thus reducing wind velocity over the baby and raising the local humidity. If the baby is not intubated and on a ventilator, it is, of course, necessary to leave a space open at the nose and mouth so that it may breathe. Alternatively, the incubator may be humidified, but in practice this is difficult to do on transport. The most practical source of additional heat for transport is a Porta Warm mattress (Marion Scientific Co., Kansas City, MO), which contains a number of compartments of supercooled liquid with a freezing point of 40°C. When the small inner packs are punctured, the liquid will begin to freeze, thus raising its temperature to 40°C. This provides a substantial amount of controlled heat during transport at a temperature that can safely be placed in contact with the baby. Hot water bags are to be avoided; if they are made too hot, they can easily burn a baby.

The contact temperature between the baby and any object that is a good thermal conductor should be less than 42°C.* A thermal insulator can be allowed to be somewhat warmer provided the heat flow to a baby never exceeds 6.3×10^{-3} watts/cm^2. It must be remembered that babies, like comatose adults, cannot complain about contact with a hot object or remove themselves from the contact before permanent damage is done. In intrahospital transport, heated water pads can be used provided the surface does not exceed 40°C; however, they usually require a source of alternating current electricity often not available during transport. By bundling up the baby, covering its head and wrapping it in a heated water pad at about 40°C, it is possible to keep almost any baby warm. This technique may be useful in some transport situations. Since the baby is dependent on the heater in the transport incubator, it is important that this heater be adequate to the task at hand.

Transport environments vary markedly in North America, and transport incubators that work well in a relatively warm environment may function poorly in a cold environment. The battery life of a transport incubator depends strongly on the environment in which it is used. Most manufacturers provide data about expected battery life as a function of ambient temperature and how well a transport incubator will keep an infant simulator warm at various ambient temperatures. Careful review of this material before purchase will allow one to purchase a transport incubator suitable for the local environment.

---

* The temperature required to burn the skin depends on the length of contact and the thickness of the skin. For very thin skin, if the time of contact is t seconds, the temperature to produce a burn is

$$0.494 \left(\frac{t}{2.5}\right)^{-.412} (31.5) + 41$$

A sensation of pain is produced in about 40% of the time it takes to produce a burn. (Stoll AM, Chawla MA, Piergalli JR: Aviat Space Environ Med 50:778–787, 1979.)

Just as it is important to remember that one can ventilate a patient using mouth-to-mouth resuscitation if a bag and mask are not available, it is important to know technqiues for keeping a baby warm in the absence of a functioning transport incubator. All adults carry a source of heat in their own skin. By placing a baby next to an adult's skin under blankets, it is possible to keep most babies warm. If the baby is transported with its mother, this technique can be used if the baby is stable enough so that close observation is not needed or if no other technique is available. Kangaroo care—placing the baby between the mother's breasts so that it is surrounded on three sides by her flesh—has been effectively used in very small infants in primitive environments. One should also remember the ambulance heater. Transporting a baby in a 98°F ambulance may be very uncomfortable for the driver and attendants but life-saving for a small infant. If during transport one needs to do procedures on an infant that cannot be done through the portholes, the ambulance should be heated as hot as possible before opening the hood of the transport incubator.

HYPOTHERMIA AND HYPERTHERMIA

The best means of treating hypothermia and hyperthermia is avoidance. By careful attention to thermal management, a baby's temperature should be maintained at appropriate levels throughout transport. If a baby becomes hypothermic for any reason, it needs to be rewarmed. The primary measure is to move the baby from an environment that is too cold to one that is the appropriate temperature. The rate at which the baby is rewarmed is not important—only that the baby's temperature is steadily increasing.

Hyperthermia, a much rarer situation in transport, is handled similarly. The baby is placed in a heat-losing environment and its temperature allowed to decrease gradually. If the baby's temperature is less than 106°F or 41°C, placing it in a heat-losing environment is adequate. If a baby's temperature is greater than 41°C or 106°F, sponging the baby with water to increase evaporative heat losses should be done. Body temperatures higher than 106°F or 41°C will result in heat stroke with damage to multiple organ systems.

Careful attention to maintenance of the equipment is critical to successful transport. Always carry back-up supplies such as temperature probes, fuses, batteries, and alternative sources of power such as Porta Warm mattresses. Most transport disasters are caused by equipment failure. Simple but common sense approaches to specific problems often will work well. For example, covering up a transport incubator with a quilt or blanket when it has to be moved through a particularly cold environment may prevent the baby's temperature from dropping.

SUMMARY

Infants on transport are very susceptible to cold stress and may die of cold exposure at temperatures that adults find comfortable. Careful attention to both thermal control and the maintenance of the thermal control equipment is critical for the safe transport of small infants.

REFERENCES

1. American National Standard Infant Incubator. Arlington, VA, AAMI, 1991.
2. American National Standard—Transport Incubators. Arlington, VA, AAMI, 1995.
3. Klaus MH, Fanaroff AA: Care of the High Risk Neonate, 3rd ed. Philadelphia, W.B. Saunders, 1986, pp 96–112.
4. Polin RA, Fox WW (eds): Fetal and Neonatal Physiology. Philadelphia, W.B. Saunders, 1992, pp 477–515.

Common Radiologic Findings in Pediatric and Neonatal Transport Patients

JEFF E. SCHUNK, M.D.
GEORGE A. WOODWARD, M.D.

Owing to the variety of transported pediatric patients, transport personnel must be able to perform an accurate (though often brief) history, physical examination, and assessment of laboratory and radiographic findings. Furthermore, they must convey this information to the receiving hospital so that decisions can be made about transport interventions, anticipated complications, and preparation for the patient's arrival at the receiving hospital. Since nearly all referring institutions have x-ray facilities and most seriously ill or injured infants and children undergo radiographic examination, adequate radiologic assessment becomes a critical element of the transport team's assessment.

Although radiographs are a frequent component of a complete patient evaluation, their interpretation is infrequently taught to nonphysician transport personnel. This is in spite of the fact that the control physician may need confirmation of radiographic findings to ensure a safe and complication-free transport. In addition, the transport team member may be asked to obtain and interpret radiographs prior to transport. The team will frequently carry (and report the results of) radiographs obtained at the referring hospital or clinic. The referring physicians may offer radiologic interpretations, but the ability of the transport team to confirm such findings is an important and often underemphasized skill. Transport personnel may need to decide whether a radiograph should be obtained before returning. Many factors go into this decision, including seriousness of illness or injury, the nature of complication that the radiograph is confirming, duration and mode of transport, and time needed to obtain radiographs. Increased awareness of what information can be obtained from a radiograph will aid the transport personnel in making such decisions.

This chapter provides a basic framework for interpretation of common radiographs and outlines some radiographic features frequently seen in pediatric and neonatal transport patients. Evaluation of plain films of the chest, skull, abdomen, neck, and extremities is discussed in addition to computed tomography (CT) scans of the head. All references to "right" or "left" refer to the *patient's* right or left side, not the right or left side of the study that is viewed.

CHEST

The chest x-ray is the most common radiograph encountered in transport. It is frequently the most important, for it can provide vital clues about the patient's cardiopulmonary status. It is crucial in that it often confirms appropriate placement of endotracheal and/or naso/orogastric tubes and central lines and may identify such potentially life-threatening conditions as pneumothorax. The standard roentgen evaluation includes an upright posteroanterior (PA) and a lateral view. However, in the seriously ill or critical patient a supine portable chest radiograph (obtained anteroposterior or AP) may be the only view available. Regardless of which view is obtained, it should include all of the chest skeletal structures and should clearly outline the diaphragm, including the costophrenic angles. In general the AP view may make the heart and mediastinal structures appear larger than on a PA view; other distinctions will not be made.

Chest x-ray interpretation should progress from the outer portion of the film to the inner details. It is easy to concentrate too quickly on the heart and lungs, thereby overlooking other significant findings. We should train ourselves to examine the soft tissues and bony structures first. Special attention should be paid to the ribs (outlining the margins of each rib) because fractures can be easily missed. This added attention is particularly important in the trauma victim because it can alert the transport team to the potential for such serious underlying conditions as a pneumothorax, pulmonary contusion, or thoracic vascular injuries (associated with upper rib or sternal fractures). It also may provide the clue that the patient is the victim of child abuse if unexplained or healing rib fractures are noted.

The lungs are examined next. A chest x-ray is shown in Figure 1. The normal chest x-ray is taken during inspiration and should reveal at least 9–10 ribs posteriorly. Inadequate inspiratory effort may make the lungs appear abnormally opacified, and the heart may appear large (Fig. 2). The main airways should be identified and their position noted. In small children, a bend to the right often is seen where the trachea enters the thorax (with the aortic arch left of the trachea), or there may be apparent tracheal buckling in this area.[1] This normal finding may be mistaken for a neck or mediastinal mass. The position of the carina and mainstem bronchi should be noted. Abnormal position of the trachea to one side of the chest may indicate either volume loss on the same side (e.g., atelectasis) or contralateral hyperinflation (e.g., pneumothorax). The left mainstem bronchus normally has a more horizontal position than the right. The lung fields show symmetric lucency, and the lung markings extend to the periphery. Asymmetric lucency may indicate increased opacity (unilateral pneumonia) or increased air (pneumothorax, unilateral hyperinflation with an aspirated foreign body). The left diaphragm (with the stomach bubble located beneath) is slightly lower than the right. Deviations from this relationship may provide a clue about increased or decreased lung volume. In the infant—not premature—the perihilar structures are less prominent, and the lungs may appear more lucent than in the older child.[2]

The mediastinal exam naturally focuses on the heart. In the infant the thymus may appear as a prominent structure in the superior portion of the mediastinum and can be mistaken for a tumor or central lung disease. The normal heart may occupy up to 60% of the thoracic width in the infant. In the older child this is usually less than 55%. The right heart border in the PA view is primarily right atrium because the ventricle lies more anteriorly. The right border of the left atrium may be seen "through" the heart to the right of the midline. The left heart border is comprised mainly of the left ventricle and, superiorly, the pulmonary

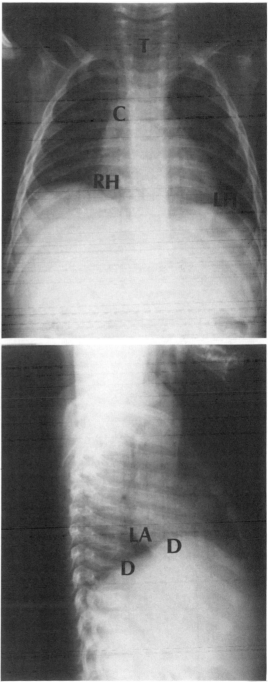

FIGURE 1. Posteroanterior (top) and lateral (bottom) chest radiographs in an infant. Note the clear heart border (right heart, RH; left heart, LH), nearly symmetric aeration, tracheal air column (T), and the carina (C). Some deviation of the tracheal air column to the right is often seen. The vertebrae can be visualized "through the heart," indicating adequate x-ray beam penetration. On the lateral film note the diaphragm leaflets (D) and the posterior portion of the heart (left atrium, LA).

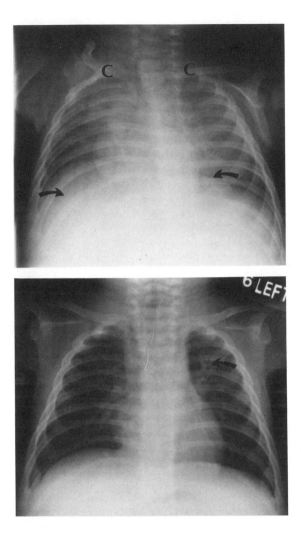

FIGURE 2. This demonstrates the effect of poor quality radiographs as the patient is rotated and captured during expiration. The asymmetry of the clavicles (C) and the terminus of the anterior portion of the ribs (arrows) are important clues in recognizing a rotated chest radiograph. Also note that the heart appears larger and the lungs more opaque in expiration. At bottom, the same patient's chest radiograph, taken with proper technique, demonstrates a small left upper lobe area of consolidation consistent with pneumonia (arrow).

artery. The aortic arch and descending aorta normally are located to the left of the midline and often can be seen "through" the left portion of the mediastinal shadow. Figures 1–5 depict the relationships of the cardiac structures.

Important in proper chest x-ray interpretation is determining whether the patient is rotated and whether the film is appropriately exposed. Comparing the ribs and clavicles can confirm the presence or absence of a rotated film. The anterior portion of the ribs should "end" at about the same region in the thorax on the right and left. The two clavicles should have similar configurations. Failure to recognize rotation may result in the inappropriate labeling of normal structures as "abnormal." Rotated and nonrotated chest radiographs are compared in Figure 2. Proper exposure can be checked by examining the thoracic spine through the mediastinal structures. Disk spaces should be readily seen and the pulmonary vessels visualized in the medial third of both sides of the chest.[3]

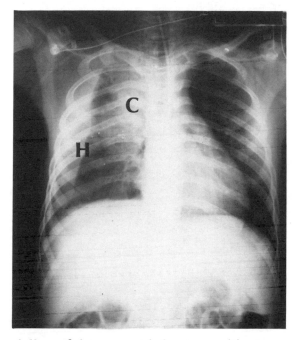

FIGURE 3.   Chest radiograph of a gunshot victim shows a hemothorax (H) in the right chest. The increased density in the upper right lung represents pulmonary contusion (C). Also note the bullet fragments and position of the nasogastric tube.

The lateral view can be especially useful to accurately locate opacities (e.g., pneumonia) hidden in the PA view and to view the heart structures. Usually the tracheal air column anteriorly and air in the esophagus posteriorly are seen on the lateral view. The leaflets of the diaphragm arch from their more distal attachment posteriorly to more proximal anteriorly. The right diaphragm is typically more superior than the left and usually can be seen in its entirety.[2] The posterior portion of the heart on this view is mainly left atrium.

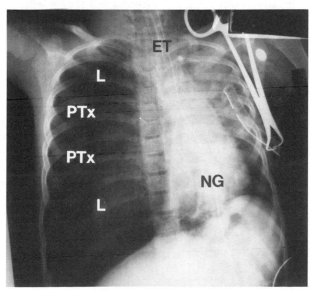

FIGURE 4.   Chest radiograph demonstrating a right tension pneumothorax (PTx) after evacuation of the left pneumothorax with a chest tube. Note the edge of the lung (L) in contrast to the air density and absence of pulmonary markings in the area of the pneumothorax. A shift of the mediastinum to the left chest is indicated by the heart position as well as the nasogastric (NG) and endotracheal (ET) tube positions.

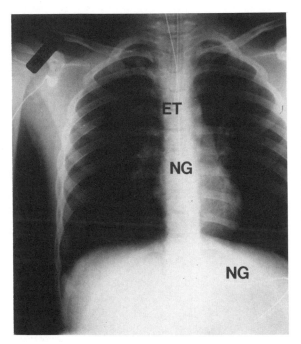

FIGURE 5. Chest radiograph of an intubated patient. Note the position of the endotracheal (ET) and naso-gastric (NG) tubes. The lungs show symmetric aeration and normal cardiac structures. This patient was intubated to assist in the management of a head injury.

Structures outside the chest also should be examined. The chest radiograph may reveal neck-related diagnoses such as an ingested foreign body or croup, abdominal conditions such as a perforated hollow viscus (with free air underneath the diaphragm in the upright chest film), or a markedly distended stomach (which may need to be decompressed prior to transport to help prevent emesis).

Although the presentation and diagnosis of specific pediatric and neonatal conditions are discussed elsewhere in this text, examples of specific findings on the chest radiograph are outlined in Figures 6–9.

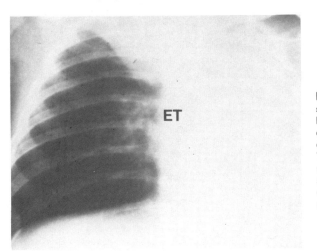

FIGURE 6. Chest radiograph shows marked density in the left lung with loss of volume. The endotracheal tube (ET) is located down the right mainstem bronchus. There is also collapse of the right upper lobe. Areas of collapse resolved after pulling back the endotracheal tube to proper position above the carina.

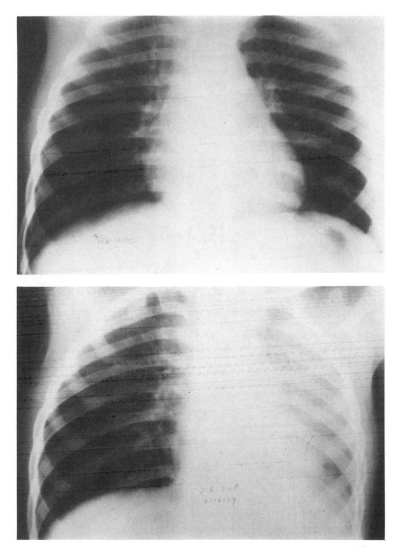

FIGURE 7. Posteroanterior chest radiographs during inspiration (top) and expiration (bottom). Note the asymmetric deflation of the right (less deflation) compared with the left (normal deflation) lung during expiration. This patient had aspirated a peanut, which was removed from the right bronchus during bronchoscopy. (From Fleisher GR, Ludwig S (eds): Textbook of Pediatric Emergency Medicine, 3rd ed. Baltimore, Williams & Wilkins, 1993, p 213, with permission.)

HEAD

Plain x-ray studies of the head are used less frequently than in the past since the advent of head CT scanning and its nearly ubiquitous availability. However, skull films are still often obtained in the trauma victim and can be particularly confusing in the pediatric patient because of growing bones and numerous suture lines. Some of the normal sutures, including the sagittal, coronal, lambdoidal, and squamosal-temporal, are shown in Figures 10 and 11. Normal suture lines may be misinterpreted as fractures. A typical nondisplaced linear skull fracture in an infant is shown in Figure 10. A skull fracture should alert one

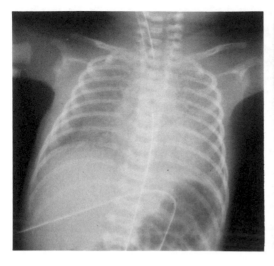

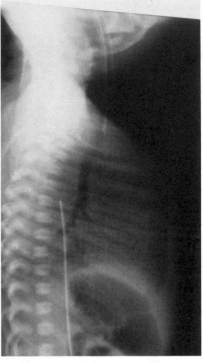

FIGURE 8. Anteroposterior (left) and lateral (right) chest radiographs of a premature infant demonstrate typical "ground glass" appearance of the lungs seen in hyaline membrane disease. The airways are especially well seen on the lateral view. Also note the normal position of the "high" umbilical artery catheter and the endotracheal tube.

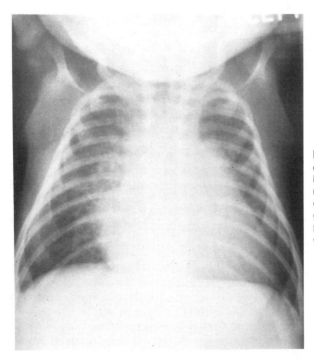

FIGURE 9. Chest radiograph demonstrates cardiomegaly with increased density in the perihilar region consistent with pulmonary congestion. This infant was in congestive heart failure secondary to prolonged supraventricular tachycardia.

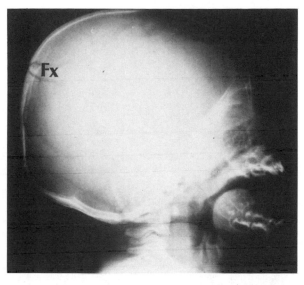

FIGURE 10. A linear skull fracture (Fx) in an infant, extending across the midline and involving the posterior portion of both parietal bones. This fracture was the result of nonaccidental trauma. Some of the normal sutures in the small child are labeled in Figure 11.

to the possibility of intracranial injury; it does indicate a significant traumatic event, but is an inadequate screen for intracranial injury. Transport personnel should not be reassured by normal skull x-ray studies if the clinical condition or history suggests more serious brain injury.

Accurate diagnosis of a depressed skull fracture has direct neurosurgical implications. Depressed skull fractures frequently need operative repair. Head CT scanning may be used to delineate further the degree of depression, the extent of the fracture, or the presence of underlying brain injury or hemorrhage. A depressed skull fracture is seen in Figure 11.

HEAD COMPUTED TOMOGRAPHY

Computed tomography has become the modality of choice for accurate examination of the head trauma victim. It clearly identifies intracranial hemorrhage and swelling and the relationships between neuroanatomic structures. It also detects most, but not all, skull fractures and determines more accurately the depth of a depressed fracture. Transport personnel are frequently presented with CT scans, and some familiarity with typical injury patterns is useful. Specific lesions that are discussed here include epidural, subdural, and intraparenchymal hemorrhage and swelling. In addition, intraventricular hemorrhage (although more frequently diagnosed by ultrasonography) is also discussed.

When CT scans are used for the evaluation of head injury, they usually are completed without contrast material. Such nonenhanced CT scans clearly demonstrate blood collections. The immediate goal of the initial head CT scan is to identify blood collection or internal injury that requires medical or surgical intervention. One view from a normal CT scan is shown in Figure 12.

An epidural hematoma is a localized, lenticular collection of blood (Fig. 13). The epidural blood is usually of arterial origin, but hematomas occurring in the infratentorial region are often venous. These are most common in children under the age of 2 years. Although they occur only in 1–2% of head injuries, they are responsible for approximately 15% of deaths, owing to rapid onset, lack of recognition, or lack of intervention.[4] Rapid medical intervention can stabilize these patients until temporizing or definitive surgical therapy occurs.

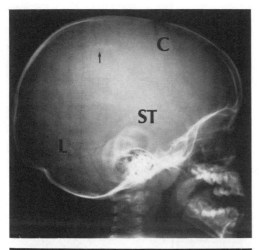

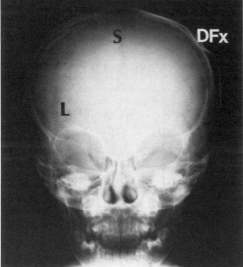

FIGURE 11. Lateral view (top) shows a depressed skull fracture in a child (arrow). The findings of increased density of overlapping bone are subtle on this view. The depression (DFx) is clearly seen on the frontal view (bottom). Some of the normal sutures in the small child are labeled as sagittal (S), coronal (C), lambdoidal (L), and squamosal-temporal (ST).

A subdural hematoma is a crescent-shaped collection of venous blood (Fig. 14) that originates from the bridging veins between the dura and the arachnoid. A subdural hematoma usually signifies more severe CNS injury than does an epidural hematoma. These are seen often in younger children; combined with a suspicious history, they may lead one to suspect nonaccidental trauma.[4,5] Once a subdural hematoma is identified, rapid medical and neurosurgical intervention is imperative. Differentiating this blood collection from the epidural may be a critical point when notifying the neurosurgical consultant prior to the arrival of the transport patient.

Intraparenchymal hemorrhage can occur from closed head injury but occurs less often than the previously mentioned intracranial hemorrhages. These hematomas often are not amenable to surgical therapy but should alert the transport team to the potential severity of the head injury and the possible need for aggressive medical intervention.

Intraventricular hemorrhages also are seen secondary to trauma but are seen more often in the premature infant in the first week of life.[5] They also are not

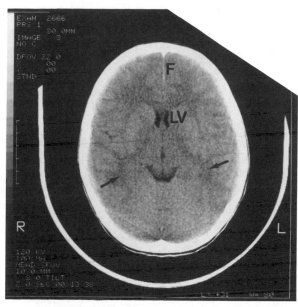

FIGURE 12.   A normal cut from a CT scan of the head. Note the symmetry of the brain structures, midposition of the midline structures such as the falx (F), the lateral ventricles (LV) of similar dimensions, and the easily differentiated gray-white matter interface (arrows).

usually amenable to immediate surgical removal, although they may lead to obstruction of CSF drainage and eventually require ventriculoperitoneal shunting. These can be diagnosed readily by ultrasound obtained through an open fontanel. Interpretation of the ultrasound study by a physician should be accomplished before transport team review.

Diffuse cerebral edema may result from a hypoxic episode or diffuse trauma. Although usually not seen in less then 24 hours after an anoxic or traumatic event, cerebral edema occasionally may be evident on CT scan within the first

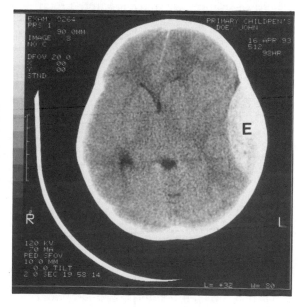

FIGURE 13.   A large epidural hematoma (E) in the temporal-parietal region of the brain. This radiograph demonstrates the typical lenticular shape of the epidural hematoma. Note also the mass effect with a shift of midline structures to the contralateral side and obliteration of the ventricle on the side of the hematoma.

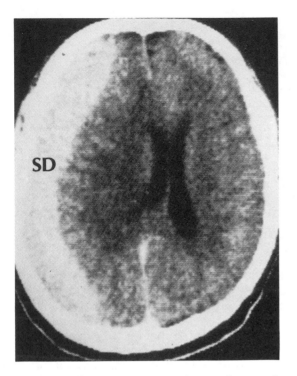

FIGURE 14. CT scan shows a very large subdural (SD) hematoma. Note the difference in shape between this intracranial hemorrhage and the one depicted in Figure 13. The subdural hemorrhage more closely follows the contour of the brain surface. There is also significant shift of structures to the contralateral side as the right lateral ventricle is pushed to the left.

few hours.[5] These CT scans show a decreased gray/white matter interface and an ablation of ventricular system structures in contrast to what is depicted in the normal CT scan in Figure 12.

NECK TRAUMA

In the trauma victim proper interpretation of cervical spine radiographs is critical. However, for the transport team, c-spine immobilization should continue until a more complete evaluation can be performed. Despite this cautionary word, since most transported trauma victims will have had c-spine radiographs, some understanding of their interpretation and limitations is essential.

The cervical spine should never be cleared radiographically with a single lateral cervical spine view. The sensitivity of this single view is only approximately 82%. A three-view radiographic series (with anteroposterior and odontoid views added) raises the fracture identification sensitivity to 93%.[6] The lateral radiograph, however, is the most common initial view and should show any persistent distortion, distraction, or cervical spine abnormality (Fig. 15). The study should be evaluated systematically, initially ensuring that the complete cervical spine is shown. This means that the C7–T1 junction should be visible on the film. The radiograph is then reviewed by applying the ABCs approach. The ABCs stand for alignment, bones, cartilage, and soft tissue and are reviewed in that order.

Normal alignment will be demonstrated by four lordotic curves: the anterior spinal line; the posterior spinal line; the spinolaminal line; and the spinous process tips (Fig. 16). It is important to remember that the spinal cord is housed between the posterior cervical line and the spinolaminal line and that any bony impingement into that space suggests spinal cord injury. Children who are in cervical collars, on a spine board (secondary to a large occiput), are less than

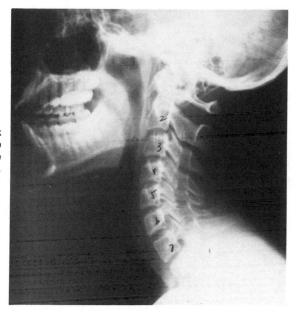

FIGURE 15. Normal lateral neck radiograph. All 7 cervical vertebrae (numbered) should be visualized. Note the normal lordotic curve of the spine.

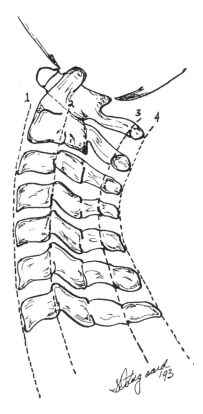

FIGURE 16. Lordotic curves used to assure normal alignment on the lateral c-spine radiograph. The lines are the anterior spinal line (1), the posterior spinal line (2), the spinolaminal line (3), and the spinous process tips (4). (From APLS: The Pediatric Emergency Course, AAP, ACEP, 2nd ed, p 108, with permission.)

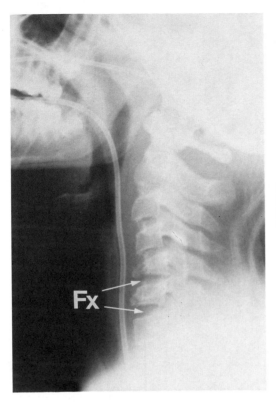

FIGURE 17.   Cervical spine radiograph in a 12-year-old bike accident victim shows several fractures (Fx) and abnormal alignment.

6 years old, have neck muscle spasm or a cervical spine injury may not demonstrate lordosis, but the cervical alignment should still be intact.

Bones are then reviewed, looking for obvious fractures or distorted relationships between the adjacent bones. Cartilage is present in abundance in the pediatric cervical spine secondary to multiple growth plates and developing bone. Unfortunately, cartilage is radiolucent on x-ray, so that fractures or dislocations can occur without direct radiographic evidence. A fracture involving the cervical vertebrae with malalignment is shown in Figure 17.

Evaluation of the soft tissue also is important. Increased size of the prevertebral space suggests blood or edema in that space secondary to underlying bone, cartilage, or ligamentous injury. One can be fooled in a child, however, by the routine variability (enlargement) of this space during expiration, crying, or neck flexion.[7,8] A true abnormality in the prevertebral space should be reproducible on repeat radiographs. The use of naso/orogastric tubes or endotracheal tubes may alter the relationships of the prevertebral space. The prevertebral space should be less than one-half to two-thirds the width of the adjacent vertebral body at levels above the glottis.[7,8] This space will double below the glottis owing to the typically airless esophagus.

A common misdiagnosis in the pediatric cervical spine is pathologic subluxation of C2 on C3.[7] It is important to remember that the cervical spine of a child has more anterior/posterior movement than an adult and that up to 4.5 mm of anterior overlap can occur with C2 on C3 and still be normal. A useful diagnostic tool to distinguish between a normal (pseudosubluxation) and abnormal C2/C3 relationship is to use the posterior cervical line depicted in

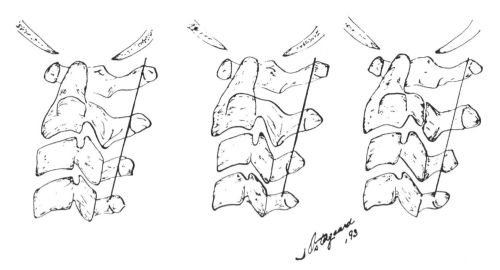

FIGURE 18. In children less than 8 years old, there may be an apparent subluxation of C2 on C3. This pseudosubluxation can be tested by checking the alignment of the lateral portion of the posterior spinous process. A line drawn between C1 and C3 should come within 1–2 mm of the lateral process of the posterior spinous process (From APLS: The Pediatric Emergency Course, AAP, ACEP, 2nd ed., 1993, p 112, with permission.)

Figure 18. A line is drawn from the cortex of the spinous process of C1 to the cortex of the spinous process of C3, and the relationship noted between the line and the cortex of the spinous process of C2. If the line passes through or within 2 mm of the cortex of the spinous process of C2, this is considered normal. If the distance is greater than 2 mm, one should be suspicious of a fracture causing the overlap of C2 on C3. This technique should be used only to evaluate anterior overlap (subluxation) of C2 on C3.

CT scans sometimes are performed as part of the cervical spine evaluation. If the providers are concerned enough to do a CT scan of a potentially injured cervical spine, then mobilization and transport care should not be influenced by the transport team's evaluation of the CT scan. It can be argued that transport team evaluation of a cervical CT scan before transport would serve only to delay the patient's arrival at the definitive treatment center and should not be attempted.

It is important to remember that children may have normal cervical spine radiographs and still have significant spinal cord damage. This syndrome is known as SCIWORA (spinal cord injury without radiographic abnormality).[9] This should reinforce to the transport team members that spinal immobilization should almost always be maintained during transport with or without radiographic changes consistent with cervical spine damage.

NECK (NONTRAUMA)

The patient presenting with acute upper airway compromise is anxiety-provoking even for experienced practitioners. The potential for complete obstruction and respiratory arrest makes accurate diagnosis and appropriate intervention essential. Soft tissue neck radiographs are obtained frequently in patients with symptoms such as hoarseness, drooling, barking cough, and stridor in association with respiratory distress and fever. Since different etiologies of upper airway obstruction suggest varied management strategies, proper interpretation of some common pediatric conditions affecting the neck region is imperative.

The normal lateral soft tissue neck study should be obtained during inspiration in a true lateral position with the neck slightly extended. This should show the easily recognized mouth structures, nasopharynx, and the air column including the hypopharynx, vocal cord, and subglottic region. In the normal individual, and of particular importance, the air column is nontapering. The air column is "shouldered" at the vocal cords on the AP view.[10] The normal configuration of the epiglottis and the narrow prevertebral space are shown in Figure 19. If the lateral soft-tissue radiograph is obtained with the neck flexed or during expiration, the soft tissue structures will be misrepresented and likely misinterpreted as abnormal. The radiographic findings in croup, epiglottitis, and retropharyngeal abscess are discussed below.

Croup, or viral laryngotracheobronchitis, causes upper airway swelling and the typical clinical presentation with stridor, barking cough, and respiratory distress. The findings on plain x-ray studies include normal epiglottis and retropharyngeal space, normal or distended hypopharynx, and narrowing of the airway distal to the vocal cords. The typical (normal) shouldering at the level of the glottis in the AP view is replaced by a more gradual widening to the normal tracheal diameter as the air progresses distally. This is referred to as "steepling" because of the resemblance to a church steeple.[11,12] Soft tissue neck radiographs in a patient with croup are shown in Figure 20.

Epiglottitis is a bacterial infection, usually caused by *Haemophilus influenzae*, affecting the epiglottic and the supraglottic region. The potential for sudden and complete upper airway obstruction is greater than in the other conditions discussed here. To determine if the epiglottis is normal, the following routine may be employed: (1) trace the anterior border of the trachea beginning inferiorly up to the level of the epiglottis (the posterior border of the epiglottis); (2) trace the contour of the tongue inferiorly into the vallecula to define the anterior

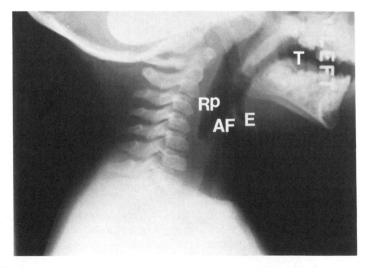

FIGURE 19.   Lateral view of normal soft-tissue structures in the neck, including epiglottis (E), aryepiglottic folds (AF), tongue (T), and retropharyngeal soft tissue (RP).

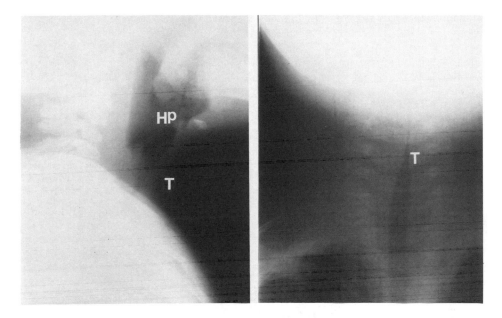

FIGURE 20. Typical radiographic findings in patients with croup include narrowing of the trachea (T) below the glottis on the lateral view (left) and the classic "steeple" sign on the AP view (right). Note also the distended hypopharynx (HP).

border of the epiglottis. Usually the epiglottis is only a few millimeters wide—a widened epiglottis suggests epiglottitis. In addition, the aryepiglottic folds will be enlarged and the vallecula small or obliterated.[13,14] The typical findings of epiglottitis are shown in Figure 21.

A retropharyngeal abscess shares some of the clinical features of croup and epiglottitis. The infection and swelling occur behind the pharynx and hypopharynx, presenting as widening of the prevertebral soft tissues (Fig. 22).[15,16] Improper technique in obtaining the lateral neck radiograph (neck is flexed or poor inspiration) will also lead, falsely, to this finding.

ABDOMINAL RADIOGRAPHS

Abdominal x-ray studies tend to be difficult to interpret and require a fair amount of experience. On the other hand, many of the radiographic findings are relatively nonspecific, even in surgical conditions such as appendicitis or intussusception. The image of the abdomen varies dramatically with the amount of gas present and the disease process. Unlike chest films, the examiner does not have a symmetry to aid the interpretation, and many normal abdominal radiographs may look remarkably different. From a practical standpoint, transport personnel are most often concerned with mechanical bowel obstruction (e.g., volvulus, intussusception), paralytic ileus (e.g., gastroenteritis), bowel perforation, congenital anomalies (often leading to obstruction), and necrotizing enterocolitis.

As with the chest radiograph, the abdominal study is not restricted to organs within the cavity but also examines the bony structures and regions outside the abdomen. Useful information about the chest may also be found on abdominal films. When examining the abdominal radiograph, attempt to locate GI

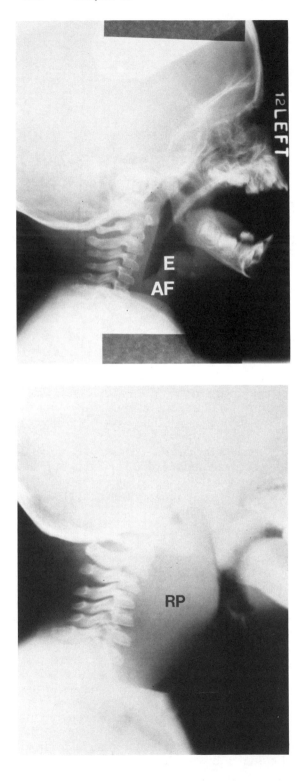

FIGURE 21. This lateral neck view shows the findings typical of epiglottitis. There is a widened epiglottic shadow (E) and swelling of the aryepiglottic folds (AF).

FIGURE 22. Lateral neck radiograph depicting the markedly increased retropharyngeal space (RP) in this patient with a retropharyngeal abscess. Compare this with normal soft-tissue lateral neck in Figure 17.

structures that have relatively stable locations and define solid organs. This would include locating the stomach, rectum, hepatic and splenic flexure of the large bowel, spleen, liver, kidneys, and bladder. This type of orderly or structured approach to the abdominal radiograph will provide a framework where increased exposure to such films will enhance interpretation skills. Some structures, such as the kidney and psoas shadow, will be seen less clearly in neonates and infants owing to lack of perinephric or retroperitoneal fat.[17] A normal abdominal series is shown in Figure 23.

The typical abdominal series offers two views. Most often these are supine and upright views. This enables the examiner to see the location and character- istics of the abdominal contents both with and without the effect of gravity. This is especially important in differentiating obstructive patterns from simple distention. Sometimes a lateral decubitus film or a cross-table radiograph may be substituted for the upright view. Unfortunately, in the critically ill or injured patient the transport team may not have the benefit of both views.

Although definitve diagnosis for bowel obstruction often requires further GI studies with air or barium, routine abdominal radiographs may provide clues about the etiology. This is especially true in the neonate, in whom some gas patterns are characteristic of certain types of congenital anomalies that frequently cause bowel obstruction (e.g., duodenal or jejunal atresia). In children 6 months to 6 years, intussusception is the most common cause of abdominal obstruction, whereas appendicitis plays a more prominent role in the older child.[18]

It is important for transport personnel to recognize abdominal gas patterns. Marked gastric distention, regardless of cause, unnecessarily puts the patient at risk for vomiting and aspiration (especially during air transport) and should always lead to consideration of naso/orogastric tube placement for proper stomach ventilation (Fig. 24). Failure to recognize the pattern of bowel obstruction not only places the patient at risk of vomiting and aspiration but also bowel perforation. In these instances, gastric ventilation is mandatory.

A few abnormal gas patterns on the abdominal x-ray should be discussed. These include the paralytic ileus, mechanical ileus, and the gasless pattern. In the gasless abdomen there may be no GI gas, or gas only in the stomach. It is the easiest to recognize and may be due to such relatively minor causes as acute gastroenteritis or to such surgical conditions as appendicitis. In paralytic ileus there is distention throughout the GI tract, with gas-filled, multiple, disorganized, dilated loops of bowel, and air-fluid levels on the upright view. This may occur in gastroenteritis as well but also can be seen in such systemic conditions as sepsis or spinal shock. The pattern of mechanical obstruction differs in that the dilated loops are more organized—sometimes even stacked—and fewer loops tend to be seen. The loops can make sharp turns on the upright view, and fluid levels tend to be at different heights on each end of the loop.[19,20] (See Figs. 23 and 25 for comparison.)

SKELETAL TRAUMA

Fractures in the transport patient infrequently have a major effect on treatment, with the exceptions mentioned previously (rib and skull fractures). Pelvic fractures, however, may signify major abdominal/pelvic trauma and can cause significant blood loss. Femur fractures infrequently cause significant blood loss in the pediatric patient, although they serve as an important marker of significant force involved in the injury. In the newborn, the most common long bone fractue involves the clavicle and is almost universally inconsequential.

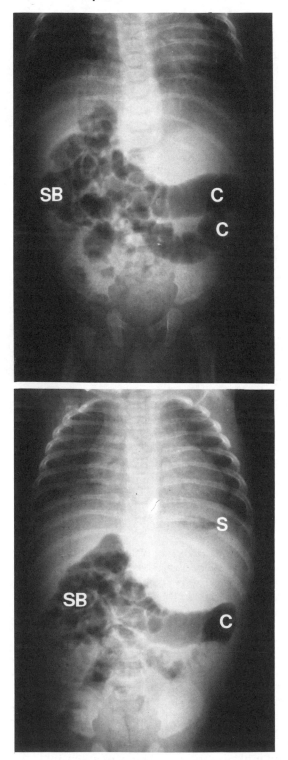

FIGURE 23. Normal two-view (supine, top, and upright, bottom) abdominal series. Note the relative distribution of gas. Gas is seen in the stomach (S), small bowel (SB), and colon (C). There is no significant bowel distention, and no air fluid levels in the upright film.

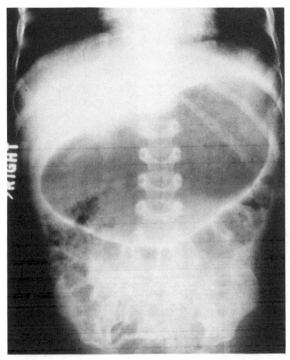

FIGURE 24. Abdominal view shows marked distention of the stomach. This may be seen in trauma patients with crying and increased air swallowing or in patients following bag-mask ventilation. Significant gastric distention increases the likelihood of emesis, limits interpretation of the abdominal examination, and can inhibit respiration.

Extremity fractures are encountered frequently in the trauma victim. For the most part, proper stabilization and immobilization are all that is required for the duration of transport. Only occasionally will neurovascular injury mandate fracture reduction or operative treatment prior to transport. There are important differences in biomechanics between the bone of a child and that of an adult.[21] These differences do allow for different types of fractures and fractures that involve areas unique to growing bone.[22,23] From a radiographic standpoint, transport personnel need only a working understanding of fracture description.

Fracture description can be divided into several parts. These include identifying the bone or bones involved, location on the bone, fracture type, proper description of the fragment relationships, and whether the fracture is open or closed.[23,24] A complete description should succinctly include all areas mentioned above. Once a fracture is noted, the search for additional injuries should not cease. This is especially true when considering injuries to the distal arm and leg, since there may be another fracture and/or dislocation present as well. A forearm fracture involving both the radius and ulna is shown in Figure 27.

Proper identification of bones involved usually is not difficult. In adults and teens, without growth plates, the fracture location with a long bone is usually identified by dividing the bone into thirds (e.g., "oblique fracture of the distal third of the femur, not involving the joint"). In children, some familiarity with the anatomy of the growing bone is needed to identify properly the growth plate (physis), epiphysis, metaphysis, and diaphysis. The anatomy of a growing long bone is pictured in Figure 28.

Fracture *type* should be noted next. Several common fracture types are shown in Figure 29. Fractures relatively unique to children include the buckle or torus fracture, the greenstick fracture, and the bowing or plastic fracture.[21,23,24]

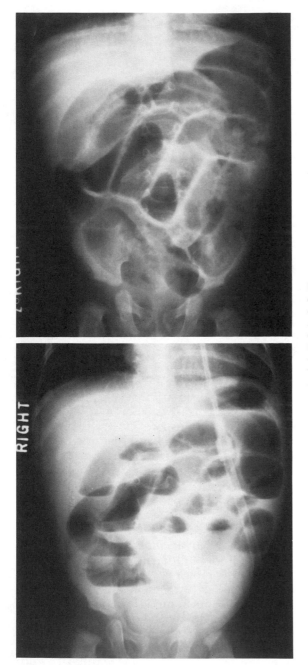

FIGURE 25. This two-view study of the abdomen shows findings typical of small bowel obstruction. In the supine view (top), note the marked distention of the loops of bowel, layered pattern, and absence of colon gas or air in the rectum. In the upright view (bottom), note the prominent air-fluid levels.

It is a frequent misconception that *all* pediatric fractures should be classified according to the Salter-Harris system. This classification is only for fractures involving the growth plate (physis)[25] and is shown schematically in Figure 30. An example of a Salter type II fracture of the distal tibia is shown in Figure 31.

Next, attention should be focused on the fragment relationships. This is often an area of confusion. Fractures involving the growth plate may occur with

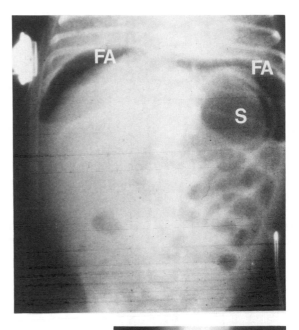

FIGURE 26. Free air (FA) beneath the diaphragm and above the stomach suggests perforation of a hollow viscus and a surgical emergency.

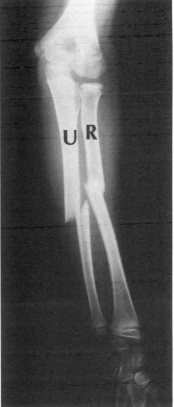

FIGURE 27. Forearm fracture involving both the radius (R) and ulna (U). See text for proper fracture description.

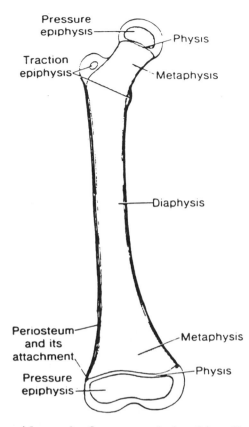

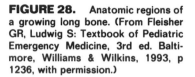

FIGURE 28. Anatomic regions of a growing long bone. (From Fleisher GR, Ludwig S: Textbook of Pediatric Emergency Medicine, 3rd ed. Baltimore, Williams & Wilkins, 1993, p 1236, with permission.)

or without the fragment relationships discussed next. Displacement refers to movement away from the line of the long axis of the bone and may occur with or without angulation. This is usually described as a percentage of width of the bone. Angulation is used to describe the amount the bone is "bent" at the fracture line. Typically the distal fragment is described in terms of the proximal fragment. As an example, if the distal portion of the radius is angled toward the palmar aspect of the hand in relation to the proximal fragment, this would be referred to as "anterior" or "ventral" angulation. Distraction implies that fragments are pulled apart in the long axis, while shortening connotes the opposite effect. A transverse fracture would have to be 100% displaced to be shortened. Examples of these fragment relationships are shown in Figure 32. As an example, the fracture in Figure 27 could be described as "closed, diaphyseal fractures of the radius and ulna. The transverse radial fracture is shortened and shows 15° of lateral angulation. The oblique ulnar fracture is displaced 80% laterally." The radiograph usually does not reveal whether the fracture is open or closed (an open fracture implies bone exposure to the environment during and/or following the injury) unless the bone clearly protrudes beyond skin shadows. This distinction is made by visual inspection and identification of wounds in the area of the fracture.

CONCLUSION

This chapter presents information to aid transport personnel in radiologic interpretation. The reader is referred to radiology textbooks (listed in the

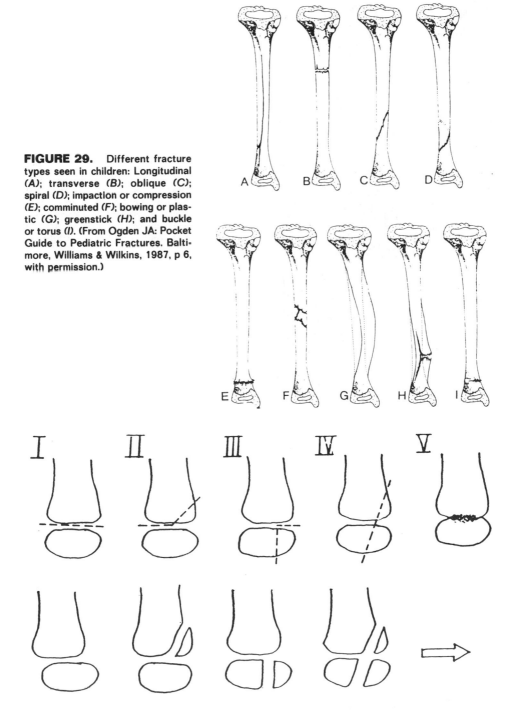

FIGURE 29. Different fracture types seen in children: Longitudinal *(A)*; transverse *(B)*; oblique *(C)*; spiral *(D)*; impaction or compression *(E)*; comminuted *(F)*; bowing or plastic *(G)*; greenstick *(H)*; and buckle or torus *(I)*. (From Ogden JA: Pocket Guide to Pediatric Fractures. Baltimore, Williams & Wilkins, 1987, p 6, with permission.)

FIGURE 30. Salter-Harris classification types I-V (without displacement) for fractures involving the growth plate. The bottom row shows fracture types I-IV with displacement in the direction indicated by the arrow.

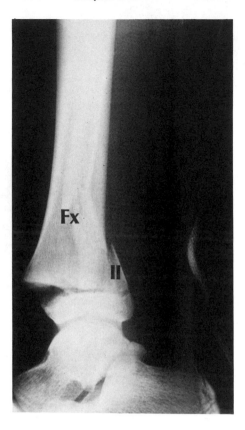

FIGURE 31. Lateral view of the ankle showing a Salter II fracture (II) of the distal tibia (with posterior displacement) and a greenstick fracture (Fx) of the distal fibula. (From Fleisher GR, Ludwig S: Textbook of Pediatric Emergency Medicine, 3rd ed. Baltimore, William & Wilkins, 1993, p 1239, with permission.)

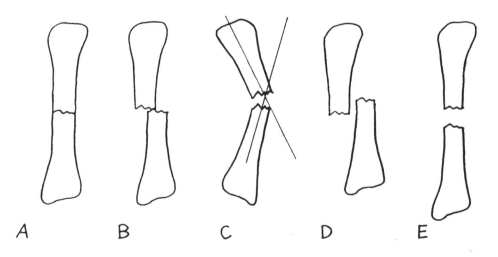

FIGURE 32. Typical fragment relationships in more complicated fractures. From the left: normal alignment (A); displacement (B); angulation (C); shortening (with complete displacement) (D); and distraction (E). Though not depicted, fractures may also be rotated.

references) for more complete discussion of all topics. In the context of the pediatric/neonatal transport patient, a basic framework for the interpretation of chest, head, neck, abdominal, and extremity radiographs will enhance the level of care provided by the transport team.

REFERENCES

1. Swischuk LE: Normal chest, normal variation and artifacts, tracheal buckling. In Swischuk LE: Imaging of the Newborn, Infant, and Child, 3rd ed. Baltimore, Williams & Wilkins, 1989, p 7.
2. Swischuk LE: Looking for pneumonia; know your normal chest first. In Swischuk LE: Emergency Imaging of the Acutely Ill or Injured Child, 3rd ed. Baltimore, Williams & Wilkins, 1994, pp 27–35.
3. Hedlund GL, Kirks DR: Chest: Ordered approach. In Kirks DR (ed): Practical Pediatric Imaging, Diagnostic Radiology of Infants and Children, 2nd ed. Boston, Little, Brown, 1991, pp 523–528.
4. Jellinger K: The neuropathology of pediatric head injuries. In Shapiro K (ed): Pediatric Head Trauma. Mount Kisco, Futura, 1983, pp 143–194.
5. Bruce D: Head injuries in the pediatric population. Curr Probl (February):66–107, 1990.
6. Streitwieser D, Knopp R, Wale L, et al: Accuracy of standard radiographic views in detecting cervical spine fractures. (July 15):74–87, 1983.
7. Swischuk LE: The spine and spinal cord. In Swischuk LE: Emergency Radiology of the Acutely Ill or Injured Child, 2nd ed. Baltimore, Williams & Wilkins, 1986, pp 556–609.
8. Fesmire F, Luten R: The pediatric cervical spine: Developmental anatomy and clinical aspects. J Emerg Med 7:133–142, 1989.
9. Pang D, Pollack I: Spinal cord injury without radiographic abnormality in children—the SCIWORA syndrome. J Trauma 29:654–664, 1989.
10. Swischuk LE: Normal anatomy of the upper airway. In Swischuk LE: Emergency Imaging of the Acutely Ill or Injured Child, 3rd ed. Baltimore, Williams & Wilkins, 1994, pp 151.
11. Fleisher GR: Infectious disease emergencies, laryngotracheobronchitis. In Fleisher GR, Ludwig S (eds): Textbook of Pediatric Emergency Medicine, 3rd ed. Baltimore, Williams & Wilkins, 1993, pp 615–617.
12. Swischuk LE: Upper airway obstruction and acute stridor, croup. In Swischuk LE: Emergency Imaging of the Acutely Ill or Injured Child, 3rd ed. Baltimore, Williams & Wilkins, 1994, pp 158–164.
13. Fleisher GR: Infectious disease emergencies, epiglottitis. In Fleisher GR, Ludwig S (eds): Textbook of Pediatric Emergency Medicine, 3rd ed. Baltimore, Williams & Wilkins, 1993, pp 617–621.
14. Swischuk LE: Upper airway obstruction and acute stridor, epiglottitis. In Swischuk LE: Emergency Imaging of the Acutely Ill or Injured Child, 3rd ed. Baltimore, Williams & Wilkins, 1994, pp 155–158.
15. Swischuk LE: Retropharyngeal abscess. In Swischuk LE: Emergency Imaging of the Acutely Ill or Injured Child, 3rd ed. Baltimore, Williams & Wilkins, 1994, pp 171–174.
16. Fleisher GR: Infectious disease emergencies, retropharyngeal abscess. In Fleisher GR, Ludwig S (eds): Textbook of Pediatric Emergency Medicine, 3rd ed. Baltimore, Williams & Wilkins, 1993, pp 614–615.
17. Swischuk LE: Abdomen. In Swischuk LE: Imaging of the Newborn, Infant, and Young Child. Baltimore, Williams & Wilkins, 1989, pp 550–552.
18. Shandling B: Intussusception. In Behrman RE, Kliegman RM, Nelson WE, Vaughan VC (eds): Nelson Textbook of Pediatrics, 14th ed. Philadelphia, W.B. Saunders, 1992, pp 958–959.
19. Swischuk LE: Abnormal intraluminal gas patterns. In Swischuk LE: Emergency Imaging of the Acutely Ill or Injured Child, 3rd ed. Baltimore, Williams & Wilkins, 1994, pp 187–197.
20. Kirks DR, Caron KH: Intestinal obstruction. In Kirks DR (ed): Practical Pediatric Imaging, Diagnostic Radiology of Infants and Children, 2nd ed. Boston, Little, Brown, 1991, pp 730–732.
21. Rang M: Children are not just small adults. In Rang M (ed): Children's Fractures, 2nd ed. Philadelphia, J.B. Lippincott, 1983, pp 1–9.
22. Rang M: Injuries to the epiphysis, the growth plate, and the perichondrial ring. In Rang M (ed): Children's Fractures, 2nd ed. Philadelphia, J.B. Lippincott, 1983, pp 10–20.
23. Bachman D, Santora S: Orthopedic trauma, general principles of pediatric orthopedics. In Fleisher GR, Ludwig S (eds): Textbook of Pediatric Emergency Medicine, 3rd ed. Baltimore, Williams & Wilkins, 1993, pp 1236–1241.
24. Ogden JA: Pocket Guide to Pediatric Fractures. Baltimore, Williams & Wilkins, 1987, pp 1–10.
25. Salter RB, Harris WR: Injuries involving the epiphyseal plate. J Bone Joint Surg 45:587–622, 1963.

Transport Equipment and Techniques

MELODY YOUNG, R.N.
CINDY O'BOYLE, R.N.
DAVID G. JAIMOVICH, M.D.

The equipment needed to provide the highest level of care during the transport of critically ill infants and children includes a wide range of components and medications. The equipment should be complete and adequate to provide continuing intensive care throughout the transport. The equipment must be dedicated to the treatment of critically ill patients, regardless of whether the team is dedicated to transport or a part of a pediatric or neonatal intensive care unit. The operation and maintenance of the equipment should be the sole responsibility of the transport team.

Portable monitoring equipment should be capable of measuring heart rate, respiratory rate, blood pressure (invasively and noninvasively), arterial saturation by pulse oximetry, and temperature. Because a large proportion of transported infants and children have respiratory problems and oxygen requirements, an oxygen analyzer should be available to assess the fraction of inspired oxygen (FiO_2).

Transport equipment should be appropriate in its size and weight, and it must be battery-powered, thereby capable of functioning independently of the electrical supply of both surface and air carriers for at least twice the anticipated transport time. All necessary parts and cables must be stored with the equipment because space limitation is a significant concern in the transport environment. Due to the nature of the transport environment, the equipment must be well-secured during the duration of the transport. This chapter discusses the various types of equipment necessary to care for a critically ill infant or child before and during transport.

In addition, critically ill infants and children may require, before or during transport, a variety of procedures to reach and maintain a point of stabilization before arrival at the tertiary care center. The decision to perform these procedures must be based on the child's immediate needs and not definitive treatment. This chapter attempts to cover a variety of these necessary procedures.

ELECTROCARDIOGRAM

Electrocardiographic (EKG) monitoring and the direct measurement of blood pressure have become standard practice during transports of critically ill patients. The EKG is used to detect electrical activity of cardiac muscle, and the device consists of a sensor system (electrodes), amplifier, and recorder.[19] Transducers are not needed because physiologic electrical activity is measured directly. Cardiac rhythms and dysrhythmias are monitored and utilized to determine the presence or absence of myocardial ischemia and/or dysfunction.

The EKG measures the electrical forces produced by the heart.[23] Cardiac cells generate electrical current by changing the charge distribution at their cell membrane. This transfer of electrical energy is detected by electrodes placed on the tissue whose electrical energy is to be measured.[19] Transport personnel must remember that the major goal of EKG tracing is to faithfully record and display the signal and to eliminate spurious or undesired signals (known as noise or artifact). Poor EKG quality is a common problem, especially during transports, but most of these problems can be corrected easily through understanding and optimizing the technique.

Proper preparation of the skin reduces the electrode resistance, thereby minimizing electrical noise and maximizing EKG signal. The skin site should first be cleansed with alcohol and then dried to provide good adhesion. Cleaning removes dead cells from the skin's surface, permitting the EKG signal to travel more efficiently to the electrode.

To reduce muscle and motion artifact, the electrodes should be placed over bony areas. During transport, however, proper lead placement may be impossible, depending on the patient's clinical state and possible thoracic involvement (e.g., chest tubes, thoracic trauma); therefore, arms and legs may be used in special situations. Muscle artifact, skin movement, and respiration also interfere with the EKG signals, compounding the motion created by the transport vehicle. When EKG tracings are questionable, the transport personnel must remember that the clinical assessment is essential in evaluating a patient's possible cardiac instability.

Another cause of artifact in pediatric and neonatal transport may be shivering from hypothermia. Therefore, it is important to maintain a euthermic environment within the transport isolette or with blankets over the small patient. Chest or abdominal wall movement due to respiration may cause artifact, but this can be minimized by repositioning the electrodes.

Electrodes used for monitoring are designed for single use only; and proper storage must be observed since the electrode gel may dry. Pre-gelled leads not stored properly can result in high-resistance skin contact, causing unstable monitor traces. Loose or eroded clips will result in poor contact between the lead wires and electrodes, increasing resistance and thereby interference. At times, simply disconnecting and reconnecting the cable between the lead wire and patient cable may improve the signal.

One must also consider the outside environment during the transport, as it can contribute to artifact and problems with EKG monitoring. One such source of environmental influence is power lines, which, depending on how close the power surface is to the transport vehicle, may result in artifact.

Adjusting the gain on the monitor will determine the size of the P wave and QRS complex. Setting the gain and amplitude of the electrical signal allows the monitor to compute the heart rate by sensing the signals. Some transport monitors have an automatic gain mechanism that can adjust the amplitude of the EKG complex internally, thereby maintaining a standard amplitude for the screen display or printout if available.

Alarms should be set for high and low limits at **10–15 beats** above and below the patient's heart rate. Alarms should always be on when the patient is attached to the monitor.

Provided that the lead placement is accurate and the monitor utilizes a suitable filtering circuit, the EKG may be recorded from the same electrodes that record respirations. Measuring electrodes are placed on either side of the chest, with the respiratory electrode placed on the manubrium or a suitable distant point. Oscilloscope display of the respiratory waveform often has a superimposed cardiac component that is easily identified if the EKG and respiratory waveforms are displayed on the same screen. The size of the respiratory waveform correlates with the depth of the patient's respirations, and the alarms are usually set to signal in the absence of respiration. The preset alarm limits are usually **6–11 seconds of apnea**, and therefore, this system may also be used as an apnea monitor.

The above-mentioned system has an incidence of 2% false-positive alarms for apnea and 0% false-negatives. The clinician must remember that even an obstructed airway may still show respiratory motion (chest wall activity), and alarms may not be triggered despite ineffective or absent respirations; therefore, clinical assessment is always the most dependable way to assess a patient's clinical state.[19] Always assess your patient by auscultation of breath sound and evaluation of the respiratory effort. One must also remember that the EKG monitor will detect bradycardia, which may be secondary to an apneic episode and thereby potentially life-threatening.

PULSE OXIMETRY

Pulse oximetry provides noninvasive, continuous information about the percentage of oxygen that is combined with hemoglobin. Pulse oximeters utilize two light-emitting diodes (LEDs) of given wavelengths: red light at approximately 660 nm and infrared light at approximately 920 nm.[21] A photodetector placed opposite these LEDs measures the intensity of transmitted light across an arterial vascular bed. The difference in the intensity of transmitted light at each wavelength is caused by the difference in the absorption of light by oxygenated and deoxygenated hemoglobin contained in the vascular bed. The determination of arterial hemoglobin saturation (SaO_2) is computed by the pulse oximeter from the amount transmitted to the photodetector.[21]

To provide reliable pulse oximetry data, it is necessary to ensure that the sensor, which contains the LEDs, is chosen and applied properly. The sensors are selected according to body weight, available application site, activity level, and expected duration of monitoring.[21] To decrease the risk of infection, disposable sensors are utilized. For proper placement, the LEDs and photodetector must be positioned directly across from each other on the chosen site with good skin contact.

Pulse oximetry is used more frequently in emergency departments and during transport for quick assessment of a patient's oxygenation state and respiratory compromise and to evaluate the response to respiratory treatments.[8] During transport, motion at the sensor site may be a problem. It can result in light absorption changes that seem like pulsatile activity. The photodetector is unable to differentiate, and therefore, inaccurately high or low values may be obtained. The transport team must be alert to this possibility when utilizing pulse oximetry.

Hypotension, hypothermia, and peripheral vasoconstriction are other clinical situations in which inaccurate measurements may occur. These situations cause a significant reduction in vascular pulsation, detected by a discrepancy between the oximeter heart rate measurement and the heart rate obtained by chest wall impedance, palpation, or auscultation.[2] Edema can scatter light from the

LEDs throughout the edematous tissue before reaching the photodetector. Positioning the sensor on nonedematous sites is suggested. However, if peripheral edema is extensive, a forehead reflectance sensor may be an acceptable alternative.

For reliable pulse oximetry readings, hemoglobin must be the dominant color species in the blood. In the case of severe anemia when hemoglobin values fall below 5 gm/dl, the pulse oximeter may be unable to provide reliable information. Adequate SaO_2 and adequate hemoglobin are necessary to estimate oxygen content accurately.[14] Different colors of nail polish (blues, greens, black, and brown-red) also have been known to interfere with the ability of the photodetector to measure light correctly.

The availability of pulse oximetry has improved the early detection of changes in systemic oxygenation, resulting in a more rapid response to adverse alterations and gas exchange.[2] Pulse oximetry is noninvasive and safe, and it can provide useful data if the health care provider is aware of the clinical and technical situations that can interfere with proper measurement. Pulse oximetry can provide misleading information. Because it detects only oxyhemoglobin and reduced hemoglobin, the presence of carboxyhemoglobin or methemoglobin may lead to overestimation of the true SaO_2.[7] Methemoglobin molecules are a type of dyshemoglobin, representing molecules that are unavailable for oxygen transport.[27] The body has an enzyme system to prevent the build-up of methemoglobin, but methemoglobinemia or endogenous build-up may result from inherited or acquired conditions. If acquired, it may be caused by exposure to certain medications, including nitrates, nitrites, phenacetin, pyridium, sulfonamides, and anilin dyes.[7]

OXYGEN-DELIVERY SYSTEMS

Indications for oxygen administration are to:
1. relieve hypoxemia
2. decrease the work of breathing
3. decrease myocardial work[26]

Many devices are available for use in infants and children, supplying varying concentrations of oxygen; however, the efficiency of any system depends on the child's acceptance and cooperation.[26]

When any of these devices is used on transport, some extra attention may be required to maintain the device and the cooperation of the child. Respiratory equipment can be one of the most important components of transport supplies. Depending on the composition of the transport teams, a respiratory therapist may or may not be present; therefore, all transport members must be familiar with the different oxygen delivery systems available.

Incubators. Closed incubators provide both oxygen and a stable thermal environment. Most incubator units are designed with air-entrainment devices, restricting the maximum FiO_2 within the unit to 0.4. Higher concentrations can be obtained by closing the air-entrainment port, allowing only oxygen to enter the incubator, and thus raising the FiO_2 up to 0.85 with the proper liter flow.[25]

Nasal Cannula. A nasal cannula is a vinyl catheter with two short prongs that fit into the nares. Oxygen gas flow enters through each prong. Nasal cannulation is useful in children who are capable of nasal breathing and require FiO_2 of ≤ 0.5. Maximum oxygen flow should not exceed 4–5 liters/min. Nasal cannulas are sometimes more comfortable than masks for children, and they can talk without altering FiO_2 delivery. One disadvantage is that when oxygen flow is too high, it may cause discomfort and drying of nasal musoca. Children who have upper respiratory disease may be mouth-breathing and reduce the effectiveness of the system.

Simple Mask. This simple vinyl mask fits over the child's nose and mouth. It has two open ports on each side to allow exhalation of carbon dioxide. These ports also allow the patient to draw in room air if gas flow in the mask does not meet peak inspiratory flow. The mask is fairly comfortable for older children. One disadvantage of the mask is that some children remove the mask frequently, making O_2 delivery inconsistent. Gas flow must be sufficient to the mask to prevent CO_2 accumulation.

Partial Rebreather Mask. A partial rebreather mask can achieve an FiO_2 of ≥ 0.6. It is similar to a simple mask but has a reservoir bag on the bottom. Oxygen is directed into and inhaled from the bag, and room air may be pulled in through ports on each side of the mask. On exhalation, a certain percentage of exhaled gas goes back into the reservoir bag. The concentration depends on the patient's size and tidal volume. This initial exhaled gas represents the portion of tidal volume that remains in the upper airways and is high in O_2 and low in CO_2. This gas mixes with the gas in the reservoir bag and is inhaled on the next breath. With this system, the gas flow must be adjusted so that the bag does not collapse during inspiration by more than one-third of its volume. The FiO_2 may be variable if the child's tidal volume changes.

Nonrebreathing Mask. A nonrebreathing mask is used in patients who require high FiO_2 concentrations. It is a facemask with a reservoir bag attached, and two valve systems are used. The first valve is found between the mask and reservoir bag, allowing one-way gas flow from the bag into the mask and preventing exhaled gas from flowing back into the reservoir. The second valve is located at the exhalation port and, when the patient inhales, closes to prevent entrapment of room air. When the patient exhales, the ports open to allow escape of CO_2-rich exhaled air. Oxygen flow is determined by the patient's inspiratory demands. Because this mask fits tightly to deliver a high FiO_2 and the patient can only breathe from the reservoir, which has one-way gas flow, the clinician must ensure that the oxygen tubing is not bent, compressed, or disconnected from the O_2 source, as any of these problems may compromise the patient's FiO_2 delivery.[26]

Face Tents. This large vinyl mask is soft and fits loosely around the patient's face. These are found only in adult sizes but may be inverted for use by children. The inversion creates a smaller reservoir and a better fit.[26] Face tents provide an oxygen concentration that is equal to the gas source's. Bag-valve-mask set-ups equipped with pressure manometers should be available if ventilation is inadequate despite oxygen administration and maintainable airways, regardless of the oxygen-delivery system.

Oxygen Toxicity. Oxygen is a drug and must be treated as such. Close monitoring of the patient's oxygen concentration is required. Arterial O_2 tension (PaO_2) can be monitored by arterial blood gases or by noninvasive monitoring with pulse oximeters ($SpaO_2$). Oxygen should be analyzed every 4 hours and with any changes of FiO_2. The most common form of oxygen toxicity in the neonate or infant is retrolental fibroplasia, in part, as a result of excessive PaO_2 delivered to the retinal artery.[26]

Pulmonary oxygen toxicity is characterized by a decrease in surfactant production, absorption atelectasis, and ventilation-perfusion abnormalities.[25] Pulmonary and systemic oxygen toxicity depend both on the oxygen concentration and duration of administration.[25] Weaning should be started as soon as monitoring parameters and the patient's clinical state allow.

INFUSION PUMPS

Infusion pumps are very useful for transports since they are lightweight, free-standing, easily transportable, usually small in size, and easy to set up, requiring minimal tubing and accessory equipment. They ensure a constant rate of infusion and volume administered per unit of time, thereby preventing volume overload in smaller infants and children and maintaining the patency of peripheral intravenous lines.

Different types of constant infusion pumps are available. The first employs peristaltic propulsion of liquid through tubing compressed by rollers. The second relies on a constant pressure on the plunger of the syringe, and the last, a low-volume filling from a volumetrically regulated cassette (i.e., slow, constant pressure infusion).

Infusion pumps may be battery-powered and electrically driven. Most infusion pumps, once charged, will run 6–8 hours and can be recharged in 20–30 minutes, making them ideal for transports. Infusion pumps can be used to infuse at rates as slow as 0.1 ml/hr and up to 999 ml/hr. Most pumps are designed to alarm for any obstruction, such as fluid flow-in, presence of air, low battery states, and completion of the infusion. These pumps cannot detect the presence of infiltration, and, therefore, the insertion site must be checked for extravasation frequently. The pump will continue to deliver fluid and medications, which may cause skin irritation and injury if infiltrated.

TEMPERATURE-SENSING DEVICES

Temperature is measured in degrees, most commonly Fahrenheit or Celsius. Both scales can be interconverted by the following equations:

$$(°C \times 9/5) + 32 = °F$$
$$(°F - 32) \times 5/9 = °C$$

The core temperature is usually measured per rectum, by mouth, or esophagus and is a reflection of basal metabolic energy production. Temperature can also be measured on skin (axillary) and at the tympanic membrane. Temperature can be monitored continuously or intermittently.

There are two commonly used thermometers, thermoexpansive and thermoresistive. The thermoexpansive thermometer is a mercury-based device in which this metal, in liquid form, expands with the increase in temperature. Mercury glass thermometers are useful for the measurement of extreme temperatures ($< 94°F$ and $> 106°F$). However, glass thermometers are fragile, making them inappropriate for the transport environment, and they should be considered only when extreme temperatures must be recorded.

The thermoresistive thermometer is based on the conduction of electricity, which is altered by changes in temperature.[16] This altered conductance will then transduce temperature, which is sensed by measuring the conductor's electrical resistance, the reciprocal of conductance.[16] For thermistors to be accurate, the probe must be in the right contact with the medium. Advantages of thermistors include that they have a rapid response, are small and lightweight, sensitive to small temperature changes, and inexpensive. Their disadvantages are instability due to resistance in the probe (which gradually increases with time), fragility due to small size, and nonisolated circuitry despite battery operation. This type of device is commonly employed in the continuous measurement probes used in servocontrolled incubators and heating blankets, as well as in standard intermittent measurements.[16]

The main difficulty of measuring temperature is inaccuracy due to the inappropriate measurement technique. If the temperature sensor is placed too close to a large blood vessel or high-flow organ (i.e., liver or stomach), it may cause a false elevation of temperature. On the other hand, a false decrease in the temperature may occur due to poor contact of the temperature probe or if the skin probe is used in the presence of severe vasoconstriction. If the accuracy of the temperature measurement is questioned, core temperature should be measured orally or rectally. If a probe is placed for continuous measurement of temperature, the skin should be checked frequently for irritation, and the probe should not be placed over an area where skin has broken down. When the temperature is checked tympanically, the clinician should ensure that the tympanic membrane is intact, the external ear canal is not occluded by infection, and the tympanic membrane is not severely dysfunctional due to a suppurative otitis media.

PRESSURE TRANSDUCERS

Although it is not common to monitor arterial or central venous pressure during transport, certain patients may be transported between institutions who have received indwelling pressure monitoring catheters in the intensive care unit. Arterial catheters are used in acute situations for patients who are hemodynamically unstable. The indwelling catheter is used for frequent blood drawing and monitoring of arterial blood gases. It may also be used to display arterial blood pressure continuously (both numerically and by waveform) and, if necessary, to provide a partial or total exchange transfusion (again, an uncommon procedure during transport).

The pressure-monitoring system consists of tubing, transducer, and monitor. The tubing should be relatively short, noncompliant (pressure tubing), and filled with liquid (saline) so that pressure changes in the blood vessels may be transmitted to the transducer. The transducer is also fluid-filled and attached to a thin diaphragm that converts mechanical energy into an electrical signal that is displayed on the monitor.

The system is calibrated to provide accurate physiologic measurements. Pressure is measured relative to a reference point, typically atmospheric pressure. This procedure is called "zeroing" and is performed with a stopcock to room air, thereby creating a zero-pressure baseline from which positive and negative pressure can be referenced.[11] After the calibration is done, the catheter tip must also be referenced to the transducer.[11] The mid-chest point is considered the reference point; if the transducer is above this level, there will be a very low pressure reading. Conversely, if placed below this level, there will be a high reading. Each inch above or below the mid-chest point will alter the measurement by approximately 1.9 mmHg.

Pressures may be recorded intermittently or continuously with the use of a fluid source (usually heparinized 0.9% normal saline; concentration, 1 U of heparin/ml of fluid). The transducer is attached to an infusion pump or a pressure bag for continuous infusion of the heparinized crystalloid.

Any indwelling catheter may be a possible source of infection, embolization, bleeding, and possible electrocution. The clinician must be especially careful to prevent air from entering the system, which may cause an air embolus, thus exposing the patient to severe morbidity or mortality. Transducers, however, reduce the risk of air entry to the patient. All electrical systems are grounded and should be treated frequently for failure.

Pressure readings may be inaccurate or the waveform "dampened" for several reasons. The clinician must first check the patient's clinical stability, check the level of the transducer, and make sure connections are secure. The catheter is then withdrawn and checked for blood return from the catheter, testing for air in the catheter, tubing, or transducer. Arterial spasm is another possible cause of misleading readings.

RADIANT WARMING DEVICES

Transportation of neonates and small infants is often done without an external source of heat, thereby increasing the potential for hypothermia. The use of isolettes for neonates (premature and full-term) and small infants is the standard of care on transports. The standard closed incubator controls the infant's temperature by recirculating warmed, humidified air.[18] There are some obvious disadvantages with this type of incubator, including loss of heat when the doors are opened and inaccessibility to the patient if an emergency should arise. Although the temperature and humidity are maintained at a constant, heat loss still occurs through the incubator walls.

Other devices include warming by radiant energy in the infrared spectrum, which is at least as effective as a standard incubator in maintaining the infant's temperature within a range that minimizes oxygen consumption and caloric expenditure.[18] A radiant warmer consists of an electrically heated element that emits infrared radiation. The elements used to produce the heat may be a quartz heating tube, a coil, or light that can be incorporated into a free-standing or fixed open incubator. The quartz heating tube is preferred due to its rapid heating time, resistance to thermal shock, insensitivity to drafts, and lack of emission of visible light. Some advantages to using radiant warmers include easy access to the patient, easy cleaning, and a more efficient servocontrol mechanism than most closed incubators. The essential factors that need to be included in radiantly warmed incubators are

1. Uniform distribution of heat to the patient;
2. Temperature alarms that cannot be silenced without evaluation of the patient; and
3. An alarm for the probe or heater.

There should be a constant display of the infant's skin temperature, and of course, all electrical connections should be checked for safety and appropriate state. Some features that make this heating source desirable include resistance to tipping, protection of the patient and personnel from a hot surface, a tilting mattress, adequate work and storage space, space for roentgenographic plates, and phototherapy lights.[18]

The incubator unit should be preheated with its own energy source so that the infant is not exposed to a hypothermic environment. A skin probe should be placed appropriately on the infant as soon as the patient is placed in the incubator so that the skin temperature can be monitored (which controls the heater output).[18] The probe should always be placed on the anterior chest or abdomen and not between the patient and the mattress, since the probe will then sense both temperatures and affect the heating device. A desired set point for temperature should be 36.5°C for term infants and 27–37.5°C for preterm infants. A double-walled hood in most most isolettes permits full visibility of the patient. Front and head access is provided by arm ports and door panels, but one must remember that opening these panels also increases heat loss.

Overheating can be the most serious complication for a radiant warming device in transport isolettes. The most tragic of complications from undetected hyperthermia can result in permanent neurologic damage and even death to the infant. The transport personnel should be able to set the temperature in the isolette to provide a warm environment for the infant, and they should be familiar with the manual and automatic control modes determining the heater output, as well as with the thermistor placement. A regular maintenance program is needed to check the overall heater system. If the transport is prolonged in duration, fluid requirements may have to be increased by 20–50%, especially if phototherapy is being utilized.

VASCULAR ACCESS

Peripheral venous access in children can be difficult and time-consuming, particularly in children presenting with cardiovascular collapse. Much of the difficulty can be explained by vessels that are fragile and small and a generous amount of subcutaneous fat. It is very important to establish and secure adequate venous access prior to transporting critically ill infants and children, so that fluid and emergency medications can be administered as necessary. Some basic tips can aid in starting peripheral intravenous (IV) lines in infants and children.[22] The hands, wrists, arms, and feet are acceptable sites for peripheral venous access. The feet in infants, particularly the saphenous vein area, are an excellent source of peripheral IV access.

Usually, IV access has been established before the transport team's arrival at the referring institution; if IV access has not been established or has been lost, it is imperative that a patent IV be established. The transport must have the appropriate equipment to start an IV (Table 1). The clinician must remember that universal precautions must also be applied with pediatric patients. All veins that are visible or palpable through the skin are "fair game" and may be catheterized for infusion of medications and fluids. At times, vascular access may be lost during transport (air or ground), and this setting may not be the ideal place to start an IV line on children, but having the proper equipment and technique may aid and simplify this procedure.

VENOUS CUTDOWN

A venous cutdown is usually performed at the referring institution's emergency department or by a specialized pediatric transport team to gain access to a vein when the patient cannot be cannulated percutaneously. This procedure is not as popular due to the resurgence of the intraosseous line (see later discussion). An number of sites can be safely and rapidly accessed for use by cutdown techniques:
   1. Cephalic and basilic veins at the antecubital region
   2. Brachial or basilic veins in the mid-arm region

TABLE 1.   Equipment Necessary to Establish Venous Access in a Pediatric Patient

22- and 24-gauge catheters for infants and small children
Tourniquet
3-cc and 5-cc syringes
Bacteriostatic normal saline
T-connector (Fig. 1)
Nonporous or hypoallergenic tape
Small arm board
Soft restraints

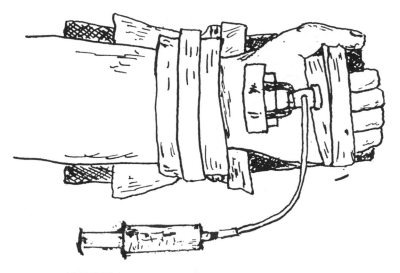

FIGURE 1.   T-connector attached to an intravenous line.

3. Cephalic vein at the deltopectoral groove
4. External jugular vein in the neck
5. Saphenous vein at the ankle and inguinal regions
6. Femoral vein in the inguinal area

The ideal site to place an elective cutdown is the operating room, but if one is needed in an emergency situation, a cutdown should be done in as sterile a procedure as possible in the emergency department.

CENTRAL VENOUS ACCESS

Central venous cannulation should not be attempted as a first choice to access a patient's circulation in an emergency situation. If central venous cannulation is chosen, attempts to access the central circulation should be done in a controlled environment and not in an ambulance or helicopter. It should also be performed by the most skilled individual available.

The four most common routes to access the central circulation are the antecubital, internal, jugular, subclavian, and femoral veins. The most direct access route to the right atrial circulation is the right internal jugular vein, followed by the left internal jugular and the left subclavian veins.[4] Again, if the patient is in need of urgent fluid resuscitation, the quickest, easiest, and most desired route of fluid administration would be the intraosseous route. For rapid central venous cannulation, the femoral and subclavian veins are the easiest to cannulate.

Single, double, or triple lumen catheters may be used; all lumina should always be flushed with heparinized saline (preferably) prior to the insertion of the catheter, thereby preventing the risk of air emboli and clotting of the respective lumen. The clinician must remember that infection control begins with proper preparation of the skin prior to the insertion of the catheter, regardless of the emergent nature of the situation. There are standard equipment and techniques that are necessary for the appropriate and successful placement of these lines, including proper positioning of the patient, depending on the site chosen. The patient should be prepped adequately with an antiseptic solution (usually an iodine-povidine solution) and draped with sterile towels. The clinician should be wearing a mask, head cover, sterile gown, and gloves to avoid accidental contamination of the catheter whenever possible.

Pain management should be considered, and preferably, sedation (benzodiazepines and/or narcotics), along with local anesthesia, should be administered if the patient can tolerate it hemodynamically. If parenteral sedation is not possible, then local anesthetics should be utilized. Usually lidocaine 1% is administered to the site and should be sufficient to control pain locally if the subcutaneous tissues are also adequately infiltrated.

These catheters are usually placed by the Seldinger technique (needle-over-wire technique). Once placement has been checked by the easy withdrawal of blood into each of the lumina and, ultimately, a chest x-ray, then the catheter should be stabilized by suturing to the skin. A sterile occlusive dressing should be placed to maintain the insertion site as surgically clean as possible.

Antecubital Venous Access

The antecubital approach utilizes the superficial location of the cephalic and basilic veins, which may be accessed percutaneously with a puncture needle-over-wire, an introducer, or by direct venous cutdown and visualization of the vessel.[4] Even though the antecubital approach has a lower rate of complications, it is very time-consuming and therefore not recommended in an emergency situation. If this approach is chosen, after cannulation the patient's arm should be stabilized on an arm board to avoid flexion at the antecubital site. Monitoring for air bubbles in the IV lines is of primary importance, because even though this site is initially peripheral, it is a central venous line and, therefore, air emboli are a potential concern.

Internal Jugular Access

The internal jugular vein is one of the safest sites to access the superior central circulation.[4] The limiting factor in the pediatric population is the short neck of the infant and small child, thereby limiting this vascular access site to the older child population. The insertion procedure is simple. The needle is placed at the junction of the lateral border of the sternocleidomastoid muscle and the external jugular vein, directing the needle toward the sternal notch.

To cannulate the external jugular vein, the vein is fixed distally with a finger to fill the vein. It is then entered with a needle and guidewire at the lateral border of the sternocleidomastoid muscle.

Subclavian Venous Access

The subclavian approach may be used, although the incidence of pneumothorax is higher, especially with a patient who may be hemodynamically unstable or intravascularly depleted. The vein exits from under the clavicle at the junction of the medial third and lateral two-thirds of the clavicle.[4] The needle is directed toward the sternal notch just under the clavicle (Fig. 2). The subclavian approach may be performed even in newborns, although there may be high rates of complications, especially when performed during an emergency.

Femoral Venous Access

The femoral venous approach involves localizing the femoral artery just below the inguinal ligament, infiltrating with local anesthetic and entering the region medial to the artery (Fig. 3).[4] The clinician must consider that this approach has a higher rate of infection and thrombosis than other vascular sites.

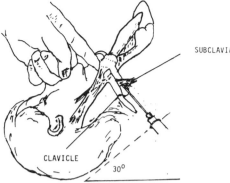

FIGURE 2. Positioning of patient and angling of needle when performing a subclavian approach for placing a central venous line.

This site is less desirable for emergency vascular access, especially in patients with trauma to the abdomen and lower extremities. In addition, a certain level of expertise is required to place central venous lines; therefore, the intraosseous route is preferable and recommended in an emergency situation in an infant or child (up to 5 years of age).

Intraosseous Vascular Access

Due to the difficulty in obtaining conventional peripheral vascular access in children, especially when they are in cardiovascular collapse, have suffered trauma, or are experiencing seizures, intraosseous lines (IO) have become more popular in the past few years. Establishing and securing an IO line are relatively easy tasks, and this approach is preferred and recommended when vascular access is required quickly in either the emergency department or transport environment. Resuscitation fluids, including blood, plasma, crystalloid, and colloid, may be infused through an IO line. Resuscitative medications and certain antibiotics may also be administered via this route.

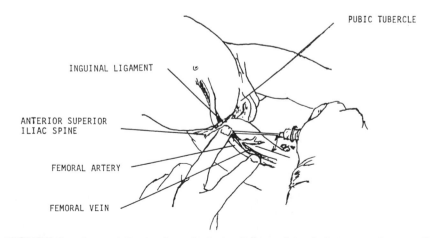

FIGURE 3. Anatomic landmarks in the femoral approach to placing a central venous line.

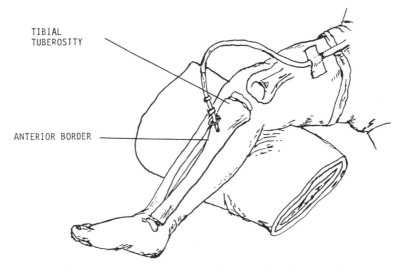

FIGURE 4. Positioning of the leg, anatomic landmarks, and preferred site for an intraosseous line.

Landmarks are important when cannulating the IO space of a developing bone. The preferred site is the anteromedial aspect of the proximal tibia approximately 1–2 cm below the tibial tuberosity (Fig. 4). The needle should be directed caudal to avoid entering the epiphyseal plate. With successful cannulation, there should be an immediate lack of resistance (or a "pop") after the needle passes thorugh the cortex. Although there are commercially available IO lines, a 16- or 18-gauge stylet needle (Seldinger, spinal, or bone marrow) may be utilized. The needle should stand upright without support, and one should be able to aspirate bone marrow to verify placement and then be able to infuse fluids freely without any subcutaneous infiltration. It is preferable to place IV fluids on an infusion pump so that accurate rates are maintained; in addition, clotting of the IO line is avoided. If the site becomes obstructed, the bone is traversed, or the line becomes dislodged, it must be placed in a new site because there will be subcutaneous infiltration from the original site if the same bone is used.

Umbilical Vessel Catheterization

In newborn infants, the umbilical artery and vein may be used to introduce a catheter into the aorta and/or inferior vena cava, respectively. In a transport situation, a delivery room, or emergency department, this route is preferred because the vessels are easily exposed in a newborn infant and the catheters can be easily introduced. Due to the high complication rate with these catheters (13.5%), some physicians no longer recommend their use in an electively emergent situation, when there is sufficient time to introduce a peripheral or central venous catheter.[12] Medications such as antibiotics, sodium bicarbonate, electrolyte solutions and replacement medications (calcium, magnesium, etc.) may be administered through the umbilical vein, but not through the umbilical artery due to the potential damage to the aorta.[12]

The equipment necessary to perform an umbilical vessel catheterization includes a single-lumen, polyvinyl chloride catheter with a 3.5 or a 5.0 French gauge (depending on the size of the infant), heparinized solution (1 U of heparin/ml of fluid), an infusion pump, a pressure transducer, and pressure monitor (if an arterial umbilical catheter is to be inserted). The procedure, as with other central vascular lines, is performed under sterile technique. Before introducing the catheter, the infant's legs and arms should be restrained; constant monitoring of the heart rate, respiration, and pulse-oximetry should be maintained.

The umbilical clamp, stump, and surrounding skin are cleansed with an antiseptic solution, and umbilical tape is placed loosely around the base of the umbilical cord, tightening only if there is bleeding. To place the catheter at the level of the third or fourth lumbar vertebra, the clinician should measure and calculate approximately 65% of the distance from the shoulder to the umbilical stump; measuring this from the tip of the catheter would give the clinician the appropriate length. A stopcock is placed at the distal portion of the catheter, and the catheter is flushed with heparinized solution. The umbilical cord is cut approximately 2–3 cm above the skin, and the clamp and cut umbilical cord are discarded. The clinician should always remember that there are two umbilical arteries and one umbilical vein in the normal newborn. Any variation from this anatomic finding should be considered abnormal; therefore, most likely the patient may exhibit other physical abnormalities.

The artery is dilated with a small forceps and the catheter is inserted into the artery, advancing until the marker on the catheter reaches the cut surface of the cord. Blood is aspirated into the catheter, confirming the intravascular placement and also avoiding any air bubbles. The catheter is flushed and then secured with #4-0 silk sutures. When the catheter is placed, one should observe the lower extremities and buttocks for cyanosis or mottling; also, the strength and quality of the femoral pulses should be examined following placement. An x-ray should be obtained to confirm the placement of the umbilical catheter at the level of L3 or L4 (Fig. 5).

ENDOTRACHEAL INTUBATION

In most transport scenarios, when an endotracheal tube is placed, it is usually in an emergent fashion.[17] However, the procedure of intubation needs to be approached in a calm, systematic, but expeditious manner for several reasons:
1. To reduce the possibility of airway trauma
2. To ensure the patient's stability
3. To ensure proper technique
4. To maintain patient oxygenation and ventilation

Indications for intubation include:
1. Apnea
2. Respiratory failure ($PaO_2 < 50$ mmHg with $FiO_2 > 0.8$; $PaCO_2 > 55$ mmHg acutely)
3. Airway obstruction (upper and lower)
4. Control of ventilation, as in deliberate hypocarbia or status epilepticus
5. Inadequate chest wall function, as seen in flail chest or neuromuscular disorders such as Guillain-Barré syndrome
6. Inability of the patient to maintain a patent airway due to inadequate airway reflex activity[17]

Procedure

Regardless of the reason for intubation, control of the airway must be established with either bag-valve-mask ventilation or standard mouth-to-mouth

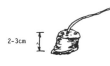

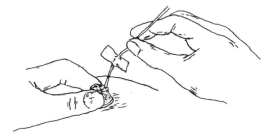

FIGURE 5. Anatomic landmarks and positioning site of an intravascular umbilical line.

technique (universal precautions should be taken), while preparation for intubation is made, making sure that all equipment is readily available and functioning. It is essential that every member of the transport team be familiar and able to identify all intubation equipment and the location of this equipment. Necessary equipment includes:

1. Laryngoscope handle
2. Appropriately sized blades (straight and curved)
3. Appropriately sized endotracheal tubes
4. Suction catheters
5. Appropriately sized masks
6. Self-inflating/anesthesia-type ventilation bag

There should be at least two trained personnel performing the intubation, one person preparing the equipment and the other monitoring the patient's cardiorespiratory status, assisting in positioning of the patient, and maintaining the airway. If possible, attempts should be made to empty all stomach contents with a nasogastric tube, but all patients should be considered a "full stomach" intubation in the emergency department and/or transport setting. The patient should be bag-valve-mask ventilated and oxygenated with FiO_2 of 1.0 for several minutes to replace alveolar air with oxygen. This will also provide an added source of oxygen should the patient become apneic.[20] Optimal saturation for intubation is 100% in a patient without pre-existing cardiac or pulmonary disease. If the patient has a history of prematurity or cyanotic congenital heart disease, then optimal saturation should be adjusted to the patient's disease (e.g., a premature infant with bronchopulmonary dysplasia would be expected to have maximum optimal saturation of 96–97% on FiO_2 of 1.0).

There are two methods of selecting an endotracheal tube. One uses the formula:

$$\text{tube size} = 16 + (\text{age in years}) \div 4$$

An easier and quicker method (which correlates well with the airway diameter) is to take the inner diameter of the endotracheal tube and compare it to the tip of the patient's small fifth digit. In children less than 8 years of age, uncuffed tubes are recommended so that unnecessary pressure is not placed on the airway mucosa, thereby creating a pressure injury. If a cuffed tube is used, it should have a low pressure cuff to minimize tracheal mucosal trauma, and Pressure-Easy™ is recommended to maintain a constant cuff pressure. The clinician should have available tubes that are a half-size smaller and a half-size larger, in case the patient's airway is not able to accept the appropriately sized tube. When choosing the laryngoscope blade, a straight blade is generally preferred in newborns due to the infant's rigid epiglottis.[20] It is safer and easier to place an oral endotracheal tube in an emergent situation; only with more expertise and time during the procedure is a nasotracheal tube recommended, and this should be done with appropriately trained personnel.

It is desirable to have established IV access prior to intubation because emergency medications may need to be administered. Atropine, 0.2 mg/kg IV, should be administered before intubation in children under 2 years of age so that vagal nerve stimulation may be blocked. This stimulation may be caused by the laryngoscopic procedure, causing bradycardia in infants and neonates. The patient's head should be in the "sniffing" position, and the person performing the intubation should be at the foot of the bed. One should avoid hyperextension of the neck, because this may obstruct the larynx of the infant or small child due to the very soft tissues of the infant's airway. An assistant may have to restrain the arms, shoulder, and head of the patient while direct flow of oxygen is administered at the patient's face. Downward pressure over the cricoid cartilage is placed while the intubation procedure is performed, because these patients should be considered a "full stomach" intubation. If during the procedure the patient develops bradycardia or begins to have desaturation of oxygen by pulse-oximetry, the patient should be bag-valve-mask ventilated with an FiO_2 of 1.0 as necessary until the heart rate and SaO_2 improve.

Once the patient is intubated, hand ventilation should be continued while an assistant checks for bilateral breath sounds at the midaxillary line and symmetrical chest expansion. If at any time there is a question as to placement, visualization of the vocal cords with the laryngoscope should be done to verify appropriate placement. It is of utmost importance to stabilize the endotracheal tube with tape, and preferably benzoin solution, and to restrain the patient so as to avoid accidental extubation.

Complications

It is important first to assess the patient's facial anatomy, range of motion of the neck and jaw, and structure of the intraoral cavity before attempting intubation, if possible. Anatomic features that can increase the difficulty of intubation include:

1. Normal neonatal anatomy
2. Inability to open the mouth fully
3. Inability to extend the neck
4. Missing or broken teeth, or intraoral appliance
5. Short, thick neck
6. Macroglossia
7. Midfacial or palatal abnormalities
8. Active bleeding in the mouth from the nasopharyngeal or lower airway

9. Airway masses
10. "Anterior larynx"[17]

If the patient is not intubated when the transport team arrives at the referring institution, and if there is a question whether the patient should be intubated to maintain the airway during transport, intubation should be undertaken prior to departing to provide the safest transfer of the patient.

SUCTIONING

Airway secretions consists of cellular debris, mucus, blood, inflammatory cells, microorganisms, water, glycoproteins, and immunoglobulins.[5] The submucosal and mucosal glands in the lungs produce these airway secretions.

The volume, consistency, color, odor, and presence of foreign substances can be of great diagnostic value.[5] There are several reasons that suctioning may be necessary. The presence of an endotracheal tube, essentially a foreign body, increases mucus production. Neurologic disorders, such as cerebral palsy, Neimann-Pick disease, and anoxic CNS injury, and certain surgical procedures which can prevent proper mobilization of secretions, such as thoracic, abdominal, or airway surgery, may increase secretions. Certain patients may have an ineffective cough and need assistance in removing secretions. When the need for suctioning is apparent, the proper equipment must be in place (Table 2).

If a patient is not yet intubated, nasopharyngeal suctioning may be temporarily beneficial by removing upper airway secretions. Place the patient in the sniffing position, hyperoxygenate, and ventilate. Hyperoxygenation and ventilation are accomplished by increasing the flow of oxygen to 5–6 liters/min and allowing or assisting the patient, prior to the suctioning, to breathe high-flow oxygen. If a patient has a history of pulmonary hypertension, an FiO_2 of 1.0 should be administered for a minimum of 1 full minute before and after each suctioning attempt.[16]

Procedure in the Nonintubated Patient

In an aseptic manner, the catheter package is opened, gloves are put on, and lubricant is applied to the catheter tip. The catheter is then inserted gently into the nares on a line parallel to the patient's earlobe.[13] If at this point the catheter will not advance, it can be twisted to change directions, and if this does not advance the catheter, it should be removed and inserted into the opposite nare. Once the catheter is inserted into the nasopharynx, it will meet resistance. Pull back approximately 1 cm and apply suction while twirling the catheter on the way out. This entire process should take no more than 5–10 seconds.[13]

Procedure in the Intubated Patient

If an endotracheal tube is present, again the appropriate-sized inflation bag should be available and connected to an inline manometer (to control inflating

TABLE 2.   Equipment Necessary for Adequately and Safely Suctioning
a Patient's Endotracheal Tube

Appropriate-size mask (in case of accidental extubation)
Inflation bag with manometer
Suction material reservoir
Appropriate-sized suction catheters
Adjustable vacuum regulator
0.9% sodium chloride solution

pressures). Appropriate-sized suction catheters should be available. All equipment should be tested before the procedure is started. When selecting an appropriate-sized catheter, multiply the patient's endotracheal (ET) tube size by two to obtain the proper size catheter.[13]

$$ET \text{ tube size} = 4$$
$$4 \times 2 = 8$$
$$8 = \text{suction catheter}$$

Again, sterile technique is used when opening the catheter package. Two gloves should be worn during the procedure; one should be kept sterile throughout the procedure, and the other is used to prevent contact with secretions. With the sterile hand, remove the catheter from the package and attach it to the suction tubing. Normal saline solution is introduced into the endotracheal tube with the unsterile hand. The patient is then ventilated manually using the inflation bag and pressure manometer as discussed earlier (usually a 10% higher concentration of oxygen is delivered). The catheter is inserted until resistance is felt; it is then withdrawn 1 cm, suction is applied, and with a twirling motion, the catheter is removed. This procedure is then repeated two more times with manual breaths between suctioning. If necessary, as with copious secretions, suctioning may need to be repeated more. With all suctioning, the patient must be observed for toleration of the procedure by monitoring vital signs, skin color, and chest excursion. Following suctioning breath sound should be assessed.

Complications of suctioning include hypoxemia, due to the removal of alveolar gas, and dysrhythmias (from vagal stimulation). Mucosal damage and atelectasis may occur if inflating pressures are too high or if an inappropriate sized catheter is used, respectively.[13] Subsequent bacterial growth is always a threat, but strict analgesic technique will minimize this possibility.

THORACENTESIS AND THORACOSTOMY

Indications for thoracentesis and chest tube placement include:
1. Pneumothorax
2. Tension pneumothorax
3. Pleural effusion
4. Hemothorax

Pneumothorax is a collection of air in the pleural cavity. This condition may be caused by penetrating or blunt trauma, by an underlying disease process causing the lungs to collapse, or by a spontaneous collapse of the lung.[24]

Tension pneumothorax occurs when air enters the pleural space but cannot escape, creating an elevation of intrapleural pressure that may lead to a mediastinal shift away from the affected side. This may either collapse the affected lung, or, if the shift does take place, it may impair ventilation of the opposite lung. Further complications of tension pneumothorax consist of hemodynamic instability and a decrease in cardiac output, thereby creating severe hypotension.

A pleural effusion is an abnormal collection of fluid beween the visceral and parietal pleura. Hemothorax is a collection of blood in the pleural space.

All of these situations may cause respiratory distress, asymmetric chest wall movement, and decreased breath sounds.[24] The symptoms and severity of the presentation will depend on the size and significance of the intrathoracic injury. In addition to the above-mentioned symptoms, if a mediastinal shift takes place with any of these conditions, a decrease in cardiac output, severe hypoxia, and possible death may occur if not treated promptly.[24]

There are two methods for removal of air or fluid from the chest: thoracentesis, as a rule, is a diagnostic tool, and chest tube placement (thoracostomy) is a treatment modality.

Thoracentesis

Thoracentesis may be done as a diagnostic measure, before placement of chest tubes, or may be performed as a therapeutic procedure. When a thoracentesis is performed, the patient is positioned so that adequate exposure is ensured. A roll may be placed under the affected hemithorax and the arm positioned superiorly.

The incision site is determined by marking the point at which tactile fremitus (the feel of vibrations due to the presence of air or fluid in the thoracic cavity) and percussion becomes dull. Prepare the skin with an antiseptic solution. Local anesthetic (usually 1% lidocaine) is infiltrated into the skin, the intercostal muscle, and deep down to the rib periosteum. A 16- or 18-gauge catheter is then inserted through the tissue into the pleural space (this will be confirmed by a "pop" felt as the needle passes through the pleura), followed by the return of air or fluid into the syringe once the intrathoracic cavity has been entered. Remove the inner needle and place a 30-ml syringe with an attached three-way stopcock to the catheter hub. This part of the procedure must be done on expiration to prevent air from entering the pleural space, with the clinician maintaining a seal over the hub of the catheter at all times when the stopcock is placed. Intravenous extension tubing may be placed to the third arm of the stopcock, and when the syringe is full, it may be emptied through the tubing into a reservoir. Caution must be taken to prevent kinking of the catheter.

When chest tubes are placed to drain fluid, they should be low in the chest, at the fifth to seventh intercostal space between the midaxillary and posterior axillary lines.[10] Lower insertion may injure the liver, spleen, or diaphragm. If a chest tube is placed for evacuation of air, it is usually placed high, at the second or third intercostal space in the midclavicular or midaxillary line, thereby avoiding the pectoralis muscle.[10] Once the appropriate-sized chest tube is chosen, the area is prepared with an antiseptic solution and anesthetized with 1% lidocaine, similar to the thoracentesis procedure. A small incision is made, and by blunt dissection, the thoracic cavity is entered. Entry should be made over the top of the rib to avoid the intercostal neurovascular bundle.[15] The tip of the chest tube is held by a curved hemostat and gently inserted into the pleural space. It is important to advance the chest tube so that all the evacuation ports are within the pleural space. The tube should be placed to a water-seal device with 20 cm H_2O of negative pressure suction.

This procedure presents a wide spectrum of possible complications ranging from very minor to life-threatening. Some of these include an incision made too high above the rib, thereby risking laceration of the intercostal vessels (artery or vein). If sterile technique is not maintained, contamination and subsequent infection (empyema) may result. Occasionally, in small infants, pressure placed on the aorta may cause distal hypoperfusion.[15]

The chest tube should be secured to the skin with heavy silk sutures and then taped to the chest. If during transport a patient has any of the conditions discussed in this section, causing an adverse clinical state, action must be taken (in most cases) to avoid severe morbidity. In a transport setting, it is most likely that thoracostomy would be the procedure of choice, since it can be done quickly and is easier to accomplish at the referring institution or in the confines of a transport vehicle.

ABDOMINAL PARACENTESIS

Hemorrhage from thoracoabdominal injuries is second only to head trauma as the leading cause of traumatic death in pediatric victims.[6] In children, blunt abdominal trauma accounts for 80% of abdominal injuries since children rarely have penetrating trauma.[6] Peritoneal lavage is an important diagnostic tool for patients who have experienced blunt abdominal trauma. It is a procedure in which the abdominal cavity is entered percutaneously to obtain diagnostic information for the differential diagnosis of ascites, peritonitis, and intraperitoneal hemorrhage.[1]

When this procedure is performed, the patient is placed in a supine position, with the head slightly elevated. The area is prepared with an antiseptic solution. The bladder should be emptied by catheterization, and the stomach should be decompressed with a nasogastric tube. A 20- or 22-gauge intracatheter needle and catheter set, perpendicular to the skin in either flank, in line with the nipples, and below or at the level of the umbilicus, is advanced until the peritoneum is entered; the needle is withdrawn, and the catheter is further advanced into the peritoneal cavity. During advancement, suction should be applied with a syringe. If the tap is unsuccessful, the needle should be withdrawn and relocated as described previously. The needle should not be manipulated while in the abdominal cavity, as this risks peritoneal organ injury.[1]

Risks encountered when performing this procedure include perforation of blood vessels and/or introduction of skin contaminants. Hematomas may form, or if large amounts of fluid are suddenly removed, fluid shifts and/or hypotension may occur.

Peritoneal lavage in the evaluation of abdominal trauma is a controversial procedure due to the possible complications and the potential for abdominal pain when the catheter is placed. Double-contrast computed tomographic scans and ultrasound scans of the abdomen are now becoming the studies of choice.[6] The skilled transport team should observe the patient for deterioration and perform peritoneal lavage only if absolutely necessary. If possible, they should wait for other means of diagnosis when they have reached the referral institution.

PERICARDIOCENTESIS

Pericardiocentesis is a technique for aspirating pericardial fluid for diagnostic or therapeutic purposes.[9] It can be life-saving when performed to relieve cardiac tamponade (the accumulation of blood in the pericardial sac). The blood accumulation must be significant (25–50 ml) to cause symptoms. The most common causes for accumulation of pericardial fluids are:

1. Penetrating trauma
2. Uremic pericarditis
3. Acute purulent pericarditis
4. Bleeding following open-heart surgery[3]

When the accumulation is significant, it compromises ventricular diastolic expansion. This then produces a decrease in cardiac output, persistent hypotension, distension of neck vessels, muffled heart sounds, and pulsus paradoxus.

The technique for the removal of fluid from the pericardial sac involves:

1. Placing the patient in a supine position with 10–15° of reverse Trendelenburg

2. Preparation and maintenance of a sterile field
3. Using a pericardiocentesis needle or spinal needle attached to a 5-ml syringe.

The needle is inserted beneath the xyphoid process at approximately 45° to the horizontal plane and 45° toward the left shoulder.[9] When performing this procedure, EKG guidance may be used by attaching chest lead (V) to the needle using an alligator clip; if the needle is inserted too far, ST-segment elevations or premature ventricular contractions will be seen.[9] When the needle has been inserted, aspirations should be done intermittently. As described, this procedure is very delicate and may not always be easily performed on transport. To minimize hazards, proper technique is essential. Risks include further bleeding into the pericardial space or laceration of a coronary vessel.

REFERENCES

1. Dammert W: Abdominal parecentesis. In Levin D, Morris F, Moore G (eds): A Practical Guide to Pediatric Intensive Care, 2nd ed. St. Louis, C.V. Mosby Co., 1984, pp 609–610.
2. Fait C, Wetzel RC, Dean JM, et al: Pulse oximetry in critically ill children. J Clin Monit 1(4):232–235, 1985.
3. Feltes T: Cardiac tamponade. In Levin D, Morris F (eds): Essentials of Pediatric Intensive Care. St. Louis, Quality Medical Publishing, 1990, pp 328–333.
4. Grassmik B: Venous and arterial access. In Victor L (ed): Manual of Critical Care Procedures. Rockville, MD, Aspen, 1989, pp 333–354.
5. Hatfield N, Rauschuber T: Suctioning. In Levin D, Morris F, Moore G (eds): A Practical Guide to Pediatric Intensive Care, 2nd ed. St. Louis, Mosby, 1984.
6. Hazinski MF: Abdomen. In Hazinski MF (ed): Nursing Care of the Critically Ill Child, 2nd ed. St. Louis, Mosby, 1992, pp 856–857.
7. Hicks D, Anas N: Oxygen saturation monitoring. In Levin D, Morris F (eds): Essentials of Pediatric Intensive Care. St. Louis, Quality Medical Publishing, 1990.
8. Kulick RM: Pulse oximetry. Pediatr Emerg Care 3(2):127–130, 1987.
9. Leonard ST, Nikaidah H: Pericardiocentesis. In Levin D, Morris F (eds): Essentials of Pediatric Intensive Care. St. Louis, Quality Medical Publishing, 1990, pp 984–987.
10. Leonard S, Nikaidob H: Thoracentesis and chest tube insertion. In Levin D, Morris F (eds): Essentials of Pediatric Intensive Care. St. Louis, Quality Medical Publishing, 1990, pp 937–944.
11. Levin DL, Mast CP: Pressure transducers. In Levin D, Morris F, Moore G (eds): A Practical Guide to Pediatric Intensive Care, 2nd ed. St. Louis, Mosby, 1984, pp 478–482.
12. Levin D, Mast CP: Vascular catheter, arterial catheters. In Shoemaker WC, Ayres S, Grenvik A, et al (eds): Textbook of Critical Care, 2nd ed. Philadelphia, W.B. Saunders, 1989, pp 490–503.
13. Lybarger C, Vinson R: Suctioning. In Levin D, Morris F (eds): Essentials of Pediatric Intensive Care. St. Louis, Quality Medical Publishing, 1990, pp 927–929.
14. Mihm FG, Halperin BD: Noninvasive detection of profound arterial desaturation using a pulse oximetry device. Anesthesiology 62:85–87, 1985.
15. Moore G, Mills L, Mast C: Thoracentesis and chest tube insertion. In Levin D, Morris F, Moore G (eds): A Practical Guide to Pediatric Intensive Care, 2nd ed. St. Louis, Mosby, 1984, pp 576–583.
16. Morris FC: Temperature sensing devices. In Levin D, Morris F, Moore G (eds): A Practical Guide to Pediatric Intensive Care, 2nd ed. St. Louis, Mosby, 1984, pp 488–489.
17. Morris F, Burns D, Vinson R: Intubation. In Levin D, Morris F, Moore G (eds): A Practical Guide to Pediatric Intensive Care, 2nd ed. St. Louis, Mosby, 1984, pp 536–541.
18. Morris FC, Grandy ME, Johnson LT: Radiant warming devices. In Levin D, Morris F, Moore G (eds): A Practical Guide to Pediatric Intensive Care, 2nd ed. St. Louis, Mosby, 1984, pp 485–490.
19. Morris FC, Mast CP: Electrocardiographic and respiratory monitors. In Levin D, Morris F, Moore G (eds): A Practical Guide to Pediatric Intensive Care, 2nd ed. St. Louis, Mosby, 1984, pp 474–478.
20. Morris F, Stone J, Butler L: Intubation. In Levin D, Morris F (eds): Essentials of Pediatric Intensive Care. St. Louis, Quality Medical Publishing, 1990, pp 888–816.
21. New W: Pulse oximetry. J Clin Monit 1(2):126–129, 1985.
22. O'Brien R: Starting IV lines in children. J Emerg Nurs 17:225–230, 1991.

23. Rakita L, Vrogel TR: Electrocardiography in critical care medicine. In Shoemaker WC, Ayres S, Grenvik A, et al (eds): Textbook of Critical Care, 2nd ed. Philadelphia, W.B. Saunders, 1989.
24. Talamonti W: Thoracentesis and chest tube insertion. In Victor L (ed): Manual of Critical Care Procedures. Rockville, MD, Aspen, 1989, pp 93–109.
25. Wade B, Elmore G: Oxygen administration. In Levin D, Morris F (eds): Essentials of Pediatric Intensive Care. St. Louis, Quality Medical Publishing, 1990, pp 884–887.
26. Walters P, Elmore G, Grandy M: Oxygen administration. In Levin D, Morris F, Moore G (eds): A Practical Guide to Pediatric Intensive Care, 2nd ed. St. Louis, Mosby, 1984, pp 551–555.
27. Zijlstra WG, Buursma A, Meeuwsen van Der Roest WF: Absorption spectra of human fetal and adult oxyhemogloibn, deoxyhemoglobin, carboxyhemoglobin, and methemoglobin. Clin Chem 37:1633, 1991.

Laboratory Values

BLOOD CHEMISTRIES

Drug	Conventional Units	Drug	Conventional Units
Alanine Aminotrans-		**Carbon Dioxide (CO_2**	
ferase (ALT)		**Content)**	
Infants	< 54 U/L	Cord blood	14–22 mEq/L
Children/Adults	1–30 U/L	Infant/Child	20–24 mEq/L
		Adult	24–30 mEq/L
Alkaline Phosphatase			
Infant	150–420 U/L	**Carbon Monoxide**	
2–10 yr	100–320 U/L	**(Carboxyhemoglobin)**	
11–18 yr male	100–390 U/L	Nonsmoker	0–2% of total
			hemoglobin
Ammonia Nitrogen		Smoker	2–10% of total
(heparinized venous			hemoglobin
specimen in ice water,		Toxic	20–60% of total
analyzed within 30 min)			hemoglobin
Newborn	90–150 µg/dl	Lethal	> 60% of total
0–2 wk	79–129 µg/dl		hemoglobin
< 1 mo	29–70 µg/dl		
Adult	15–45 µg/dl	**Chloride**	96–109 mEq/L
Amylase		**Creatine Kinase (Crea-**	
Newborn	0–44 U/L	**tine Phosphokinase)**	
Adult	0–88 U/L	Newborn	10–200 U/L
		Adult male	0–175 U/L
Aspartate Aminotrans-		Adult female	10–55 U/L
ferase (AST)			
Newborn/Infant	20–65 U/L	**Creatinine (Serum)**	
Child/Adult	0–35 U/L	Cord	0.6–1.2 mg/dl
		Newborn	0.3–1.0 mg/dl
Bicarbonate		Infant	0.2–0.4 mg/dl
Premature	18–26 mEq/L	Child	0.3–0.7 mg/dl
Full term	20–25 mEq/L	Adolescent	0.5–1.0 mg/dl
> 2 yr	22–26 mEq/L		
		Fibrinogen	200–400 mg/dl
Bilirubin (Total)			
Cord	Preterm: < 1.8 mg/dl	**Gamma-glutamyl**	
	Term: < 1.8 mg/dl	**Transferase (GGT)**	
0–1 day	Preterm: < 8 mg/dl	Cord	19–270 U/L
	Term: < 6 mg/dl	Premature	56–233 U/L
1–2 days	Preterm: < 12 mg/dl	0–3 wk	0–130 U/L
	Term: < 8 mg/dl	3 wk – 3 mo	4–120 U/L
3–7 days	Preterm: < 16 mg/dl	> 3 mo males	5–65 U/L
	Term: < 12 mg/dl	> 3 mo females	5–35 U/L
7–30 days	Preterm: < 12 mg/dl	1–15 yr	0–23 U/L
	Term: < 7 mg/dl	16 yr – adult	0–35 U/L
Thereafter	Preterm: < 2 mg/dl		
	Term: < 1 mg/dl	**Glucose (Serum)**	
Adult	0.1–1.0 mg/dl	Premature	20–65 mg/dl
		Full term	20–110 mg/dl
Bilirubin (Conjugated)	0–0.4 mg/dl	1 wk – 16 yr	60–105 mg/dl
		> 10 yr	70–115 mg/dl
Calcium (Total)			
Premature < 1 wk	6–10 mg/dl	**Ketones**	
Full Term < 1 wk	7.0–12.0 mg/dl	Qualitative	Negative
Child	8–10.5 mg/dl	Quantitative	0.5–3.0 mg/dl

(Table continued on following page.)

BLOOD CHEMISTRIES (Continued)

Drug	Conventional Units	Drug	Conventional Units
Lactate		**Phosphorus** (*Cont.*)	
Capillary blood		1–5 yr	3.5–6.8 mg/dl
Newborn	< 27 mg/dl	Adult	2.7–4.5 mg/dl
Child	5–20 mg/dl	**Porcelain**	10–25 mg/dl
Venous	5–18 mg/dl		
Arterial	3–7 mg/dl	**Potassium**	
		< 10 days of age	3.5–6.0 mEq/L
Lactate Dehydrogenase		> 10 days of age	3.5–5.0 mEq/L
(37°C)			
Neonate	160–1500 U/L	**Sodium**	
Infant	150–360 U/L	Premature	130–140 mEq/L
Child	150–300 U/L	Older	135–145 mEq/L
Adult	100–250 U/L		
		Urea Nitrogen	5–25 mg/dl
Magnesium	1.5–2.0 mEq/L		
		Uric Acid	
Methemoglobin	(0–1.3% of total hg)	0–2 yrs	2.0–7.0 mg/dl
		2–12 yrs	2.0–6.5 mg/dl
Phosphorus		12–14 yrs	2.0–7.0 mg/dl
Newborn	4.2–9.0 mg/dl	14 yrs–adult male	3.0–8.0
1 yr	3.8–6.2 mg/dl	Adult female	2.0–7.0 mg/dl

AGE-SPECIFIC INDICES

Age	Hgb (gm%)	Hct (%)	MCV (fl)	MCHC (gm/% RBC)	WBC/mm³	Platelets (10³/mm³)
26–30 wk gestation	13.4	41.5	118.2	37.9	4.4	254
32 wk	15.0	47	118	32.0	—	290
1–3 days	18.5	56	108	33.0	18.9	192
1 mo	13.9	44	101	31.8	10.8	—

Erythrocyte Sedimentation Rate		Partial Thromboplastin Time Activated (APTT)		Prothrombin Time (PT)	
Newborn (0–48 hr)	0–4 min/hr			Preterm	17 (range, 12–21) sec
Child	4–20 mm/hr	Preterm	70 sec	Full-term	16 (range, 13–20) sec
Adult male	0–10 mm/hr	Full-term	45–65 sec	Child/adult	13 (range, 12–14) sec
Adult female	0–20 mm/hr	Child/adult	30–45 sec		

BLOOD COMPONENT REPLACEMENT
Approximate Blood Volume

Age	Total Blood Volume	Age	Total Blood Volume
Premature infants	90–105 ml/kg	> 1 yr	68–88 ml/kg
Term newborns	78–86 ml/kg	Adult	68–88 ml/kg
> 1 mo	78 ml/kg		

Ref: Nathan DG, Oski FA: Hematology of Infancy and Childhood. Philadelphia, W.B. Saunders, 1993, pp 29, 1916.

Required Packed Cell Volume: Infuse no faster than 2–3 ml/kg/hr or in 10 ml/kg aliquots over several hours.

$$\text{Vol of cells (ml)} = \frac{\text{Est blood vol (ml)} \times \text{desired Hct change}}{\text{Hct of PRBC}}$$

The usual Hct of PRBC is 65%.

Platelet Transfusions: Platelet counts > 50,000/mm³ advisable for lumbar puncture. One unit of platelets/m² raises platelet count 10,000/mm³

$$\text{Platelet increment/mm}^3 = \frac{30,000 \times \text{(number of units)}}{\text{Est blood vol (L)}}$$

Treatment Algorithms and Charts

NEWBORN INFANT IN DISTRESS

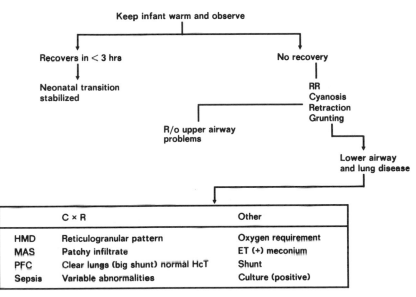

Keep infant warm and observe

Recovers in < 3 hrs / No recovery

Neonatal transition stabilized

RR
Cyanosis
Retraction
Grunting

R/o upper airway problems

Lower airway and lung disease

	C × R	Other
HMD	Reticulogranular pattern	Oxygen requirement
MAS	Patchy infiltrate	ET (+) meconium
PFC	Clear lungs (big shunt) normal HcT	Shunt
Sepsis	Variable abnormalities	Culture (positive)

CENTRAL CYANOSIS IN A NEWBORN INFANT

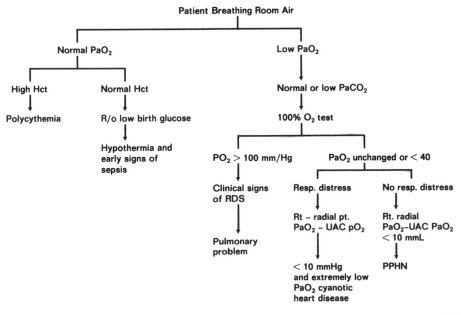

Patient Breathing Room Air

Normal PaO$_2$ / Low PaO$_2$

High Hct / Normal Hct

Polycythemia

R/o low birth glucose

Hypothermia and early signs of sepsis

Normal or low PaCO$_2$

100% O$_2$ test

PO$_2$ > 100 mm/Hg / PaO$_2$ unchanged or < 40

Clinical signs of RDS

Resp. distress / No resp. distress

Pulmonary problem

Rt – radial pt. PaO$_2$ – UAC pO$_2$

Rt. radial PaO$_2$–UAC PaO$_2$ < 10 mmL

< 10 mmHg and extremely low PaO$_2$ cyanotic heart disease

PPHN

493

MANAGEMENT OF SICK NEONATE
BY BLOOD PRESSURE MONITORING

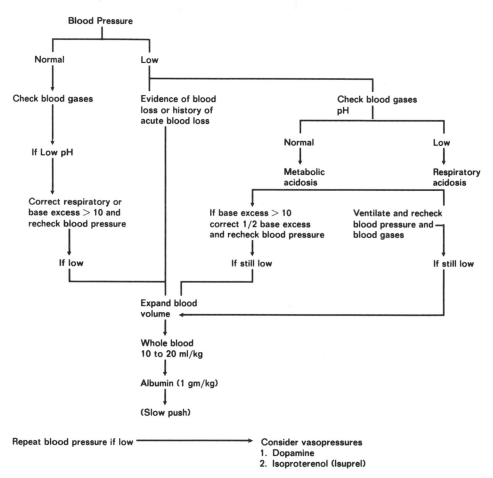

Blood Pressure

Normal — Low

Check blood gases

If Low pH

Correct respiratory or
base excess > 10 and
recheck blood pressure

If low

Evidence of blood
loss or history of
acute blood loss

Check blood gases
pH

Normal — Low

Metabolic
acidosis

Respiratory
acidosis

If base excess > 10
correct 1/2 base excess
and recheck blood pressure

Ventilate and recheck
blood pressure and
blood gases

If still low

If still low

Expand blood
volume

Whole blood
10 to 20 ml/kg

Albumin (1 gm/kg)

(Slow push)

Repeat blood pressure if low ⟶ Consider vasopressures
1. Dopamine
2. Isoproterenol (Isuprel)

ELECTRICAL DEFIBRILLATION

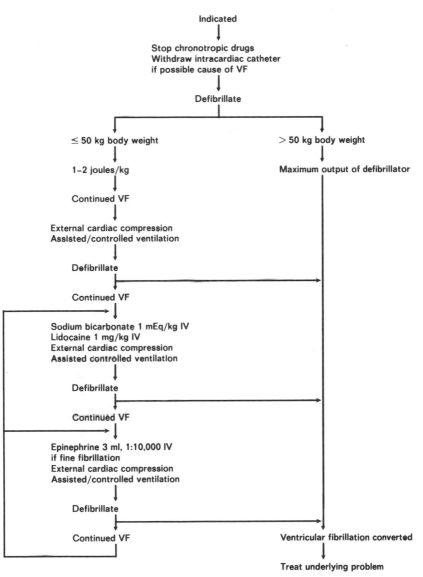

SMOKE INHALATION

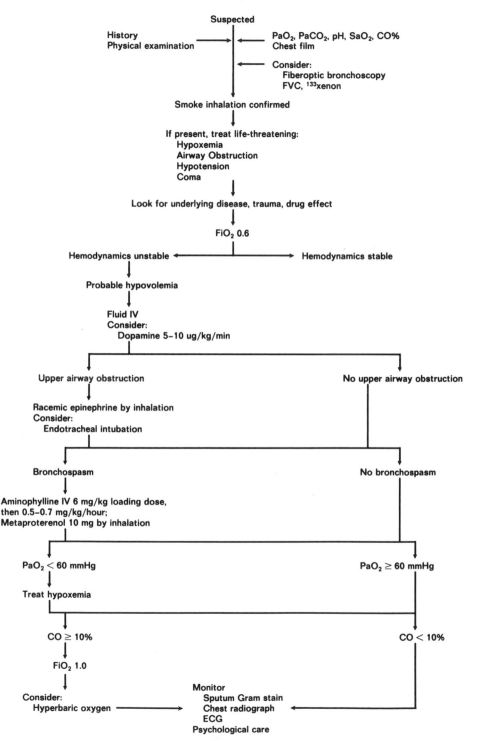

Suspected

History
Physical examination → ← PaO$_2$, PaCO$_2$, pH, SaO$_2$, CO%
Chest film

← Consider:
Fiberoptic bronchoscopy
FVC, [133]xenon

Smoke inhalation confirmed

If present, treat life-threatening:
Hypoxemia
Airway Obstruction
Hypotension
Coma

Look for underlying disease, trauma, drug effect

FiO$_2$ 0.6

Hemodynamics unstable ←→ Hemodynamics stable

Probable hypovolemia

Fluid IV
Consider:
Dopamine 5–10 ug/kg/min

Upper airway obstruction   No upper airway obstruction

Racemic epinephrine by inhalation
Consider:
Endotracheal intubation

Bronchospasm   No bronchospasm

Aminophylline IV 6 mg/kg loading dose,
then 0.5–0.7 mg/kg/hour;
Metaproterenol 10 mg by inhalation

PaO$_2$ < 60 mmHg   PaO$_2 \geq$ 60 mmHg

Treat hypoxemia

CO $\geq$ 10%   CO < 10%

FiO$_2$ 1.0

Monitor
Sputum Gram stain
Consider: →   Chest radiograph   ←
Hyperbaric oxygen   ECG
Psychological care

DRUG OVERDOSE

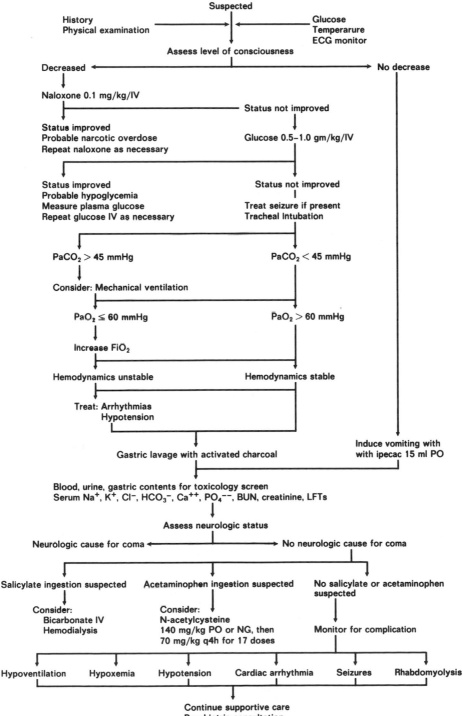

Suspected

History
Physical examination

Glucose
Temperarure
ECG monitor

Assess level of consciousness

Decreased ← → No decrease

Naloxone 0.1 mg/kg/IV

Status not improved

Status improved
Probable narcotic overdose
Repeat naloxone as necessary

Glucose 0.5–1.0 gm/kg/IV

Status improved
Probable hypoglycemia
Measure plasma glucose
Repeat glucose IV as necessary

Status not improved

Treat seizure if present
Tracheal Intubation

$PaCO_2 > 45$ mmHg

$PaCO_2 < 45$ mmHg

Consider: Mechanical ventilation

$PaO_2 \leq 60$ mmHg

$PaO_2 > 60$ mmHg

Increase FiO_2

Hemodynamics unstable

Hemodynamics stable

Treat: Arrhythmias
Hypotension

Gastric lavage with activated charcoal

Induce vomiting with
with ipecac 15 ml PO

Blood, urine, gastric contents for toxicology screen
Serum Na^+, K^+, Cl^-, HCO_3^-, Ca^{++}, PO_4^{--}, BUN, creatinine, LFTs

Assess neurologic status

Neurologic cause for coma ← → No neurologic cause for coma

Salicylate ingestion suspected

Acetaminophen ingestion suspected

No salicylate or acetaminophen
suspected

Consider:
Bicarbonate IV
Hemodialysis

Consider:
N-acetylcysteine
140 mg/kg PO or NG, then
70 mg/kg q4h for 17 doses

Monitor for complication

Hypoventilation   Hypoxemia   Hypotension   Cardiac arrhythmia   Seizures   Rhabdomyolysis

Continue supportive care
Psychiatric consultation

SEIZURE DISORDER

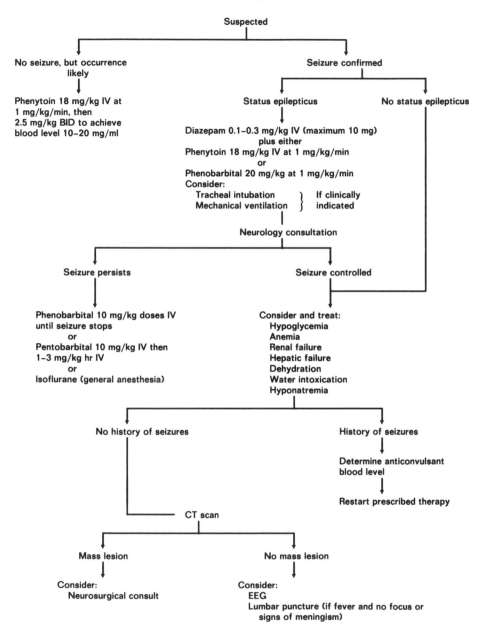

Suspected

No seizure, but occurrence likely

Phenytoin 18 mg/kg IV at 1 mg/kg/min, then 2.5 mg/kg BID to achieve blood level 10–20 mg/ml

Seizure confirmed

Status epilepticus

No status epilepticus

Diazepam 0.1–0.3 mg/kg IV (maximum 10 mg) plus either
Phenytoin 18 mg/kg IV at 1 mg/kg/min
or
Phenobarbital 20 mg/kg at 1 mg/kg/min
Consider:
   Tracheal intubation   } If clinically
   Mechanical ventilation } indicated

Neurology consultation

Seizure persists

Phenobarbital 10 mg/kg doses IV until seizure stops
or
Pentobarbital 10 mg/kg IV then 1–3 mg/kg hr IV
or
Isoflurane (general anesthesia)

Seizure controlled

Consider and treat:
   Hypoglycemia
   Anemia
   Renal failure
   Hepatic failure
   Dehydration
   Water intoxication
   Hyponatremia

No history of seizures

History of seizures

Determine anticonvulsant blood level

Restart prescribed therapy

CT scan

Mass lesion

Consider:
   Neurosurgical consult

No mass lesion

Consider:
   EEG
   Lumbar puncture (if fever and no focus or signs of meningism)

DIFFERENTIAL DIAGNOSIS OF RESPIRATORY DISTRESS
IN SOME SPECIFIC STATES

	RDS	PPHN	GROUP G STREP	TTN	MAS
Gestation	Usually preterm	Often term	Preterm or term	More often term	Usually post-term
Clinical features	Grunting with gradual deterioration	Cyanosis main feature with sudden deterioration	Shock, early apnea, and pulmonary hemorrhage	RR > 60, mild distress	Meconium staining, overexpanded chest, progressive deterioration
Effect of oxygen	Improvement	Cyanosis unchanged	May improve	Improvement	May improve
Blood gases	Hypoxemia raised PCO_2, mixed acidosis	Marked hypoxemia, low or normal PCO_2, metabolic acidosis with R radial/UAC PO_2 difference	Hypoxemia, metabolic or mixed acidosis	Mild hypoxemia, low or normal PCO_2, mild metabolic acidosis	Hypoxemia, metabolic acidosis
Chest X-ray	Underinflation, reticulogranular, pattern, air bronchogram	Overinflation, clear lung fields, cardiomegaly	Coarse infiltrates collapse or mimic RDS	Overinflation, streaking, pulm. vasc., pulm. edema, S1 cardiomegaly	Coarse infiltrates, overinflation ± pneumothorax
Treatment	CPAP helpful, IPPV	CPAP unhelpful, mechanical ventilation	Penicillin blood transfusion ± mechanical ventilation	Oxygen, IPPV (rarely)	Airway suction at birth, may need IPPV, CPAP unhelpful
Outcome (mortality)	< 5%, low	–20%, high	–40%, high	0%, very low–none	–30%, high if PPHN

Modified from Holliday H, et al: Handbook of Neonatal Intensive Care. Philadelphia, W.B. Saunders.

ALTITUDE CHART

Altitude	Barometric Pressure	FIO_2 Required to Maintain Consual PaO_2								
16000	412	0.41	0.59	0.78	0.98					
14000	446	0.37	0.53	0.71	0.89					
12000	483	0.34	0.49	0.65	0.81	0.98				
10000	523	0.31	0.45	0.60	0.75	0.90				
8000	564	0.29	0.41	0.55	0.69	0.83	0.96			
6000	609	0.27	0.38	0.51	0.63	0.76	0.89			
4000	656	0.24	0.35	0.47	0.58	0.70	0.82	0.94		
2000	707	0.23	0.32	0.43	0.54	0.65	0.76	0.86	0.97	
Sea level	760	0.21	0.30	0.40	0.50	0.60	0.70	0.80	0.90	1.0

1) As compared to that required at sea level.
Modified from Neonatal/Pediatric Respiratory Care, Editor Dana F. Oakes, B.A., R.R.T.
Health Educator Publications Inc.
1580 Kirkland Road
Old Town Main 04468

APPENDIX III

Drug Therapy

DRUG THERAPY

Drug	Route	Dose
Acetaminophen	PO/PR	10–15 mg/kg/dose PO/PR q 4–6° hr. Do not exceed 5 doses in 24 hr.
Activated charcoal	PO	1 gm/kg, max 50 gm.
Adenosine	IV	PALS dose for treatment of SVT, 0.1 mg/kg; if not effective give 0.2 mg/kg; maximum single dose 12 mg. For rapid bolus IV use: only give over a few seconds, administer at IV site closest to patient; follow each bolus with normal saline flush.
Adrenaline	IV or intra-osseus	First dose: 0.01 mg/kg of 1:10,000 solution. Subsequent doses: 0.1 mg/kg of 1:1000 solution. Can be repeated q 3–5 min as needed.
	ET	0.1 mg/kg of 1:1000 solution.
	Aerosol	0.25–0.5 ml of 2.25% of racemic epinephrine solution diluted in 3 ml normal saline.
Aminophylline	IV	Loading dose: 4–6/kg over 20–30 min. Continuous infusion: 1 mg/kg/hr.
Amrinone infusion	IV/IO	0.75 mg/kg IV bolus over 2–3 min, followed by maintenance infusion 5–10 μg/kg/min.
Ampicillin in meningitis	IV/IO	Birth–8 weeks: 200 mg/kg/day q 6°. 8 wk–5 yr: 200 mg–400 mg/kg/day q 4°–6°
Atropine sulfate	IV/IO	0.01 mg/kg (minimum dose 0.1 mg). Maximum dose 2 mg.
	ET	0.02 mg/kg; follow with 2–3 ml normal saline.
	Aerosol	0.03–0.05 mg/kg nebulized; maximum 2 mg.
Bretylium	IV	Treatment of V-Fib: PALS guidelines, initial dose 5 mg/kg. Then attempt defibrillation if ventricular fibrillation persists. May repeat as needed to a total of 30 mg/kg.
Calcium chloride	IV	20–50 mg/kg/dose. Administer slowly.
Cardioversion Unstable tachy-arrythmias		0.5–1 watt sec/kg (synchronized)
Ceftriaxone sodium	IV/IO	Loading dose: 75 mg/kg/dose. Maintenance: 50–75 mg/kg/day q 12–24°.
Chloramphenicol	IV	50–75 mg/kg/day divided q 6°; maximum daily dose 4 gm/day.
Chlorpromazine	IV	0.05–1 mg/kg/dose. Profound drop in B/P may occur.
Defibrillation		2-watt-sec/kg first attempt; 4-watt-sec/kg thereafter.
Diphenhydramine	IV-IM	5 mg/kg/day q 6–8°, not to exceed 300 mg/day.
Dexamethasone	IV	0.5–2 mg/kg/day q 6°
Dextrose	IV/IO	200–500 mg/kg/dose. Infuse 12.5% peripherally 25% central line. DO NOT INFUSE 50% GLUCOSE TO A CHILD.
Diazepam	IV/IO	Infants: 0.05–0.3 mg/kg/dose q 15–30 min. Maximum 5 mg given over 2–3 min. 5 yr–adolescents: 0.05–0.3 mg/kg/dose q 15–30 min. Maximum 10 mg.
Dobutamine	IV/IO	IV infusion Neonates: 2–15 μg/kg/min; titrate to desired response. Children: 2–20 μg/kg/min; titrate to desired response. Maximum 40 ×g/kg/min.

Table continued on following page.

DRUG THERAPY (Cont.)

Drug	Route	Dose
Dopamine	IV/IO	Neonates: 2–15 μg/kg/min; titrate to desired response. Children: 1–20 μg/kg/min; maximum 50 μg/kg/min.
Fentanyl	IV	Children: 1–12 years, 1–2 μg/kg/dose. May repeat 30–60 min intervals. Continuous infusion: Initial bolus 1–2 μg/kg; then 1 μg/kg/hr; titrate upward 1–3 μg/kg/hr.
Furosemide	IV/IM	Premie and NB infants: 1–2 mg/kg q 12–24°. Children: 1–2 mg/kg/dose in divided doses q 6–12° up to 6 mg/kg/day.
Hydrocortisone	IV/IM	1–2 mg/kg/dose bolus; then 25–150 mg/day in divided doses.
Insulin	IV	NO LOADING DOSE IN PEDIATRIC PATIENTS. Continuous infusion: 0.1 unit/kg/hr. (Range 0.05–0.2 unit/kg/hr depending upon the rate of decrease of serum glucose. Optimum rate of serum glucose decrease 80–100 mg/dl/hr.) *NOTE*: TOO RAPID DECREASE OF SERUM GLUCOSE MAY LEAD TO CEREBRAL EDEMA.
Isuprel	IV/IO	0.05–2 μg/kg/min.
Lidocaine HCl	IV	Loading: 1 mg/kg/dose, maximum 100 mg. Infusion: 20–50 μg/kg/min. Renal or hepatic impairment: decrease dose by 50%.
Lorazepam	IV/IO	Infants–children: 0.1 mg/kg slow IV over 2–5 min. Do not exceed 4 mg/ single dose. May repeat 2nd dose in 10–15 min.
Mannitol	IV	Initial: 0.5–1 gm/kg. Maintenance: 0.25–0.5 gm/kg q 4–6 hr.
Metaproterenol	Aerosol	0.01–0.02 ml/kg of 5% solution. Maximum dose 0.3 ml.
Morphine sulfate	IV	0.1–0.2 mg/kg/dose q 2–4°; maximum 15 mg/dose.
Midazolam HCl	IV/IO/IM	0.05–0.15 mg/kg. May be repeated frequently.
Naloxone HCl	IV/IM	0.1 mg/kg every 2–3 min as needed.
Nitroprusside (sodium)	IV	Continuous infusion: 0.3–0.5 μg/kg/min; titrate to effect. Usual dose 3 μg/kg/min; max 10 μg/kg/min.
Nitroglycerin infusion	IV	Continuous infusion: start 0.25–0.5 μg/kg/min, and titrate by 0.5–1 μg/ kg/min every 3–5 min as needed. Usual dose 1–3 μg/kg/min; maximum up to 20 μg/kg/min.
Norepinephrine infusion	IV/IO	Initial 0.05–0.2 μg/kg/min; titrate to desired effect. Maximum dose 1–2 μg/kg/min.
Pancuronium	IV/IO	0.04–0.2 mg/kg q 30–60 min as needed.
Penicillin G	IV/IO	25,000–50,000 units/kg/day divided doses q 4–6°.
Phenobarbital	IV/IO	Loading: 20 mg/kg slowly at 1 mg/kg/min, max 30 mg/min. Maintenance: 6–8 mg/kg/day, divide q 12°.
Phenytoin	IV	Loading: 15–18 mg/kg slowly at 1 mg/kg/min; max 50 mg/min. Maintenance: 5–7 mg/kg/day, divided q 12°
Sodium bicarbonate	IV/IO	1 mEq/kg initially. May repeat as indicated by the patient's acid-base status. NB–0.5 mEq/kg.
Succinylcholine	IV/IO	1–2 mg/kg/dose.
Terbutaline	Aerosol	0.01–0.3 ml/kg minimum dose; 0.1 ml maximum dose, 2.5 ml dilute; 1–2 ml normal saline q 4–6 hr.
Vancomycin	IV	40–60 mg/kg/day q 6°.
Vecuronium	IV/IO	Initial: 0.08–0.2 mg/kg/dose. Maintenance: 0.5–0.1 mg kg q hr as needed. Continuous infusion: 0.1 mg/kg/hr. (May cause hypotension if administered too rapidly.)
Verapamil	IV	< 1 year not indicated. 1–16 years: 0.1–0.3 mg/kg/dose over 2–3 min; maximum 5 mg/dose. May repeat dose once in 30 min if adequate response not achieved.
Vitamin K	IV	2.5–10 mg/dose; may repeat in 6–8 hr. May cause hypotension if administered rapidly.

Index

Page numbers in *italics* refer to illustrations; page numbers followed by "t" refer to tables.